ALLERGY

Slide Atlas

A Slide Collection of Allergy, based on the contents of this book, is available. In the slide atlas format, the material is split into volumes, each of which is presented in a binder, together with numbered 35mm slides of each illustration. Further information can be obtained from:

Gower Medical Publishing,
Middlesex House
34–42 Cleveland Street
London W1P 5FB
UK

Raven Press Ltd
1185 Avenue of the Americas
New York
New York 10036
USA

ALLERGY

Stephen T Holgate
MD, DSc, FRCP
MRC Clinical Professor of Immunopharmacology,
University of Southampton;
Honorary Consultant Physician,
Southampton and SW Hampshire District Health Authority,
Southampton, UK

Martin K Church
MPharm, PhD, DSc
Professor of Experimental Immunopharmacology,
University of Southampton,
Southampton, UK

Foreword by K Frank Austen, MD
Theodore Bevier Bayles Professor of Medicine,
Harvard Medical School;
Chairman, Department of Rheumatology and Immunology,
Brigham and Women's Hospital,
Boston,
Massachusetts, USA

Gower Medical Publishing
LONDON • NEW YORK

Distributed in the USA and Canada by:
Raven Press Ltd
1185 Avenue of the Americas
New York
New York 10036
USA

Distributed in the rest of the world by:
Gower Medical Publishing
Middlesex House
34–42 Cleveland Street
London W1P 5FB
UK

Project Managers: Lucy Hamilton
Robert Whittle
Zak Knowles

Design: Judith Gauge
Anne-Marie Woodruff
Jane Brown
Richard Prime

Illustration: Judith Gauge
Anne-Marie Woodruff
Jane Brown
Richard Prime
Mark Willey

Index: Nina Boyd

Production: Susan Bishop
Adam Phillips

Publisher: Fiona Foley

Cataloguing in Publication Data:

Catalogue records for this book are available from the US Library of Congress and British Library.

ISBN 0–397–44725–6

Type set on Apple Macintosh®
CRC output by The Text Unit
Text set in New Century School Book;
legends and tables set in Frutiger.
Origination by Colourscan, Singapore.
Printed in Hong Kong.
Produced by Imago Services, Hong Kong.

Foreword

Allergy, the 'brainchild' of Professors Stephen Holgate and Martin Church, establishes a new standard for a 'user-friendly' textbook of quality. The text is developed with a thoughtful progression from preclinical to applied bioscience, and with a presentation form readily acceptable to individuals entering the field as well as to established practitioners who seek a convenient state-of-the-art update.

The past ten or fifteen years have provided truly novel insights into the molecular and cellular pathobiology of allergic disease. The focus is no longer limited to the environmental insult or to the specific immune response, but has now grown to include an understanding of the cellular mechanisms that elicit the clinical signs and symptoms appropriate to future intervention. The fact that mast cells arise from progenitors in bone marrow, travel in an unrecognized form to tissues for site-specific proliferation and differentiation has critical functional and therapeutic implications. The findings that more than half-a-dozen recombinant cytokines can modulate mast cell proliferation and phenotype may provide the basis for understanding tissue-specific mast cell heterogeneity. At the same time, the recognition that mast cells themselves elaborate cytokines as well as secretory granule-derived and membrane-derived lipid mediators indicates that this tissue cell has a biological capability second to none, in terms of initiating and sustaining an inflammatory response involving additional diverse cell types, both constitutive and infiltrating. The appreciation that the mast cell, the basophil, and the eosinophil are the principal sources of the cysteinyl leukotrienes highlights a system capable of constricting smooth muscle and altering vascular permeability, a system now amenable to therapeutic intervention.

Whether cytokine regulation of mast cells is autocrine in part, or entirely the purview of the T cell, remains to be determined, but still emphasizes the complex cellular interaction in sustained reactions falling within the clinical definition of allergy. That definition is extended by the observation that mast cells and eosinophils may profoundly alter connective tissue and elicit proliferative responses relevant either to tissue remodelling or pathobiological fibrosis. These are but a few of the insights now being gained as regards the effector cell functions of systems recruited by the specific immune response relevant to allergic disease. Although certain of these interactions have been appreciated in *in vitro* culture systems, they appear to have been validated by morphological, molecular biological and immunochemical analysis of lesional tissue from patients with allergic conditions. Thus, a major advance has been the validation of preclinical concepts at the clinical level.

The presentation of these important complexities is facilitated by the creative style used throughout this volume. The detailed, yet coherent, text, which accompanies the high quality photographs and schema, unravels the complexities and presents them in a format that is easily appreciated. The result is a comprehensive text directly pertinent to the basic science and clinical practice of allergy. The illustrative presentation style, with appropriate text, the integration of one chapter with another due to editorial influence, and the sequence with which the critical aspects of modern allergy are introduced and developed provide the reader with an enjoyable, yet profound, educational experience.

K Frank Austen, MD
Theodore Bevier Bayles Professor of Medicine,
Harvard Medical School;
Chairman, Department of Rheumatology and Immunology,
Brigham and Women's Hospital,
Boston,
Massachusetts, USA

Preface

Allergic diseases, including asthma, rhinitis, conjunctivitis, dermatitis and food allergies are major contributors to morbidity and, less frequently, to mortality in the civilized world. Their incidence and severity seem to be rising and yet our methods of treatment still stem from empirical and serendipitous findings rather than from a scientific base. The main reason for this is that, while basic and clinical immunology have made great strides over the past two decades, it is only in the last five years or so that techniques, such as bronchial biopsy in asthmatics, and reagents, such as monoclonal antibodies to adhesion proteins or gene probes for cytokines, have been available to study the detailed pathogenesis of allergic disease at the cellular and mediator level. This has led to a state of rapidly expanding knowledge, so changing the concept of allergy, along with the broader framework of immunology, especially in relation to disease processes and treatment. It is truly an exciting time to be involved in allergic disease research.

It is against this background that we undertook the preparation of an entirely new text on allergic diseases and their mechanisms, based as much on specially designed, clear and informative diagrams as on textural information. We believe that such an approach, initially adopted by Ivan Roitt, Jonathan Brostoff and David Male in their textbook, Immunology, also published by Gower, has allowed us to present a text which finds a unique niche between the heavy reference texts and the more superficial guides. We have invited leading research workers in the fields of immunology, cell biology and clinical medicine to contribute.

The book first introduces the reader to the individual cells that participate in the allergic response and then builds on this information to prepare detailed synopses of the histopathological features, diagnoses and treatment of allergic reactions occurring in all major organs. The balance of text and diagrams, we hope, will make this a compulsive book, presenting easily digestible state-of-the-art information to practising clinical immunologists, organ-based specialists, allergists and other clinicians with an interest in this field. In addition, we believe that portrayal of clear clinical information will help the postgraduate researcher to understand the clinical context of this rapidly expanding field of immunology.

The availability of a complementary slide set will make this book an ideal teaching base for many aspects of allergic disease. The division of the book into sections on cellular and antibody mechanisms, which constitute the basis of the allergic response, and clinical descriptions of the pathogenesis, diagnosis and treatment of all aspects of allergic disease ensure a comprehensive coverage of the discipline.

In preparing this book, we have asked our contributing authors to construct their chapters in a novel way, so that the text embellishes the diagrams rather than the reverse. We know that this was not an easy task and we thank them for all the effort that they have made in the many excellent chapters. As it was not our intention to produce a full bibliography for each chapter, but rather a short reading list, may we take this opportunity to extend our sincere thanks to all the scientists and clinicians whose work has formed the backbone of the book, but who have not received specific acknowledgement. May we also offer our thanks to our colleagues and secretarial assistants within Southampton General Hospital for their help. Finally, may we thank Fiona Foley, for giving us the inspiration to undertake this work, and her Gower team of Zak Knowles, Robert Whittle, Lucy Hamilton and Judith Gauge, who worked so hard with the artwork and layout of the text.

As readers, we hope that you will appreciate the novelty of our approach to allergy and that you find the result refreshing and enjoyable to read. If you have views on the book, then please let us know, for only through feedback can we strive for further improvement.

STH
MKC

CONTRIBUTORS

Dr N Franklin Adkinson
Johns Hopkins University School of Medicine,
Johns Hopkins Asthma and Allergy Center,
Baltimore,
Maryland, USA

Dr Cheryl R Adolphson
Dept Immunology,
Mayo Clinic and Foundation,
Rochester,
Minnesota, USA

Professor Ross StC Barnetson
Dept Dermatology,
University of Sydney,
Sydney, Australia

Mr Roger J Buckley
Contact Lens and Prosthesis Dept,
Moorfields Eye Hospital,
London, UK

Dr Peter GJ Burney
Dept Public Health Medicine,
United Medical and Dental Schools of Guy's and
St Thomas's Hospitals,
London, UK

Professor Robert J Davies
Dept Respiratory Medicine,
St Bartholomew's Hospital,
London, UK

Dr Judah A Denburg
Dept Medicine,
McMaster University,
Hamilton,
Ontario, Canada

Dr John P Caulfield
Syntex Research,
Division of Syntex USA Inc,
Palo Alto,
California, USA

Professor Martin K Church
Immunopharmacology Group,
University of Southampton,
Southampton, UK

Dr Christopher J Corrigan
Dept Allergy and Clinical Immunology,
National Heart and Lung Institute,
London, UK

Dr Patricia A Duffy
University of Texas Southwestern Medical Center,
Dept Internal Medicine, Division of Allergy,
Dallas,
Texas, USA

Dr Gerald J Gleich
Dept Immunology,
Mayo Clinic and Foundation,
Mayo Medical School,
Rochester,
Minnesota, USA

Professor Hannah J Gould
Division of Biomolecular Sciences,
King's College,
University of London,
London, UK

Dr Christine Jenkins
Institute of Respiratory Medicine,
Royal Prince Alfred Hospital,
Sydney, Australia

Dr David B Jones
Dept Pathology,
University of Southampton,
Southampton, UK

Dr David J Gawkrodger
University Dept Dermatology,
Royal Hallamshire Hospital,
Sheffield, UK

Professor Christopher Haslett
Respiratory Medicine Unit,
Dept Medicine,
University of Edinburgh,
Edinburgh, Scotland

Professor Stephen T Holgate
Immunopharmacology Group,
University of Southampton,
Southampton, UK

Dr Richard F Horan
Harvard Medical School and
Brigham and Womens Hospital,
Boston,
Massachusetts, USA

Professor Anthony B Kay
Dept Allergy and Clinical Immunology,
National Heart and Lung Institute,
London, UK

Dr Donald A Kennerly
University of Texas Southwestern Medical Center,
Dept Internal Medicine, Division of Allergy,
Dallas,
Texas, USA

Dr Stephen Lane
Guy's and St Thomas's Hospitals,
Division of Medicine,
London, UK

Professor Rona M MacKie
Dept Dermatology,
University of Glasgow,
Glasgow, Scotland

Dr Frances Lawlor
Institute of Dermatology,
St Thomas's Hospital,
London, UK

Professor Tak H Lee
Guy's and St Thomas's Hospital,
Division of Medicine,
London, UK

Professor Maurice H Lessof
Dept Medicine,
United Medical and Dental Schools of
Guy's and St Thomas's Hospitals,
London, UK

Professor Susan Lightman
Institute of Ophthalmology,
Moorfields Eye Hospital,
London, UK

Dr Anthony D Ormerod
University Dept Dermatology,
Aberdeen Hospitals,
Aberdeen, Scotland

Dr Clive P Page
Dept Pharmacology,
King's College,
University of London,
London, UK

The Late Dr Ulf Pipkorn
Dept Otorhinolaryngology,
University of Lund,
Lund, Sweden

Dr Jacqueline A Pongracic
Johns Hopkins University of Medicine,
Johns Hopkins Asthma and Allergy Center,
Baltimore,
Maryland, USA

Dr Lars K Poulsen
Medical Dept, Allergy Unit,
State University Hospital,
Copenhagen, Denmark

Dr Duncan A F Robertson
Dept Medicine,
Royal United Hospital,
Bath, UK

Dr John E Salvaggio
Clinical Immunology Division,
Tulane Medical School,
New Orleans,
Louisiana, USA

Dr Albert L Sheffer
Harvard Medical School and
Brigham and Women's Hospital,
Boston,
Massachusetts, USA

Dr Geoffrey A Stewart
Clinical Immunology Research Unit,
Princess Margaret Hospital Children's Medical
Research Foundation,
Subiaco,
Western Australia

Dr Philip J Thompson
University Dept Medicine,
Sir Charles Gairdner Hospital,
Nedlands,
Western Australia

Dr Cecilia Trigg
Dept Respiratory Medicine,
St Bartholomew's Hospital,
London, UK

Dr Bent Weeke
Medical Dept, Allergy Unit,
State University Hospital,
Copenhagen, Denmark

Professor Ann J Woolcock
Institute of Respiratory Medicine,
Royal Prince Alfred Hospital,
Sydney, Australia

User Guide

The following cells appear regularly in the book.

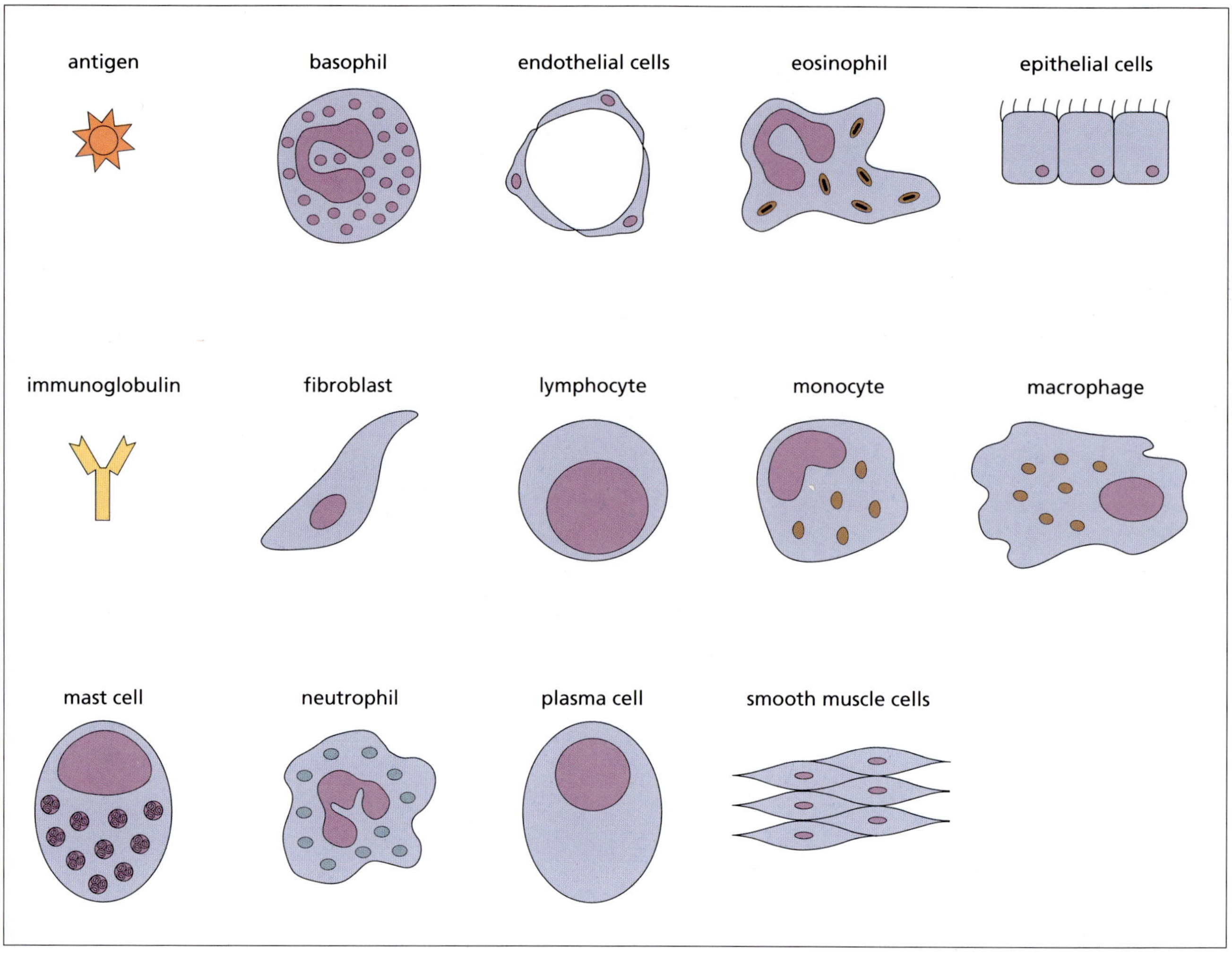

Acknowledgements

The authors would like to acknowledge the following for their kind permission to reproduce or adapt material:

Bettler B et al. *J Biol Chem* 1992;**267:**185-191 [Fig. 2.11];
Leiferman KM, Fujisawa T, Gray BH, Gleich GJ. *Lab Invest* 1990;**62**:579–589 [Fig. 6.19];
Jefferey PK et al. *Am Rev Respir Dis* 1989; **140**:1745–1753 [Fig. 8.13];
Burrows B. *Chest* 1986;**90(4)**:481–482 [Fig. 14.17];
Mygind N, Weeke B. *Allergic and Vasomotor Rhinitis: Clinical Aspects.* Munksgaard: Copenhagen, 1985 [Fig.17.12];
Ferguson H et al. *Respir Medicine* 1991;**3**:247–249 [Fig. 17.14];
Mygind N, Pipkorn U, Dahl R. *Rhinitis and Asthma.* Munksgaard: Copenhagen, 1990 [Fig. 17.16];
Professor M Greaves, Institute of Dermatology, United and Medical Dental School, University of London [photograph, Fig. 22.10];
Dr J Harvey, Imperial Cancer Research Fund, London [Fig. 25.7];
Olof Kalm, MD, Sweden [*cover*: CT scan];
Mr S Robertson, Institute of Dermatology, St John's Centre, London, UK [*cover*: urticarial lesions];
Science Photo Library, UK [*cover*: pollen grain, house dust mite].

The authors would also like to thank the following for their assistance:

Daniella Metz, for help in the preparation of the illustrations for Chapter 19;
Miss J Foster, for preparation of the manuscript for Chapter 25;
The Coeliac Trust, for funding of research at Southampton on T-cell populations in the gut [Chapter 25].

Contents

Chapter 1

Allergens

Introduction

This chapter is concerned with substances (antigens=allergens) which cause Type I immediate hypersensitivity reactions, resulting from two temporally distinct processes:

- the sensitization stage, or antibody induction process, in which inhaled, injected, or ingested allergen is presented to the immune system where it is recognized as being foreign, and in susceptible individuals, causes IgE antibody to be produced;
- the second stage, sometimes weeks or years later, when allergen is again internalized and encounters immune cells which possess allergen-specific IgE antibodies on their surface. When several IgE molecules bind the allergen, inflammatory mediators are released and the characteristic features of allergic disease follow (Fig. 1.1).

The World Health Organization recognizes rhinitis, sinusitis, asthma, hypersensitivity pneumonitis, extrinsic allergic alveolitis, conjuctivitis, urticaria, eczema, dermatitis (contact and atopic), anaphylaxis and angioedema, allergic and migraine headache, and certain gastrointestinal disorders as diseases in which IgE-mediated allergy may be involved.

The Diversity and Abundance of Allergens

The most complex sources of allergens are fungi, pollen, and mites; the least complex are animal dander and urine extracts. Of the many proteins in such sources, 20–60 per cent are allergenic when tested on sensitized patients. A sensitized patient will recognize more than one allergen from a particular source, but the precise number reflects both the genetic capability of the host, the complexity of the source, and the assay used to determine allergenicity. Individuals will not necessarily recognize the same allergens but the ones more often recognized are termed the 'major allergens', while the remainder are termed the 'minor allergens'.

Factors Influencing Allergenicity

Most major allergens are either proteins or haptens and do not posses physicochemical properties which distinguish them from other antigens. However, it is thought that they may possess certain characteristics which may facilitate a protein becoming an allergen in a susceptible host. They include:

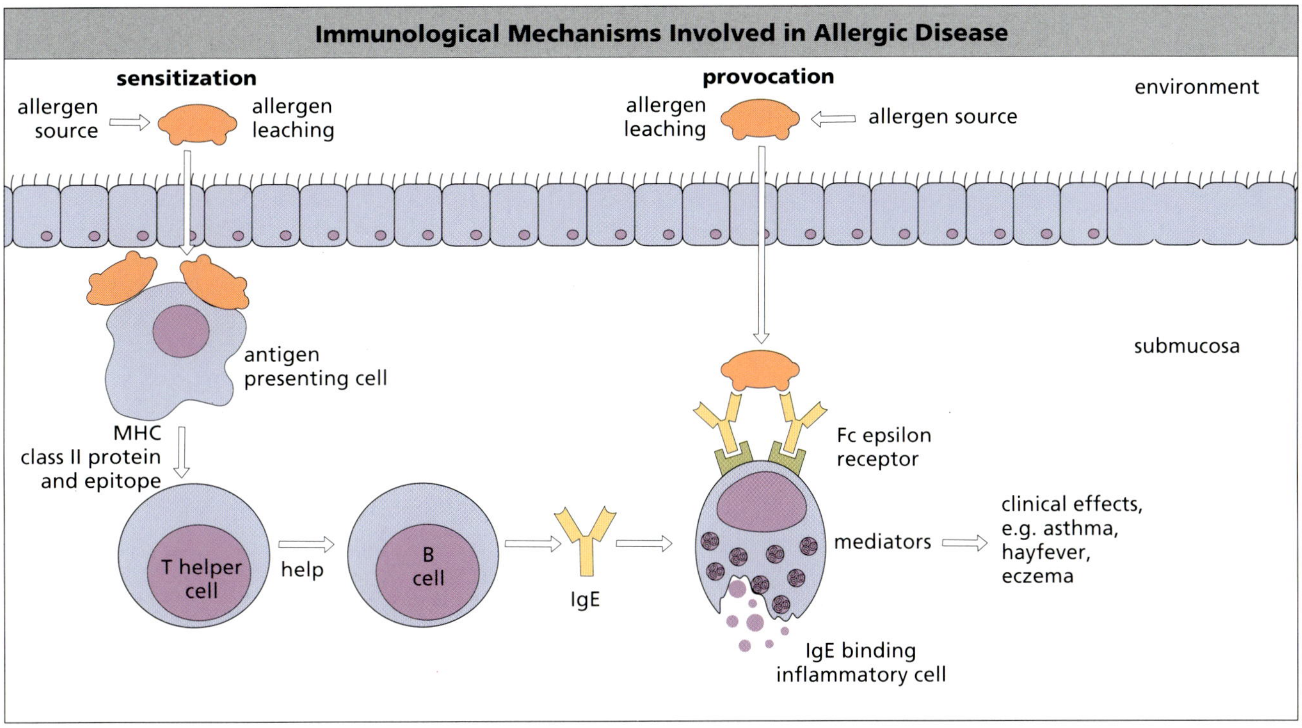

Fig. 1.1 Immunological mechanisms involved in allergic disease.

- its ability to breach physical defence mechanisms and gain access to the immune system;
- its molecular complexity;
- its concentration;
- its solubility;
- its foreignness;
- its stability;
- its biochemical characteristics; and
- the genetic predisposition of the host.

Before an allergen can stimulate IgE production, it must gain access to sites patrolled by the immune system. Most allergens are able to cross mucous membranes following inhalation or ingestion; some gain access by direct contact or injection. The lungs, nose, and eyes are the prime sites for allergic reactions, and so the ability of an allergen to become airborne is of particular importance.

Generally the more concentrated the allergen exposure, the more likely it is to induce an allergic response. To gain access to immune cells, the allergen usually needs to be soluble and stable in body fluids. The foreignness and the size of a protein will influence its immunogenic potential. The larger a molecule, the more likely it is to contain epitopes which will be recognized as foreign.

The genetic characteristics of the host are also important in determining whether an allergic response occurs. For example, the capacity to produce IgE antibodies to certain low molecular weight minor allergens from pollen sources such as *Ambrosia artemisiifolia* (ragweed) and *Lolium perenne* (rye grass) are associated with products of both class I (HLA-A,B,C) and class II (HLA-D) genes, the latter being particularly important in presenting antigen fragments (epitopes) to T helper cells for subsequent antibody production. For example, responses to rye grass allergens *Lol p* I, II, and III allergens are associated with the presence of the haplotype DR3, while responses to the ragweed allergens *Amb a* V and VI are associated with the presence of DR2/Dw2 and DR5 respectively. Genetic analysis of the IgE response to these allergens represents an important model for studying the regulation of the immune response in general. At present, such studies are providing direct information concerning the region on the Class II molecule (desetope) of the host antigen presenting cell (APC) which binds to a processed allergen fragment (Fig. 1.2). In addition, information on the region of the allergen fragment (agretope) which binds to the desetope and the region of the fragment (epitope) which binds to the T-cell receptor or antibody combining site (paratope) is increasing rapidly due to the availability of techniques for sequencing and epitope mapping.

A number of extrinsic factors may facilitate sensitization by altering normal homeostatic defence mechanisms, e.g. exposure to allergen concomitantly with industrial pollutants, cigarette smoke, or viral infections may enhance the immunogenicity of allergens, presumably in part by increasing epithelial permeability and increasing allergen access.

Epitope, T Cell and APC Binding

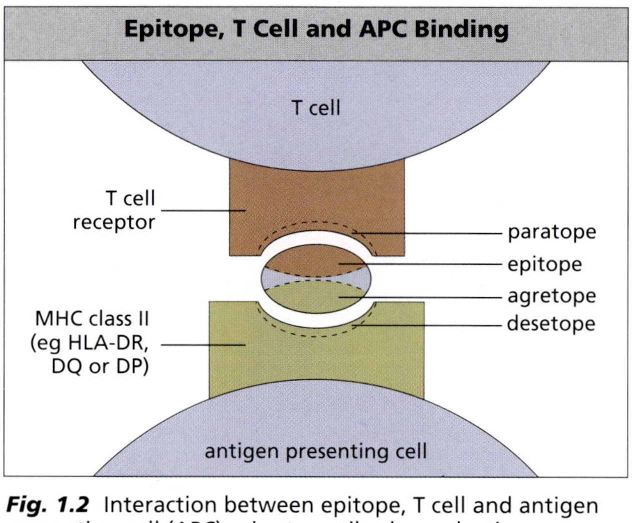

Fig. 1.2 Interaction between epitope, T cell and antigen presenting cell (APC) prior to antibody production.

Source of Allergens

Pollen Allergens

Plant pollens represent some of the most clinically important allergen sources (Fig. 1.3) and may account for 10–20 per cent of allergic disease in the community, usually presenting as rhinitis. The archetypal pollens implicated include those from *Lolium perenne* (rye grass), *Ambrosia artemisiifolia*

Common Allergen Sources

Group	Examples
Airborne	
pollens	
grasses	rye, couch, wild oat, timothy, Bermuda, Kentucky blue, cocksfoot
weeds	ragweed, parietaria, plantain, mugwort
trees	alder, birch, hazel, beech, Cupressae, oak, olive
moulds	*Aspergillus* spp, *Cladosporium* spp, *Alternaria* spp, Basidiospores, Ascomycetes
cereal grains	wheat, rye, oat
animal dander and urine	cat, dog, horse, rabbit, guinea pig, hamster
bird feathers	budgerigar, parrot, pigeon, duck, chicken
house dust mite	*Dermatophagoides pteronyssinus, D. farinae, Euroglyphus maynei*
insects	cockroach, fly, locust, midge
Oral	
foods	seafood, legumes, peanuts, nuts, cereals, dairy products, eggs, fruits, tomatoes, mushrooms, alcoholic beverages, coffee, chocolate
drugs	penicillins, sulphonamides and other antibiotics, sulphasalazine, carbamazepine
Injected	
insects	bee and wasp stings, ant and mosquito bites
drugs	blood products, sera, vaccines, contrast media, drugs (including anti-asthma, drugs and antibiotics)

Fig. 1.3 Common allergen sources and examples (see also Fig 1.7).

(ragweed) and *Betula verrucosa* (birch tree). Pollen grains are the male gametes produced by flowering plants and are produced in very large amounts to ensure contact with the pistil of the female flower of the corresponding species. The shape, size and botanical features of pollen grains vary from plant to plant. The major allergenic pollens are those derived from the wind-pollinated (anemophilous) rather than insect-pollinated plants, and the pollen produced is characterized by its buoyant density, ease of dispersion, and profusion. Pollen grains from individual species vary in size, ranging from 5 to over 200 μm, but in wind-borne pollen the size range varies from 17-58 μm. Although the pollen grain is thought to be the primary source of allergen, studies have shown that at least some allergens may be associated with submicronic particles. Pollens are absent from the atmosphere on wet days and are frequently released when hot dry conditions prevail. As a consequence, pollen release and atmospheric loading is usually seasonal with late spring and summer being common. The contents of individual pollen grains (protoplast) are held together by a two-walled structure comprising an inner wall (intine) and an outer wall (exine) which contributes to the characteristic appearance of certain pollen types (Fig. 1.4).

Allergic reactions ensue in susceptible individuals when the pollen grains fall on to respiratory epithelia and their contents are released. The number of pollen grains required to provoke disease is unclear but studies indicate that the number required varies with prior exposure. Thus, the amount of pollen required to initiate symptoms at the beginning of the hay fever season is greater than at the end of the season, an effect known as priming. Empirical studies suggest that between 10 and 50 grains per cubic metre represent threshold exposure concentrations.

Fungal Allergens

Theoretically, fungal allergens should be highly significant, because fungal spores are the most abundant airborne particles. Their size is often under 10 μm, small enough to penetrate deep into the respiratory tree. Comparison of species reveals that the conditions influencing the release of spores is highly variable but can be extremely specific for a given species, e.g. *Didymella exitalis* and basidiospores, which release spores at night after rain, and may be the cause of increased asthma after thunderstorms.

Fungal spores may also be a major source of allergen inside the home. Several species have been studied in detail, and species belonging to the Deutermycotina are important worldwide (Fig. 1.5). The Basidiomycotina spp (mushrooms, puffballs, rusts, smuts and bracket fungi) are also thought to represent significant allergen sources. Both groups use airborne spore dispersal and are often produced in very large quantities.

Animal- and Bird-derived Allergens

The incidence of positive skin tests in an unselected population where pets are common is approximately 5

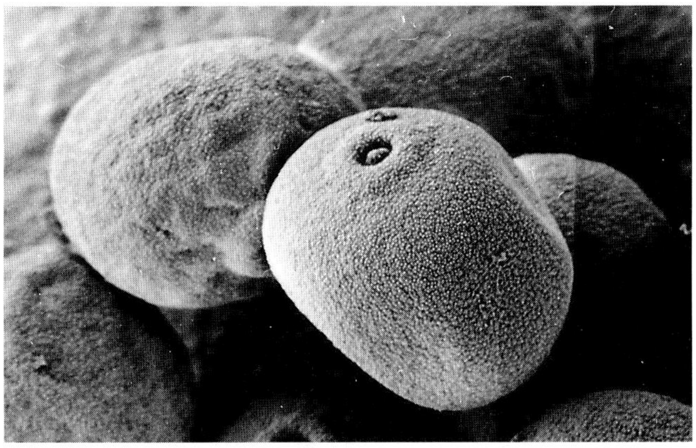

Fig. 1.4 SEM of pollen grains from *Lolium perenne* (rye grass), showing clearly the aperture through which the pollen tube grows. Each pollen grain is about 20 μm in length. (Courtesy of Prof. B Knox and Dr P Taylor, Department of Botany, University of Melbourne.)

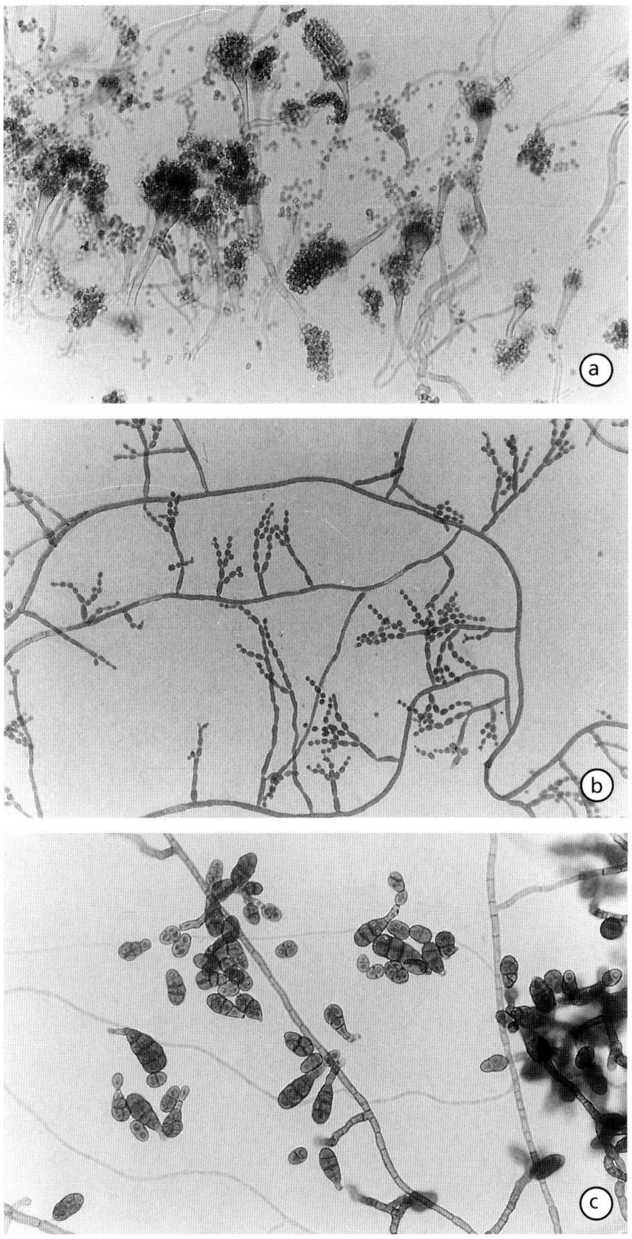

Fig. 1.5 Fungi commonly involved in allergic disease: (a) *Aspergillus fumigatus*, (b) *Cladosporium*, (c) *Alternaria*. (Courtesy of R McAleer, State Health Laboratories, Western Australia.)

per cent which rises to over 30 per cent in atopic asthmatics. Cats and dogs are most commonly involved, but allergy to rats, horses, rabbits, mice, gerbils and guinea pigs have been described. The allergens include dander, epithelium, fur, urine, and saliva, although it is possible that the allergens originate from the same source, e.g. saliva or urine on the fur.

Arthropod Allergens

Arthropod allergen sources are mainly in the Classes Insecta and Arachnida, and are usually injected or inhaled. Some of these allergens, such as the house dust mite, are strongly associated with asthma; others, such as the venom from stinging insects, are associated with life-threatening anaphylaxis.

Insect allergens

The major families of stinging insects associated with allergic reactions belong to the Orders Hymenoptera and Diptera (e.g. bees, wasps, hornets, ants and mosquitos). Of these, allergens from the honey bee appear to be the most clinically important and anaphylaxis is commonly observed. The venom from bees, wasps, hornets, and paper wasps are similar in that they contain vasoactive amines and peptides, and several enzymes such as phospholipase, hyaluronidase and acid phosphatase.

There are a number of inhalent insect allergens, including those from the cockroach, the Chironomid midges, moths and butterflies and locust. Allergy to these insects may arise either through environmental contact or through contact in the workplace such as scientific institutions where they are reared. In these situations, they may cause allergic disease in up to a third of workers.

Arachnid allergens

The major allergen source in the Class Arachnida is the house dust mite (Subclass: Acari); which represent the most clinically important allergen sources worldwide (Fig. 1.6). Mites are ubiquitous, but the most important are those in domestic dwellings or in food storage areas. The major house dust mites belong to the Family: Pyroglyphidae and include the species *Dermatophagoides pteronyssinus*, *D. farinae* (and its sibling species *D. microceras*) and *Euroglyphus maynei*. The storage mites belong to the Families Acaridae and Glycyphagidae, and include the species *Acarus siro* and *A. farris*, *Tyrophagus putrescentiae*, *T. longior*, *Glycyphagus domesticus* and *Lepidoglyphus destructor*. The house dust mites live in carpets, soft furnishings and mattresses. Mite growth is dependent on microclimatic conditions and they proliferate best when the ambient temperature is around 25°C and the relative humidity is 80 per cent. It is because of their association with allergic rhinitis and asthma that mites and their allergens have been studied in detail. Of all the potential allergens in the environment associated with asthma, allergy to the house dust mite alone is the most common independent risk factor for the development of the disease.

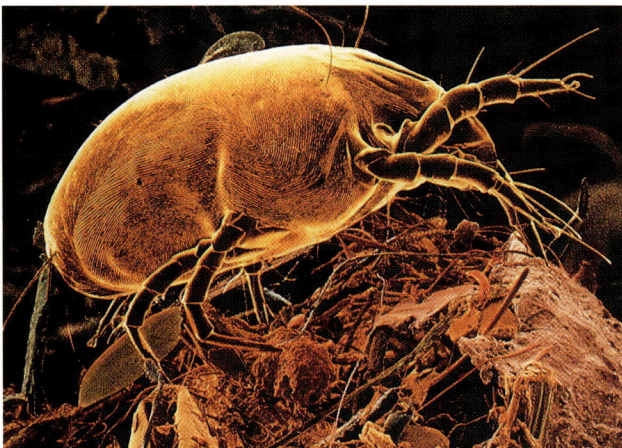

Fig. 1.6 SEM of *Dermatophagoides pteronyssinus*, a house dust mite (× 500). (Courtesy of Science Photo Library, Australia.)

Food Allergens

The frequency, severity, and variety of diseases caused by food intolerance is controversial. A precise definition of food allergy is lacking and the number of double-blind placebo-controlled trials is limited. There are many mechanisms involved, including Types I–IV hypersensitivity responses, direct release of inflammatory mediators from cells following exposure to food products, and the presence of inflammatory mediators in food. Food intolerance causes a variety of clinical entities, including anaphylaxis, and neurological, gastrointestinal, cutaneous, and respiratory disorders. Alcohol also causes allergic responses, probably more frequently than realized. It is usually immediate and more commonly causes upper respiratory tract and eye symptoms. The cause of this is as obscure as with food, and for similar reasons. Diagnosis of food allergy is difficult and food extracts for skin testing are not well characterized.

Drug Allergens

Most drugs associated with allergic disease are of low molecular weight and act as haptens by combining with host proteins. Typical drugs involved in immediate hypersensitivity include antibiotics and anaesthetics. Reactions may occur with subtherapeutic doses. Severe reactions such as anaphylaxis are usually associated with injected drugs.

Contact Allergens

Contact allergens usually cause dermatitis which is generally restricted to the area of contact, although secondary eczema is not uncommon. Contact dermatitis is thought to be a Type IV reaction in which the T lymphocytes become sensitized, and so will not be discussed further.

Occupational Allergens

Workers may become sensitized to substances in the workplace and, on subsequent exposure, experience respiratory and dermatological problems. Occupational allergens range from low molecular weight chemicals of relatively simple structure through to complex proteins (Fig. 1.7). Exposure usually affects only a few individuals in the workforce.

The response time between exposure and symptoms may be delayed by many hours, so that the subject may have left the workplace and be at home when symptoms occur, thus complicating the diagnosis. Recurrent exposure may lead to chronic disease with little variability being discernible, so making it difficult to associate disease with exposure. A number of predisposing factors for occupational allergy have been investigated including: prior atopic status, duration of exposure and smoking.

Allergen Nomenclature

Recently, guidelines have been introduced by the Allergen Nomenclature Subcommittee of the International Union of Immunological Societies (IUIS) to facilitate the consistent naming of purified allergens. In particular, this scheme was introduced for those allergens which were isolated from complex allergen sources comprising several individual allergens. The system has been used throughout this chapter. The naming of one of the major allergens from the house dust mite *Dermatophagoides pteronyssinus* will be used as an example.

This allergen, previously described by several authors as Pl, Dpt12 and Dp42, is now referred to as *Der p* I. The designation is constructed by taking the first 3 italicized letters of the genus (i.e. *Dermatophagoides*) together with the first italicized letter of the species (i.e. *pteronyssinus*) and combining it with a Roman numeral, often reflecting the order in which the allergen was isolated and described. However, the obviously recognizable major allergen in any extract is always given priority in the numbering order. Similar allergens from different species within a genus will use the same numbering arrangement as seen with the structural equivalents of *Der p* I from the mites *D. farinae* and *D. microceras*, which are referred to as *Der f* I and *Der m* I respectively. Collectively, such related allergens are often referred to as belonging to a group, e.g. the group I mite allergens.

Isolation and Characterization of Allergens

Individual allergens are usually isolated from aqueous extracts of the original allergenic source material. As most allergens are protein or glycoprotein, any of the physicochemical techniques available for isolating proteins in general will suffice. In addition, monoclonal antibody methodology and recombinant DNA technology are being utilized in the isolation and characterization of allergens.

Determination of Allergenicity

Several techniques have been developed to monitor the allergenicity of both allergen source and individual allergens, all of which rely on detecting the binding of allergen-specific IgE to the material under investigation. Before the discovery of IgE, the only methods available were biological, such as the skin test reaction where the putative allergenic material was injected in the forearms of appropriately sensitized volunteers and the resulting weal and flare reaction recorded. Although the direct demonstration of IgE binding has, in the main, supplanted the biological assays in monitoring fractionation procedures, it is still thought necessary to confirm allergenic activity in at least one biological assay.

Radioallergosorbent assay

The allergen or allergen extract is immobilized on to an insoluble matrix such as plastic, cellulose nitrate, cellulose (paper) or agarose beads and incubated with sera from allergic patients. The IgE antibody then binds to the immobilized allergen and the complex is detected by incubating it with an antibody specific for IgE which may be complexed to one of several markers such as a radioisotope (usually ^{125}I) or enzymes

Common Occupational Allergens

Source	Examples	Industry
Low molecular weight chemicals		
metals and their salts	platinum, aluminium, vanadium, nickel and chromium salts	metal refining, plating, boiler cleaning, welding
chemicals	chloramine T, colophony (pine resin), polyvinyl chloride, isocyanates, anhydrides, ethylenediamine	brewing, soldering, meat wrapping, plastics and chemical
drugs		
antibiotics	pencillin, tetracycline, cephalosporins	manufacture
miscellaneous	salbutamol, methyldopa	manufacture
animal proteins		
miscellaneous – mammalian	dander, urine, serum, feathers, droppings	research, breeding
miscellaneous – invertebrate	scales, somatic debris, body fluids	research, breeding
	mites	farming, grain handling
enzymes	trypsin, pepsin, amylase, lysozyme, lipase	manufacture
plants		
vegetable dust	wood, cereals, legumes	carpentry, baking, milling, processing
enzymes	papain, bromelain, pectinase, cellulase, amylase	pharmaceuticals, food processing
bacterial		
enzymes	alcalase (protease) esperase (protease)	detergent

Fig. 1.7 Common occupational allergens.

such as horseradish peroxidase or alkaline phosphatase. The degree of IgE binding is determined by measuring the bound radiolabel or measuring the conversion of an appropriate substrate spectrophotometrically. In this method, the greater the binding, the greater the allergenicity.

A useful variant of this method is RAST-inhibition (Fig. 1.8) where varying concentrations of the allergens are mixed with aliquots of the allergic serum before incubation with the matrix-bound allergen. If the soluble allergen has bound IgE in the serum, this is reflected in decreased IgE binding to the matrix. The results are expressed in terms of the amount of allergen required to give 50 per cent inhibition of maximum binding. In addition, the slope of the inhibition curve obtained gives information regarding the range of allergens contained within an extract and this technique is regularly used in studies aimed at standardizing allergen extracts.

Crossed radioimmunoelectrophoresis

In this technique, the allergen extract is electrophoretically separated in an agarose gel. At the conclusion of the electrophoresis, the gel is rotated 90 degrees and the separated proteins electrophoresed into agarose containing an antiserum raised against the allergen extract. The proteins migrate into the gel until they meet their homologous IgG antibody which, because of the chosen conditions , remains stationary. Once sufficient antibody and homologous antigen have interacted, a precipitate forms which can be visualized either by eye or by protein staining. Multiple precipitin bands are formed which provide information on the number of antigens contained within a mixture, and is termed crossed immunoelectrophoresis (CIE).

To determine which of the precipitated proteins are allergenic, the unstained CIE plate is washed and incubated with allergic serum. Allergen-specific IgE binds to remaining epitopes on the precipitate, and the bound IgE is detected using radiolabelled anti-IgE (Fig. 1.9). The allergens are then visualized by autoradiography; this technique is crossed radioimmunoelectrophoresis (CRIE).

This technique provides both qualitative and semiquantitative information, and may be modified to study other aspects of allergen structure such as carbohydrate composition using intermediate gels containing insoluble lectins. Cross-reactivity studies may also be performed using intermediate gels containing appropriate antisera or by analysing two extracts of interest using adjacent wells. In addition, CIE can be combined with other physicochemical techniques such as isoelectric focusing and polyacrylamide gel electrophoresis, and the separated components tested for allergenicity as described. Thus, the physicochemical characteristics of individual allergens can be established without their actual isolation. Other quantitative immunoelectrophoretic methods have also been used in the study of allergens but primarily in the quantitation of individual allergens once the allergen of interest has been isolated

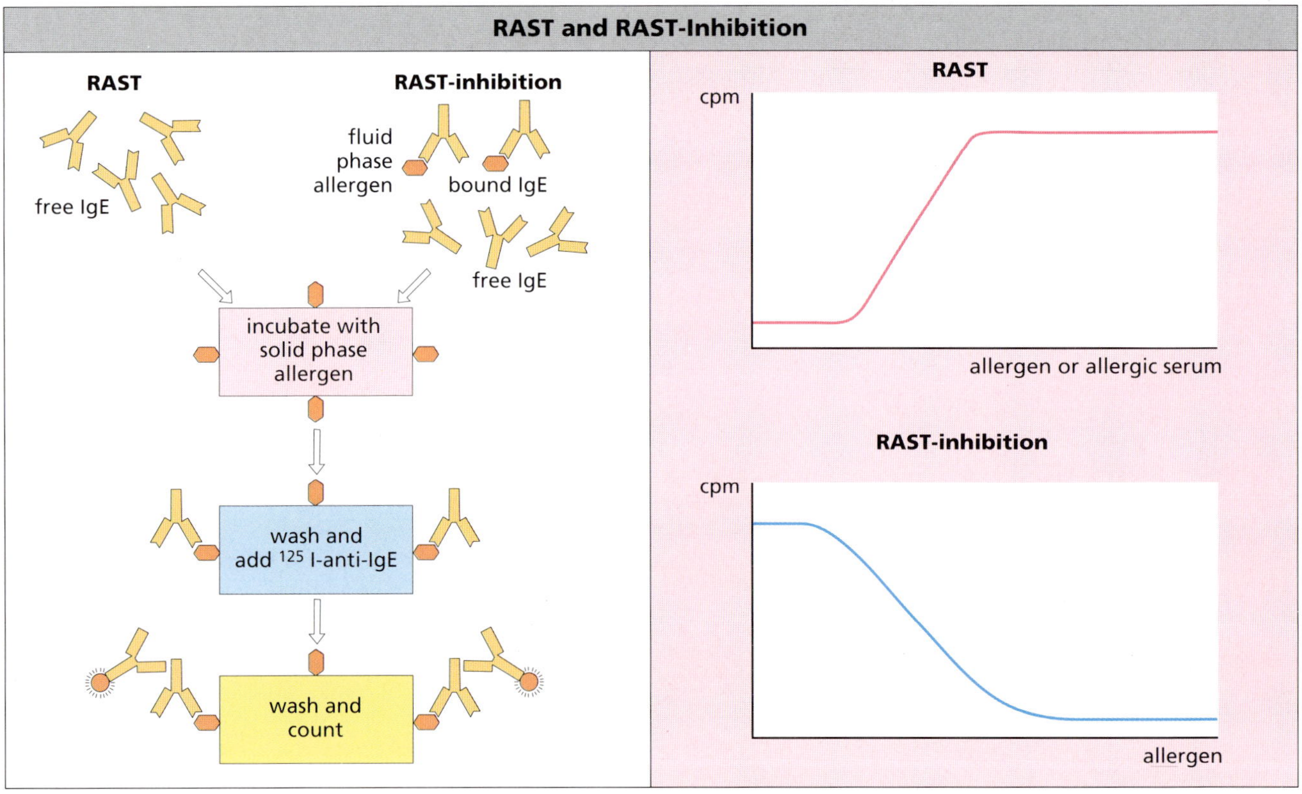

Fig. 1.8 Outline of the steps involved in RAST and RAST-inhibition assays. In RAST, increasing concentrations of allergen are coupled to a solid phase and then incubated with serum from an allergic donor. The amount of IgE bound thus increases with allergen concentration, giving rise to a positive dose response curve [right, above]. In RAST-inhibition, the serum is incubated with fluid phase allergen prior to incubation with solid phase allergen. The more potent the fluid phase allergen, the less free IgE is available to bind to the solid phase allergen. This gives rise to a negative dose response curve [right, below].

and used to prepare a monospecific antibody. Such techniques include single radial immunodiffusion and rocket immunoelectrophoresis. These immunochemical techniques are only as good as the antisera used, in that if the antiserum does not recognize a particular allergen then this component will not be detected.

Immunoblotting

This technique is performed after sodium dodecyl sulphate polyacrylamide electrophoresis (SDS-PAGE). The individual protein components of an allergen extract are electrophoresed after reduction of both intra- and inter-chain disulphide bonds. The proteins separate out on the basis of their molecular weight in descending order. After electrophoresis, the proteins are transferred to a cellulose nitrate membrane which is then treated with allergic serum. The IgE bound to individual allergens is then detected using an enzyme or radiolabelled anti-IgE reagent and the reactivity detected after appropriate treatment (see Fig. 1.10).

Immunoblotting provides information regarding the apparent molecular weights of individual allergens, and the number of allergens in an extract. Its drawbacks include the possibility that the denaturing conditions used in SDS-PAGE may destroy the allergenicity of certain allergens; to minimize this possibility, such experiments are also performed in the absence of reducing reagents. Furthermore, the covalently and non-covalently-bound chain structure of complex allergens may be missed.

Allergen Isolation and Structure

Cloning of allergens

Recombinant DNA technology has facilitated the sequencing of allergens from mites, wasps, grass and tree pollen, and the cloning of other allergens is being pursued. In this technique, messenger RNA is isolated from the allergen source, and complementary DNA prepared by transcribing the RNA using the enzyme reverse transcriptase. The single-stranded copy DNA (cDNA) produced is then converted into double-stranded DNA with the enzyme DNA polymerase and the resulting material inserted into appropriate vectors, such as plasmids, using restriction endonucleases, and cloned. The array of cDNA reflecting the starting RNA represents the library which is then screened to isolate the cDNA coding for the allergens of interest (Fig. 1.11). Screening may be accomplished by hybridization using oligonucleotide probes synthesized on the basis of amino acid sequences obtained by conventional protein sequencing of known allergens

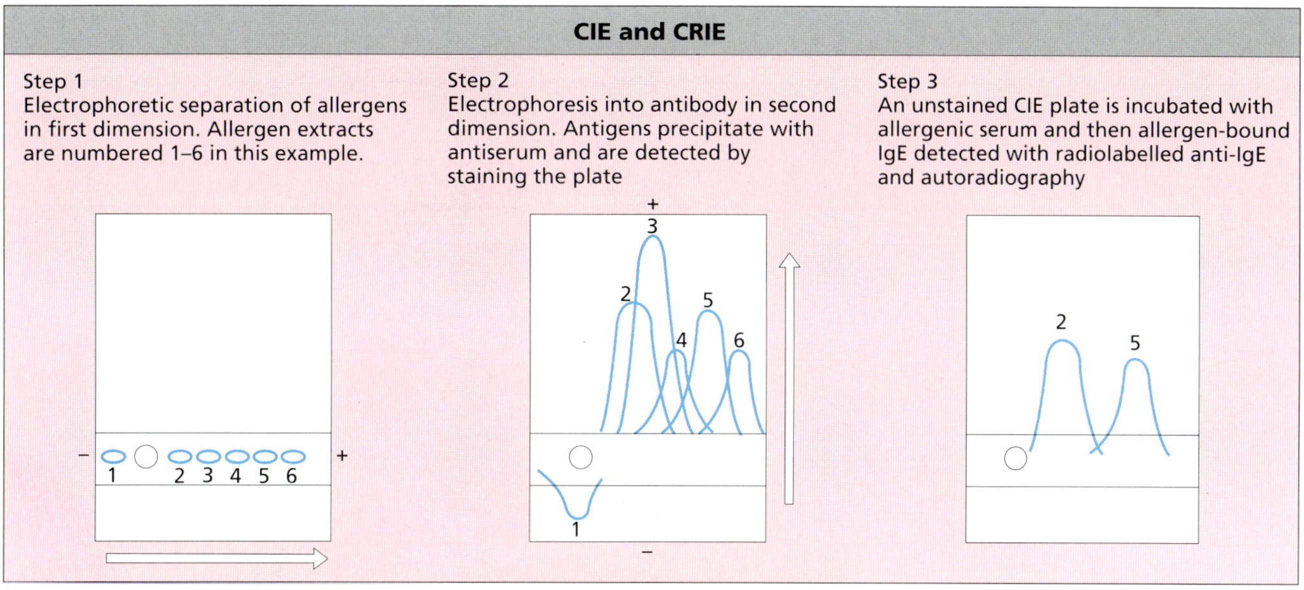

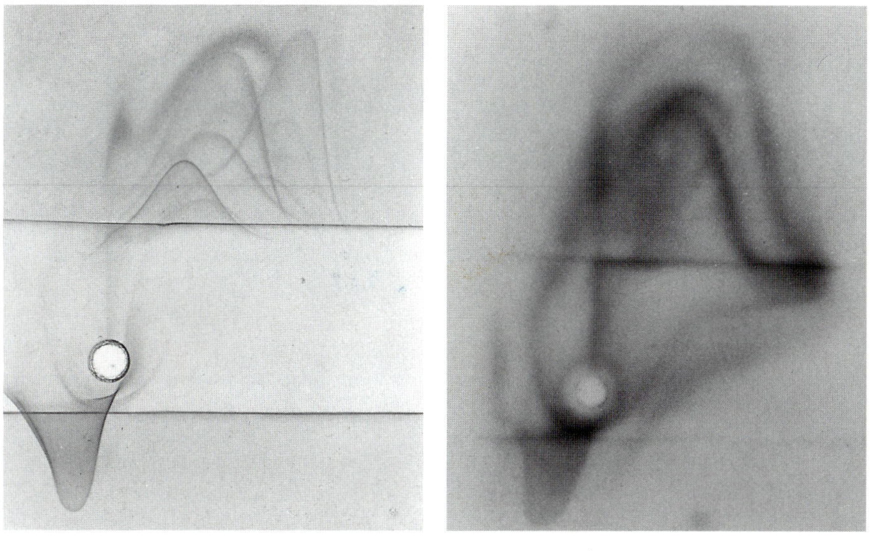

Fig. 1.9 Crossed immunoelectrophoresis (CIE) and crossed radioimmunoelectrophoresis (CRIE) analysis of allergen extracts, with CIE [below, left] and CRIE [below, right] analyses of *Lolium perenne* pollen extract.

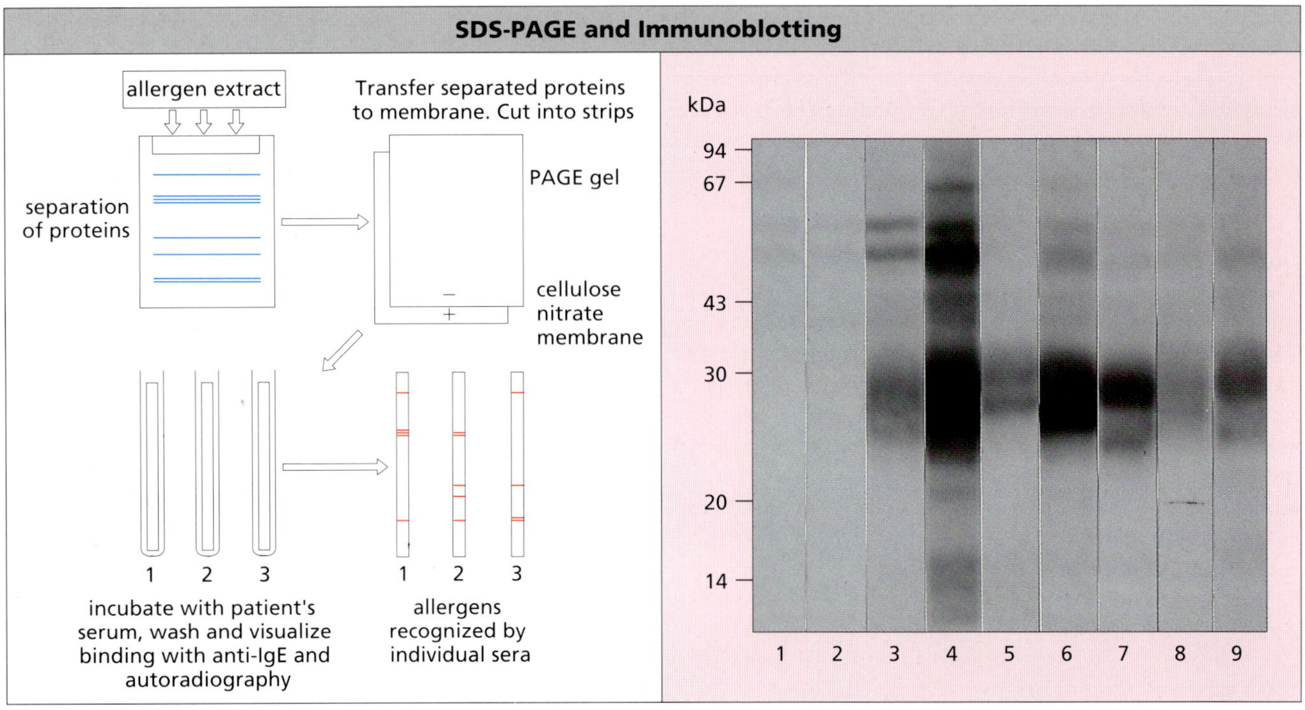

Fig. 1.10 SDS-PAGE and immunoblotting analysis of allergen extracts [left]. SDS-PAGE-IgE immunoblot of *Lolium perenne* pollen extracts [right], demonstrating the responses obtained with sera from seven atopic individuals (1–7) and two non-atopic individuals (8, 9). The molecular weights of appropriate markers, in kDa, are shown. The intensely staining bands in the region of 30 kDa represent responses to the group I allergens.

or, alternatively, by using sera from allergic individuals. The latter technique is used when direct sequence information of the allergens is unavailable and use is made of vectors, termed expression vectors, which direct the synthesis of the allergen. The protein produced is detected using anti-IgE reagents as described above for immunoblotting. Once cloned, the cDNA is sequenced and the DNA data converted to the amino acid sequence and checked to see if the allergen shows homology with any other protein thus far sequenced. Such information may well be useful in determining the role played by the allergen within the original source.

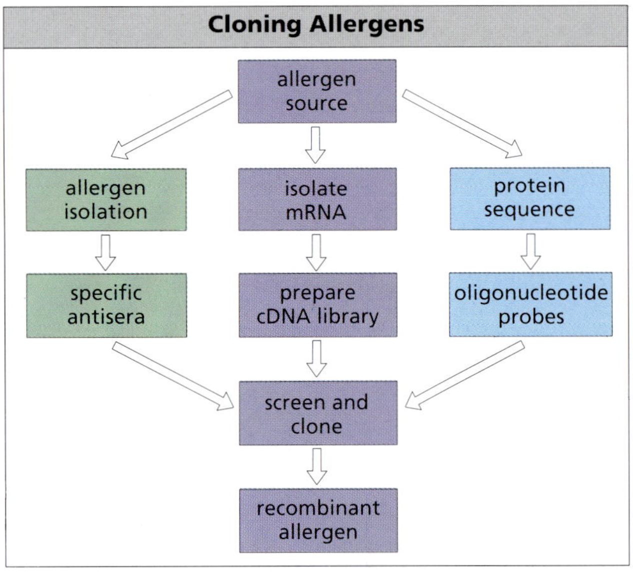

Fig 1.11 Schematic outline of the steps involved in cloning allergens.

In addition, the availability of the cDNA clone for a particular allergen facilitates epitope mapping studies to be performed. In this procedure, the gene is fragmented randomly by physicochemical techniques or at

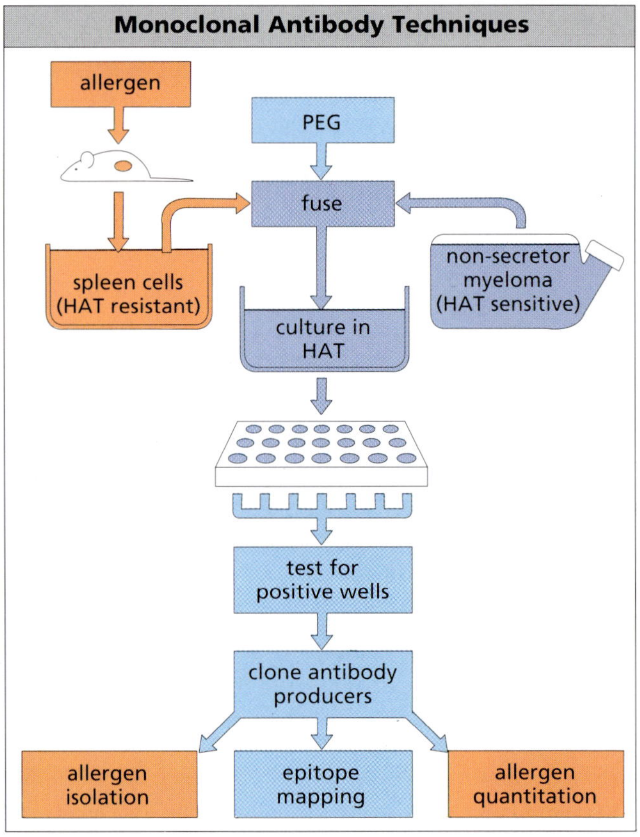

Fig. 1.12 The production of monoclonal antibodies to allergens and their subsequent uses. (Modified from Roitt, IM, Brostoff J, Male DK. *Immunology.* Gower Medical, 2nd Edn, 1989.)

specific sites with appropriate restriction endonucleases, and the resulting fragments cloned into expression vectors. The immunogenicity of the resulting products is then determined and the epitopes mapped.

Monoclonal antibody techniques
In these techniques, mice are immunized with the allergen and spleen cells from the immunized mouse are fused with plasmacytoma cells. The resulting hybridoma represents the sum of the characteristics of the plasmacytoma cell: the capacity to synthesize and secrete antibody, and to divide continuously; and the antibody specificity of the B cell from the immune animal. Both the non-fused plasmacytoma cells (which are metabolically deficient with regard to certain enzymes and thus die in the presence of a selective medium) and the B cells from the immune animal die gradually. However, the fused cells proliferate because they have inherited both the B cell's machinery to overcome the inherent metabolic deficiency of the plasmacytoma cell, and the plasmacytoma cell's capacity to proliferate in tissue culture and produce antibody. The hybridomas are subsequently cloned after establishing the specificity of the antibody produced. Such hybridomas represent a potentially immortal supply of antibody which can be used for a variety of purposes.

With regard to allergens, they are used to isolate, and purify allergens from sources such as mites and grass pollen; to map epitopes; to determine allergen concentrations in the environment and to standardize the concentration of allergens in extracts from different manufacturers (Fig. 1.12).

Identification and Characterization of Specific Allergens

Pollen Allergens

Grass pollen allergens
Of the grass allergens, those from rye grass, timothy grass (*Phleum pratense*), June grass (*Poa pratensis*), orchard grass and Bermuda grass (*Dactylis glomerata*) have been described. However, the most detailed information concerning grass pollen allergens relate to rye grass and the data obtained have been used to interpret those from the other grass pollens (Fig.1.13). The original studies showed that rye grass pollen contained several allergens. Initially, four of the most important allergens, originally designated

Characteristics of Common Plant and Fungal Allergens

New nomenclature	Old nomenclature	Molecular weight (Da)	Isoelectric point (pI)
***Lolium perenne* (rye grass)**			
Lol p I	I	27–35 000	4.0–6.0
Lol p II	II	11 000	5.0
Lol p III	III	11 000	9.0
Lol p IV	IV	57 000	9.0
Lol p V	V	25–30 000	5.0–7.0
Lol p X	X**	12 000	>9.0
***Ambrosia artemisiifolia* (short ragweed)**			
Amb a I	AgE	37 800	5.0
Amb a II	AgK	38 200	5.9
Amb a III	Ra3	12 300	8.5
Amb a V	Ra5	5 000	9.6
Amb a VI	Ra6	11 500	>7.0
Tree pollen			
Betula verrucosa (birch)			
Bet v I	Bv-23	17 000	5.2
Alnus glutinosa (alder)			
Aln g I	Ag-5	17 000	5.2
Corylus avellana (hazel)			
Cor a I	Hla	12–18 000	5.4
Fungal			
Alternaria alternata			
Alt a I	Alt1, Ag1	14–28 000	4.2
Alt a II	basic peptide	6 000	9.5–9.8
Cladosporium herbarium			
Cla h I	Ag32	13 000	3.4–4.4
Cla h II	Ag54	22 000	5.0
Aspergillus fumigatus			
Asp f I	Ag3	24 000	4.5
Asp f II	Ag7	150 000	
Aspergillus oryzae			
*	amylase	56 000	
Saccharomyces cerevisiae			
*	enolase	43 000	
Candida albicans			
*	enolase	43 000	

* Not yet assigned
**This allergen has been shown to be biochemically identical to cytochrome C

Fig. 1.13 Characteristics of common allergens: plant- and fungus-related (see also Fig.1.14).

Groups I–IV, were characterized, but subsequent studies have revealed that rye grass pollen extracts contain other allergens including, for example, cytochrome C and another allergen with an apparent molecular weight similar to the group I allergen. The major allergen is the Group I allergen, now referred to as *Lol p* I, this is recognized by 80–95 per cent of rye allergic individuals. It is an acidic glycoprotein protein of molecular weight 27 kDa and is found in the outer wall and cytoplasm of the pollen grain. *Lol p* I comprises 5 per cent of the total pollen protein and contains about 5 per cent carbohydrate although this moiety is not allergenic *per se*. There is extensive immunological cross-reactivity between the Group I allergens from many grass species in the subfamily Festucoideae. Several monoclonal and polyclonal antibodies to this allergen have been produced and are currently being used to map the IgE and T cell binding epitopes. This allergen has also been cloned.

The rye grass group II and III allergens are non-glycosylated proteins of similar size and each contains 97 amino acid residues. They share 59 per cent sequence identity and demonstrate extensive immunological cross-reactivity. The group IV allergens are relatively high molecular weight basic protein allergens whereas the group V allergens are acidic to neutral proteins. The group X allergens are low molecular weight allergens which have been shown to be biochemically identical to cytochrome C.

Weed pollen allergens

Wind-pollinated weeds are common sources of hay fever in the northern hemisphere: *Artemisia vulgaris* (mugwort) and *Parietaria judaica* (wall pellitory) are the most important in Europe while *Ambrosia artemisiifolia* (short ragweed) and *A. trifida* (giant ragweed) dominate in the USA. Several allergens from short ragweed have been isolated and in certain instances sequenced (see Fig. 1.13). *Amb a* I and *Amb a* II are the two most important allergens from ragweed and represent 6 per cent and 3 per cent of the pollen protein respectively. They demonstrate

Characteristics of Common Insect, Food and Animal Allergens

New nomenclature	Old nomenclature	Molecular weight (Da)	Isoelectric point (pI)
Insects, order Hymnoptera			
Apis mellifera (honey bee)			
Api m I	phospholipase A2	19 500	10.5
Api m II	hyaluronidase	43 000	>10.0
Api m III	mellitin	2 840	Basic
Api m IV	acid phosphatase	49 000	4.0–5.0
Api m V	allergen C	23 000	
Vespula germanica (common wasp)			
Ves g I	phospholipase A_2/B	37 000	Basic
Ves g II	hyaluronidase	43 000	Basic
Ves g V	Ag5	23 000	Basic
Polistes annularis (paper wasp)			
Pol a I	phospholipase A_2/B	37 000	Basic
Pol a II	hyaluronidase	43 000	Basic
Pol a V	Ag5	23 000	Basic
Food			
Gallus domesticus (hen egg white)			
Gal d I	ovomucoid	31 500	4.1
Gal d II	ovalbumin	43 000	4.6
Gal d III	conalbumin	77 000	4.7–6.0
Gadus callarias (cod fish)			
Gad c I	allergen M (parvalbumin)	16 200	4.7
cows' milk	beta lactoglobulin	35 000	
Vegetable dust			
Triticum spp (wheat)			
*	amylase inhibitor	15 000	
*	salt soluble fraction (albumin, globulin)		
*	trypsin inhibitor		
*	agglutinin	34 000	
Ricinus communis (castor bean)			
Ric c I	2S storage albumin	11 000	
Ric c II	crystalloid protein (doublet)	47 000 51 000	5.9
Animal dander			
Felis domesticus (cat)			
Fel d I	Cat1, Ag4	32 000	3.8
Rattus norvegicus (rat)			
Rat n I	prealbumin	20 000	4.5

* Not yet assigned

Fig. 1.14 Characteristics of common insect, food and animal allergens.

immunological cross-reactivity. *Amb a* III is an intermediate, basic protein allergen whereas *Amb* a V and VI are minor, low molecular weight, basic protein allergens.

Tree pollen allergens

The major allergens from trees in temperate zones appear to be structurally and immunochemically similar and are referred to as the group I allergens (see Fig. 1.13). All are acidic proteins (pI 4–6) with molecular weights of about 20 kDa, and there is marked amino acid sequence identity between the allergens from different species (80–90 per cent). The cDNA coding for the group I allergen from the birch has been cloned and sequenced.

Fungal Allergens

Several fungal allergens have been characterized and include those from the major species listed (see Fig. 1.13). A problem confounding research is the fact that extracts prepared by the same methodology can result in considerable variability in the concentration of the major allergen. Such findings have made it difficult to determine if extensive immunological cross-reactivity exists between the different fungal species. Major allergens have been isolated from *Aspergillus fumigatus*, *Alternaria alternata*, and *Cladosporium herbarium*; these are distinct allergens with little or no immunological cross-reactivity. Several fungal allergens such as *Cla h* II are heavily glycosylated but studies in which this moiety has been enzymatically removed indicate that the major IgE-binding epitopes are associated with the protein portion alone. Other allergens have been isolated from *Aspergillus oryzae*, *Saccharomyces cerevisiae* (Bakers yeast, Class: Ascomycotina), and *Candida albicans*, and have been shown to be enzymes such as amylase and enolase. They represent important occupational allergens, particularly in the baking industry.

Animal Allergens

The most important allergens from dogs and cats are derived from epithelium, serum, and saliva. The major allergen associated with the cat is *Fel d* I which is derived from the saliva and epithelium. It is an acid glycoprotein which exists as a dimer, each having a molecular weight of about 18 kDa. Other dog and cat allergens include serum albumin and gamma globulin and it is these allergens which represent the cross-reacting allergens found in such extracts. There do not appear to be any differences between breeds although quantitative differences have been reported.

The primary source of allergens from rodents is the urine; several allergens have been described. The major mouse allergen is the mouse urinary complex, and has a molecular weight of about 17 kDa; it is found in the prealbumin fraction of urine. A similar situation has been found for rat urine allergens, but as well as the prealbumin, a euglobulin is also allergenic. Both these are low molecular weight allergens. Although of similar molecular weights, the rat and mouse prealbumins do not cross-react.

Arthropod Allergens

Insect allergens

Bees and Wasps. The enzymes contained in bee and wasp venom are allergenic and within related species often cross-react (Fig. 1.14). In addition, cross-reactivity between different allergens from different genera may vary. For example, the hyaluronidase from the honey bee (*Apis mellifera*) cross-reacts with that from the wasp (Genus Vespula), but the phospholipases show limited cross-reactivity, and the group V allergens show none at all. In addition to these enzymes, the venom from these insects contain other allergens, the biochemical activities of which have not been determined.

The major allergen from the honey bee is the phospholipase (*Api m* I) whereas in the vespids, it is the component previously designated antigen 5 (e.g. *Pol a* V) which appears to be the most important. A group V allergen from the white-faced hornet (*Dolichovespula maculata*) has been cloned and sequence studies reveal homology with scorpion neurotoxin and with a pathogenesis-related protein from the tobacco leaf.

Chironomid midges. The larvae from *Chironomus thummi thummi* are used commercially as fish food and it was during a study of allergy induced in patients handling this material that haemoglobin was found to be the major allergen (*Chi t* 1). The major allergen in the non-occupational setting is again haemoglobin and exposure to it is thought to arise through contact with the adults which have been shown to retain a certain proportion of haemoglobin during metamorphosis. The various haemoglobins from different species of midges are immunologically cross-reactive.

Cockroach. The major species are *Blatella germanica*, *Periplaneta americana* and *Blatta orientalis*. Individual allergens derived from any species have yet to be isolated and characterized; however, it has been established that extracts of these insects contain several allergens ranging in molecular weight from 12 to 120 kDa. The major allergens correspond to the relatively high molecular weight components (with molecular weights in the region of 70 kDa).

Arachnid allergens

House dust mite allergens. CRIE and immunoblotting have revealed that mite extracts are complex and contain many allergens, several of which have been isolated and characterized. However most emphasis has been directed toward studying the allergens known as *Der p* I and *Der p* II, proteins with molecular weights of about 26 kDa and 15 kDa respectively. Both allergens are recognized by more than 80 per cent of mite-allergic individuals.

Der p I, one of the first allergens to be cloned and sequenced, is a protease belonging to the group of enzymes which have an essential cysteine residue in the catalytic site (see Fig. 1.15). Cysteine proteases in this group include the mammalian proteases cathepsin B and H, and the plant proteases actinidin (from the Chinese gooseberry or Kiwi fruit) and papain. *Der p* I is proteolytically active, and such activity can be

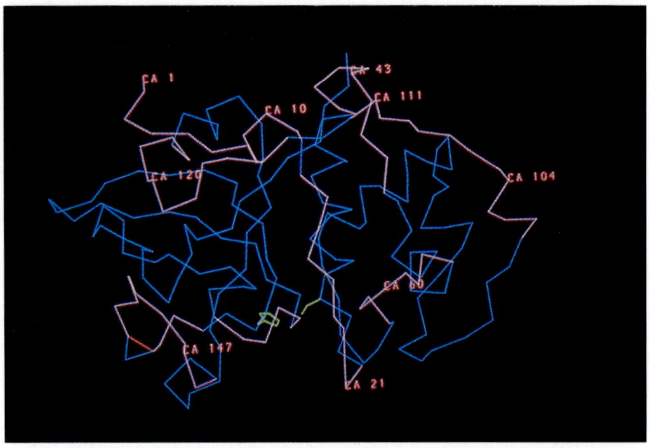

Fig. 1.15 A computer-generated model of the cysteine protease, actinidin, which shows significant homology to the mite allergen, *Der p* I. The sections coloured pink represent IgE/G binding epitopes. The yellow regions indicate the amino acid residues involved in catalysis. (Courtesy of Dr E Baker, Massey University, New Zealand.)

demonstrated in house dust samples. The allergen demonstrates immunological cross-reactivity with both *Der f* I, *Der m* I and possibly *Eur m* I. It is found in the faecal pellet which is about the same size as a pollen grain and becomes airborne during domestic activity. The biochemical identity of the group II allergens remains unknown. Studies have revealed that the recently described group III (e.g. *Der f* III and *Der p* III) and Group IV (e.g. *Der p* IV) allergens correspond to trypsin and amylase respectively. Faecal pellets contain other enzymes involved in digestion, such as chymotrypsin, glycoamylase, lysozyme, lipase, esterase and a variety of glycosidases, but their allergenicities are unknown. In summary, it appears that the majority of house dust mite allergens are enzymes involved in digestion which become entrapped within the faecal pellet (Fig. 1.16).

Storage mites. Our knowledge regarding the storage mites is not as extensive as that for the house dust mites, but RAST-inhibition and immunoblotting studies have been performed which show that such mites are allergenically complex and that, in extracts derived from mites such as *Lepidoglyphus destructor*, the major allergens have apparent molecular weights of 16 kDa and 18 kDa. Cross-reactivity studies indicate that the storage mites are more closely related to each other than they are to the house dust mites. It is possible that these data indicate that the storage mites produce allergens which are biochemically similar to those found in the house dust mites and cross-react weakly because their sequences have diverged during evolution. Alternatively, given that digestive enzymes are inducible and reflect the major food source, and that primary food sources of storage mites are different from those of the house dust mite, it is possible that storage mite allergens represent proteins which do not have counterparts in the house dust mites. It is likely that both explanations have merit.

Biochemical Characteristics of Mite Allergens

Group	Molecular weight (Da)	Carbohydrate	Enzyme activity
I	25 371	probably	cysteine protease
II	14 131	no	not known
III	30 000	unknown	trypsin
IV	56 000	unknown	alpha amylase

Fig. 1.16 Biochemical characteristics of mite allergens.

Food Allergens

As outlined earlier, it is difficult to identify relevent allergens, but the allergens listed in Fig. 1.14 have been described at the biochemical and molecular level.

Occupational allergens

Vegetable dust and flour

Several vegetable dusts and flours have been shown to be potent aeroallergen sources and include cereal flours, castor beans, green coffee beans, cotton seed, Ispaghula and soya beans. Several individual allergens from these sources, particularly cereals and castor beans, have been described in detail (see Fig. 1.14). Flour from wheat (*Triticum* spp), rye (*Secale cereale*) and barley (*Hordeum vulgaris*) have been shown to be significant sources of aeroallergens. In industries such as baking, the frequency of positive skin tests to wheat components may be as high as 30 per cent. The allergens to which bakers become sensitized include not only those associated with the flour, but also with the additives; these include amylase derived from *Aspergillus oryzae* and the enzyme enolase derived from *Saccharomyces cerevisiae* (see fungal allergen section above).

The major allergens in cereals are found in the water-soluble fraction, and there is extensive cross-reactivity amongst the cereals but not between the cereals and the grasses. The major allergens include proteins with amylase and trypsin inhibitory activities, and wheat germ agglutinin.

Other vegetable dusts which cause sensitization are those derived from legumes such as *Ricinus communis* (castor beans) and soya bean. Two allergens from *R. communis* have been described: a low molecular weight storage protein (an albumin), and a higher molecular weight crystalloid protein which appears as a doublet on SDS-PAGE-immunoblot analyses.

Another common group of occupational allergens are hydrolytic enzymes derived from animals, plants, and bacteria. They include enzymes such as proteases, cellulases, amylases, lipases and lysozyme. Their detailed physicochemical characteristics are to be found in most biochemical textbooks and will not be discussed here.

Allergen Usage and Standardization

Allergens are used diagnostically and to desensitize patients. Most allergen extracts used for these purposes are crude, in that they contain not only allergens but also irrelevant antigens. They have a finite shelf life and there may be wide variation in potency between the same type of extract produced by different manufacturers. Attempts have been made to standardize allergen extracts.

Standardization is important if accurate diagnosis, treatment and research are to be pursued (Fig. 1.17). To standardize extracts on qualitative and quantitative criteria, it is necessary to:

- ensure that the allergen source is derived from the correct species;
- ensure that the allergen source is not contaminated with other allergen sources;
- establish that a spectrum of major allergens is present (expanding the spectrum of allergens to include the full complement of minor allergens does not appear to offer significant diagnostic advantages);
- measure and standardize the total allergen content;
- determine the concentration of selected major allergens where assays are available; and
- ensure that the extract is biologically active.

Recently, the WHO and the IUIS Allergen Standardization Subcommittee initiated a program to produce International Reference Preparations to aid researchers and commercial manufacturers to prepare and use standardized extracts.

Monitoring Allergen Exposure

Monitoring the allergen source or individual allergen concentration can prove useful in several situations. For example, monitoring atmospheric pollen concentrations can warn people at risk of seasonal allergies. Monitoring atmospheric concentrations of pollen and fungi require skill in the recognition of these agents, and such monitoring should include a precise identification of the airborne particles so as to distinguish between fungal spores and grass pollen, since there may be a non-parallel variation in the concentrations of the allergenic and non-allergenic types.

Specific allergen concentration monitoring may also be useful to determine whether atmospheric concentrations constitute a risk in the workplace or in the home. With regard to the latter, it has been proposed that the measurement of a single allergen, namely *Der p* I, reflects the total house dust mite allergen concentration. The concentration of this allergen has been monitored in dust from mattresses, soft furnishings and carpet, and found to vary (0–100 μg/g of fine dust, and it has recently been proposed that approximately 2 μg of *Der p* I correspond to 100 whole mites. It has been suggested that allergen concentrations of 2 μg/g and 10 μg/g of fine dust probably represent risk factors for allergic sensitization and provocation respectively.

Measuring allergen concentrations may also be useful for assessing the effectiveness and timing of allergen avoidance measures.

Criteria Used to Standardize Allergen Extracts

Parameter	Method
Qualitative	
purity of source material	taxonomic identification of species, determination of contaminants (e.g. fungal spores in pollen preparations)
allergenicity of source material	RAST, RAST-inhibition, skin test
spectrum of major allergens	CRIE, immunoblotting
Quantitative	
total allergenicity	RAST-inhibition
individual allergen content	RAST-inhibition, CRIE, RIA, ELISA
stability	RAST-inhibition, CRIE, RIA, ELISA

Fig. 1.17 Criteria used to standardize allergen extracts.

Allergen Avoidance

One approach to reducing allergen-induced disease is to avoid the allergen source. This has had some success but, in many instances, total avoidance proves impossible. The simple way is to change jobs or move residence, but this is not often practical because of the costs involved and the possibility of other allergens in the new location showing cross-reactivity with the allergen being avoided. It is also possible to remove the source completely, e.g. by relinquishing the family pet, killing mites with acaracides, or installing high-efficiency filters to remove allergens from the atmosphere. A more recent approach is to attempt to modify the allergen itself so as to render it non-allergenic, e.g. by chemically modifying allergens such as those from the mite with tannic acid.

Allergens Used in Immunotherapy

Allergens are often used in immunotherapy, despite our lack of understanding of the mechanisms underlying the clinical benefit observed. One explanation offered is that the injection of allergen stimulates the production of allergen-specific IgG antibodies which out-compete IgE for the allergen, thus inhibiting interaction with sensitized mast cells. Several techniques to modify allergens have been developed which facilitate the production of allergen-specific IgG without increasing the risk of anaphylaxis which may occur when native allergen is injected into a sensitized recipient. Such techniques include polymerising the allergen with cross-linking reagents such as glutaraldehyde or polyethylene glycol.

Future Directions

Over the next few years, progress in allergen research is likely to be considerable. The main areas in which advances will be made are:

- the further purification and characterization of allergens using both cDNA cloning and sophisticated protein chemistry techniques;
- the refinement of methods for detecting and quantifying specific allergens in the environment;
- the development of more specific and reproducible methods for assessing the allergens recognized by individual patients;
- the clarification of the role, if any, of the biochemical activity of allergens with respect to enhancing or initiating allergic responses;

- a definition of specific epitopes on allergens of major clinical importance and perhaps an exploitation of such information in the development of novel immunotherapeutic reagents.

All these developments should contribute significantly to our understanding of the nature of allergens and how they interact with the mechanisms involved in the disease process and, ultimately, in better management of allergic conditions.

Further Reading

Aas K. What makes an allergen an allergen? *Allergy* 1978;**33:** 3.

Allergy: Which allergens? Pharmacia Publication (1985) Pharmacia, Uppsala, Sweden.

Baldo BA, Tovey ER, eds. *Protein Blotting: Methodology, Research and Diagnostic Applications.* Karger, Basel, Switzerland, 1989.

Chapman MD. Allergen specific monoclonal antibodies: New tools for the management of allergic disease. *Allergy* 1988; **43:**7.

Chua KY, Stewart GA, Thomas WR, Simpson RJ, Dilworth RJ, Plozza TM, Turner, KJ. Sequence analysis of cDNA coding for a major house dust mite allergen, Der p 1 Homology with cysteine proteases. *J Exp Med* 1988;**167:**175

Drebourg S,Einarsson R, Longbottom J. The chemistry and standardization of allergens. In: *Handbook of Experimental Immunology in Four Volumes,* Vol. 1, 10.1. Weir DM ed. Blackwell Scientific Publications, Oxford, 4th Ed., 1986.

Gutman A. Allergens and other factors important in atopic disease. In: *Allergic Diseases: Diagnosis and Management.* Paterson R ed. J B Lippincott Co. Philadelphia, 3rd Ed., 1985.

International Workshop Report. Dust mite allergens and asthma: A worldwide problem. Bull. WHO. 1988;**66:**769.

IUIS Subcommittee for Allergen Standardization. *Allergen Nomenclature.* Bull. WHO. 1986; **64:**767.

Kurth R, ed. *Regulatory Control and Standardization of Allergenic Extracts. Fifth International Paul Ehrlich Seminar, September 2-4, 1987, Frankfurt.* Gustav Fischer Verlag, Stuttgart, 1988.

Lake FR, Ward LD, Simpson RJ, Thompson PJ, Stewart GA. House dust mite-derived amylase: allergenicity and physicochemical characterization. *J Allergy Clin Immunol* 1991; **87:**1035.

Lowenstein H. Quantitative immunoelectrophoretic methods as a tool for the analysis and isolation of allergens. *Prog Allergy* 1978; **25:**1.

Lowenstein H, Ipsen H, Lind P, Mattheisen F. The physicochemical and biological characteristics of allergens. In: *Allergy: An International Textbook,* Lessof MH, Lee TH, Kemeny DM, eds. John Wiley and Sons, Chichester, 1987; 87–104.

Marsh DG. Allergens and genetics of allergy. In: *The Antigens,* Vol. 3. Sela M, ed. Academic Press, London, 1975;271–359.

Marsh DG. In: *Genetic and Environmental Factors in Clinical Allergy.* Marsh DG, Blumenthal MN, eds. University of Minnesota Press, 1989.

Platts-Mills TAE, Chapman MD. Dust mites: immunology, allergic disease, and environmental control. *J Allergy Clin Immunol* 1987;**80:**755.

Registration of Allergen Preparations: Nordic Guidelines. Nordic Council on Medicines, Uppsala, Sweden, 2nd Ed., 1989.

Said El Shami A, Merrett T G, eds. Allergy and Molecular Biology. Proceedings of the DPC First International Symposium on Allergy and Molecular Biology. *Adv.Biosciences* 1989; **74:**1.

Stewart GA, Thompson PJ, Simpson RJ. Protease antigens from house dust mite. *Lancet* 1989;**2:**154.

Solomon WR. Aerobiology of pollinosis. *J Allergy Clin Immunol* 1984; **74:**449.

Tovey ER, Chapman MD, Platts-Mills TAE. Mite faeces are a major source of house dust allergens. *Nature* 1981;**289:**592.

Valanta R, Duchêne M, Pettenburger K et al. Identification of profilin as a novel pollen allergen; IgE autoreactivity in sensitized individuals. *Science* 1991; **253:** 485.

Chapter 2

IgE Structure, Synthesis and Interaction with Receptors

Introduction

Immunoglobulin (Ig) E is the primary antibody involved in the initiation of immediate allergic responses, alternatively named type I hypersensitivity reactions. Like other antibodies, IgE may be subdivided into two functional regions: an Fc region by which it attaches to effector cells and an Fab region which is responsible for its interactions with allergen. There are two types of cell surface receptor specific for interaction with the Fc region of IgE. Mast cells and basophils have a high affinity (K_a = 10^{-10}/M) receptor for IgE, termed $Fc_\epsilon R1$, which sensitizes them for their subsequent release of histamine, eicosanoids (which initiate the symptoms of the early phase response), and cytokines (which initiate allergic inflammation). A second receptor for IgE, $Fc_\epsilon R2$, is found on inflammatory cells, including NK cells, macrophages, eosinophils and platelets, B and T cells, Langerhans' cells and follicular dendritic cells. $Fc_\epsilon R2$ has a lower affinity for IgE (K_a=10^{-7}/M), and is implicated in IgE antibody-dependent cell cytotoxicity (ADCC), as well as in allergic inflammation. This receptor is, moreover, a multifunctional lymphokine, which induces the growth and differentiation of activated B cells, and acts as a co-factor for the IL-4 induced heavy chain switching to IgE expression. The binding of IgE-antigen complexes to the receptor on B cells, and subsequent internalization, contributes to antigen presentation. When first identified on lymphocytes, this molecule was termed CD23. It was subsequently found to be identical to $Fc_\epsilon R2$, and the names are now used synonymously. The name $Fc_\epsilon R2$ will be used here. The essential properties of IgE and its receptors are summarized in Figs 2.1–2.3.

Essential Characteristics of Human IgE	
cell distribution	committed and selected B cells
sub-unit structure (no. of amino acids)	two (κ or λ) light chains, two ϵ-heavy chains (556 for IgE MD)
post-translational modifications	six glycosylation sites
isoforms	secreted IgE (IgE), membrane-bound (mIgE)
regulation	IL-4: commitment (switching), $Fc_\epsilon R2$: selection (cell growth), unknown factors: splicing to generate IgE or mIgE

Fig. 2.1 Essential characteristics of human IgE.

Essential Properties of Receptors for Human IgE		
	$Fc_\epsilon R1$	$Fc_\epsilon R2$
other names	high affinity receptor	low affinity receptor, CD23
affinity for monomeric IgE	Ka=10^{-10}/M	Ka=10^{-7}/M
cell distribution	mast cells, basophils	B cells, T cells, eosinophils, platelets, macrophages, NK cells, follicular dendritic cells
sub-unit composition (number of amino acids)	α-chain (260), β-chain (263)* two γ-chains (86)	trimer (321)
orientation of polypeptide chains (extra-cellular)	N-terminus	C-terminus
structural motifs	two Ig domains per α-chain	animal C-type lectin domain, α-helical coiled-coil stalk, RGD adhesion sequence, trafficking signals
post-translational modifications	serine, threonine and tyrosine phosphorylation sites in α-chain 7 carbohydrate sites in α-chain	one N-glycosylation site per chain three protease processing sites per chain
isoforms	one known	$Fc_\epsilon R2a$ and $Fc_\epsilon R2b$ (see Fig. 2.3)
function	cell degranulation	growth and/or differentiation factor for haempoietic cells, anti-apoptosis, antigen presentation, IgE expression, IgE-ADCC
associated disease states	immediate hypersensitivity	inflammation, EBV transformation of B cells

Fig. 2.2 Essential properties of the two receptors for human IgE (* determined for rat β-chain).

Comparison of the Two Isoforms of $Fc_{\epsilon}R2$

	$Fc_{\epsilon}R2a$	$Fc_{\epsilon}R2b$
N-terminal sequence	MEEGQYS	MNPPSQ
cell distribution	B cells	B cells, T cells, macrophages, eosinophils
regulation	B-cell constitutive	IL-4 inducible
function	growth/ differentiation factor, antigen presentation	growth/ differentiation factor, regulation of IgE synthesis, immunity to parasites

Fig. 2.3 Comparison of the two isoforms of human $Fc_{\epsilon}R2$.

Covalent Structure of Human IgE

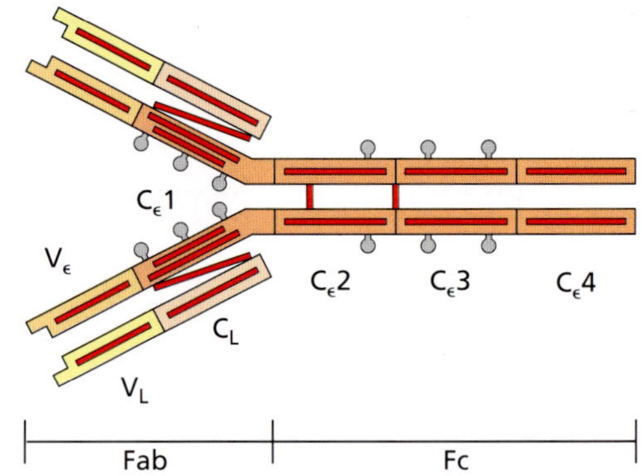

Fig. 2.4 The covalent structure of human IgE. The light and heavy chains, the variable (V), constant (C), Fab and Fc regions, the disulphide bonds (red) and N-linked glycosylation sites (grey) are shown.

Myeloma IgE 'ND' ϵ-chain

common sequence	1	(Q T Q L V Q S G A E V R K P G A S V R V S C K A S	25
	26	Q Y T F I D S Y I H W I R Q A P G H G L E W V G W	50
	51	I N P N S G G T N Y A P R F Q G R V T M T R D A S	75
	76	F S T A Y M D L R S L R S D D S A V F Y C A K S D	100
	101	P F W S D Y Y N F D Y S Y T L D V W G Q G T T V T	125
	126	V S S) (A S T Q S P S V F P L T R C C K N I P S N A	150
	151	T S V T L G C L A T G Y F P E P V M V T C D T G S	175
	176	L N G T T M T L P A T T L T L S G H Y A T I S L L	200
	201	T V S G A W A K Q M F T C R V A H T P S S T D W V	225
	226	D N K T F S) (V C S R D F T P P T V K I L Q S S C D	250
	251	G G G H F P P T I Q L L C L V S G Y T P G T I N I	275
	276	T W L E D G Q V M D V D L S T A S T T Q E G E L A	300
	301	S T Q S E L T L S Q K H W L S D R T Y T C Q V T Y	325
	326	Q G H T F E D S T K K C A) (D S N P R G V S A Y L S	350
	351	R P S P F D L F I R K S P T I T C L V V D L A P S	375
	376	K G T V N L T W S R A S G K P V N H S T R K E E K	400
	401	Q R N G T L T V T S T L P V G T R D W I E G E T Y	425
	426	Q C R V T H P H L P R A L M R S T T K T S) (G P R A	450
	451	A P E V Y A F A T P E W P G S R D K R T L A C L I	475
	476	Q N F M P E D I S V Q W L H N E V Q L P D A R H S	500
	501	T T Q P R K T K G S G F F V F S R L E V T R A E W	525
	526	E Q K D E F I C R A V H E A A S P S Q T V Q R A V	550
	551	S V N P	
secretory		. . . . G K)	
membrane – long form		. . . . (G L A G G S A Q S Q R A P D R V L C H S G	575
	576	Q Q Q G L P R A R G G S V P H P R C H C G A G R A	600
	601	D W P G P P E L D V C V E E A E G E A P W T W T G	625
	626	L C I F A A L F L L S V S Y S A A L T L L M) (V Q R	650
	651	F L S A T R Q G R P Q T S L D Y T N V L Q P H A)	
membrane – short form		(E L D V C V E E A E G E A P W T W T G L C	575
	576	I F A A L F L L S V S Y S A A L T L L M) (V Q R F L	600
	601	S A T R Q G R P Q T S L D Y T N V L Q P H A)	

immunoglobulin domains

transmembrane segments

cytoplasmic sequences, presumed to be involved in signal transduction and cellular trafficking

( ) exon boundaries

N potential N-glycosylation sites

Fig. 2.5 Structural organization of secreted and membrane-bound forms of the human ϵ-chain: [above] the complete sequence of the ϵ-chain of a myeloma IgE; [below] ϵ-chain sequences translated from the mIgE expressed in B cells. (Data adapted from Peng C et al, *J Immunol*, 1992; **148**:129–136.)

IgE is the least abundant of all the antibody classes, and is present in serum at only about 0.1–0.3 μg/l, as against 5–15 g/l for IgG. After antigenic stimulation, however, the newly synthesized IgE antibodies make up a higher proportion of the total pool of IgE than do IgG antibodies of total IgG. This may be due in part to its short half-life in serum namely two days, as compared with 20 days for IgG. The result is that specific IgE antibodies can compete more effectively with non-specific IgE for binding to cell receptors, and are more likely than IgG antibodies to elicit degranulation of mast cells and basophils and initiate the cascade of later reactions. Its high affinity for the receptor, $Fc_{\epsilon}R1$, on these cells (K_a is greater by at least an order of magnitude than that of IgG for its high affinity receptor, $Fc_{\epsilon}R1$), also assists its efficacy at low concentrations. The IgE system is at once extremely sensitive and liable to overshoot with undesirable consequences – hence the term hypersensitivity. The physiological controls that normally operate are evidently inadequate in individuals predisposed to allergy.

In this chapter, the state of knowledge about the structures of IgE, $Fc_{\epsilon}R1$ and $Fc_{\epsilon}R2$, and the nature of their interactions will be reviewed first. Then there will be consideration of the mechanisms which control the concentrations and activities of these components, with reference mainly to the human system.

The Structure of IgE

Like other immunoglobulins, IgE has two heavy (H) and two κ- or λ-light (L) chains, each with variable (V) and constant (C) regions, organized into globular domains of about 110 amino acids and stabilized by one or more intra-chain disulphide bonds (Fig. 2.4). IgE differs from other heavy chain classes in possessing ϵ-heavy chains, distinguished from other heavy chains by their C region sequence (Fig. 2.5). The two identical light chains are both made up of one V (V_L) and one C (C_L) domain. The ϵ-chains comprise a single V (V_{ϵ}) domain and four C domains, termed $C_{\epsilon}1$, $C_{\epsilon}2$, $C_{\epsilon}3$ and $C_{\epsilon}4$. IgE contains four inter-chain disulphide bonds, those between C_L and $C_{\epsilon}1$ uniting the light and heavy chains and those between the $C_{\epsilon}2$ domains, the two ϵ-chains. IgE is cleaved by papain between $C_{\epsilon}1$ and $C_{\epsilon}2$ into two Fab fragments and one Fc fragment. Each Fab contains one light chain, covalently linked to the N-terminal fragment of the ϵ-

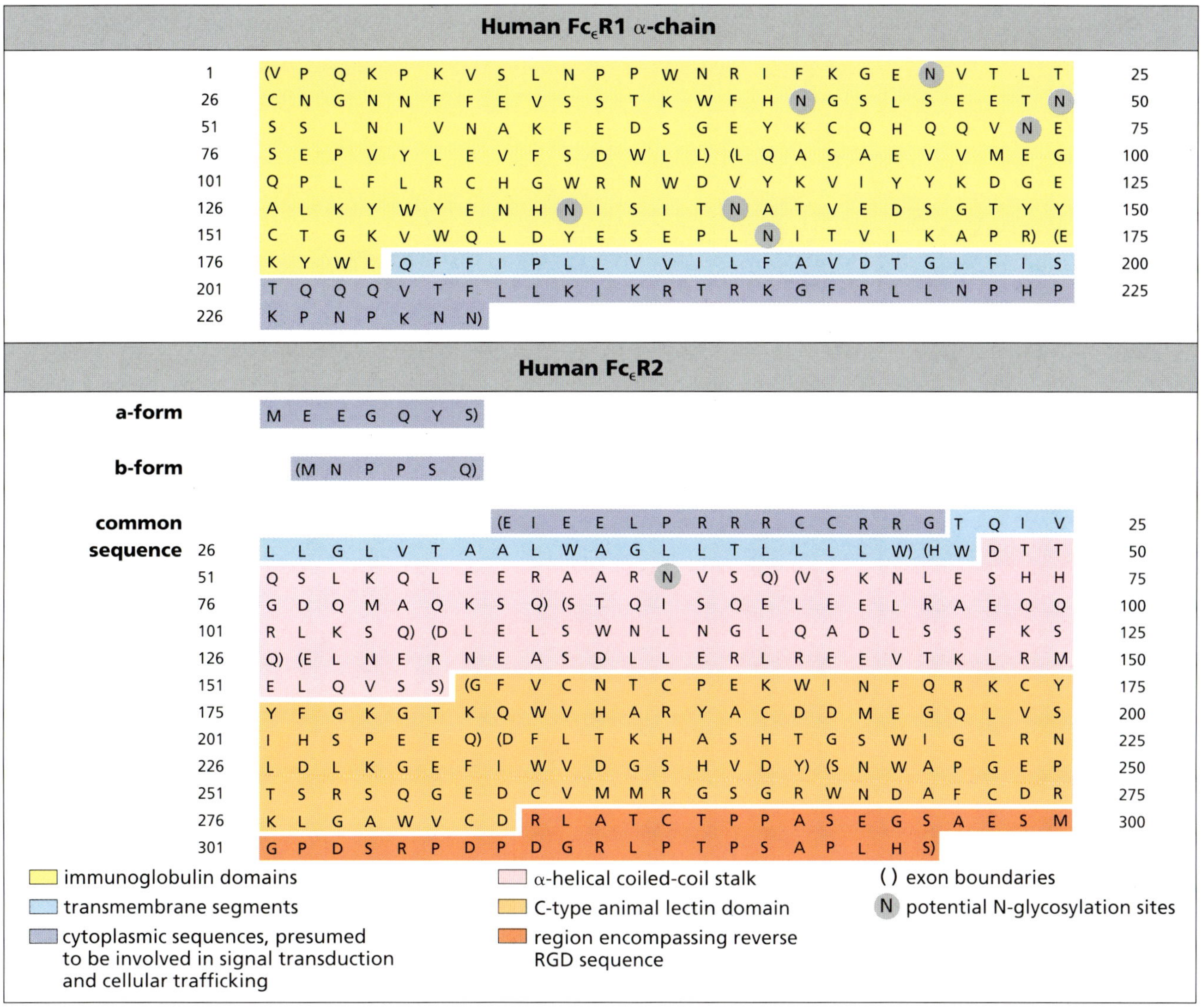

Fig. 2.6 Structural organization of human $Fc_{\epsilon}R1$, $Fc_{\epsilon}R2a$ and $Fc_{\epsilon}R2b$.

chain, and retains full affinity for antigen. The Fc is a dimer of the C-terminal ϵ-chain fragments, linked by the two disulphide bonds in $C_\epsilon 2$; this retains full binding affinity for both receptors.

Immunoglobulins are the prototypic members of the immunoglobulin superfamily (see Fig. 2.9), which includes all antibodies, many cell receptors, cell adhesion molecules, and other proteins, containing one or more immunoglobulin domains. The domain structure is the basis for the function of these molecules in molecular recognition. These domains have a number of general features (Fig. 2.7). They consist of compact, independently folding units, connected by stretches of extended polypeptide chain. The conformations of the units are similar, although not identical; all consist of two anti-parallel β-pleated sheets, connected by loops of variable length. Interaction between the two β-sheets is stabilized by one or more intra-chain disulphide bonds. Sequences that form this β-sheet structure are characterized by alternating hydrophobic and hydrophilic side chains that dictate the orientation of the β-sheets towards the solvent or interior of the domain. In an immunoglobulin domain, the two hydrophobic faces are apposed, and the two cysteines that form the disulphide bond linking the β-sheets are conserved. The differences between the conformations of different domains relate principally to the lengths of the strands and the degree of twist in the sheets, and are most marked between V and C domains in IgG (compare V_L and V_γ with $C_\gamma 1$ in Fig. 2.7).

The immunoglobulin domains make relatively few contacts with one another along each chain, but they associate in pairs between chains in a conserved manner that determines the gross shape common to all antibodies. In IgE these pairs comprise V_L/V_ϵ, $C_L/C_\epsilon 1$, $C_\epsilon 2/C_\epsilon 2$ and $C_\epsilon 4/C_\epsilon 4$ domains. In contrast, the two $C_\epsilon 3$ domains probably do not make contact and are separated by the conserved carbohydrate attached to Asn 394.

The three-dimensional structure of IgE is unknown, but the structure of a part of the Fc ($C_\epsilon 3$ and $C_\epsilon 4$) has been predicted (Fig. 2.8) on the basis of its sequence similarity with the Fc fragment of IgG_1, for which a crystal structure exists. $C_\epsilon 3$ is modelled on the homologous $C_\gamma 2$ domain, and $C_\epsilon 4$ on $C_\gamma 3$. In

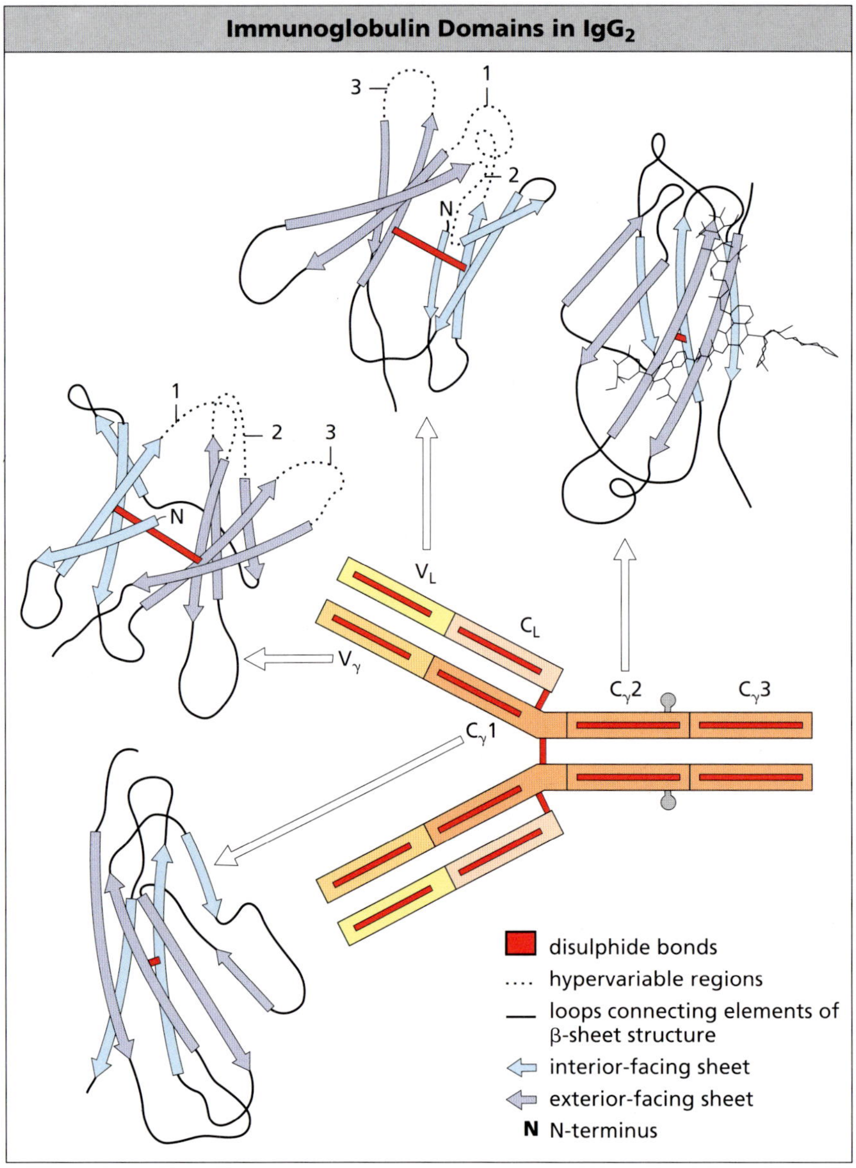

Fig. 2.7 Folding of immunoglobulin domains in IgG_1. The face in $C_\gamma 2$ which is homologous to $C_\epsilon 3$ is partially covered by a branched oligosaccharide chain, but it forms the domain pair interface in $C_\gamma l/C_L$ and $C_\gamma 3/C_\gamma 3$. In Vγ and VL, the hypervariable regions of the sequence (numbered 1, 2, 3 from the N-terminus) form the antigen-binding site. (Adapted from Dwek RA et al, *Biochem Soc Symp* 1984; ***49***:123–36).

IgG, the hinge region replaces $C_\epsilon 2$, and hence there is no structure on which to model this domain in IgE.

The points of attachment of the carbohydrate residues in IgE are indicated in the amino acid sequence (see Fig. 2.5). The two sugar-linked asparagines – at positions 265 and 371 of the Fc region – are unique to IgE, while that at position 394 is conserved in other immunoglobulin classes and probably plays a role in determining the shape of the molecule (see Fig. 2.8 – note that these residues are at positions 274, 380 and 403 in the sequential numbering scheme shown in Fig. 2.5). Glycosylation is unnecessary for the recognition of IgE by its receptors, and may indeed interfere with it (see below).

The presence of linker regions between immunoglobulin domains in antibodies, allows the domains a measure of freedom (differing with the lengths of the link between different pairs of domains and between those in different antibody classes) to rotate and bend relative to each other. Various physical techniques have been employed to study the shapes and flexibility of antibodies in solution. The X-ray scattering profiles and frictional properties of IgE suggest that its average conformation is bent. This is consistent with measurements of fluorescence energy transfer between donor and acceptor probes attached at the extremities of the chain. These indicate a rigidly bent form for IgE both in free solution and when bound to the cell through $Fc_\epsilon R1$ (see Figs 2.12 and 2.15).

Antibodies are first expressed on the cell membrane, where they function in signalling for the clonal expansion of B cells on interaction with antigens. The membrane-bound immunoglobulin (mIg) differs from the secreted protein in its C-terminal sequence, which is determined by differential splicing of precursor mRNA. Splicing favours the membrane-bound form of the immunoglobulin before, and the secreted form after, antigenic stimulation of B cells. The C-terminal sequence of the membrane-bound form of IgE (mIgE) possesses a canonical hydrophobic sequence to anchor the protein in the cell membrane (see Fig. 2.5). On the extracellular side of the membrane anchor is a unique sequence, rich in anionic side chains, which is probably therefore quite extended and flexible. To the cytoplasmic side are the sequences that presumably engage in signal transduction for survival and differentiation of the cell.

The Structure of $Fc_\epsilon R1$

The high affinity receptor, $Fc_\epsilon R1$, contains four transmembrane polypeptide chains, an α-, a β- and two γ-chains (Fig. 2.9), with the IgE-binding function contained within the α-chain. The $Fc_\epsilon R1$ α-chain, like the Fc receptors for IgG and IgA, belongs to the immunoglobulin superfamily (Fig. 2.10). It consists of two N-terminal immunoglobulin-like domains that project out of the cell, a single membrane spanning segment and a cytoplasmic C-terminal sequence. It is loosely associated with the β- and γ-chains in the cell membrane. These chains are required for insertion of the α-chain into the cell membrane and for signal transduction following allergen interaction with IgE.

Little is known at present about the structure of the extracellular element of the $Fc_\epsilon R1$ α-chain. Of all immunoglobulin receptors, $Fc_\epsilon R1$ is most similar to $Fc_\gamma R3$ for IgG because of the sequence similarities between their two α-chains. Also both share the same β- and γ-chains. The α-chain of $Fc_\epsilon R1$ is glycosylated at seven sites (see Figs 2.5 and 2.9), but this glycosylation is unnecessary for the binding to IgE.

Although the structure of $Fc_\epsilon R1$ is still unknown, there is some evidence that a reversible conformational transition is required to allow it to bind to IgE. The evidence comes from the kinetics of interaction with IgE, which reveal that the association rate constant does not depend on IgE concentration. This suggests that IgE interacts with a normally unpopulated conformation of the receptor (see Fig. 2.15) and,

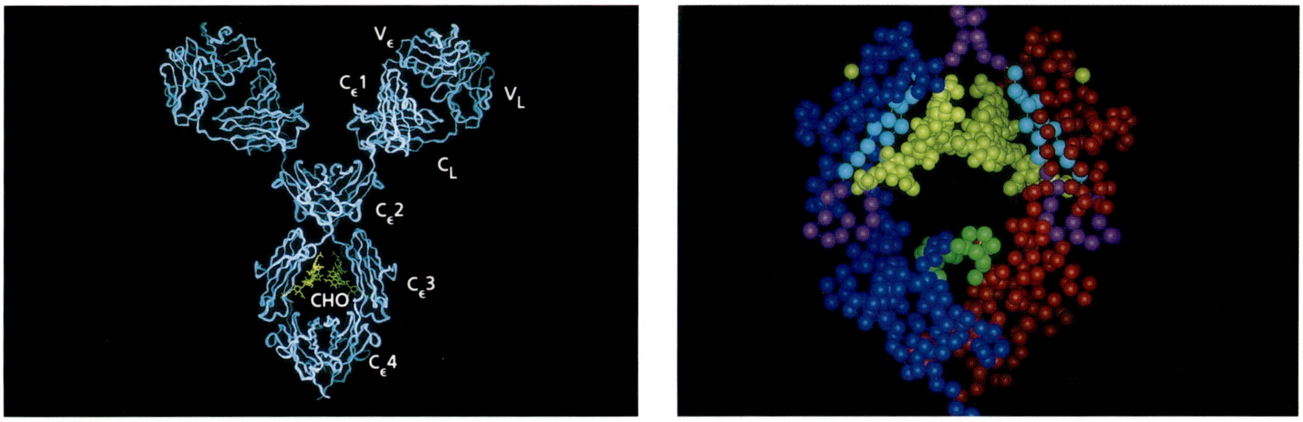

Fig. 2.8 Models of the three-dimensional structure of human IgE. [left] α-carbon backbone of whole IgE, modelled on IgG_1 (courtesy of Dr BJ Sutton). An IgG_1 Fab has been grafted onto the Padlan and Davies model for the $C_\epsilon 2$–$C_\epsilon 4$ domains of IgE (*Mol Immunol* 1986 **23**:1063). The carbohydrate in $C_\epsilon 3$ is labelled CHO. [right] Space-filling model of the α-carbon atom backbone of the $C_\epsilon 3$ and $C_\epsilon 4$ domains of IgE, based on the Padlan and Davies coordinates. The Asn 394 carbohydrate chain (fully described) and Asn 371 glycosylation site are in yellow, the solvent-exposed and buried parts of the first two β-strands of $C_\epsilon 3$ in magenta and blue, respectively, and the epitopes in $C_\epsilon 4$ of an antibody which blocks IgE binding to cell surface $Fc_\epsilon R1$ in green. Note that the two epitopes are predicted to lie on the concave and convex surfaces of the bent IgE molecule (see text). The two ε-chains are coloured in blue and red to highlight the contacts between the two $C_\epsilon 4$ domains.

if true, it carries the implication that the structure of the free receptor may not reveal the surface to which IgE binds.

The Structure of $Fc_{\epsilon}R2$

$Fc_{\epsilon}R2$ is unique among immunoglobulin receptors in that it is not a member of the immunoglobulin superfamily. Instead it shares a homology with animal C-type lectins, such as the asialoglycoprotein receptor, Kupffer cell receptor and mannose binding protein, and, lower in the scale of evolution, with echinoidin, a sea urchin protein. While the name lectin (Latin: *lectus*, to select) was given to these proteins to refer to their role in discriminating between the sugar substituents on different glycoproteins, $Fc_{\epsilon}R2$ recognizes a motif in the polypeptide structure of IgE, rather than its attached carbohydrate.

$Fc_{\epsilon}R2$ is oriented with its C-terminus outside the cell and its N-terminus in the cytoplasm. It is, therefore, also classified as a type II integral membrane protein, a category that embraces several of the animal C-type lectin membrane proteins, and a few other transmembrane proteins.

$Fc_{\epsilon}R2$ can be divided into several functional domains, which, unlike those in antibodies described above, exhibit a variety of structural motifs. These are depicted in Fig. 2.11 (see also Fig. 2.6). At the C-terminal end of the protein is a sequence of 36 amino acids including the tripeptide, DGR (Asp-Gly-Arg), which is the reverse of the RGD (Arg-Gly-Asp) sequence that functions in cell adhesion and homing. Interestingly, antibodies against an epitope consisting of the RGD sequence in fibronectin cross-react with $Fc_{\epsilon}R2$ and a synthetic peptide with the RGD sequence inhibits the activity of $Fc_{\epsilon}R2$ in causing cell aggregation. Contiguous with this is the domain of 121 amino acids that is homologous to the C-type lectins. This homology is established from the presence of conserved amino acids in the sequence, including notably the cysteines that form the intrachain disulphide bonds, required to maintain the native, IgE-binding conformation. Like all other calcium-regulated C-type lectins, binding is calcium-dependent.

The lectin domain is separated from the transmembrane segment by a sequence of 109 residues. The latter contains three (imperfectly) repeated sequences of 21 amino acids, each encoded by separate exons in the gene. Closer inspection reveals that this represents a higher order repeat of a basic heptad periodicity. This is characterized by hydrophobic side chains at positions one and four of each repeat, and ionic side chains at positions two and seven, and is characteristic of fibrous proteins,

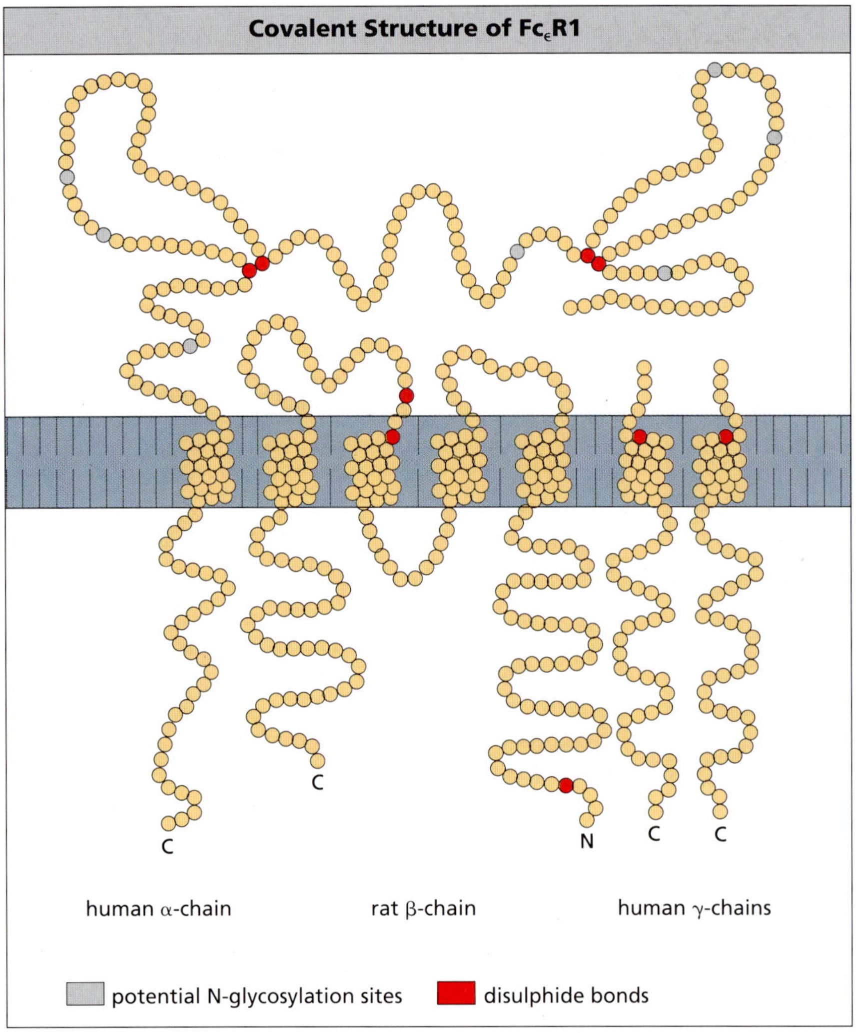

Fig. 2.9 Covalent structure of $Fc_{\epsilon}R1$. Sequences shown are the human α- and γ-chains and the rat β-chain. The β-chain is required for the surface expression and function of the rat receptor. Recent evidence suggests that it may be dispensable, or replaceable by a different protein sub-unit in the case of the human receptor.

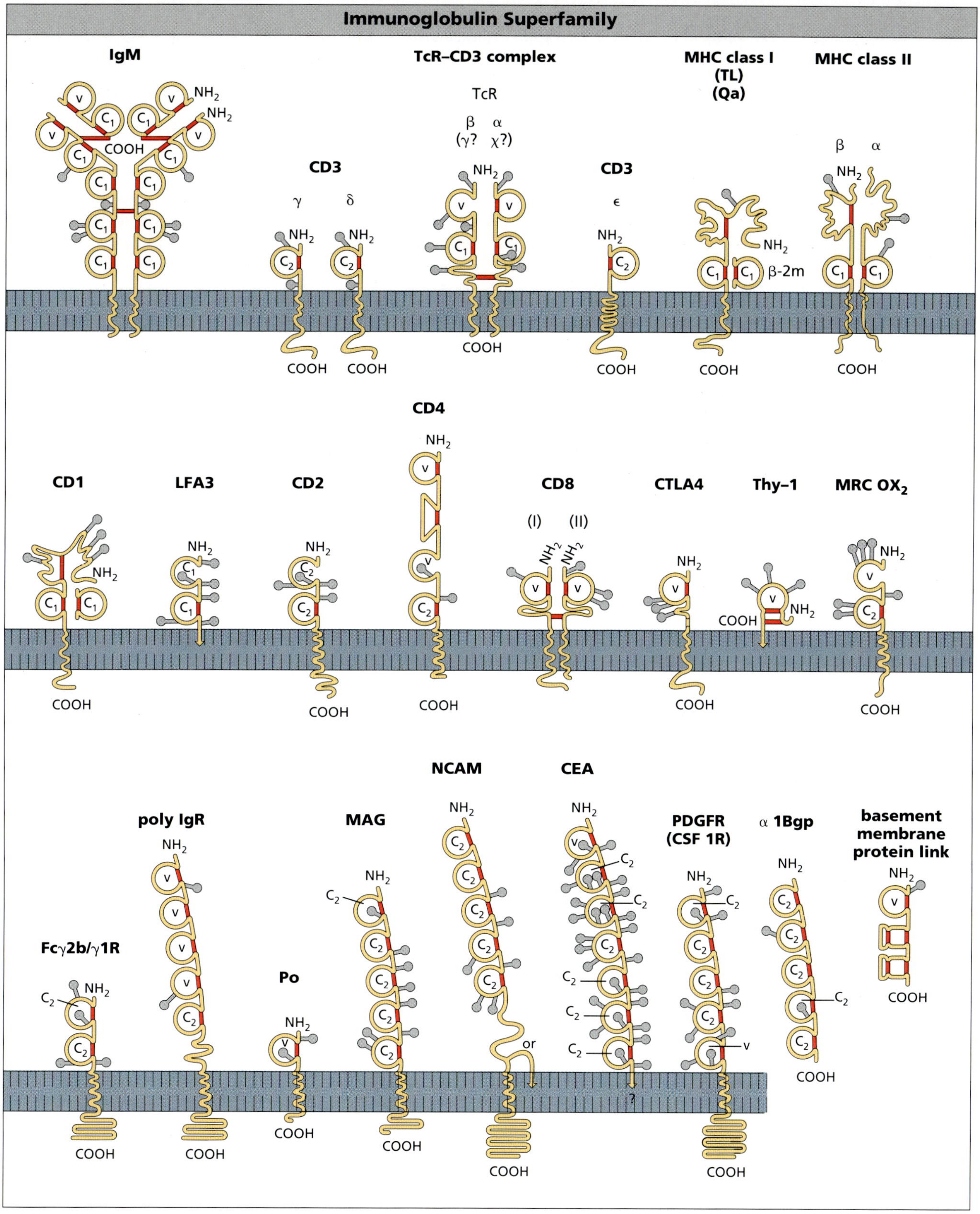

Fig. 2.10 Models for molecules in the Ig superfamily. A model is shown for each main molecular type from one species, and suffices for additional structures named in brackets. The circles show sequence segments that form, or are predicted to form, immunoglobulin domains. V, C_1 and C_2 denote different categories of immunoglobulin domains. α, β, γ, χ are the names given to different protein sub-units. IgM represents an immunoglobulin (like IgE with five heavy chain domains). TcR:CD3 is the T cell receptor complex with the accessory proteins CD3; MHC = major histocompatibility complex (TL and Qa types); β2m = β-microglobulin; CD1 = a distinct type of protein containing a β-microglobulin subunit; LFA3 and CD2 = T cell adhesion molecules; CD4, CD8 and CTLA4 = T subset antigens; Thy-1 and MRC OX-2 = brain/lymphoid antigens; Fcγ2b/γ1R and poly IgR = immunoglobulin receptors (note that Fcγ2b/γ1R may also represent the structure of $Fc_{\epsilon}R1$); Po = a myelin protein; MAG = myelin associated glycoprotein; NCAM = neural adhesion molecule; CEA = carcinoembryonic antigen; PDGFR = platelet-derived growth factor receptor; CSF1R = colony stimulating factor-1 receptor; a1B gP = non-cell surface glycoprotein; link = basement membrane link protein. (Adapted from Williams AF, Barclay NA. *Ann Rev Biochem* 1988; **6**: 381–406.)

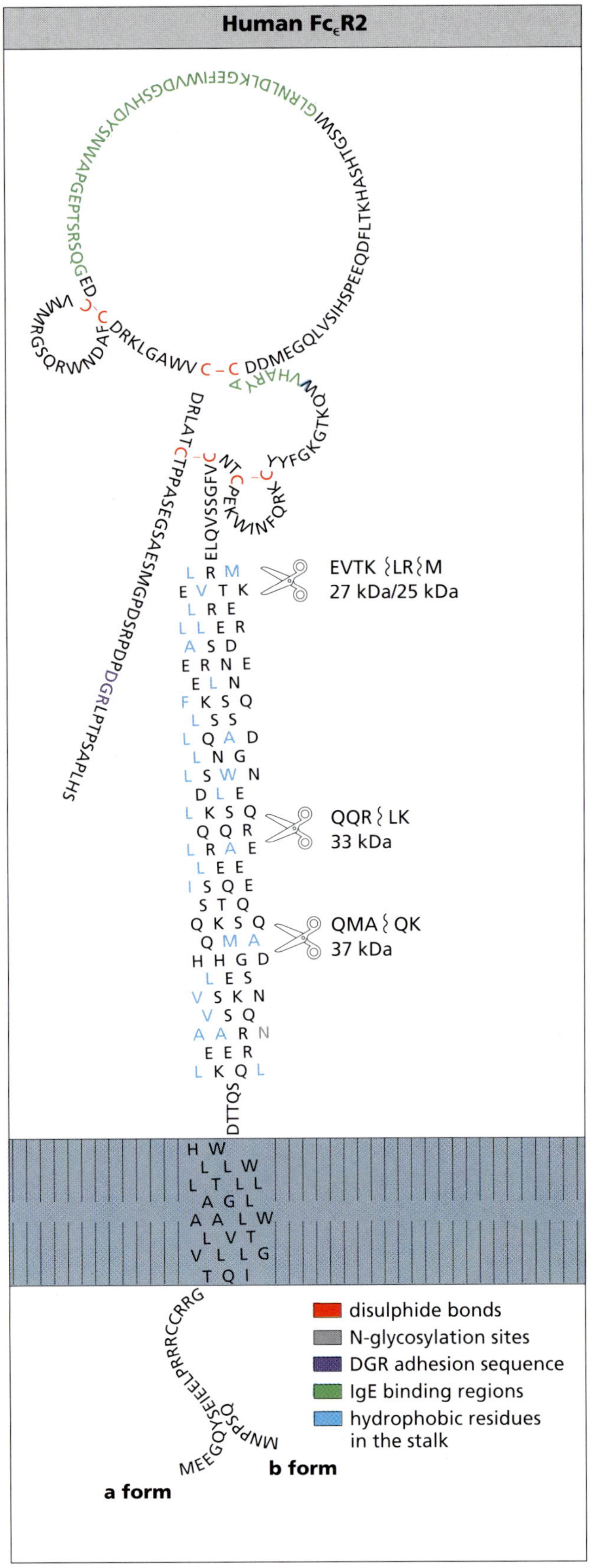

Fig. 2.11 Sequence and structural features of human Fc$_\epsilon$R2. The sites of proteolytic cleavage, the molecular weights of the soluble fragments and the locations of the cleavage sites are shown. The sequence of human Fc$_\epsilon$R2 (residues 53–150) is arranged in heptads to illustrate the alignment of hydrophobic residues, required to form the stalk which consists of three chains (see also Fig. 2.12). (Adapted from Fig. 4 of Gould HJ et al, in Gordon J (ed) *Monographs in Allergy* 1991; **29**: 28–41).

such as tropomyosin, in which α-helical chains are associated in the form of a coiled coil. Short linker regions connect the stalk with the lectin domain at its C-terminal end and with the transmembrane segment at its N-terminal end.

The α-helical coiled-coil structure implies that Fc$_\epsilon$R2 should be a dimer or trimer, and protein–protein cross-linking experiments in fact indicate that it is a trimer, as represented in Figs 2.12 and 2.13. The coiled-coil region forms a 15 nm stalk, at the end of which the ligand-binding lectin domain and the DGR adhesion sequence are presented to the extracellular milieu.

The coiled-coil acts as a rigid stalk, but is also the focus of metabolic activity; for within it are three physiologically important sites of proteolytic cleavage, as shown in Fig. 2.11. The first cleavage is at the base of the stalk and scission here releases a 37 kDa C-terminal fragment; the second site of attack is in the middle of the stalk and the third at the end. Cleavage at the end of the stalk releases a relatively stable 25 kDa fragment, but this eventually gives rise to a 12 kDa fragment. The stalk also contains the single site of N-glycosylation (Figs. 2.6 and 2.11). It has been shown that this glycosylation affords a degree of protection against proteolytic cleavage, slowing the release of soluble fragments. The carbohydrate is near to the site of cleavage and may impede the approach of proteases.

The single transmembrane segment is taken to be the highly hydrophobic sequence shown in Figs. 2.6 and 2.11. On the cytoplasmic side of this sequence is a highly basic sequence. There are two forms of Fc$_\epsilon$R2 differing in their N-terminal six/seven amino acids. These sequences are transcribed from different promoters in the gene, which are under separate genetic control. Fc$_\epsilon$R2a is constitutive to B cells, while

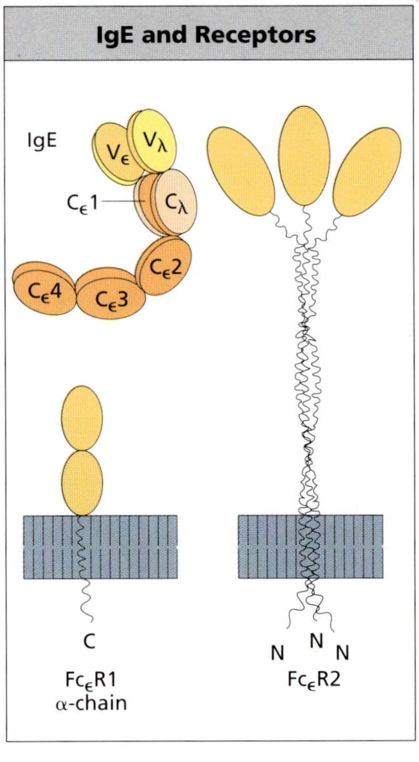

Fig. 2.12 Schematic diagrams of IgE, Fc$_\epsilon$R1 and Fc$_\epsilon$R2, drawn to the same scale. IgE is drawn as a bent molecule, while the α-chain of Fc$_\epsilon$R1 is drawn erect (see also Fig. 2.15) and simplified by omitting the β- and γ-chains (see also Fig. 2.9). Fc$_\epsilon$R2 is illustrated as a trimer in accordance with the results of protein-protein cross-linking studies (Courtesy of R Edmeades, unpublished.)

$Fc_\epsilon R2b$ is transcribed in response to IL-4 in B cells and monocytes (Fig. 2.3). Differential use of promoters may control the ability to act in antigen presentation, since a signal sequence for transport to endosomes via coated pits is present in form a, but not b. The IgE binding site is formed from two regions of the lectin domain, as shown in Fig. 2.11.

The diverse domains of $Fc_\epsilon R2$ are encoded by eleven exons, which are therefore probably assembled from many parts of the genome to create the gene for a multi-functional protein. It is likely that its affinity for IgE may have accrued at a late stage in its evolutionary history, almost certainly after the evolution of immunoglobulins themselves in vertebrates. Extending the analysis of the repeated sequences of $Fc_\epsilon R2$ to other members of the animal C-type lectin family, it appears that these too may form α-helical coiled-coils. The proteins that fall into this category are shown in Fig. 2.13.

The Interaction between IgE and $Fc_\epsilon R1$

One approach to the study of the interaction between IgE and $Fc_\epsilon R1$ has been to map the complementary binding sites in the sequences of IgE and its receptor. Studies of the kinetics of association and dissociation also provide clues to the mechanism of the interaction.

Several strategies have been used to map the $Fc_\epsilon R1$ binding site in IgE, all of which give broadly concordant results. The original papain cleavage experiment, referred to above, located the receptor

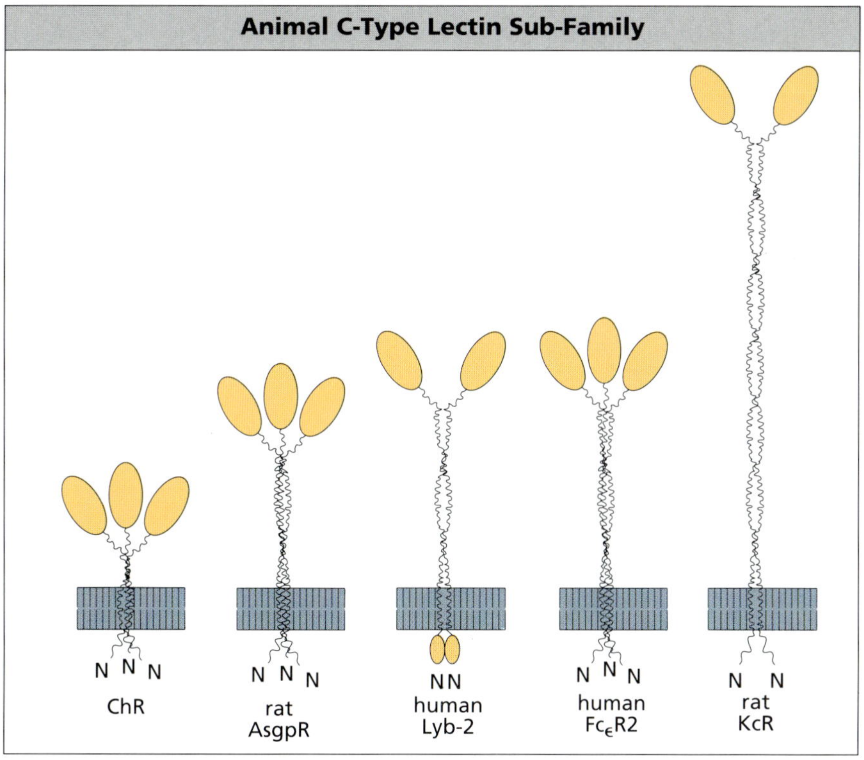

Fig. 2.13 Animal C-type lectin sub-family with α-helical coiled-coil stalks. Left to right: chicken hepatic lectin receptor (ChR); asialoglycoprotein receptor (AsgpR); human differentiation antigen (Lyb-2); human $Fc_\epsilon R_2$; rat Kupffer cell receptor (KcR). ChR, AsgpR and $Fc_\epsilon R_2$ have been shown to be trimeric. Since α-helical coiled-coil stalks, thought to be present in all these molecules, must be dimeric or trimeric, Lyb-2 and the KcR are represented as dimers. (Adapted from Beavil A et al. *Proc Natl Acad Sci USA* 1992; **89**; 753–757.)

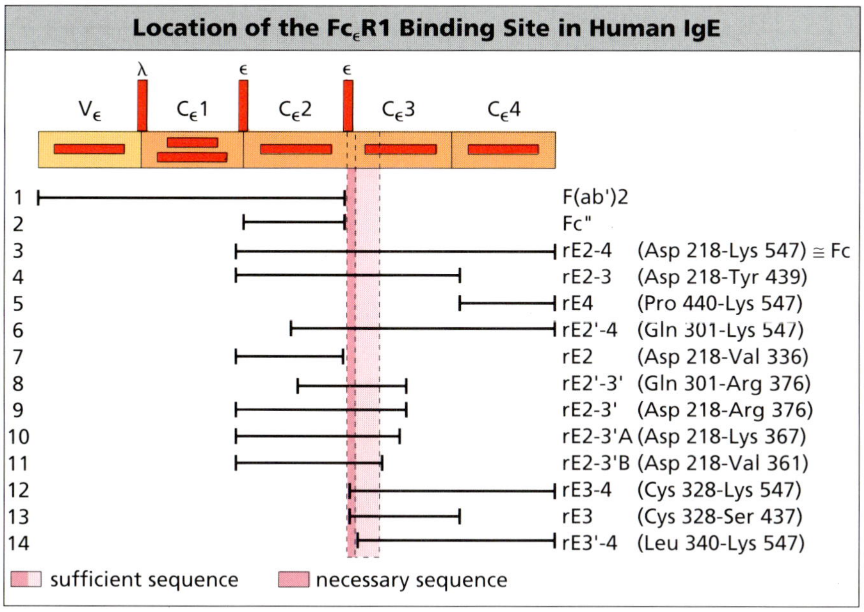

Fig. 2.14 Mapping of the $Fc_\epsilon R1$ binding site in IgE with recombinant peptides. The site has been localized to the N-terminal sequence of $C_\epsilon 3$ by testing binding to cells bearing the receptor or the sensitization of mast cells or basophils for the release of mediators, stimulated by antigen or anti-IgE. All peptides containing the sufficient sequence were found to be active. Ones in which the necessary sequence has been deleted are inactive, revealing the requirements of at least part of this sequence for activity. (Adapted from Gould HJ, in Holgate ST, ed. *Genetics of Asthma,* in press.)

binding site in the Fc fragment. No further active fragments were found by proteolytic enzyme digestion of IgE, but the use of recombinant peptides has located the site more precisely in the ϵ-chain (Fig. 2.14). These peptides were assayed either for direct binding to FcϵR1, or for their capacity to inhibit IgE binding to the receptor. The site thus identified lies in the N-terminal sequence of $C_\epsilon 3$, close to the junction with $C_\epsilon 2$. Mapping has also been performed by measuring the competition for binding to $Fc_\epsilon R1$ between IgE and unrelated proteins, such as proteases or monoclonal antibodies, whose target sites in IgE are known. For example, it was found that a region of rat IgE protected from trypsin cleavage when the IgE is bound to $Fc_\epsilon R1$ on rat basophilic leukaemia cells, lies at the junction of $C_\epsilon 2$ and $C_\epsilon 3$. Monoclonal antibodies against defined epitopes in the ϵ-chain have been tested for their ability to interfere with the binding of IgE to $Fc_\epsilon R1$, but such studies have not provided detailed information about the location of the binding site for topological reasons (see below).

For the receptor α-chain, peptide mapping experiments have only recently been made possible by gene cloning. The use of antibodies suggests, however, that the site is likely to lie, at least in part, in the second immunoglobulin-like domain (numbered from the N-terminus).

Enough is now known about IgE and $Fc_\epsilon R1$ to justify the construction of a low resolution model of the complex. IgE is a compact immunoglobulin, probably containing a rigid bend between $C_\epsilon 1$ and $C_\epsilon 2$ and between $C_\epsilon 2$ and $C_\epsilon 3$. IgE binds to $Fc_\epsilon R1$, probably through the solvent-accessible region of $C_\epsilon 3$, near to the junction with $C_\epsilon 2$. The separations between the the ends of the Fab arms, $C_\epsilon 2$, and the C-terminus, and the cell membrane (see Fig. 2.15) imply that the convex side of the IgE bend faces the membrane. The location of the binding site is such that it may be inaccessible to the receptor at the concave face of IgE, and approachable only from the convex face, or from the side. The extracellular part of the receptor contains the two immunoglobulin-like domains. Nothing is known about its orientation; it could be perpendicular to the membrane or tilted. The IgE binding site on $Fc_\epsilon R1$ may be in the second immunoglobulin domain. An orthogonally oriented receptor could attach to bent IgE on either side, whereas an angled receptor could bind at the middle, but only on the convex surface (Fig. 2.15). Consideration of the symmetry properties of a bent IgE molecule eliminates one of these options. If the $Fc_\epsilon R1$ binding sites are at the sides, both should be equally accessible for receptor binding, but, if they are on opposite surfaces of the bend, one may be masked. The observation that IgE can bind only a single $Fc_\epsilon R1$ α-chain is compatible only with the model shown in Fig. 2.15(b).

As stated above, the kinetics of the interaction between IgE and $Fc_\epsilon R1$ are unusual in that the rate of association does not depend on the concentration of IgE, as in a typical bimolecular process. This has been interpreted to suggest that a conformational change in either the IgE or the receptor, probably the latter, is the rate-limiting step in the association. Fig. 2.15 may be adopted here to symbolize (a) the inactive and (b) active forms.

The ability of fragments of IgE or antibodies to inhibit the interaction between IgE and $Fc_\epsilon R1$ can be exploited to block the allergic response *in vivo*. The peptides inhibit by virtue of their capacity to occupy the binding sites on the cell receptor, the antibodies by associating with IgE and blocking receptor binding.

Because of the large size of antibodies, they might be expected to obstruct the IgE-receptor interaction on the surfaces of mast cells and basophils, even when their epitopes are remote from the receptor-binding site. The only requirement is that they should either bind near to the receptor site, in the three-dimensional structure, or to a site on the same side of IgE as the epitopes. In such a case, the antibodies may block the IgE-receptor interaction merely by impeding the approach of IgE to the receptor, since their long dimension exceeds the maximum possible protrusion of the receptor from the membrane surface. (Note that the same argument cannot apply to $Fc_\epsilon R2$.) Certain antibodies which were thought to block receptor binding by competing for the IgE binding site may actually act in this manner, yet may be useful for blocking the IgE-receptor interaction *in vivo*. This would require that the second epitope be sequestered in the concave surface of the IgE molecule to prevent the antibody from triggering mast cell degranulation by binding to IgE-receptor complexes. Antibodies that can bind to only one of the two epitopes in IgE have been described by a number of authors.

IgE–FcϵR1 Interaction

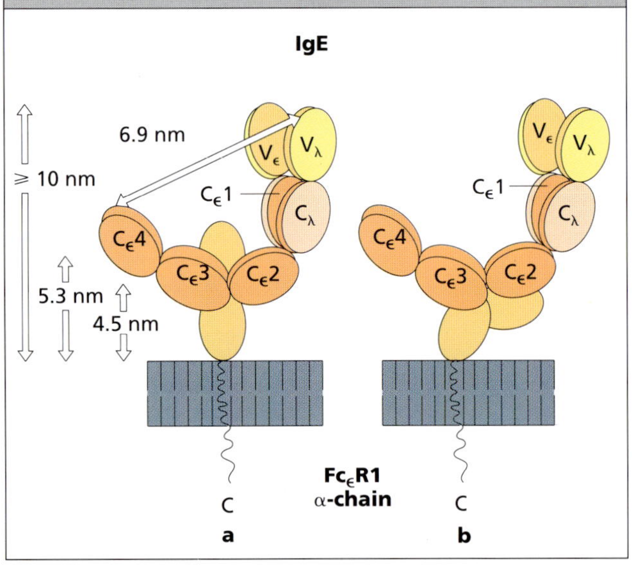

Fig. 2.15 Alternative models of the IgE interaction with $Fc_\epsilon R1$: (a) receptor contracting IgE 'from the side'; (b) receptor contacting IgE on the convex surface. This may require the receptor to bend in order that IgE may contact the receptor domain nearest the membrane. (Adapted from Gould H, in Holgate ST, ed, *Genetics of Asthma,* in press.) Distances have been revealed by fluorescent energy transfer experiments (Adapted from Zheng Y et al. *Biochem* 1991; **30**: 9125–9132.)

A soluble fragment containing the extracellular sequence of $Fc_\epsilon R1$ blocks the binding of IgE to cell-bound receptors. This is the basis of an alternative strategy for blocking allergic reactions *in vivo*.

The Interaction between IgE and $Fc_\epsilon R2$

The $Fc_\epsilon R2$ binding site on IgE has been mapped to the $C_\epsilon 3$ domain using recombinant peptides and monoclonal antibodies. The $C_\epsilon 3$ domains must be present in a dimeric chain for detectable binding. It seems likely therefore that two of the three lectin domains in $Fc_\epsilon R2$ each bind to a separate $C_\epsilon 3$ domain, as shown in Fig. 2.16 and that the formation of two $C_\epsilon 3$-lectin complexes within a single IgE–$Fc_\epsilon R2$ complex greatly enhances the strength of the interaction. $Fc_\epsilon R2$ or its trimeric 37 kDa fragment may bind similarly to mIgE.

IgE is not likely to be the only ligand of $Fc_\epsilon R2$. The presence of the DGR sequence has already been mentioned, and may lead to the attachment of cells expressing the $Fc_\epsilon R2$ to cell matrix receptors. The homology to animal C-type lectins suggests that $Fc_\epsilon R2$ may also have a carbohydrate ligand, although none has yet been identified. Furthermore, the 12 kDa fragment of $Fc_\epsilon R2$ does not retain the capacity to bind to IgE, but may still act as an autocrine growth factor for B cells. This implies the existence of yet another receptor.

The affinity of the 25 kDa fragment for IgE is about ten times lower than that of the intact (45 kDa) $Fc_\epsilon R2$ molecule. Presumably the binding of the two $C_\epsilon 3$ domains by trimeric $Fc_\epsilon R2$ gives a more stable complex than the binding of one $C_\epsilon 3$ domain by the monomer (Fig. 2.16a). Site-directed mutagenesis on the lectin domain has implicated two separate regions of the sequence in binding IgE (see Fig. 2.11).

Synthesis of IgE

In B cell differentiation, somatic recombination first creates a μ-chain gene by recombination of multiple V, D (diversity), and J (joining) gene segments and the gene encoding C_μ, the constant region of a μ-chain, as found in IgM . The recombined gene is transcribed and the mRNA translated and cytoplasmic, μ-chains appear in the cytoplasm of pre-B cells. The multiple V and J segments in the light chain gene loci then recombine with the C_L gene segments to express a light chain that can assemble with the μ-chain into

Interactions Between IgE and $Fc_\epsilon R2$ or a Vaccine Antibody

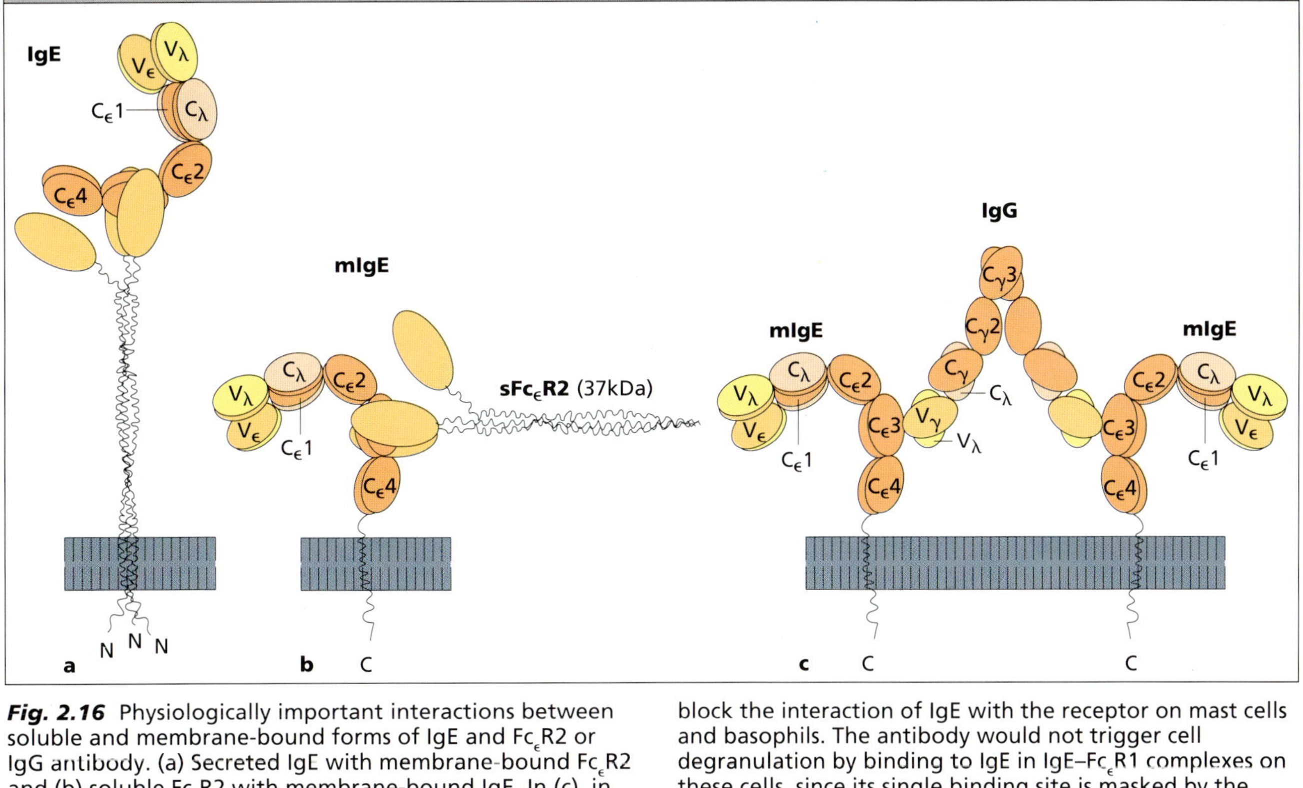

Fig. 2.16 Physiologically important interactions between soluble and membrane-bound forms of IgE and $Fc_\epsilon R2$ or IgG antibody. (a) Secreted IgE with membrane-bound $Fc_\epsilon R2$ and (b) soluble $Fc_\epsilon R2$ with membrane-bound IgE. In (c), in contrast to $Fc_\epsilon R2$ in (b), an IgG antibody against IgE is readily able to cross-link two membrane-bound IgE molecules on the surface of a B cell expressing IgE. The antibody is directed against an epitope within the $C_\epsilon 3$ domain of IgE. The epitope is present on both the convex and concave sides of IgE, but is accessible to the antibody only on the convex side, as shown. Cross-linking of mIgE by the antibody may downregulate IgE synthesis by generating a signal that arrests cell growth. The antibody may also compete with $Fc_\epsilon R1$ for binding to IgE and thus block the interaction of IgE with the receptor on mast cells and basophils. The antibody would not trigger cell degranulation by binding to IgE in IgE–$Fc_\epsilon R1$ complexes on these cells, since its single binding site is masked by the receptor. Peptides that constitute an epitope such as the one represented in (c) may provide a safe vaccine against allergy. A similar strategy has been suggested by Chang and co-workers (*Biotechnology* 1990; **8**: 122–139). These authors have generated monoclonal antibodies against the sequence which is specific to the membrane form of IgE (see Fig. 2.5). These antibodies should act selectively on the synthesis of IgE, without directly interfering with IgE effector functions.

an immunoglobulin molecule. The mRNA splicing mechanism at this stage favours formation of mIgM, which is presented on the cell surface. In the presence of antigens and in the relevant compartment (lymph node germinal centres; see below), B cells expressing specific antibodies are selected, and others are eliminated by apoptosis, a form of programmed cell death, within a few days. Further optimization of the antibody for high-affinity binding to antigen results from somatic mutations in the recombined gene and selection of cells expressing the mutant immunoglobulins. In addition, somatic recombination transposes the VDJ gene cassette, originally attached to the C_μ gene, into a downstream heavy chain gene encoding the constant region of another class. This heavy chain switch diversifies the effector function of antibodies by enabling them to bind to specific receptors, differentially expressed on different types of effector cells, e.g. $Fc_\epsilon R1$, found only on mast cells and basophils (see Fig. 2.2).

Switching is predominantly to a gene segment encoding one of the four γ-chain subclasses. The direction of switching, however, is determined by lymphokines, secreted by T helper (TH) cells, and changes in their relative concentrations affect the direction of switching. The lymphokines that have been mainly implicated in this control mechanism are IL-2 together with interferon (IFN) and IL-4. The former are secreted by TH_1 cells and the latter by TH_2 cells, which can be distinguished in rodents by their surface antigens. Not only does IFN enhance switching to IgG, but it antagonizes switching to IgE, and it is thought that the lymphokines bind to receptors on the B cell. Here, they send different signals to the nucleus, where germline gene transcription is initiated in response to the binding of specific proteins to response elements in the promoters of transcription. These proteins must be synthesized or activated in response to the relevant signals received at the cell surface. The signalling pathways, the identity of the DNA binding proteins and response elements, and the nexus between transcription and recombination have yet to be elucidated. The recombination enzymes (either for the $VDJC_\mu$ or for the heavy chain switch) remain to be identified.

A second signal required for IgE expression is delivered, wholly unexpectedly, by a soluble fragment of $Fc_\epsilon R2$. This fragment may act by selecting the committed IgE precursor cells, following the heavy chain switch in germinal centres, where follicular dendritic cells, which express high levels of $Fc_\epsilon R2$, are densely packed together with the B cell precursors. It maybe envisaged that the short-lived 37 kDa fragment of $Fc_\epsilon R2$ could have a paracrine hormone-like activity in this milieu. The ability of the 37 kDa fragment to bind to mIgE (see Fig. 2.15) in the immature, nascent IgE-expressing B cells, may be important for this activity. Interestingly, IL-4 leads to rapid up-regulation of $Fc_\epsilon R2$ expression on cell surfaces (within minutes), so that the co-factor does not limit the growth of cells after the later switching event.

In contrast to soluble $Fc_\epsilon R2$, antibodies against IgG would be expected to cross-link mIgE on the surface of B cells (see Fig. 2.15c) and thus suppress IgE synthesis. The same antibodies might also cross-link IgE bound to the high affinity receptor on mast cells and basophils and cause anaphylaxis. The judicious choice of an epitope on the IgE molecule, e.g. one which is not accessible to antibody present in mIgE, but not secreted IgE (see Fig. 2.5), might however, provide a useful agent for modulating the IgE response *in vivo*.

Regulatory Loops

As mentioned, IgE regulation is essential for keeping the levels of these antibodies within physiologically desirable limits. IgE synthesis is influenced by the nature of the antigen, the nature of the adjuvants (as when animals are artificially immunized), the route of entry of antigen, and the histocompatibility type of the individual. It is not yet possible to relate these features to the cellular and molecular events described above – it is only now becoming possible to relate the cellular and molecular events to each other. It would appear that the ratio of different cell types

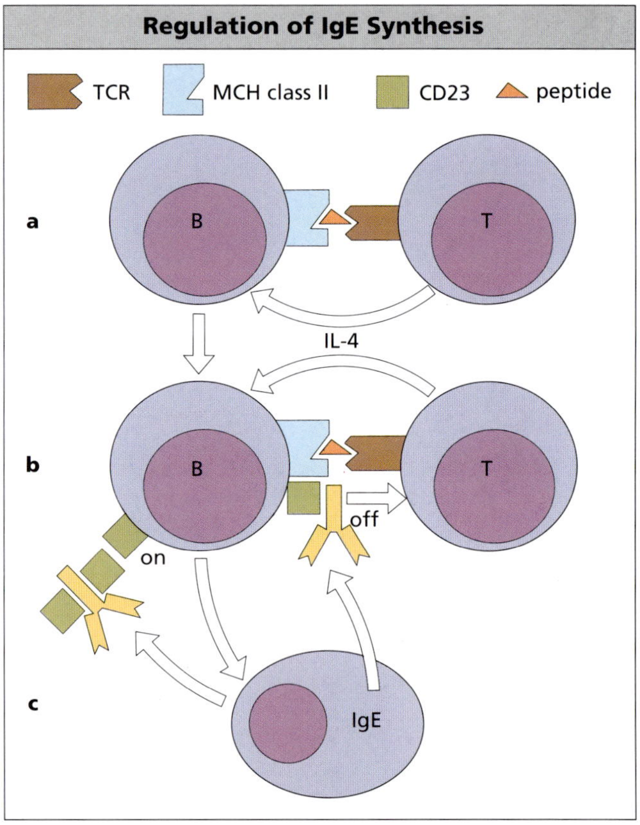

Fig. 2.17 A model for IgE feedback regulation on IgE synthesis. (a) B cells present processed antigen to T cells, leading to IL-4 production from the T cells and $Fc_\epsilon R2$ (CD23) induction of the B cell. (b) Induced $Fc_\epsilon R2$ then provides a co-stimulatory signal to amplify T-B cooperation, which eventually (c) leads to the generation of IgE plasma cells. With antigen eliminated and IgE in excess, free IgE will bind to surface $Fc_\epsilon R2$ at this stage and prevent further recruitment of B cells toward IgE production. Soluble $Fc_\epsilon RII$ would be able to promote IgE production by binding IgE in solution and preventing the blocking of the co-stimulatory signal. (Adapted from Gordon J et al, in *Monog Allergy* 1991, **29**:156–158.)

may regulate the production of IFN compared with IL-4 and thus the relative proportions of IgG and IgE antibodies synthesized. The pathological tendency of some individuals to excess IgE production is also correlated with a genetic pre-disposition to respond to the antigens which preferentially elicit an IgE response. One way in which this condition could be exacerbated is through antigen presentation mediated by IgE; this has been likened to the role of adjuvant.

Conjectural mechanisms for the termination of the IgE response may be put forward. It has been observed that the interaction of IgE with $Fc_{\epsilon}R2$ inhibits proteolysis and the release of the 37 kDa fragment from cells. Since the soluble fragments are required to induce IgE expression, the saturation of IgE binding sites on $Fc_{\epsilon}R2$ would provide an economical mechanism for aborting the life of new cells synthesizing IgE antibodies. A high proportion of the soluble $Fc_{\epsilon}R2$ in allergic individuals occurs in complexes with IgE, supporting the suggestion that IgE concentrations can reach the levels required to neutralize the activity of the receptor *in vivo.* Formation of soluble IgE–$Fc_{\epsilon}R2$ complexes may dampen the immune response generally, since soluble $Fc_{\epsilon}R2$ promotes the growth and differentiation of both myeloid and lymphoid precursors. These interactions may be represented in the form of a feedback loop (Fig. 2.17). It has also been suggested that the formation of soluble complexes of IgE with $Fc_{\epsilon}R2$ may increase the rate of metabolic clearance of IgE, thus explaining its relatively short half-life, in comparison to other immunoglobulin classes.

A further level of regulation is exercised through the enhancement or suppression of glycosylation, at least in rodent cells. There, soluble IgE-binding proteins are secreted from T cells and act as glycosylation-enhancing and -inhibiting factors (GEF and GIF). It was expected that these factors would be identical with $Fc_{\epsilon}R2$, but cDNA cloning and sequencing revealed otherwise. The results suggest that the mechanism of control of IgE production in the rodent and human systems may differ in detail.

Both IgE and the two IgE receptors are glycoproteins. It was originally thought that glycosylation would be important, at least for the recognition of IgE by $Fc_{\epsilon}R2$. In actuality, the opposite appears to be the case, for unglycosylated or deglycosylated IgE binds with an affinity to $Fc_{\epsilon}R2$ ten times higher than native IgE. The glycosylation state of the receptor also influences its activity, since carbohydrate interferes with the release of soluble $Fc_{\epsilon}R2$ from the cell surface by proteases. Thus, glycosylation of both IgE and affinity to $Fc_{\epsilon}R2$ act in the same sense to suppress the release of soluble affinity to $Fc_{\epsilon}R2$ from cells – glycosylation of IgE by opposing its binding to the receptor, where it prevents proteolytic enzyme activity, and glycosylation of the receptor which directly masks the site of attack. Glycosylation of IgE *in vivo* is heterogeneous, and may be subject to the kind of regulation that occurs in rodent cells.

Future Prospects

It should be clear from this presentation that studies of the structure of IgE and its receptors can provide valuable insight into the underlying causes of allergy. We may look forward to the time when the complete structures of these molecules are known, as well as those of their complexes. Little is now known about the mechanisms by which ligand binding to the receptors, including of course mIgE, is coupled to the signalling pathways in the cell, with such specific consequences for cellular activity in lymphocytes, macrophages and cytotoxic cells. Now that the genes for all the receptors are cloned, it will be possible to determine the protein sequence requirements for cell signalling and, with this prospect in view, attempts to work out the biochemical basis of signalling have intensified. When the second messengers are known, however, there will still be components of the signalling pathways to identify, not least of all those which are responsible for changing the patterns of gene expression following the events at the cell surface.

Further Reading

Burton DR. The conformation of antibodies. In: *Fc Receptors and the Action of Antibodies*. Metzger H, ed., American Society for Microbiology, 1990; 31–56.

Chang TW et al. Monoclonal Antibodies specific for Human IgE-producing B cells: a potential therapeutic for IgE-mediated allergic diseases. *Biotechnology* 1990; **8**: 122–126.

Esser C, Radbruch A. Immunoglobulin class switching: Molecular and cellular analysis. *Ann Rev Immunol* 1990; **8**: 717–735.

Gordon J. CD23: A novel multifunctional regulator of the immune system that binds IgE. *Monogr Allergy* 1991; **29**.

Gould, HJ. The interaction between immunoglobulin E and its high affinity receptor. In: *Genetics of Asthma*. Holgate ST, ed., in press.
Ishizaka K. Regulation of immunoglobulin E biosynthesis. *Adv Immunol* 1989; **47**: 1–44.

Kikutani H, Kishimoto T. Molecular genetics and biology of two different species of $Fc_{\epsilon}R2$. *Res Immunol* 1990; **1**: 59–108.

Kinet JP, Metzger H. Genes, structure, and Actions of the high-affinity receptor for immunoglobulin E. In: *Fc Receptors and the Action of Antibodies*. Metzger H, ed., American Society for Microbiology, 1990; 239–259.

Marcelletti JF et al. Emerging importance of IgE and Fc receptors for IgE ($Fc_{\epsilon}R$) in the regulation of B cell activity. *Contrib Microbiol Immunol* 1989; **11**: 188–205.

Ortega E et al. Kinetics of ligand binding to the type I Fc_{ϵ} receptor on mast cells. *Biochem* 1991; **30**: 3473–3483.

Stanworth DR et al. Allergy Treatment with a peptide vaccine. *Lancet* 1990; **336**: 1279–1281.

Williams AF. A year in the life of the immunoglobulin superfamily. *Immunol Today* 1987; **8**: 298–303.

Chapter 3

Cytokine Networks in Allergic Disease

Introduction

Cytokines comprise a large group of molecules which form the basis for complex networks of cell-to-cell signalling in homeostasis and pathology in all higher organisms. Cytokines include categories of proteins referred to as lymphokines, monokines, interleukins, haemopoietic or peptide growth factors, and neuropeptides, the precise name depending on the order of discovery and/or the mechanisms of action described. It is now clear that cytokines represent a ubiquitous biological syntax, allowing for uniformity, diversity, and specificity of cellular responses and the orchestration of more global physiological and pathological processes. As in many areas of medicine, cytokines have recently become crucial to the understanding of mechanisms underlying allergic reactions and diseases.

Haemopoietic growth factors, peptide growth factors, interleukins, interferons, and neuropeptides are among the classes of cytokines which probably play important roles in allergic disease. For example, haemopoietic growth factors control the production in bone marrow of the formed elements of blood, including effector cells in allergic responses. These haemopoietic growth factors stimulate the proliferation and differentiation of immature ('early', 'pluripotent') or more mature ('late', 'oligopotent') progenitor (stem) cells, which can also circulate in the blood and populate peripheral tissues, allowing their maturation along specific lineages or pathways (Fig. 3.1). Included among these growth factors are several of the interleukins, many of which retain names related to their observed activities (see Figs 3.2, 3.3, and 3.4). The peptide growth factors and neuropeptides, discovered through various *in vitro* and *in vivo* observations, are important in regulating tissue growth and repair as well as in mediating nervous stimulation of tissues cells. Some of the cytokines have mainly inhibitory or cytolytic functions (see Fig. 3.5), implicitly pointing to their role in homeostasis.

Cytokines of each catergory have been sequenced at the protein (amino acid) level and most of the genes encoding these proteins have been cloned – the genes for human haemopoietic growth factors are shown in Fig. 3.3. We shall review the importance of these with regard to acute and chronic inflammation and immune responses, with specific focus on IgE

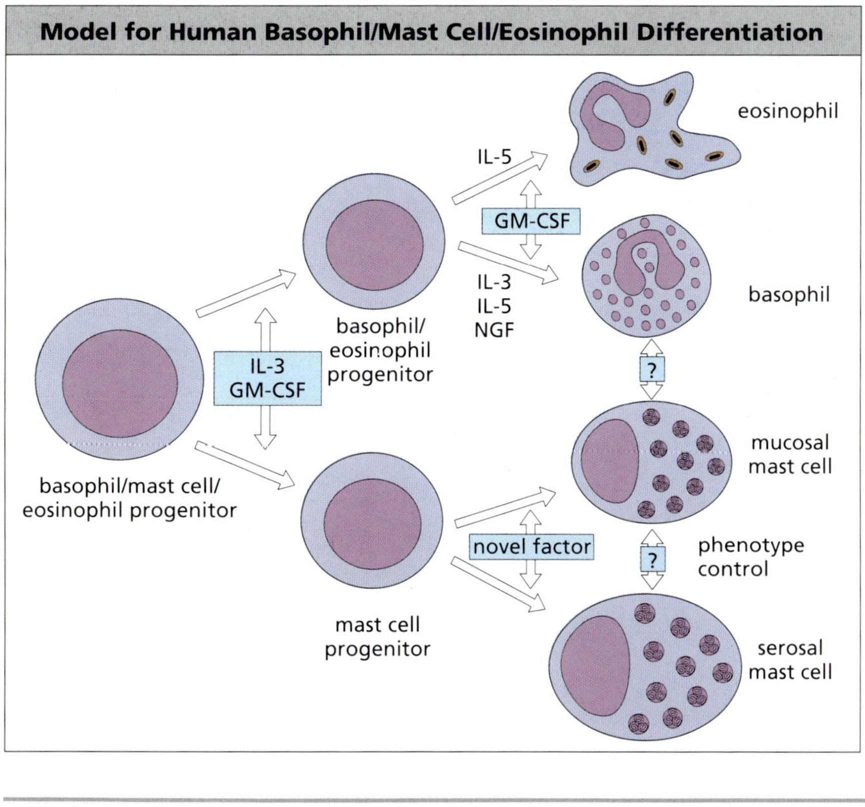

Fig. 3.1 The haemopoietic differentiation of allergic effector cells, including basophils, mast cells and eosinophils, mediated by growth factors, is depicted here. A putative common progenitor arising from the bone marrow and circulating in the peripheral blood can, under the influence of the pluripotent haemopoietic growth factors IL-3 and GM-CSF, differentiate further to mature cells. IL-5 is a specific eosinophil growth and differentiation factor and IL-3 stimulates the basophil lineage from a common basophil/eosinophil progenitor. GM-CSF probably synergizes in both basophil and eosinophil differentation. The derivation of either mucosal or serosal mast cells from a putative common progenitor in man is not yet clear, nor is the lineage interrelationship between the two subtypes of mast cell. Novel factors derived from fibroblasts may be important in mast cell development.

Interleukins			
Cytokine	**Synonym(s)**	**Cytokine**	**Synonym(s)**
Interleukin-1 (IL-1)	lymphocyte activating factor T cell replacement factor	Interleukin-6 (IL-6)	hepatocyte stimulating factor hybridoma growth factor interferon-β_2 B cell stimulating factor II megakaryocytopoietin
Interleukin-2 (IL-2)	T cell growth factor	Interleukin-7 (IL-7)	pre-B cell growth factor
Interleukin-3 (IL-3)	mutli-CSF mast cell growth factor histamine cell producting factor erythroid burst-promoting activity	Interleukin-8 (IL-8)	monocyte-derived neutrophil chemotactic factor neutrophil activating factor (peptide)
Interleukin-4 (IL-4)	B cell stimulating factor B cell growth factor mast cell growth factor II T cell growth factor II	Interleukin-9 (IL-9)	erythropoietic co-factor mast cell enhancing factor (MEA) T cell growth factor III
Interleukin-5 (IL-5)	B cell growth factor II eosinophilopoietin eosinophil differentiation factor	Interleukin-10 (IL-10)	cytokine synthesis inhibitory factor B-cell derived T-cell growth factor mast cell growth co-factor

Fig. 3.2 Interleukins and synonyms for the same substances.

Principal Human Haemopoietic Growth Factors				
		Characteristics		
Factor	**Cell source**	**Molecular Weight**	**Gene**	**Actions**
GM-CSF	fibroblasts epithelium endothelium T cells	14 – 35 kDa	5q 23 - 31	stimulates growth and differentiation of haemopoietic stem cells of all lineages (except erythroid) activates mature granulocytes
G-CSF	fibroblasts epithelium endothelium other	18 – 22 kDa	17q 11 - 21	stimulates growth and differentiation of granulocyte stem cells activates neutrophils and eosinophils
M-CSF	fibroblasts endothelium other	70 – 90 kDa	5q 33	stimulates growth and differentiation of monocyte/macrophage stem cells
IL-3	T cells	14 – 28 kDa	5q 23 - 31	stimulates growth and differentiation of stem cells of all lineages promotes basophil/eosinophil differentiation and activates eosinophils and basophils
IL-5	T cells	25 – 50 kDa	5q 23 - 31	stimulates growth and differentiation of eosinophil (and basophil) stem cells activates eosinophils and prolongs eosinophil survival
erythropoietin	renal mesangium	34 – 39 kDa	7q 11 - 22	promotes growth and differentiation of erythroid precursors
IL-9	T cells	40 kDa	unknown	promotes growth and differentiation of erythroid precursors enhances mast cell growth
IL-10	T cells B cells	20 kDa	unknown	inhibits synthesis of cytokines from TH_1-subtype T cells enhances expression of MHC II on B cells co-factor in mast cell growth and differentiation (with IL-4 and IL-3) T cell growth factor activity
IL-11	stromal cells	24 kDa	unknown	megakaryocytopoietin (synergy with IL-3)
stem cell factor (c-kit ligand; steel locus factor	stromal cells	18.5 kDa	unknown	promotes growth and differentiation of early myeloid and erythroid pregenitors synergizes with other hemopoietic growth factors enhances mast cell growth and differentiation

Fig. 3.3 Characteristics and actions of human haemopoietic growth factors.

Factor	Cell source	Molecular weight	Actions
IL-1	ubiquitous: primarily monocytes macrophages	17 kDa	activates T cells pro-inflammatory at many levels initiates cellular transcription of many genes
IL-2	T cells	14 – 16 kDa	T cell proliferation and clonal amplification
IL-4	T cells	20 kDa	co-factor in T cell activation promotes B cell growth and differentiation (IgG1 and IgE class switch) rodent connective tissue mast cell growth/co-factor (with IL-3)
IL-6 (IFNβ_2)	ubiquitous; primarily macrophages fibroblasts	22 – 29 kDa	hepatocyte stimulating factor promotes B cell growth and differentiation (including myeloma cells) acts as an interferon (β_2) stimulates transcription and synthesis of many genes of pro-inflammatory proteins in acute phase response megakaryocytopoietin
IL-7	stromal cells	15 – 25 kDa	early B cell differentiation
IL-8	macrophages	10 kDa	neutrophil chemotaxis co-factor in granulocyte differentiation
IFNα	fibroblasts	20 – 25 kDa	inhibits T cell growth inhibits stem cell growth
IFNγ	T cells	20 – 25 kDa	inhibits viral replication inhibits B cell differentiation
LIF	granulocytes	10kDa	inhibits stem cell proliferation induces cholinergic neuron growth

Other Human Interleukins and Interferons and Cytokines

Fig. 3.4 Characteristics and actions of human interleukins, interferons and other cytokines.

and the allergic response. Instances of cytokine actions in allergy and their relationship to allergic disease, as well as future directions of diagnostic and therapeutic importance related to cytokine networks in allergy, will also be discussed.

Cytokines in Inflammation

The principal pro-inflammatory cytokines include interleukins 1 and 6 (IL-1 and IL-6), and tumour necrosis factor (TNF). After tissue damage or antigen presentation, these pro-inflammatory cytokines initiate a cascade of effects, including

- the stimulation of gene expression for acute phase proteins
- the production of acute-phase proteins
- the activation of inflammatory cells through secondary release of haemopoietic growth factors
- chronic tissue reparative or damaging processes such as fibrosis, which in turn involve further actions of cytokines such as peptide growth factors.

Generally, IL-1 and IL-6 are derived from macrophages or monocytes. These cells are stimulated to synthesize these groups of molecules upon antigen presentation (see Figs 3.6 and 3.7). T cells are activated and brought into the process, thus conferring specificity to the immune response directed against an initiating stimulus. As a by-product of these interactions, T-cell-derived cytokines such as IL-3 and IL-5, as well as other haemopoietic growth factors arising from both stromal cells and T cells, initiate a cascade of events culminating in inflammatory cell ingress, activation, and prolonged survival in tissues, as well as their differentiation from progenitors, thus further amplifying the sequence: this can be construed as a microenviromental process occurring in target tissues (see Fig. 3.8).

Cytokines with Inhibitory or Cytolytic Properties
transforming growth factor
leukaemia inhibitor associated factor
haemoregulatory peptide
negative regulatory protein
inhibin
IL-1and IL-1RA
tumour necrosis factor
IL-10
IFN-γ

Fig. 3.5 A partial list of cytokines which exercise an inhibitory or cytolytic effect

Some of the peptide growth factors, such as transforming growth factor (TGF_β), serve to effect a physiological down-regulation of chronic inflammatory processes in this sequence; more recently described negative regulators, such as inhibin and related factors, may also subserve a regulatory function in this regard (see Fig. 3.9). Lineage specificty for the type of inflammatory cell differentiation or activation can be conferred during this process, since it is clear that some cytokines, e.g. IL-5, specifically increase the production and prolong the survival of eosinophils, while IL-3 appears to be a basophil lineage-specific factor (see Figs 3.1, 3.2, and 3.3).

Not to be ignored among the intiating stimuli are neuropeptides, such as substance P which, after release from appropriate nerve endings in tissues, can lead to increased gene transcription, and to synthesis and secretion of secondary factors involved in

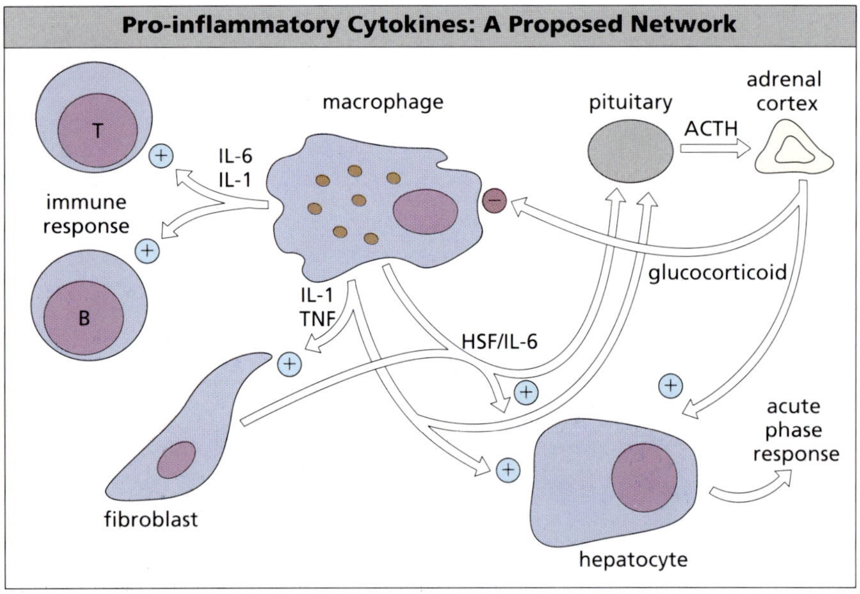

Fig. 3.6 The principle pro-inflammatory cytokines include IL-6, IL-1, and TNF. The cascade illustrated is a network of interactions, which take place after antigen processing, whereby macrophages signal to fibroblasts as well as immunocompetent T and B cells. IL-6 induces acute-phase protein responses in the liver; both IL-1 and IL-6 act at the pituitary level, and possibly at the higher cortical level, to induce adrenocortical responses, including the production of glucocorticoids which feed back in the process illustrated.

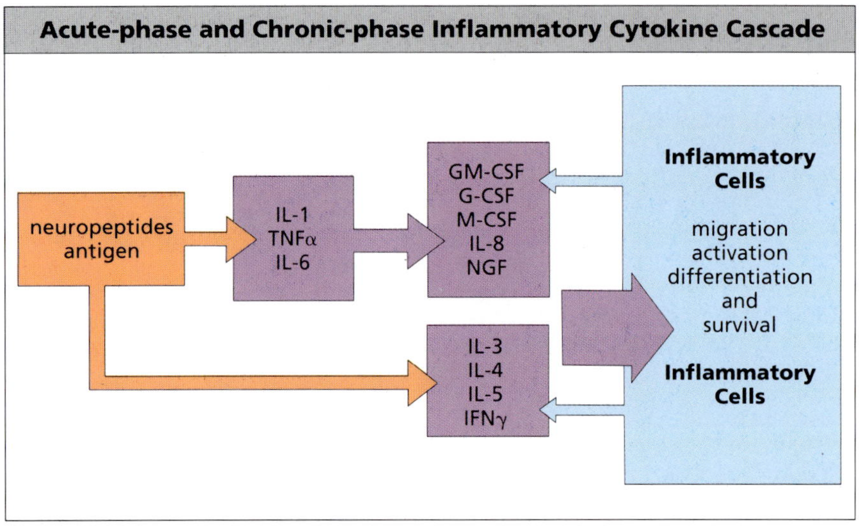

Fig. 3.7 The primary events, initiating signals, second signals, and secondary events in the acute- and chronic-phase inflammatory cytokine cascade. Inflammatory effector cells themselves can produce cytokines which may amplify the process at allergic tissue sites.

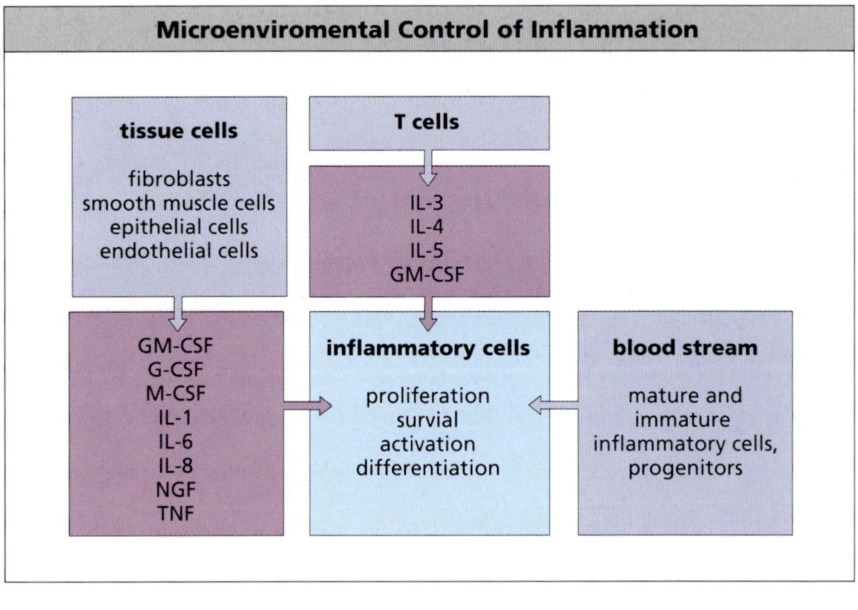

Fig. 3.8 Microenvironmental processes in inflammation, including structural cell cytokines. Mature and immature cells from the bloodstream access the tissues and become involved in a process of structural cell-determined cytokine interactions (tissue-driven response). This in turn leads to proliferation, activation, survival, and differentiation of inflammatory effector cells at the tissue level. This process is normally regulated, but when regulation is defective it leads to disturbances such as chronic inflammation and allergy.

inflammatory cell differentiation and ingress (see Figs 3.7 and 3.10). Thus, nerve release of substance P can stimulate production of granulocyte-macrophage colony-stimulating factor (GM-CSF) as well as G-CSF and M-CSF from stromal cells, thereby leading to the ingress, adherence, and activation of neutrophils, basophils, eosinophils, and macrophages (Fig. 3.8).

The effects of cytokines, including the haemopoietic growth factors, on mature granulocytes (and possibly on their immediate progenitors) include increased expression of cell-surface molecules (integrins), important in adherence to tissues and cell surfaces (Fig. 3.10). The adherence to cell surfaces involves appearance of the integrin family of molecules, such as CD11/18, and their binding to respective ligands, ICAM-I and iC3b, on tissue structural cells. Through these processes (obviously oversimplified in the above paradigm), the cells relevant to acute and chronic inflammation become involved in both immune and inflammatory responses following an initiating stimulus such as antigen, and can effectively deposit in tissues.

Cytokines in Immune Responses

The T-cell-specific cytokines IL-2 (known previously as T-cell growth factor) and IL-4 are principally involved in antigen-specific immune responses. Their actions lead to T-cell clonal amplification via increased expression of IL-2 receptors, and also to the growth and differentiation of B-cells and T-cell subsets, which also involves IL-5, -6, -7,and -10 (see Figs 3.2 and 3.4). IL-4, -5, -6, and -7 are responsible for immunoglobulin class (isotype) switching, clonal amplification of B-cell responses, and class- or subclass-specific immune responses. For example, IL-4 is a key molecule in initiating IgG1 and IgE class switching, and thus it assumes a central role in the development of IgE-dependent allergic responses (Fig. 3.9).

Secondary T-cell-derived cytokines such as IL-3 and IL-5 have haemopoietic effects on the cells involved in allergic responses – eosinophils, mast cells, and basophils; these, as well as the IgE response, can be reciprocally regulated by interferons, especially interferon-γ (IFN-γ) (see Chapter 2). A model of mast cell hyperplasia which is T-cell-dependent, stimulated by IL-3, and accompanied by IgE synthesis, is seen in nematode-parasitized rats; this model serves as an experimental counterpart to human allergic reactions involving mast cells, basophils, and eosinophils (Fig. 3.11). There is evidence that specific subpopulations of T cells may be involved in the secretion of each of the T-cell-derived cytokines, and that these in turn can be associated with classes and subclasses of T cells marked by variations in arrangements and sequences on the T-cell antigen receptor. Thus, cytokine specificity may represent an additional level of complexity in the immune response by T cells over and above that of antigen specificity. It has been pointed out that, in delayed-type hypersensitivity responses, as well as in class-specific responses such as those involving IgE, distinct subpopulations of T cells interacting with class II MHC molecules on antigen-presenting cells, themselves induced by specific cytokines (see Fig. 3.9), determine the nature and extent of the reaction. This may be mediated by specific glycosylation, which can either enhance or inhibit factors, and act in concert with IL-4 and IFN-γ in the case of IgE response (see Chapter 2). Specific populations of T cells secreting IL-3, IL-5, and GM-CSF are involved in asthma and related conditions (Figs 3.8 and 3.12). These T cells may differ from those producing IL-2 and IFNγ.

Cytokine Regulation of Immunoglobulin Isotope Switching and MHC Expression

Cytokine(s)	Immunoglobulin isotypes	MHC
IFN-γ	IgG2a	class II
IL-4	IgG1, IgE	class II
IL-5, TGF-β	IgA	–
IFNs, TNF	–	class I
IL-10	–	class II

Fig. 3.9 Cytokines closely linked with the immune response.

Cytokines in Allergy

Allergy as Inflammation

If an allergic response were to be considered as a subtype of an acute inflammatory response, it is indeed possible to implicate the same mechanisms mentioned above for the types of tissue pathology seen. Specifically, neuropeptides released in relation to

Cytokine Activation of Allergic Effector Cells

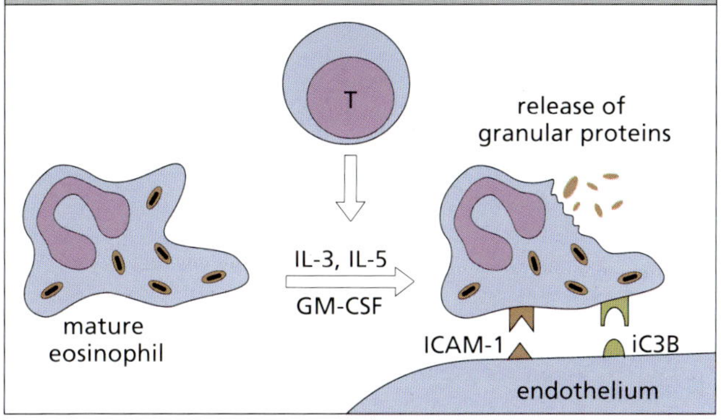

Fig. 3.10 IL-3, IL-5, and GM-CSF can induce cell-surface expression of integrin molecules, which are involved in cell adhesion, on mature inflammatory cells including eosinophils. Moreover, expression of some molecules, such as EG-2, is associated with enhanced survival of these effector cells, and also causes release of granules by activating the cells under conditions of antigen or IgE stimulation. Eosinophils become hypodense in this process, and can thus be readily detected in peripheral blood by certain immunochemical and physico-chemical properties associated with their activation. Receptors for leucocyte integrins, ICAM-1, and iC3b, are found on endothelial and related structural cells in inflamed tissues.

nerve stimulation/growth by peptide growth factors such as NGF, can initiate the production of IL-1, IL-6, TNFα, and IL-8 from structural cells such as fibroblasts, epithelial cells and endothelium (see Fig. 3.8). In addition, these structural cells may, upon further stimulation by pro-inflammatory cytokines, produce increased amounts of GM-CSF, G-CSF, and M-CSF; these, together with T-cell-derived IL-3 and IL-5, cause eosinophil, basophil, and mast cell differentiation and activation at allergen-provoked, mucosal tissue sites (Fig. 3.12). There are synergistic actions of cytokines demonstrable *in vitro* which are

Mast Cell Hyperplasia in Nematode-Infected Rats

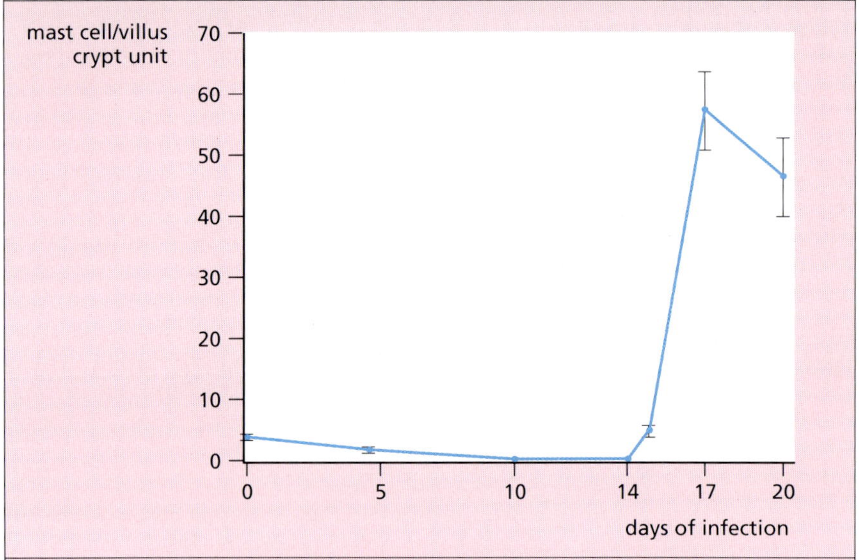

Growth of Mast Cells from Mesenteric Lymph Node

	Normal	Immune		
stimulus		day 14	17	20
none	1.0	1.0	9.3	19.0
PHA (1μg/ml)	1.0	1.0	21.8	35.6
antigen (10 worm equivalents)	0.5	1.0	13.0	−9.0*

* suppression at day 20

Fig. 3.11 In response to the nematode, *Nippostrongylus brasiliensis*, a massive mast cell hyperplasia, shown as toluidine blue-positive metachromatic cells populating the intestinal mucosa, is induced in rats after 14 - 17 days of infection. As shown in the graph and table, the expansion of mast cells is exponential over a short period of time; supernatants of cultures of lymph-node cells taken from nodes adjacent to the intestine (e.g. mesenteric) are populated with progenitors of mast cells and with T-cells which produce mast cell growth factors, including IL-3. An inhibitory effect of antigen-stimulated lymph-node culture supernatant upon *in vitro* mast cell growth is observed after the peak of *in vivo* mast cell hyperplasia, implying the existence of regulatory (homeostatic) molecules in this process. This rodent parasite model is useful in understanding human allergic responses, involving antigen and IgE, at mucosal surfaces.

Nasal Polyp or Rhinitis Histology, with Proposed Cytokine Cascade

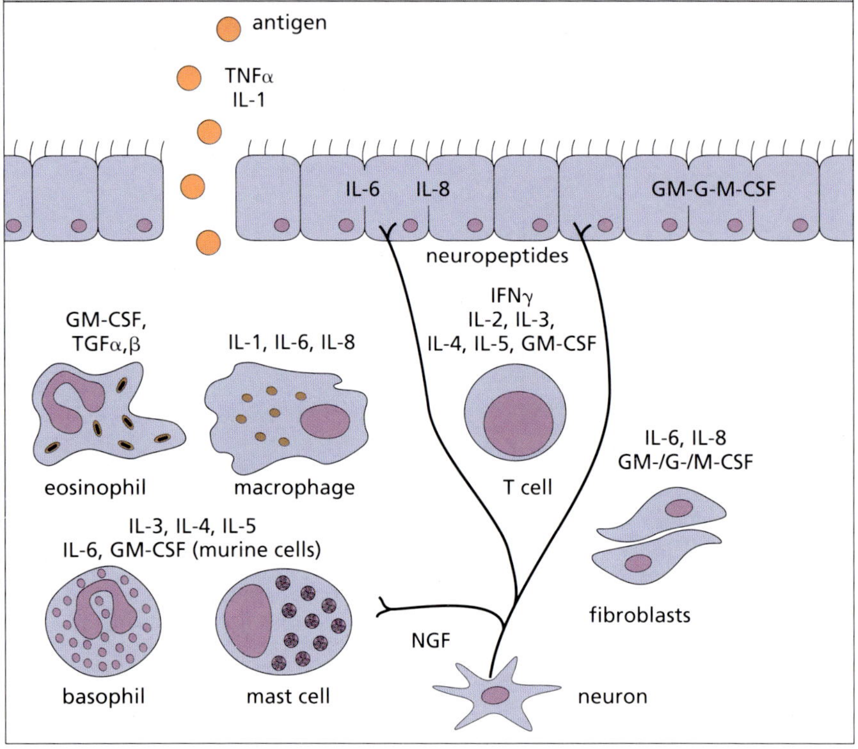

Fig. 3.12 Nasal polyp or allergic rhinitis mucosal histology, with proposed cytokine interactions. Within the damaged epithelium after allergen challenge direct access of cells to the underlying tissues is possible. These include: antigen-presenting cells (macrophages), T cell subpopulations secreting various cytokines, as well as epithelial cells, fibroblasts and endothelial cells. Cytokines as well as neuropeptides from nerves abutting upon or innervating epithelial and subepithelial structures (including T-cells) can also be involved in the cascade of events after antigenic challenge. The various cytokines depicted at various levels of the nasal polyp or allergic rhinitis mucosa are secreted preferentially, but not exclusively, by certain cell types: e.g. IL-2, -3, -4, -5 by T-cells and/or basophil/mast cells; IL-1, -6, -8, by macrophages and/or structural cells; TNFα, GM-CSF, G-CSF, M-CSF primarily by structural cells. Different types of mast cells populate the stromal and epithelial layers respectively.

most probably crucial in the ultimate outcome of a given event *in vivo*. NGF, for example, can synergize with GM-CSF in haemopoiesis, while a number of the haemopoietic growth factors synergize with each other and/or with other interleukins such as IL-4 and IL-6 (Fig. 3.13). The nature and extent of these synergistic activities *in vitro*, let alone *in vivo*, are not fully understood; clarification of these may provide keys to the understanding of regulation of the acute inflammatory response, its development into a chronic response, and the specificity of the 'language' or 'syntax' provided by these putative interactions. Moreover, the physiological or regulatory functions of inhibitory cytokines in preventing or delaying the development of inflammatory reactions must be fully understood before our reconstruction of these interactions can be considered complete.

Allergy as an Immune Response

Upon antigen presentation, T-cell-specific cytokines provide the basis for clonal amplification of T cells, B cells, and inflammatory cells such as mast cells, basophils, and eosinophils. Here too, as in inflammation, synergistic actions may determine the extent and severity of a reaction to antigen and, as initimated in the discussion on cytokine specificity of T cell populations (Fig. 3.12), whether or not IgE synthesis and thus the hallmark of an allergic response is to take place (see Chapter 2). Synergism between IL-3 and IL-5 or among IL-3, IL-5, and IL-1 has been documented; likewise, IL-2, IL-3, IL-4 and/or IL-10 synergize not only in T-cell-specific responses stimulating B cell growth and differentiation, but also in the development of mast cells (Fig. 3.13; see also Figs 3.2, 3.3, and 3.4). Recently, it has been found that mast cells themselves (at least mast cells from rodents) and perhaps basophils produce a large variety of cytokines, thus providing a possible stimulatory or positive feedback loop for perpetuating allergic tissue responses (Fig. 3.12).

Synergistic Actions of Cytokines: A New Language for Inflammation and Immunity

Synergy	Effects(s)
IL-1, IL-3, IL-5	granulocyte production eosinophilopoiesis
IL-3, IL-6	haemopoiesis
IL-4, IL-6	haemopoiesis
IL-2, IL-4; IL-3,IL-4, IL-10	T-cell amplification B-cell differentiation mast cell production
NGF, GM-CSF; NGF, IL-5	granulocyte production basophil/mast cell and eosinophil production
IL-3, IL-11	megakaryocytopoiesis

Fig. 3.13 Some cytokines which have synergistic effects in the immune response.

Cytokines in Disease

The study of the role of cytokines in specific human allergic disorders has recently begun. The hypothesis known as 'microenvironmental differentiation' or 'tissue-driven response' has been used to explain the development and chronicity of upper and lower respiratory tract allergic and related symptomatology, such as is expressed in allergic rhinitis, nasal polyposis, urticaria, and asthma (see Fig. 3.8). Stromal cell production of haemopoietic growth factors has been demonstrated, with effects upon mature inflammatory cells and their respective peripheral blood progenitors, which appear to be a hallmark of allergic disease (Fig. 3.14). Such progenitors give rise to basophils, eosinophils, and possibly mucosal mast cells in tissues where relatively large concentrations of haemopoietic growth factors as well as T cells, and presumably IL-3 and IL-5, are present. These derangements are also found in atopic dermatitis (see Fig. 3.15). The growth factors possess several activities in addition to their haemopoietic properties, including activation of basophils and eosinophils, as

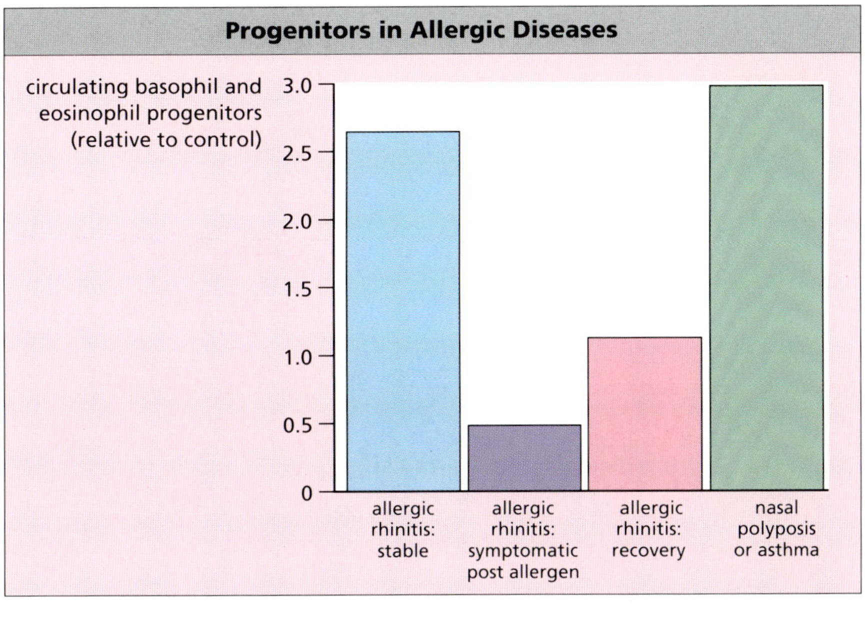

Fig. 3.14 There are varying levels of circulating basophil/eosinophil progenitors in allergic disorders. In stable, out-of-season allergic rhinitis, a large number of circulating progenitors is evident; levels fall on natural allergen exposure and with the occurrence of symptoms during seasonal allergy. With recovery, the level begins to return to its previous elevated state. Nasal polyposis and asthma are characterized by chronic elevations of these progenitors.

well as prolongation of eosinophil survival (IL-3, IL-5, GM-CSF).

Haemopoietic progenitors for eosinophils and basophils are elevated in the peripheral blood of atopic individuals. They fluctuate inversely with symptoms and signs of allergic rhinitis and asthma, and can be stimulated to differentiate *in vitro* by factors derived from nasal fibroblasts or epithelial cells (Fig. 3.16). The phenotype of such structural cells appears to be related to the severity of tissue reactivity; in nasal polyposis and allergic rhinitis, the intrinsic proliferative rate of fibroblasts and epithelial cells, as well as their production of certain cytokines, is higher than in normal controls (Fig. 3.16). In addition to bioassays for structural cell-derived cytokines, immunoassays and analysis of gene expression have confirmed that GM-CSF and IL-6 are produced in increased amounts in cells taken from allergic airways or from those with nasal polyposis/chronic rhinitis syndrome (Fig. 3.15). Even inflammatory cells themselves may produce cytokines in tissue; for example, eosinophils produce TGF and GM-CSF (Fig. 3.12). Thus conditions such as nasal polyposis (and perhaps asthma) may be expressions of cytokine imbalance or overproduction. Indeed, there is evidence for abnormal fibroblasts in biopsies from asthmatic subjects.

Cytokines in Allergic Disease

Condition	Cytokine(s) Involved	Source(s)	Assay method(s)
allergic rhinitis	GM-CSF, IL-2 IL-3, IL-5, IL-6, IL-8, IFNγ	nasal epithelium nasal fibroblasts nasal lavage nasal mucosal biopsy	haemopoietic assays immunoassay bioassay immunohistochemistry
nasal polyposis	GM-CSF, G-CSF IL-2, IL-3, IL-4, IL-5, IL-6, IL-8 TGFβ, IFNγ	nasal epithelium nasal fibroblasts T-cells nasal mucosal biopsy	haemopoietic bioassay eosinophil survival bioassay immunoassay mRNA assay (northern blot) *in situ* hybridization
asthma	GM-CSF, IL-1 IL-2, IL-3, IL-4, IL-5, IL-6, IFNγ, TFNα	alveolar macrophages bronchial epithelium bronchial fibroblasts bronchial lavage bronchial biopsy blood mononuclear cells	haemopoietic bioassay eosinophil survival therapy (indirect) immunoassay *in situ* hybridization polymerase chain reaction
atopic dermatitis	IFNγ, GM-CSF, IL-2, IL-3, IL-4, IL-5	T cells keratinocytes skin biopsy	bioassay immunoassay *in situ* hybridization

Fig. 3.15 Cytokines involved in specific allergic diseases. While probably many cytokines interact in the allergic inflammatory reaction, not all have been definitively demonstrated by *in vitro, ex vivo* or *in vivo* studies. The prinicipal cytokines are listed here according to disease and method of demonstration; however, in this rapidly expanding field, such a list cannot be exhaustive.

Effect of Structural Cell Cytokines on Basophil, Mast Cell, and Eosinophil Growth and Differentiation

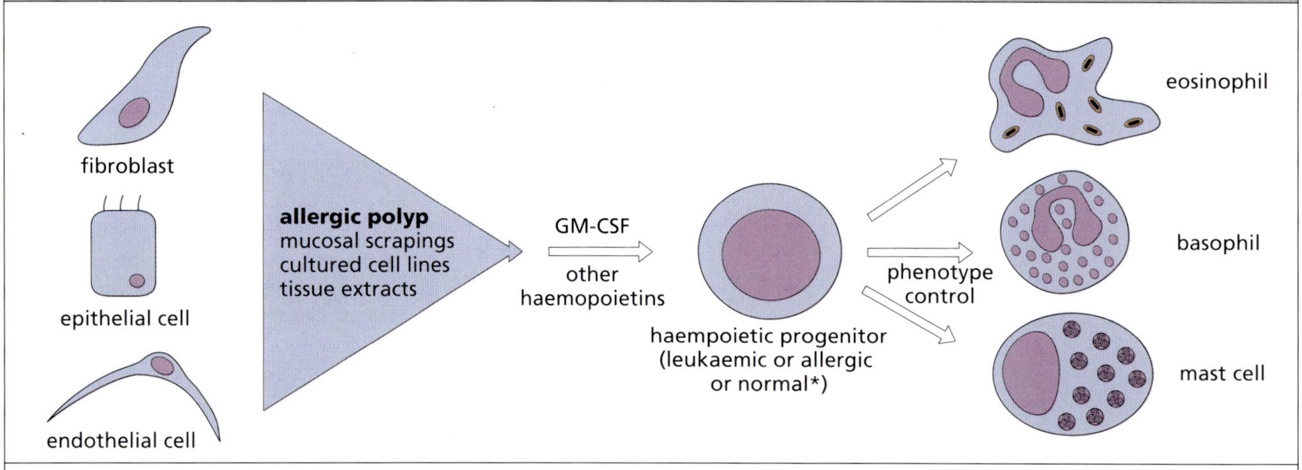

* Allergic patient progenitors are increased in circulation and more susceptible to effects than normal progenitors

Fig. 3.16 The structural cells involved in basophil/mast cell and eosinophil accumulations in tissues are shown here, based on several lines of experimental and clinical evidence. Allergic or nasal polyp mucosal scrapings, cultured cell lines or tissue extracts from fibroblasts, epithelial cells and/or endothelial cells can be shown to produce various cytokines, included among which are GM-CSF, IL-6, and IL-8. These act upon haemopoietic progenitors from allergic, normal or leukaemic donors and can be assayed for effects on differentiation to basophil, eosinophil and possibly mucosal mast cell lineages.

Moreover, peptide growth factors such as insulin-like growth factor (IGF) or NGF have been shown to be involved, respectively, in nasal polyposis and in *in vivo* accumulations of mast cells ; the latter is particularly important in mast cell hyperplasia during reactions to parasites, which may represent the developmental harbinger of an allergic response. Neuropeptides may upregulate the expression of a number of the haemopoietic growth factors and the neutrophil chemoattactant, IL-8, from structural cells derived from allergic airways diseases tissues (see Fig. 3.8). Furthermore, neuropeptides can be shown to be released in substantial amounts into nasal fluids of patients with upper airway allergic disease (Fig. 3.15), leading to a sequence of events which may well determine epithelial cell function, modulation of response to allergen, and the subsequent chronic inflammatory process.

Future Directions

Diagnostic Considerations

The role of cytokine networks in allergic disease *in vivo* has yet to be fully worked out. Analysis of tissues by *in situ* hybridization and/or gene expression for cytokines may lead to a better understanding of the processes delineated above. Of specific importance might be the diagnostic categorization of allergic diseases into disparate groups based upon cytokine profiles: for example, nasal polyposis may in fact be the result of unopposed, locally acting GM-CSF, IL-4, and IL-5, given the abundance of IgE-bearing plasma cells, mast cells, and eosinophils in this hamartomatous condition associated with asthma, rhinitis and aspirin intolerance (Fig. 3.17).

The delineation of principal cytokine processes in allergic disease may allow for the development of *in vitro* assays for naturally occurring inhibitors of cytokines, of which there are beginning to be quite a few with specific regulatory functions (see Fig. 3.5). In addition, novel factors which may stimulate subtypes of cells, such as basophils or mast cells at mucosal surfaces, or lead to specific activation profiles of inflammatory cells, may be discovered and lead to a better appreciation of the complexity of these networks.

Therapeutic Considerations

The beneficial effects of various therapeutic agents in allergic disease can be studied with a view to understanding their effects on cytokine production. For example, corticosteroids appear to cause changes in inflammatory cell numbers, which may reflect either direct cytolytic actions or complex interactions upon T cells, structural cells, and cytokines derived from them which influence cell differentiation (Figs 3.18 and 3.19). Indeed, corticosteroids may suppress eosinophil production as well as mast cell development in rodents, an action which may be due to

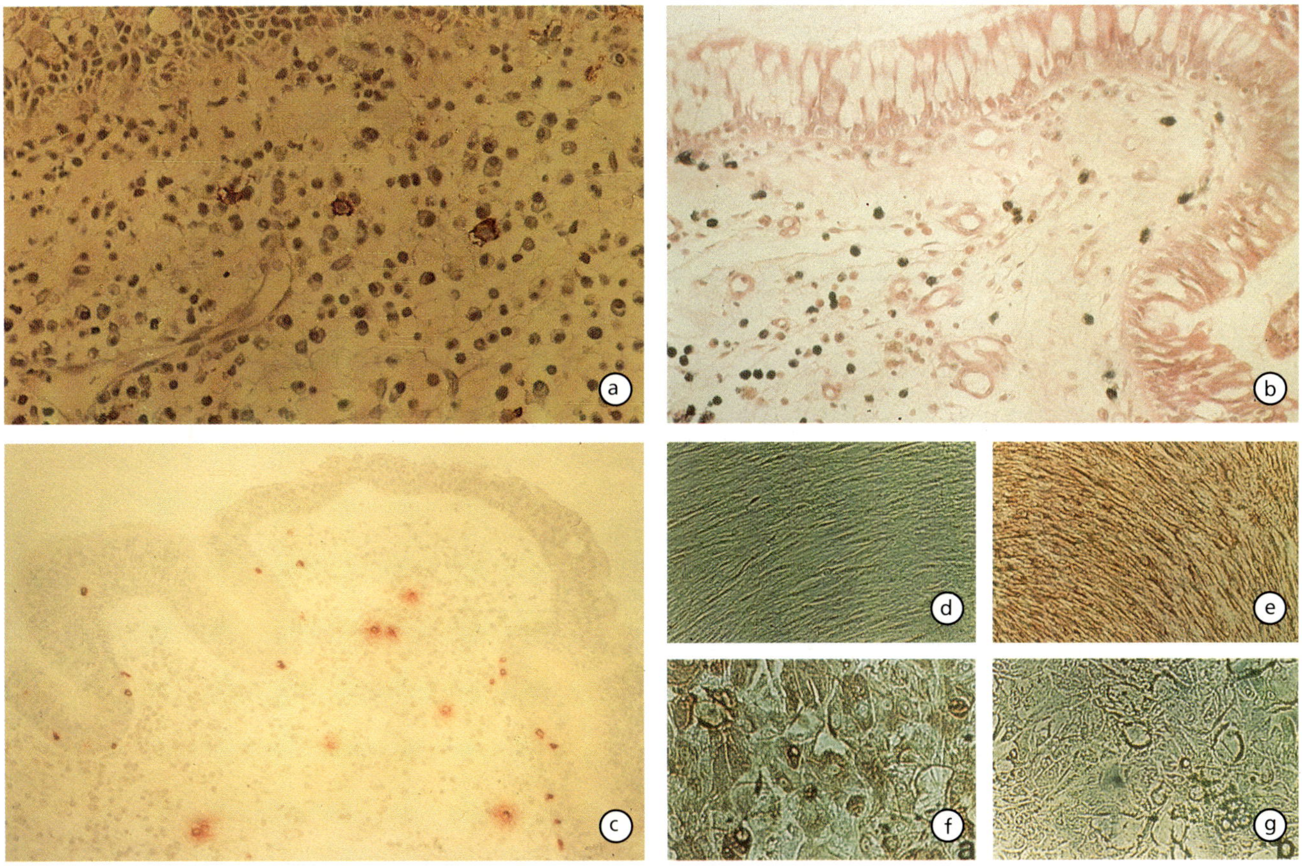

Fig. 3.17 Nasal polyp histology. (a) IgE secreting plasma cells; (b) activated eosinophils, using the EG-2 marker; (c) mast cells, using a tryptase marker; and cultured polyp fibroblasts (d,e) and epithelial cells (f,g) which secrete growth factors such as GM-CSF and IL-6 are shown here. The fibroblasts stain specifically with vimentin (d) while the epithelial cells stain specifically with keratin (g).

inhibition of synthesis or secretion of IL-3, IL-5 or GM-CSF (Fig. 3.20). Recently, it has been noted that topical corticosteroids inhaled by asthmatics in exacerbation lead to changes in circulating mature inflammatory cells as well as their progenitors which may not be accounted for by systemically absorbed levels of the drug (Fig. 3.20). This is consistent with the view that corticosteroids, when topically administered, may down-regulate the production of haemopoietic growth factors by structural cells such as epithelial cells and fibroblasts. Indeed, cells taken from the airways and subjected *in vitro* to corticosteroids at concentrations which may be eqivalent to those topically adminsitered *in vivo* cause inhibition of gene expression of GM-CSF by epithelial cells or fibroblasts, as well as direct and indirect *in vitro* effects on differentiation of eosinophils and basophils.

Probes for cytokine gene expression as well as immunoassays for cytokine production are now becoming available for use in understanding the mechanisms of action of corticosteroids and other agents which are effective in allergic disease, as well as in diagnosis of putative cytokine/disease entities (above). These may lead to the development of newer and more potent medications. Closely related to this is the projected development of analogues or competitive inhibitions of cytokines which perpetuate inflammatory cell responses including effects such as bronchial hyper-responsiveness and late phase cutaneous reactions. Indeed, newer cytokine antagonists, some analogous to cyclosporin A, the IL-2 inhibitor used in transplantation and autoimmune diseases, are now being developed and tested in allergic disease. Finally, specific antibodies to known or novel cytokines may be in future used topically to target therapy to a given location and process, leading to more specific amelioration of allergic symptomatology and even abrogation of the response for prolonged periods.

Effects of Corticosteroids on Allergic-Type Inflammation

- decreased eosinophil numbers and activity
- increased eosinophil granule leakage
- decreased mast cell protease production
- decreased mast cell response to parasites
- decreased mast cell numbers
- inhibition of basophil/mast cell mediator release
- inhibitory effects on eosinophil and basophil chemotaxis and adherence
- inhibition of basophil/eosinophil differentiation

Fig. 3.18 Cellular effects of corticosteroids when given to allergic subjects.

Effects of Topical Corticosteroids on Nasal Stromal Cell Cytokines

- inhibition of production of basophil/eosinophil differentiating factors by nasal epithelial cells and fibroblasts
- inhibition of transcription and production of GM-CSF, IL-6, and IL-8 by nasal epithelial cells and fibroblasts

Fig. 3.19 Effects of corticosteroids on cytokine production when given topically to allergic subjects.

Effects of Costeroids on Progenitors in Asthma

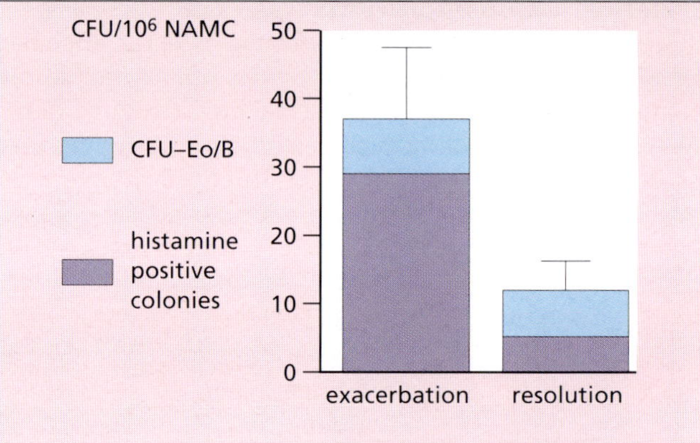

Fig. 3.20 The effects of corticosteroids on progenitors (CFU-Eo/B) in asthma are shown here. Circulating levels of eosinophils, basophils and their progenitors are increased during asthma exacerbation and fall upon resolution after inhalation of topical corticosteroids. Such an effect is not seen when topical corticosteroids are given to non-asthmatic patients with allergic rhinitis by inhalation into the lower airway. These studies suggest that airway inflammatory processes may be accompanied by the production of cytokines spilling over into the circulation and causing progenitor increases and/or fluctuations. A model similar to this has been examined in primates injected with IL-3 and GM-CSF, in which basophils/eosinophils and progenitors rise just as they do in the asthmatic patient population in

Further Reading

Austen KF, Galli SJ, eds. *Mast Cell and Basophil Differentiation and Funtion in Health and Disease.* New York: Raven Press, 1989.

Denburg JA. Phylogeny and ontogeny of basophils, mast cells and eosinophils. In: Holgate ST, ed: *Mast Cells Mediators and Disease*. London: Kluwer Academic Publishers, 1988:1–27.

Denburg JA, Dolovich J, Harnish D. Basophil/mast cell and eosinophil growth and differentiation factors in human allergic disease. *Clin Exp Allergy* 1989; **19**:249–254.

Groopman JE, Molina J-M, Scadden DT. Hematopoietic growth factors: biology and clinical applications. *N Engl J Med* 1989; **321**:1449–1459.

Balkwill FR, Burke F. The cytokine network. *Immunol Today* 1989; **10**:299–304.

Chapter 4

Activation Mechanisms of Mast Cells and Basophils

Introduction

This chapter provides a brief status report regarding IgE-mediated mast cell and basophil activation. After reviewing the repertoire of signalling elements present in nearly all cells, specific observations in mast cell models, particularly those associated with exocytosis, will be addressed.

The Problem of Cellular Communication

One fascinating biological feature of multicellular organisms is the exquisite co-ordination achieved between and within different cells. The need for well-regulated communication between cells is obvious and is largely achieved by bio-informational small molecules synthesized by one tissue and subsequently recognized by others. Structural and functional diversity demands that each cell have the potential to recognize a large subset of these molecules in the extracellular milieu, and translate an extracellular binding event into an amplified intracellular biochemical signal that causes an appropriate cellular response (Fig. 4.1).

Responsiveness requires the ability of a target cell to recognize the relevant molecule by expressing a specific cell surface or intracellular receptor. Cells must also distinguish between receptors that are occupied by the ligand and those that are not; finally, a cell must translate recognition of receptor occupancy into a meaningful response.

Receptors tend to fall into three broad categories, those that:
(1) directly translate signals,
(2) open ion channels or activate ion pumps and
(3) interact with an intermediate transducer such as GTP-binding proteins (G-proteins).

These signalling mechanisms cause rapid changes in the intracellular levels of regulatory molecules, termed second messengers.

Second messengers function to amplify receptor-mediated signals, and exert their influence by rapidly altering the activity of one or more enzymes or non-enzymatic proteins (Fig. 4.2). The levels of these second messengers are tightly regulated, and elucidating the biological pathways involved in their formation and removal are critical to understanding the events of cell activation. In contrast to the wide variety of agonists and hormones, the repertoire of second messenger molecules is somewhat restricted.

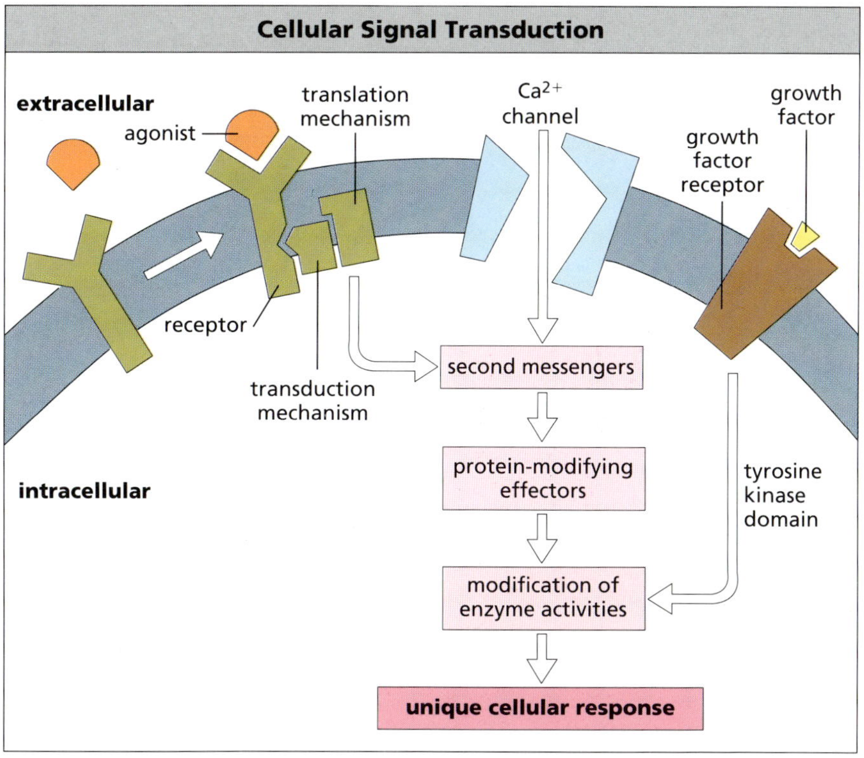

Fig. 4.1 Receptor-initiated intracellular signalling. Cells have evolved a variety of mechanisms to perceive and respond to changes in the extracellular environment. Signalling is initiated by binding of an extracellular agonist to its appropriate cell surface receptor. Subsequent conformational changes in the receptor transduce the signal across the bilayer and it is translated to form a variety of intracellular second messenger molecules. Some receptors themselves are effectors (tyrosine kinases) while others generate second messengers directly (ion channels) or indirectly (G-protein-coupled receptors).These changes result in responses that include: exyocytosis, cytokine synthesis, cell differentiation and proliferation.

Second messengers include:

- cyclic AMP (cAMP)
- cyclic GMP (cGMP)
- inositol 1,4,5-triphosphate (IP3)
- diacylglycerol (DAG)
- Ca^{2+}
- arachidonic acid (AA)
- phosphatidic acid (PA).

Receptor-mediated activation causes the genesis of a 'signal' that is defined by a specific pattern of changes in the levels of a subset of the available second messengers and effectors. Because different patterns of changes in second messenger levels probably result in different cellular responses, knowledge regarding the mechanisms of signal transduction is important to understand the regulation of mast cells and provide an important framework for developing strategies of pharmacological regulation in hypersensitivity states.

Mast Cell Activation

Mast cells and basophils release preformed granule-associated mediators and newly synthesized lipid-derived mediators when antigen (Ag) cross-links IgE bound to its high affinity receptor ($Fc_{\epsilon}R1$). Purification of rodent mast cells, human mast cells and basophils, and the establishment of immortal cell lines (RBL and PT-18) have enabled investigation of the intracellular biological mechanisms that control mediator release. The biochemical events that occur during mast cell/basophil activation may be broken down into at least five broad categories:

(1) antigen-induced receptor activation;
(2) signal transduction;
(3) signal translation and amplification;
(4) activation of target/effector proteins; and
(5) secretion of granules (Fig. 4.3).

Although mast cell activation is also associated with enhanced expression of cellular oncogenes (*myc, fos, jun,* and *ras*) and robust synthesis of important regulatory cytokines (interleukins 3, 4, 5 and 6), the mechanisms involved in this process are only now emerging and will not be addressed here.

Exocytosis and the Functional Anatomy of Membranes

Biologically relevant membranes are formed from phospholipids and cholesterol, and have a characteristic bilayer structure as a consequence of their amphipathic nature. Membranes are important biochemical barriers in the cell. They allow functional compartmentalization in cells and their organelles, but they also obstruct the flow of information. Peripheral and integral membrane proteins allow different membranes to function in a specific manner.

Mast cells and basophils, in common with all secretory cells, have the regulated ability to release

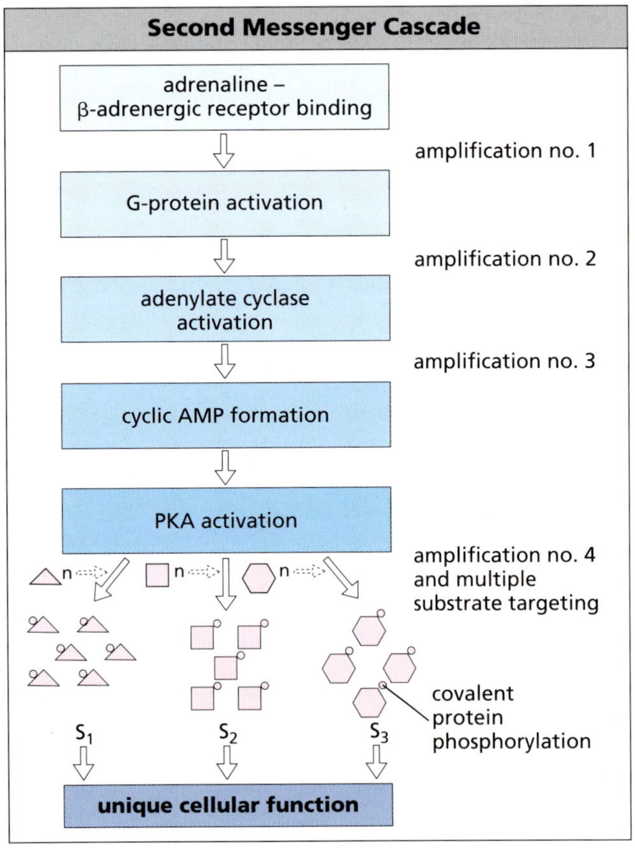

Fig. 4.2 Second messenger cascade. Intracellular second messengers are molecules that function to transmit and amplify an extracellular signal to a variety of intracellular targets. In the classic example of the β-adrenegic receptor, adrenaline binds to this receptor and activates a relevant subset of G-proteins. Each receptor activates several G-proteins that in turn each activate several adenylate cyclase enzymes that each produce many molecules of the second messenger cyclic AMP. Cyclic AMP then activates protein kinase A (PKA) which exerts its regulatory effect by selectively phosphorylating a subset of target proteins.

Biochemical Events in Mast Cell/Basophil Activation	
I	$Fc_{\epsilon}R1$-cross-linking $Fc_{\epsilon}R1$ interaction with cytoskeleton
II	Signal transduction Serine esterase activity GTP-binding proteins Membrane depolarization/repolarization
III	Signal translation and amplification A. Formation of second messengers PLC (DAG/IP3), PLD (PA/Lyso-PA), PLA_2 (AA/eicosanoids), adenylate cyclase (cyclic AMP) Ion transport (Ca^{2+}) B. Intermediate second messengers IP3 response element (Ca^{2+}) C. Effects of second messengers ↑ protein kinase C (PKC) ↑ protein kinase A (PKA) ↑ Ca^{2+}/calmodulin dependent proteins Altered polymerization of F-actin
IV	Cellular responses Exocytosis – membrane fusion, preformed mediator release Lipid mediator formation and release eicosanoid biosynthesis PAF biosynthesis Cytokine generation

Fig. 4.3 Biochemical events in mast cell and basophil activation. Antigen cross-linking of IgE bound to the high affinity ($Fc_{\epsilon}R1$) receptor on mast cells or basophils begins a complex series of intracellular biochemical events.

preformed secretory granule constituents to the extracellular environment as the result of fusion of the granule membranes with the plasma membrane. As this process is highly energetically unfavourable, it takes place only at a very slow rate in unstimulated cells. In order to overcome this energy hurdle, cells must synthesize either specialized proteins or lipids that can form non-bilayer membrane structures which facilitate membrane fusion, but do not result in loss of integrity of either the plasma membrane or granule membrane. Recent work suggests that a number of physiologically relevant lipids, called 'fusogens', can act in this capacity.

Second Messenger/Effector Systems

Receptors

With the exception of cytosolic and/or nuclear receptors, most receptors are plasma membrane proteins that span the bilayer. The extracellular portion contains the ligand binding domain, and the intracellular part contains the signal transducing domain. Interaction of an agonist with the extracellular ligand binding domain causes a conformational change in an intracellular signal transducing domain – the process of signal transduction.

However, mast cell activation by IgE/antigen interactions is considerably more complex. This evolves out of the need of mast cells to remain quiescent despite binding of IgE to $Fc_\epsilon R1$, but to become explosively activated when $Fc_\epsilon R1$ are physically approximated by multivalent antigens recognized by antigen-specific IgE bound to their receptors. Thus, the degree of receptor/receptor interaction, rather than the frequency of ligand binding to receptors, is the physiologically relevant parameter in mast cell activation. Mast cells or basophils can also be stimulated via receptors that simply recognize ligand binding (fMLP and C3a).

G-proteins

Many receptors translate information regarding ligand occupancy by utilizing a 'translation mechanism' employing a family of related proteins called GTP-binding proteins or G-proteins (Fig. 4.4). These proteins have inherent GTPase activity. Classical G-proteins involved in receptor signalling are a family of similar oligomeric heterotrimers, each consisting of one alpha, one beta, and one gamma subunit, which interact with the intracellular signal transducing domain of receptors. The beta and gamma subunits ($G_{\beta\gamma}$) are structurally very similar and functionally interchangeable among members of the G-protein family. The alpha subunit contains the guanine nucleotide binding region and GTPase activities, and provides specificity with regard to the ability of a given G-protein to interact with specific receptors and specific second messenger generating proteins. As a result, classification of G-proteins is based upon the identity of the distinct alpha subunits (G_α).

The ability to alter pharmacologically the ability of G-proteins to facilitate or antagonize signal transduction pathways enables investigators to determine if GTP-binding proteins play a role in various signal transduction pathways. Pre-treatment of cells with bacterial toxins cause ADP ribosylation of a variety of G_α subunits affecting their ability to function properly. The failure to inhibit signal transduction by toxins does not automatically rule out a role for G-proteins in that toxin-insensitive G_α subunits have been described. GTP and GDP analogues are of value in determining a role for low molecular weight GTP binding proteins (*ras*, *rho* and others) or classic G-proteins in the process of interest.

G-Protein-Mediated Signal Transduction

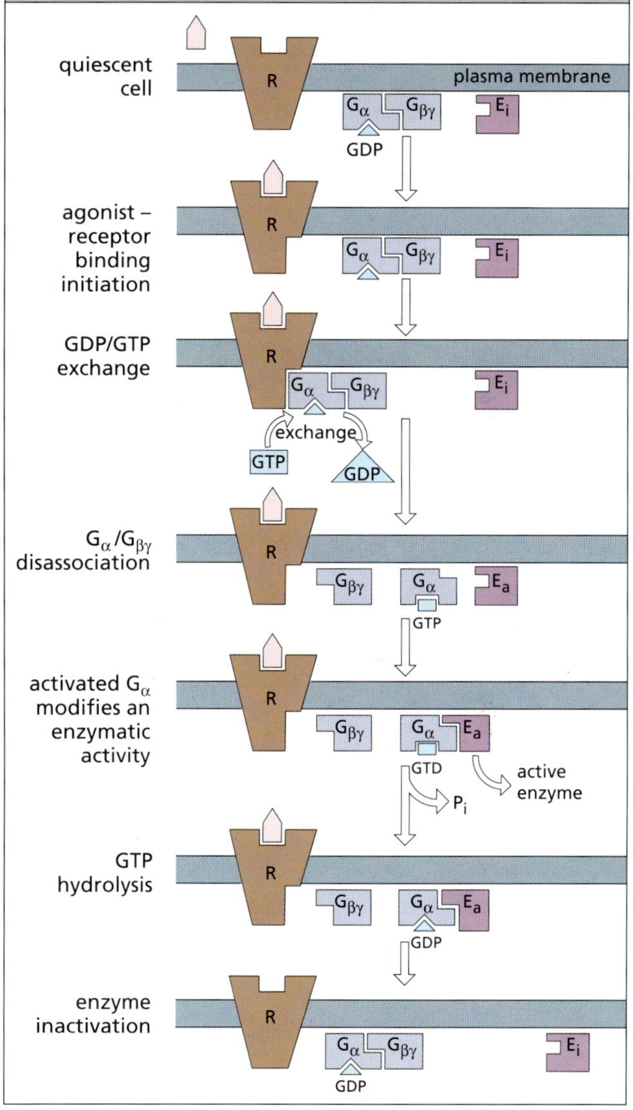

Fig. 4.4 Model of G-protein regulation of receptor-mediated signalling. Classical G-proteins consist of a heterotrimeric α,β,γ, structure with the GTP hydrolytic activity confined to the G_α subunit. Agonist binding promotes the disassociation of GDP and subsequent binding of GTP on the G_α subunit which is followed by the dissociation of the active G_α and $G_{\beta\gamma}$. Free G_α-GTP then influences the activity of an enzyme (E). As illustrated above, the G_α subunit activates E ($E_{inactive}$ to E_{active}), however different G_αs have also been shown to inhibit rather than increase enzyme activity. The subsequent hydrolysis of GTP to GDP inactivates the G_α which in turn negatively impacts the activity of E. The disassociation of the G_α/E_a complex leaves G_α free to reassociate with the $G_{\beta\gamma}$ as seen in the resting state.

Control of Cellular Processes by Regulation of Target Proteins

Adenylate cyclase and cyclic AMP

One of the best characterized signal transduction systems is the increased formation and accumulation of cyclic AMP as the result of stimulation of the β-adrenergic receptor. As a result of receptor/ligand interaction, $G_{\alpha 3}$ activity is enhanced through the dissociation of $G_{\alpha 3}$/GTP from $G_{\beta\gamma}$ and causes subsequent activation of adenylate cyclase – the enzyme catalyzing the synthesis of cyclic AMP (see Fig. 4.4). The activity of adenylate cyclase can be reduced in an analogous and receptor-dependent fashion by $G_{\alpha i}$, an inhibitory G-protein. The high energy cyclic phosphate, cyclic AMP, is converted to inactive AMP by the constitutive activity cyclic AMP phosphodiesterase.

Cytosolic Ca^{2+}

Although the $[Ca^{2+}]_{extracellular}$ is in the millimolar range, resting cells maintain a submicromolar concentration in the cytoplasm, by pumping Ca^{2+} either out of the cell or into organelles, such as endoplasmic reticulum or calciosomes, where Ca^{2+} is sequestered by calcium-binding proteins.

Because of the large concentration gradients involved, regulated changes in the activity of specific calcium channels associated with the plasma membrane, calciosomes or sarcoplasmic reticulum can dramatically increase $[Ca^{2+}]_{cytosol}$ (Fig. 4.5). Two principal mechanisms for channel activation have thus far been described:

(1) voltage-regulated Ca^{2+} channels in the plasma membrane of electrically sensitive tissues;

(2) IP3-mediated activation of channels present in calciosomes.

Phosphoinositide-derived inositol phosphates

Receptor-mediated changes in the metabolism of PI has been demonstrated to occur in virtually every cell type examined. Receptor-dependent $G_{\alpha q}$-mediated activation of a phosphoinositide-specific phosopholipase C (PI-PLC) results in the hydrolysis of the minor phospholipid PIP_2, releasing its water-soluble head group, IP3, into the cytosol. IP3 functions as a critical second messenger in regulating $[Ca^{2+}]_{cytosol}$, particularly in cells with modest expression of voltage-dependent Ca^{2+} channels. Although a role for IP4 (the phosphorylation product of IP3) at the plasma membrane has been suggested in sustaining rises in $[Ca^{2+}]_{cytosol}$, the many other inositol phosphate isomers have not been associated with second messenger functions (see Fig. 4.8).

Diacylglycerol

In many cell types, including the mast cell, receptor-mediated cell activation leads to a significant increase in the mass of 1, 2 diacylglycerol (DAG). In addition to acting as a second messenger in the regulation of protein phosphorylation, a role for DAG in membrane fusion has recently been suggested since it can facilitate the formation of nonbilayer structures in membranes that are thought to be fusion intermediates.

The mechanism by which DAG is formed has largely focused on receptor-dependant activation of phospholipases–enzymes capsule of hydrolysing phospholipids (Fig. 4.6). Mechanisms proposed to be involved in the formation of DAG (Fig. 4.7) include:

- PI-PLC in the 'PI Cycle' (see Fig. 4.8);
- hydrolysis of PC by PC-PLC;
- the two step formation of DAG by PC-PLD and PA-PHase, the 'indirect pathway' (see Fig 4.14).

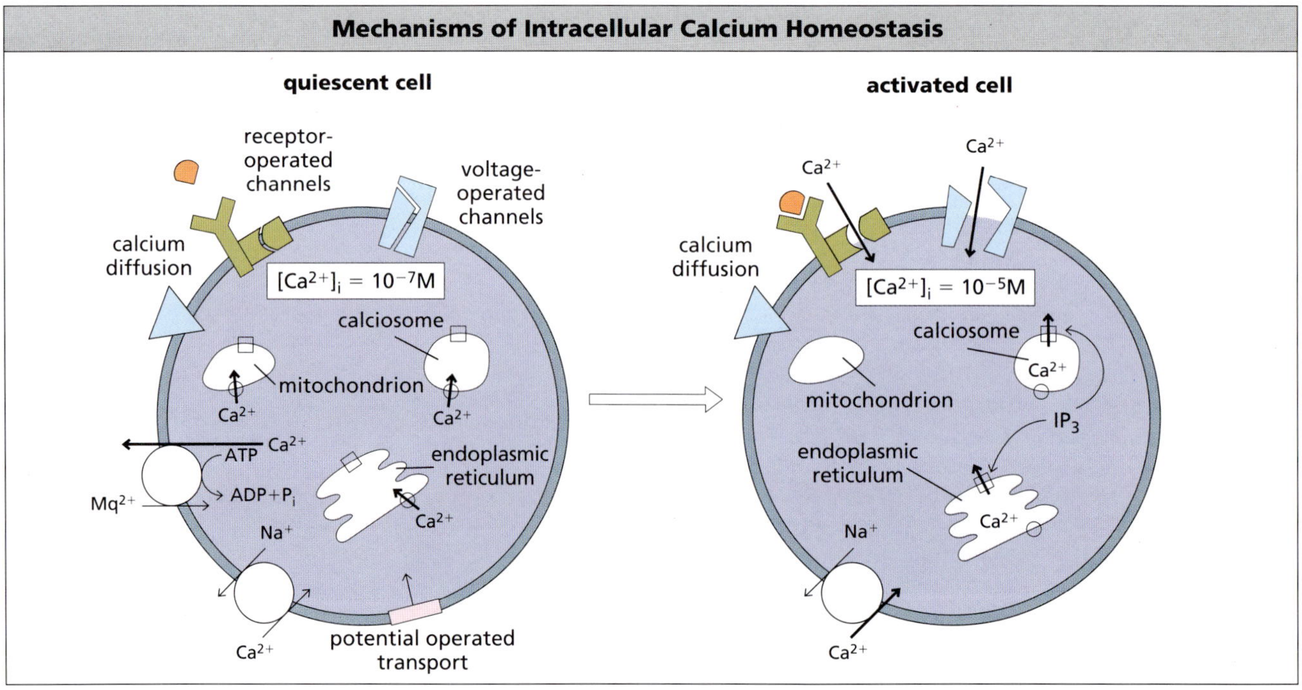

Fig. 4.5 Basic mechanisms of intracellular calcium homeostasis. Resting cells maintain a very low level of ionized intracellular Ca^{2+} (10^{-7}M) by sequestering of Ca^{2+} by Ca^{2+}- binding proteins in a variety of organelles and the active transport of Ca^{2+} out of the cell. Activation of cells can lead to 10–100 fold increases in $[Ca^{2+}]_{cytosol}$ as the result of a variety of mechanisms illustrated above.

Although early support for the importance of PI-PLC was generated by the ubiquity of receptor-dependent PI-PLC and its ability to generate two second messengers that regulated PKC (IP3→Ca^{2+} and DAG), recent data from an increasing number of laboratories suggest that pathways involving PC hydrolysis are likely to be quantitatively more important in DAG formation.

Membrane potential
Because lipid bilayers are largely impermeable to a wide variety of ions, concentration gradients result in electrochemical gradients that generate a transmembrane potential. Changes in the permeability of ions not only results in ion fluxes, but also dramatic changes in membrane potential. In general, depolarization results in excitation and secretion while hyperpolarization has opposite effects.

Products of phospholipase A_2 (PLA_2) activation
Hydrolysis of phospholipids by PLA_2 causes the release of arachidonic acid (AA) which is of both functional and regulatory interest. AA is the obligate substrate for the biosynthesis of eicosanoids – a family of, autocoids that includes prostaglandins and leukotrienes (see Fig. 4.9). Further, AA can act as the lipid activator for some PKC isoforms in the absence of changes in DAG. Less certain is its role as a fusogenic lipid and a regulator of PLD in some systems.

The specific phospholipid substrate that is of principal importance in the liberation of AA has been of considerable interest. Initial enthusiasm for PI as a substrate for PLA_2 (as the result of the high frequency of AA in its *sn*-2 position) waned as more careful studies in a variety of cells suggested that it was derived from PLA_2 hydrolysis of 1,alkyl-PE and/or 1,alkyl-PC.

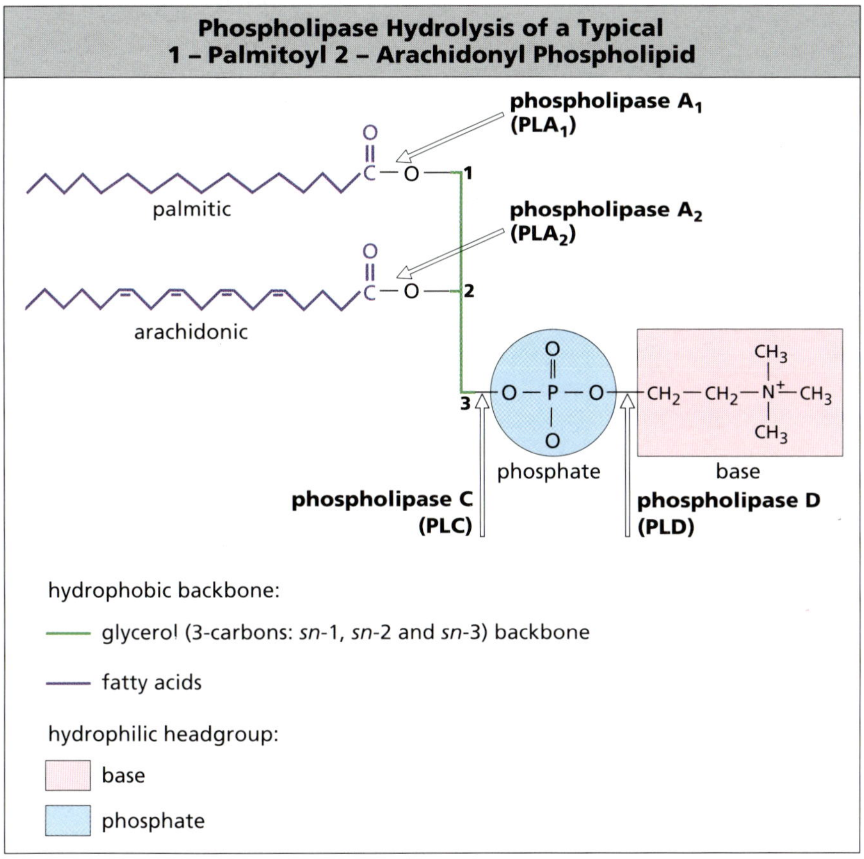

Fig. 4.6 Phospholipid hydrolysis by different phospholipases. The hydrophobic region of prototypic phospholipid has fatty acids linked to the *sn*-1 and *sn*-2 carbons of glycerol. The *sn*-1 position contains largely saturated fatty acids attached through acyl (ester), alkyl (ether) or alk, 1-enyl (plasmalogen) linkages. In contrast, fatty acids esterified at the *sn*-2 position are frequently unsaturated. The hydrophilic base is attached at the *sn*-3 position via a phosphodiester linkage. PLA_1 hydrolyzes acyl linkages at *sn*-1 position, releasing a fatty acid and a 1-lyso, 2-acyl-phospholipid. PLA_2 removes the *sn*-2 fatty acid, leaving a 1-acyl, 2-lyso-phospholipid. PLC and PLD hydrolyze phosphodiester bonds associated with the polar headgroup. PLC hydrolysis at *sn*-3 leaves diglyceride and a phosphorylated base while PLD action removes the base leaving phosphatidic acid.

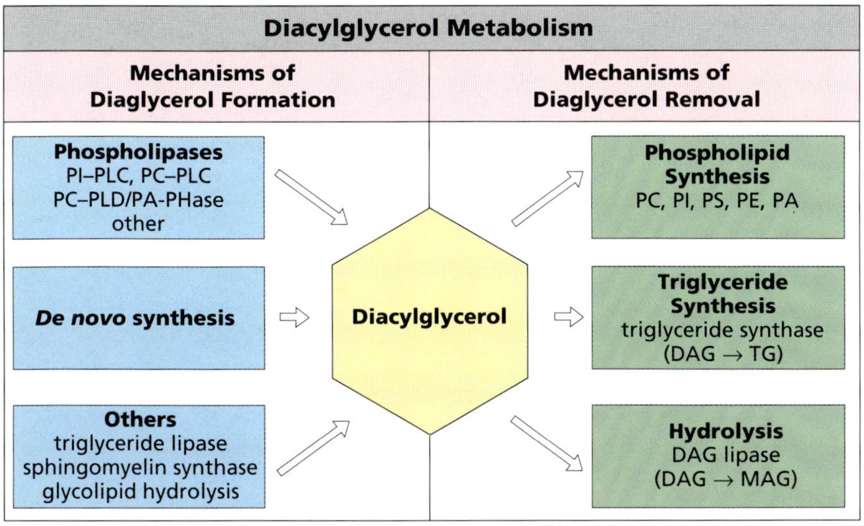

Fig. 4.7 Diacylglycerol metabolism. DAG is normally a quantatatively minor lipid in cells, but plays central roles both in the synthesis of glycerol-based phospholipids and as a second messenger in signal transduction. Data suggest that receptor-dependent activation of phospholipases play the principal role in changes in DAG formation. Since the presence of DAG is likely to be important, assessing the mechanisms of DAG removal is also important in determining its ambient level.

Phosphoinositide Cycle and Second Messenger Generation

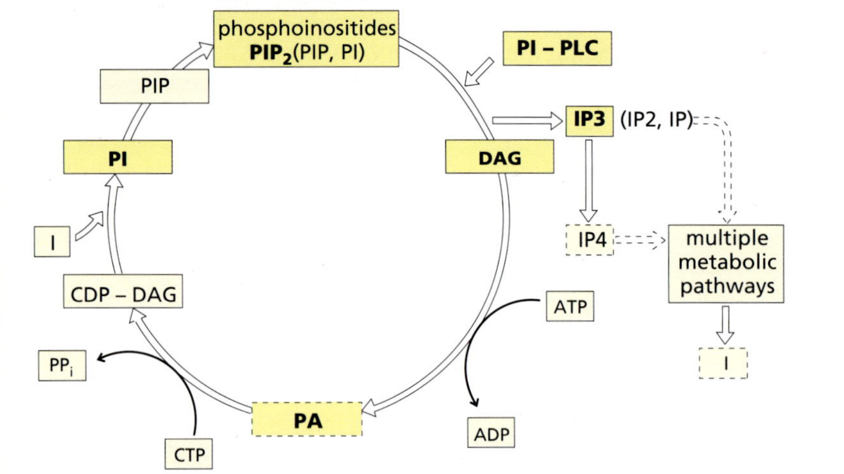

PIP_2, PIP, PI = phosphoinositides
PI–PLC = PI specific phospholipase C
IP4 = inositol 1, 3, 4, 5 tetrakisphosphate
IP3 = inositol 1, 4, 5 trisphosphate
IP2 = inositol 1, 4 bisphosphate
IP = inositol 1 phosphate
I = inositol
DAG = diacylglycerol
PA = phosphatidic acid
CDP – DAG = cytidinediphosphate diacylglycerol

Second Messenger: Functions

Documented		Proposed	
DAG	co-activator of protein kinase	PA	regulation of PA dependent protein kinases
IP3	calcium release from intracellular stores	IP4	regulation of plasma membrane Ca^{2+} influx

Fig. 4.8 The PI cycle as a second messenger generating pathway. The classic bifurcating pathway of signal transduction is initiated by the hydrolysis of PIP_2 by phospholipase C(PI-PLC). This generates two second messengers: diacylglycerol (DAG) and inositol triphosphate (IP3). The metabolism of IP3 is highly complex. IP3 may undergo further phosphorylation and/or dephosphorylation resulting in a variety of isomers of IP2, IP3 and IP4.

PLA_2 also catalyzes formation of potentially important lysophospholipids (phospholipids deacylated at the *sn*-1 or *sn*-2 position). First, recent evidence suggests that lysophosphatidic acid (lyso-PA) may act as a second messenger by contributing to the regulation of $[Ca^{2+}]_{cytosol}$. Second, lysophospholipids have been shown in some artificial membrane sytems to act as fusogens to promote bilayer fusion. Third, lyso-PC has been shown to substitute weakly for phosphatidylserine (PS) during protein kinase C activation. Finally, PLA_2 hydrolysis of 1-O-alkyl,2-acyl-PC results in the formation of the critical precursor (1-O-alkyl,2-lyso-PC)

Lipid-Derived Mediators of Mast Cells and Basophils

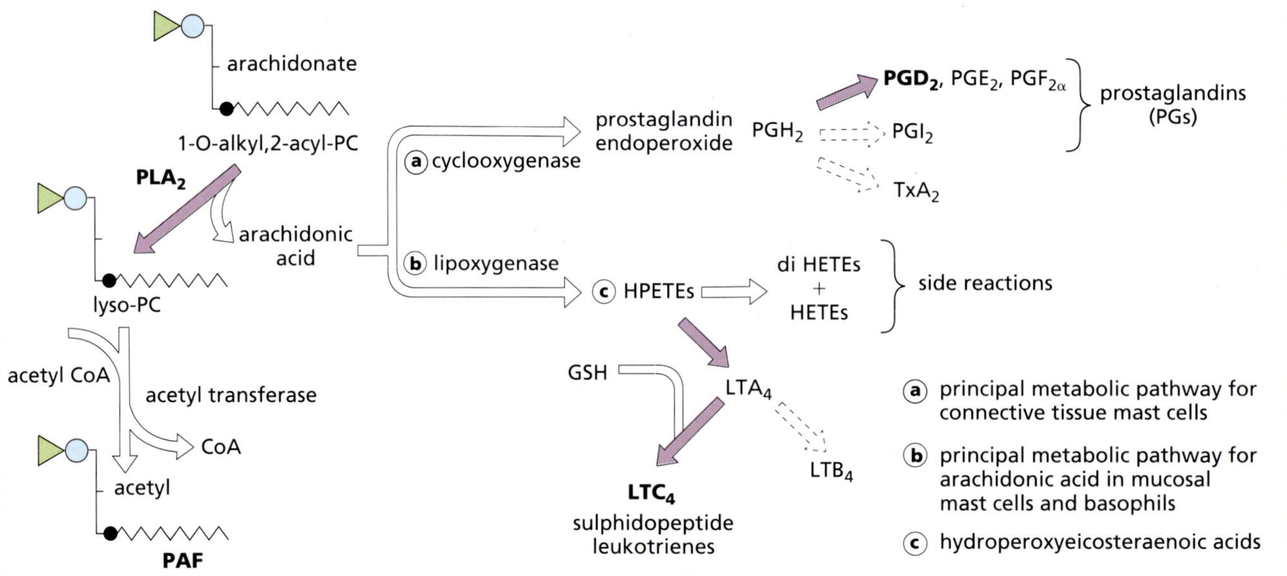

Fig. 4.9 Lipid mediators derived from PLA_2 products. Platelet activating factor (PAF) and eicosanoids (PGs, HETEs, and LTs) are the principal lipid-derived mediators produced subsequent to IgE receptor-mediated activation. PLA_2 hydrolysis of 1,alkyl-2,acyl-PC with arachidonate esterified at the second carbon generates two important products: 1,alkyl-2,lyso-PC and arachidonic acid, from which all mast cell lipid-derived mediators may be formed. 1,alkyl-2,lyso PC (lysoPAF) is acetylated at the *sn*-2 position of glycerol to generate PAF. AA may be metabolized by either the cyclooxygenase or lipoxygenase pathways.

for the biosynthesis of platelet activating factor (PAF; 1-O-alkyl,2-acetyl-PC) by PAF acetyl transferase.

Cyclic GMP

Although receptor-dependent guanylate cyclases have been demonstrated and a cyclic GMP-dependent protein kinase exists, the importance of cyclic GMP in physiological responses remains to be demonstrated in tissues other than the retina.

Phosphorylation of Regulatory Enzymes by Protein Kinases

Post-translational modification of proteins by phosphorylation is an important mechanism in the regulation of enzyme activity, and hence many cellular processes. By changing the conformation of target proteins, enzymatic or binding activity can be dramatically altered. Protein kinases fall into two main groups:

(1) those that phosphorylate serine or threonine residues on target proteins;

(2) those that phosphorylate tyrosine residues.

Cyclic AMP-dependent protein kinase (PKA)

PKA is an ubiquitous cytosolic protein which mediates most of the regulatory effects of cyclic AMP. PKA is normally inactive as the result of its physical association with an inhibitory protein – a situation that is reversed by cyclic AMP binding to the inhibitory protein, as this causes both a conformational change and the release of active PKA (Fig. 4.10).

Protein kinases C (PKC)

In contrast to PKA, activation of PKC requires two different second messengers, DAG and Ca^{2+}. Given an appropriate membrane surface containing PS, membrane-associated DAG causes PKC to translocate from the cytosol to the membrane, and to increase its affinity for Ca^{2+}, so that at permissive and physiologically relevant $[Ca^{2+}]_{cytosol}$ PKC becomes active. Different isoenzymes of PKC have variable tissue expression and respond to different regulatory molecules, including AA (Fig. 4.11). Phorbol myristate acetate (PMA or TPA) is a water-soluble plant-derived compound which mimics DAG and can artifically activate PKC. Activated PKC phosphorylates a subset of protein targets that may or may not also be substrates for PKA.

Calmodulin and calmodulin-dependent protein kinases

Changes in $[Ca^{2+}]_{cytosol}$ cause changes in the activity of a large number of enzymes. Rather than direct allosteric interactions with these enzymes, Ca^{2+} usually exerts its effects through a ubiquitous cytosolic calcium-binding protein named calmodulin. As $[Ca^{2+}]_{cytosol}$ rises, increased occupancy of high affinity Ca^{2+} binding sites on calmodulin causes a dramatic conformational change, rendering the Ca^{2+}/calmodulin complex capable of interacting with a variety of Ca^{2+}/calmodulin sensitive proteins. Among these responding proteins are two Ca^{2+}/calmodulin dependent kinases (I and II) which are able to phosphorylate a variety of target proteins at specific serine/threonine residues.

Tyrosine kinases

Unlike the family of G-protein-dependent plasma membrane receptors already discussed, another group of cell surface growth factor receptors primarily act through direct tryosine phosphorylation. These receptors consist of an extracellular ligand binding domain, a single transmembrane spanning region, and an intracellular tyrosine kinase domain. Ligand binding results in enhanced tyrosine phosphorylation not only of a set of effector proteins but also of the receptor itself. Some of the recently described oncogenes produce mutant

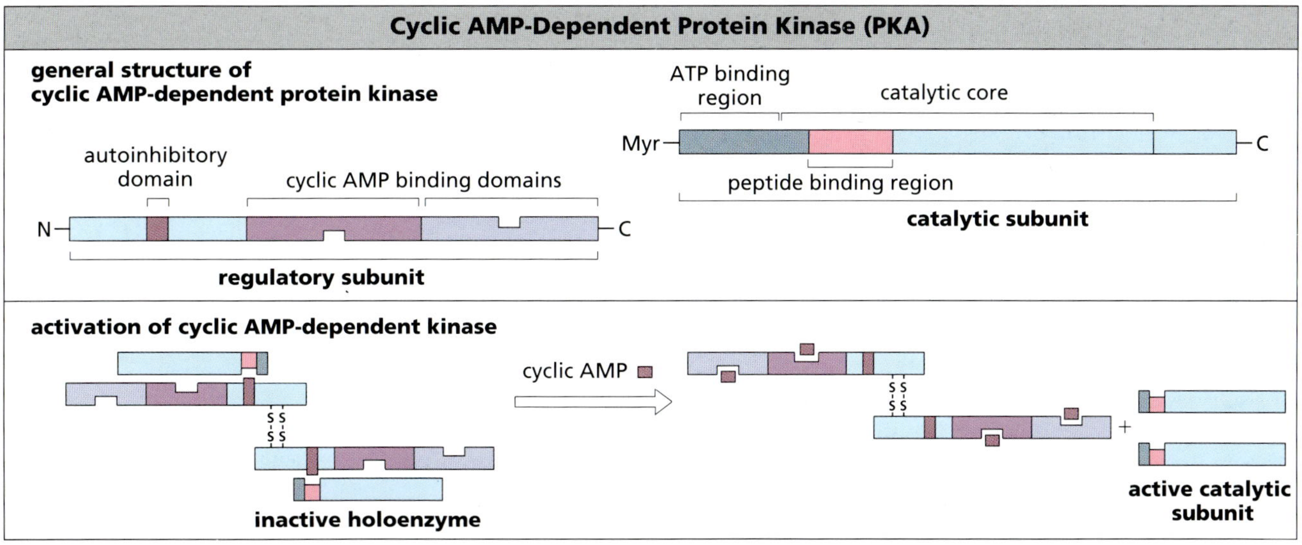

Fig. 4.10 Cyclic AMP-dependent kinase (PKA).
[above] As with many protein kinases, PKA is composed of a regulatory subunit and kinase subunit, each on different polypeptide chains. The regulatory subunit has two cyclic AMP binding domains and an autoinhibitory domain which prevents PKA activity. The catalytic peptide contains the ATP binding region and a substrate binding region.
[below] The inactive holoenzyme consists of two regulatory subunits disulfide linked near the N-terminus, and each associated with one inactive catalytic subunit. When permissive cyclic AMP levels are reached, cyclic AMP binds to sites on the regulatory subunit and the induction of a conformatinal change allows the release of active catalytic subunits of PKA.

Protein Kinase C		
Mammalian Isoenzymes		
Subspecies	**Activators**	**Tissue expression**
α	PS + DG + Ca^{2+}; AA + Ca^{2+}	universal
βI	PS + DG + Ca^{2+}	some tissues and cells
βII	PS + DG + Ca^{2+}	many tissues and cells
γ	PS + DG + Ca^{2+}; AA	brain and spinal cord
δ	PS + DG + Ca^{2+}	many tissues
ε	PS + DG + Ca^{2+}	brain
ζ	PS + DG + Ca^{2+}	many tissues

Prototypic PKC Isoenzymes

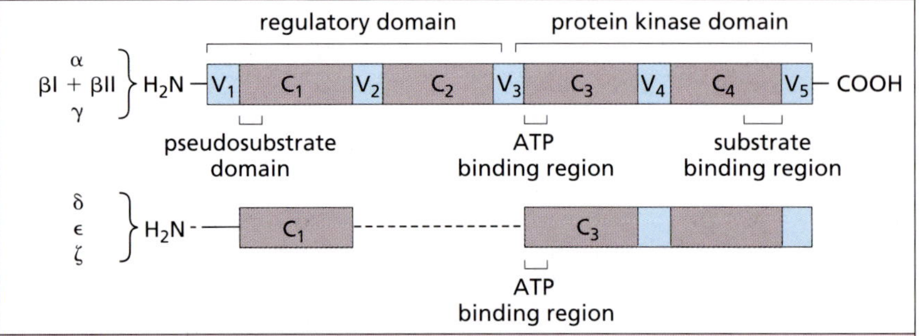

PKC Activity at a Membrane Surface

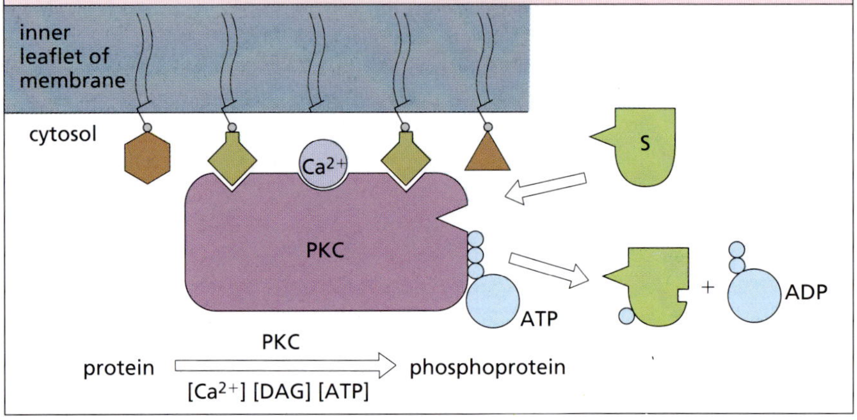

Fig. 4.11 Protein kinase C isoenzymes. [above] Mammalian cells express more than one form of PKC. Each type requires different activation conditions *in vitro* (presumably also *in vivo*) and may be expressed at different levels in the same cells. [below] Isoenzymes of PKC are derived from different genes, except for βI and βII which are alternative splice variants of the same gene. Alpha, beta and gamma are related by similar exon structure containing four constant (C) domains and five variable (V) domains. The pseudosubstrate region contained within the C1 domain is thought to downregulate PKC by mimicking substrate and blocking the substrate binding site. The ATP binding region has been localized to the amino terminal region of the C3 domain. (Data for top and centre adapted from Nishizuka Y, *JAMA* 1989; **262** (13): 1826–1833.)

growth factor receptors having constitutive tyrosine kinase activity that cause unregulated growth.

Integration of Signals

Increasing information is being acquired regarding the manner in which second messengers and their effector mechanisms interact in a complex system. The term 'cross-talk' is frequently used to refer to this type of communication between different second messenger/effector pathways. The best characterized interaction is the frequently antagonistic relationship between Ca^{2+} and processes regulated by cyclic AMP.

Since many target proteins have phosphorylation sites for both PKA and Ca^{2+}/calmodulin-dependent protein kinases, these forces can compete. Specifically, Ca^{2+}/calmodulin and/or Ca^{2+}/calmodulin-dependent kinases can alter the activity of adenylate cyclase, cyclic AMP phosphodiesterase, and PKA. Reciprocally, PKA can alter the activity of some Ca^{2+} channels.

Downregulation of Receptor Responsiveness

In order for cells to respond briskly to introduction of an extracellular agonist, but not excessively to a chronic increase in the presence of the same agonist, cells have developed a variety of mechanisms to alter the sensitivity of the system – a process known as 'desensitization' or 'adaptation'. Desensitization often involves either feedback phosphorylation of the receptor by the relevant second messenger-dependent protein kinase, or autophosphorylation by tyrosine kinase-containing receptors. Responsiveness to a ligand may be reduced simply by phosphorylation of the receptor that results in either effectively inhibiting enteraction with appropriate G-proteins or promoting their removal from the cell surface by endocytosis. Second messenger-dependent modification of G-proteins themselves may also be important in some processes of desensitization.

Signalling Events During Mast Cell Activation

In the sections that follow, knowledge regarding the specific signal transduction processes for mast cells, and/or basophils will be reviewed.

Activation through $Fc_{\epsilon}R1$ Receptors

Unique to cells of the immune system is the expression of surface Fc receptors. Rather than responding simply to receptor occupancy by a relevant ligand, it appears that for Fc receptors the state of their aggregation or immobilization is important. Aggregation of $Fc_{\epsilon}R1$ is induced when two or more associated IgE molecules bind to a multivalent antigen molecule.

Serine 'esterase' and Mast Cell Activtion

Studies in the 1960s suggested that activation of a membrane-associated enzyme with a catalytic serine in its active site was a critical early component of mast cell activation. Diisopropyl fluorophosphate (DFP), a potent irreversible inhibitor of enzymes bearing an activated (nucleophilic) serine, was found to inhibit IgE-dependent increases in cyclic AMP, Ca^{2+} influx and histamine release. Because DFP was required to be present during Ag activation and was not effective if added and washed out prior to stimulation, it seemed likely that the critical target of DFP is an enzyme that becomes activated only as the result of $Fc_{\epsilon}R1$-stimulation. Because addition of inhibitors of chymotrypsin and trypsin inhibited the same events, the activation of a membrane-associated DFP-sensitive protease was suggested. However, nucleophilic serine residues has also been demonstrated in active sites in a variety of hydrolytic enzymes outside the protease family, suggesting that the DFP-sensitive target may catalyze cleavage of substrates other than proteins. Despite these early observations, the identity of the DFP-sensitive enzyme has remained elusive.

G-Proteins in $Fc_{\epsilon}R1$-Dependent Activation

Although recent work has shown that PI hydrolysis in $Fc_{\epsilon}R1$-stimulated RBL is inhibited by pertussis toxin, there is little data in intact cells suggesting a role for classic G-proteins in regulating $Fc_{\epsilon}R1$-initiated mast cell activation. In recent studies, GTP-binding proteins were inhibited by $GDP_{\beta}s$ (introduced by reversible permeabilization), and $Fc_{\epsilon}R1$-mediated activation appeared to occur normally in both serosal and mucosal mast cells – data that seriously undermine an essential role for both signal-transducing G-proteins and low molecular weight GTP-binding proteins in $Fc_{\epsilon}R1$-mediated mast cell activation.

In contrast, a role for GTP-binding proteins in exocytosis is supported (in detergent-permeabilized mast cells) by the observation that $GTP_{\gamma}s$ introduced into mast cells caused histamine release in the presence of Ca^{2+} and ATP. Data suggest that GTP-binding proteins may play a role in signal transduction by other receptors (thrombin and fMLP) involving distinct signal transduction.

Phospholipid Methylation

Although membrane-associated methyltransferases have been suggested to play a role in signal transduction in a variety of cells, a consensus in this controversial area is developing that this mechanism is not critical to mast cell activation. Early studies in cultured human basophils and in human and mouse mast cells show that IgE-receptor cross-linking caused increased conversion of the membrane phospholipid phosphatidylethanolamine (PE) to phosphatidylcholine (PC) by the action of cellular methyltransferases. Although, methyltransferase inhibitors blocked mediator release, ability of these inhibitors to directly affect other second messenger pathways, coupled with the absence of confirmation of PE methylation, has eroded early enthusiasm regarding the importance of this signal transduction pathway.

Cyclic AMP and PKA – Uncertain Roles

Adenylate cyclase was suggested to play a role in mast cell signal transduction, in that antigen-induced $Fc_{\epsilon}R1$ stimulation caused a dramatic, rapid, and transient rise in levels of intracellular cyclic AMP in mast cells and basophils (Fig. 4.12). Interestingly, secretory agonists not using $Fc_{\epsilon}R1$ (such as 48/80) not only failed to cause an increase in cyclic AMP, but induced a modest decrease in cyclic AMP levels in serosal mast cells.

Further undermining a critical role for cyclic AMP in causing exocytosis is the observation that pharmacological agents that increased cellular cyclic AMP levels either have no effect or inhibit exocytosis, suggesting that the function of cyclic AMP is more likely to negatively regulate pro-exocytotic pathways initiated by $Fc_{\epsilon}R1$ activation.

Cytosolic Ca^{2+} – A Driving Force for Exocytosis

Studies using Ca^{2+}-sensitive fluorescent probes have shown that the $[Ca^{2+}]_{cytosol}$ increases upon $Fc_{\epsilon}R1$ stimulation. This change is likely to result in both release of Ca^{2+} from intracellular stores (regulated by IP3) and an influx of extracellular Ca^{2+} . The release of Ca^{2+} from intracellular stores seems to precede the influx of extracellular Ca^{2+}, and some observations have linked membrane depolarization with Ca^{2+} influx. However, patch clamp studies of mast cell models have failed to reveal any Ca^{2+} channels in the plasma membrane.

The increase in $[Ca^{2+}]_{cytosol}$ may have several regulatory functions including:

- activation of Ca^{2+}-dependent enzymes, including protein kinase C;
- regulation of enzymes controlled by Ca^{2+} or Ca^{2+}/calmodulin-dependent protein kinases;
- a role in membrane depolarization.

As several artificial procedures that raise intracellular Ca^{2+} (use of the calcium ionophore A23187, fusion of Ca^{2+}-containing liposomes, and direct microinjection) all cause exocytosis and new mediator synthesis, significant increases in $[Ca^{2+}]_{cytosol}$ seem to represent a sufficient activation signal. Studies have demonstrated that increased intracellular Ca^{2+} from intracellular stores is sufficient to cause suboptimal histamine release from serosal mast cells. However, in basophils, murine bone marrow-derived mast cell cultures (BMMC) and IL-3-dependent mast cell lines, $Fc_{\epsilon}R1$-mediated activation cannot occur in the absence of extracellular Ca^{2+}, implying the importance of both

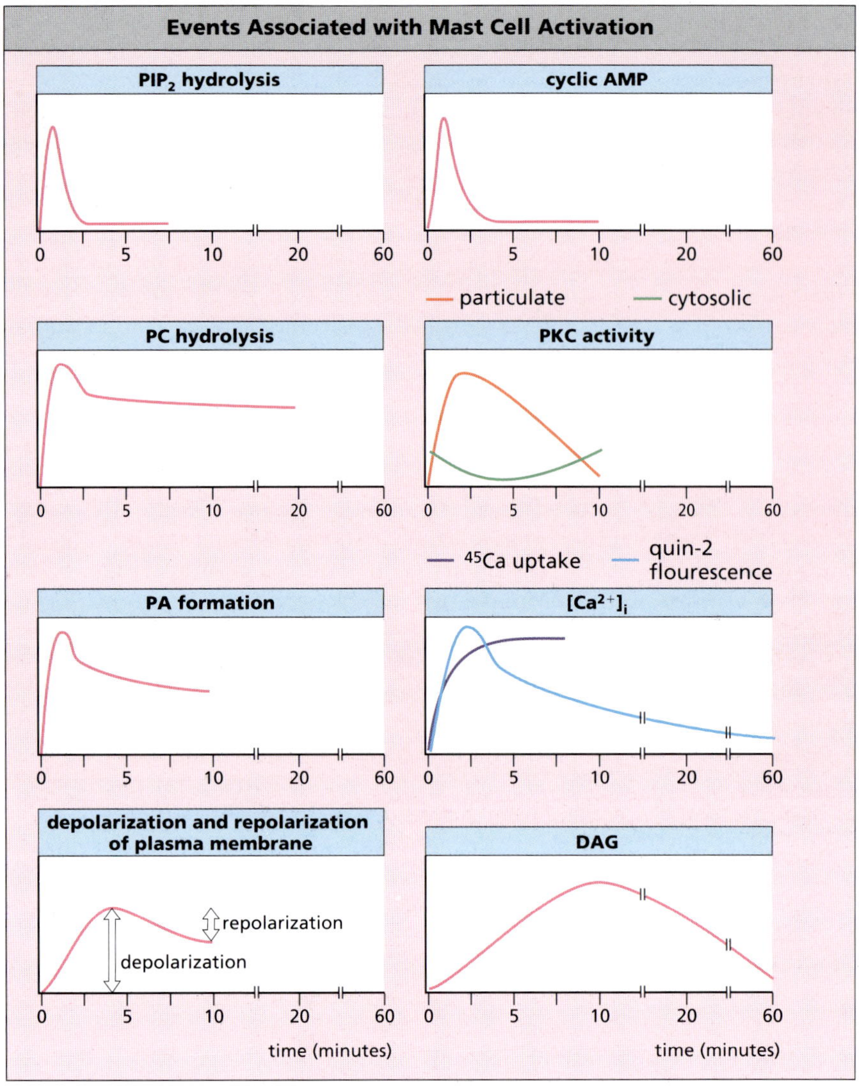

Fig. 4.12 Events associated with mast cell activation. Data from rodent mast cell models (RBL, PT-18, BMMC and rat serosal mast cells) have been integrated to provide a simplified view of their kinetic relationships. Investigators have shown that PIP_2 hydrolysis and cyclic AMP levels rise rapidly and transiently after activation. Signals that also rise rapidly but persist longer include PC hydrolysis, PA accumulation, depolarization of plasma membrane, PKC activity, $[Ca^{2+}]_{intracellular}$ and DAG. In contrast, gene activation events are considerably delayed (c-*fos* activation peaks at 30 minutes).

intracellular stores and extracellular Ca^{2+}. It has become increasingly evident that the roles of intracellular Ca^{2+} mobilization versus the influx of extracellular Ca^{2+} differ, depending on the mast cell phenotype and species.

Phosphoinositide Metabolism – An Uncertain Role

Early studies in the mast cell demonstrated that all secretory agonists initiated rapid increases in PA and PI labelling by ^{32}Pi – a reflection of the activation of the PI cycle (Fig. 4.8). These changes were coincident with the onset of exocytosis and modified in parallel by physical conditions or pharmacological agents that altered $Fc_{\epsilon}R1$-dependent exocytosis. PI hydrolysis was addressed more directly in a variety of mast cell and basophil models using cells prelabelled with $[^3H]$glycerol or $[^3H]$inositol. In serosal mast cells prelabelled with $[^3H]$glycerol, cross-linking $Fc_{\epsilon}R1$ primarily caused an increased hydrolysis of PI and PIP, and surprisingly little change in PIP_2 hydrolysis. In RBL, BMMC and basophils vigorous $Fc_{\epsilon}R1$ receptor-dependent PIP_2 hydrolysis was shown. The requirement for PI hydrolysis in mast cell exocytosis has recently been questioned since several agents that reduce PI-PLC failed to block $Fc_{\epsilon}R1$-induced histamine release. The apparent importance of Ca^{2+} in exocytosis, however, makes it difficult to dismiss PI-PLC mediated liberation of IP3 as being of little consequence.

Protein Kinase C – An Evolving Role

$Fc_{\epsilon}R1$ stimulation results in a rapid increase in both membrane-associated and total PKC activity. Inhibitors that preferentially antagonize PKC reduce $Fc_{\epsilon}R1$-dependent exocytosis. Experiments which demonstrate that activating PKC by the addition of phorbol esters cause little or no exocytosis are, however, dampening enthusiasm for a central role of PKC in regulating mast cell activation. It seems likely that PKC may be an important, but not sufficient, component of $Fc_{\epsilon}R1$-dependent mast cell activation.

Phosphatidylcholine Hydrolysis

Increasing attention has focused on metabolism of PC, since it has the potential to generate several messengers (DAG and PA) and/or requisite substrates (lyso-PAF and arachidonic acid) for the synthesis of newly formed lipid mediators, PAF and eicosanoids (Fig. 4.13). $Fc_{\epsilon}R1$ activation of mast cells prelabelled with ^{32}Pi leads to rapid and sustained increases in PC labelling, suggesting that at least some of DAG is metabolized to PC in a 'PC cycle' analogous to that of

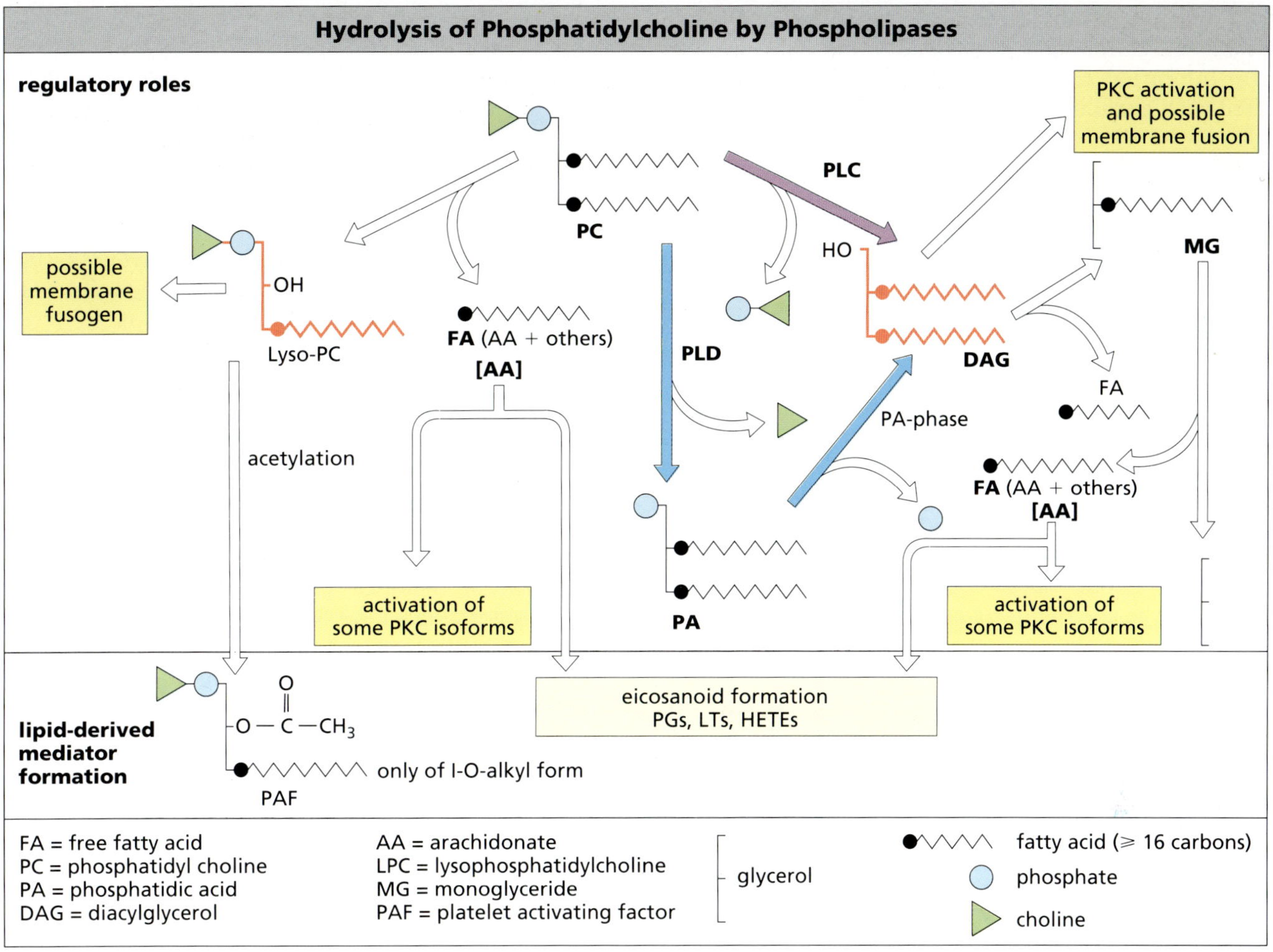

Fig. 4.13 Hydrolysis of phosphatidylcholine by phospholipases. Phosphatidylcholine (PC) can be hydrolyzed by a variety of phospholipases and subsequently metabolized to generate lipids that have important regulatory roles or can be converted to inflammatory mediators in mast cells. Preliminary studies suggest that PA, an intermediate in the PLD-initiated *indirect pathway*, may regulate a unique PA-dependent protein kinase. In certain cell models, adding PA or lyso-PA has been associated with cell activation, Ca^{2+}-induced membrane phase changes and substitution for PS for PKC binding to membranes. In recent experiments, lyso-PA, the product of PLA_2-catalyzed hydrolysis of PA and a frequent contaminant of preparations of PA, has been shown to act as a second messenger by liberating Ca^{2+} from intracellular sites. In the mast cell, $Fc_{\epsilon}R1$ stimulation results in increased accumulation of labelled lyso-PA in $^{32}P_i$ prelabelled cells. Lipid-derived mediators (eicosanoids and PAF) having important extracellular functions are also generated as a result of phospholipase activation.

PI (Fig. 4.14). Lipid fingerprinting, a technique used to examine the precursor/product relationship of lipids, has shown that most of the DAG accumulating after $Fc_{\epsilon}R1$ stimulation could not be derived from PI; instead it bears a strikingly close resemblance to PC – a finding suggesting that $Fc_{\epsilon}R1$-dependent PC hydrolysis is more important than PI hydrolysis in $Fc_{\epsilon}R1$-dependent DAG accumulation. *De novo* synthesis is unlikely to contribute significantly to the rapid rise in DAG mass and the potential contribution of the other pathways remains to be investigated.

DAG can be derived from PC by several mechanisms:

- a direct pathway involving PLC; and/or
- an indirect pathway initiated by PLD (Fig. 4.14).

Receptor-dependent activation of PLD was demonstrated in mast cells by the ethanol-dependent, PLD-mediated formation of labelled phosphatidylethanol in fatty acid prelabelled cells and a rapid rise in the mass of intracellular choline. The presence in mast cells of significant phosphatidate phosphohydrolase (PA-PHase) activity further advances the candidacy of the indirect pathway in the formation of DAG during mast cell activation. In addition, the formation of PA by PC-PLD has received increasing interest since PA may itself act as a second messenger.

Phospholipase A_2 Activation – A Role in Both Lipid Mediator Biosynthesis and Signal Transduction

The release of AA from cellular phospholipids probably principally involves activation of PLA_2 (Figs 4.9 and 4.13), although the ability of the mast cell to liberate AA from DAG has also been shown (via a two step reaction involving DAG lipase and monoglyceride lipase; Fig. 4.13). The hydrolysis of 1-O-alkyl,2-acyl-PC by PLA_2 is also of interest in that it also generates the PAF precurser 1-O-alkyl,2-lyso-PC (lyso-PAF). Connective tissue mast cells principally generate mainly PGD_2 while the mucosal mast cells synthesize predominately LTC_4 and PAF. Recent evidence suggests that PLA_2-mediated hydrolysis of phospolipids other than PC also may play a potentially important role in exocytosis. Specifically, $Fc_{\epsilon}R1$

stimulation results in the accumulation of lyso-PI and lyso-PE in addition to lyso-PC, and pharmacological inhibition of PLA_2 has been found to be associated with parallel inhibition of granule secretion.

Other Ion Channels and Membrane Potential

Rapid changes in membrane potential occur early during antigen stimulation (Fig. 4.12), and may be important in regulating exocytosis. $Fc_\epsilon R1$-dependent depolarization is dose dependent with respect to exocytosis, but not with the degree of cross-linking of receptor-bound IgE. Depolarization is abolished when both Na^+ and Ca^{2+} are absent, but can be restored by either cation alone. Replacing extracellular Na^+ with membrane-impermeable monovalent cations markedly decreases exocytosis in RBL-2H3 cells, as does amiloride (an inhibitor of Na^+ channels, Na^+/H^+ antiport and Na^+/Ca^{2+} antiport). Thus, Na^+ permeability and its contribution to the membrane potential and regulation of Ca^{2+} permeability appear important to the regulation of exocytosis.

Adenosine Facilitates Mast Cell Activation

Mast cells have surface adenosine receptors which, when stimulated, potentiate preformed mediator exocytosis from cells stimulated by $Fc_\epsilon R1$ cross-linking. Although adenosine increases cyclic AMP concentrations, the fluctuations in cyclic AMP metabolism do not correlate well with mediator release. This suggests that adenosine acts through a mechanism other than PKA. Augmented exocytosis by adenosine appears to exert at least some of its effects through a G-protein sensitive to pertussis toxin. Depleting mast cells of PKC abrogates adenosine responsiveness, suggesting that adenosine receptors and/or down-stream regulatory elements may be PKC dependent.

Role of Cytoskeletal Elements in Mast Cell Secretion

Changes in the morphology of RBL-2H3 and serosal mast cells are coincident with exocytosis, and a role for contractile proteins and F-actin depolymerization and its repolymerization have been proposed. The mechanism by which these cytoskeletal changes may effect granule mobility, granule/granule interaction, or granule/plasma membrane association is uncertain. The ability of cytoskeletal changes to take place normally in the absence of extracellular Ca^{2+} and Na^+ (which block exocytosis) suggest that these changes may be necessary, but not sufficient, for exocytosis.

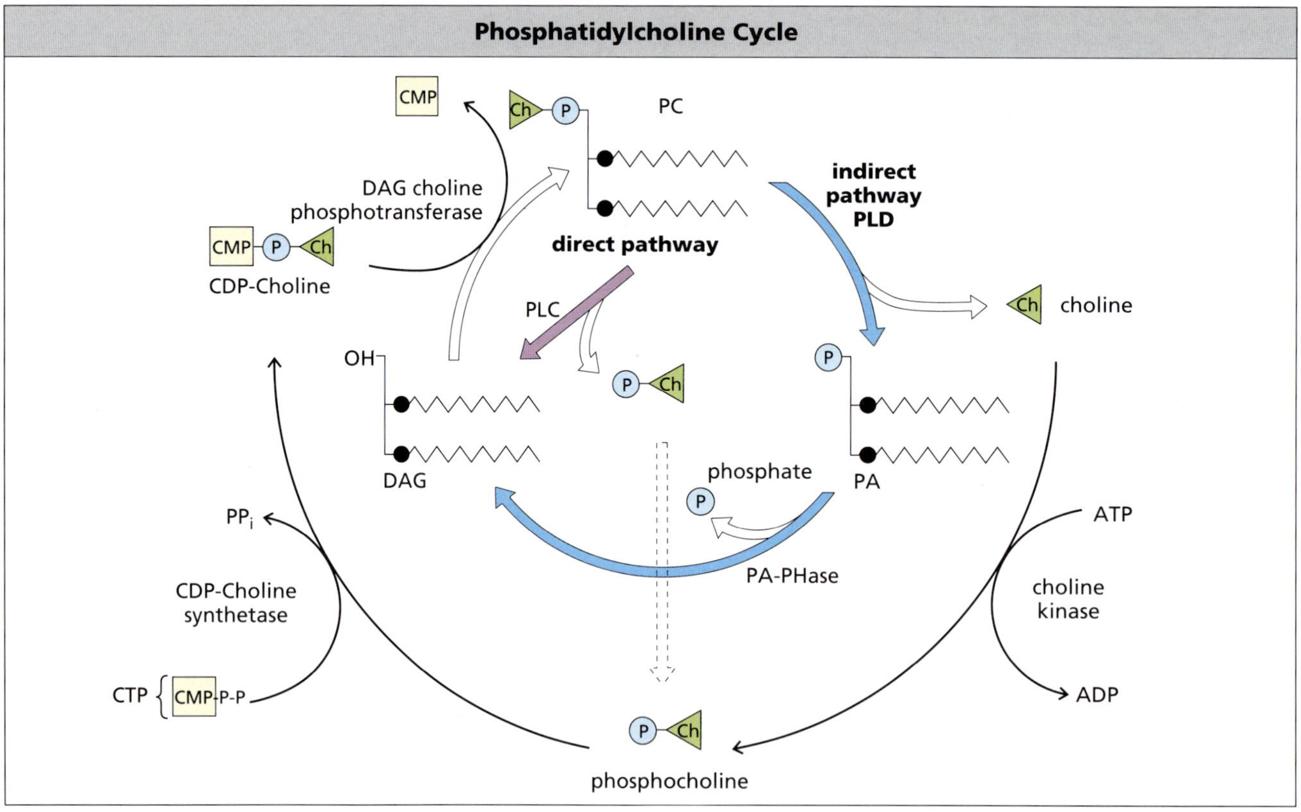

Fig. 4.14 The phosphatidylcholine cycle. IgE receptor-mediated activation of mast cells causes an increased turnover of PC. $Fc_\epsilon R1$ activation of a PC cycle is consistent with observations that have suggested a metabolic relatedness between the increased DAG mass, PC hydrolysis, and increased $^{32}P_i$ incorporation into PC. The PC cycle actually involves two interdependent cycles, one for choline and another for DAG. Evidence in mast cell and other cell models suggests that DAG may be formed from PC by either 1) a *direct pathway* in which PLC hydrolyzes PC to form DAG and phosphocholine or 2) an *indirect pathway* initiated by PLD hydrolysis of PC to form choline and PA and followed by PA is hydrolysis to DAG and phosphate by phosphatidic acid phosphohydrolase (PA-PHase). The degree to which either pathway is utilized seems to be cell model-dependent. In experiments to distinguish these two alternatives, it was shown in serosal mast cells that the levels of intracellular choline (a reflection of the PC-PLD initiated *indirect pathway)* increased dramatically as the result of $Fc_\epsilon R1$ stimulation while the levels of phosphorylcholine (a reflection of the activity of the PC-PLC-initiated *direct pathway)* actually declined. These studies suggest that the $Fc_\epsilon R1$ mediated stimulation activates primarily the *indirect pathway*. In contrast, preliminary studies in RBL cells (a mucosal cell model) suggest that a combination of the two may be utilized.

Tyrosine Kinase Activation

Recent studies demonstrate that tyrosine kinase activity is increased as the result of $Fc_\epsilon R1$ stimulation, and encourage a systematic assessment of both the role of this tyrosine phosphorylation in regulating mast cell activation, and the presence of tyrosine kinase activity associated with $Fc_\epsilon R1$.

Desensitization

Concomitant with cell activation is the initiation of an active process, termed desensitization, that counters further exocytosis. As has been shown in other cells, mast cells and basophils become transiently refractory to $Fc_\epsilon R1$ stimulation, either as the result of prior $Fc_\epsilon R1$ stimulation (associated with submaximal exocytosis) or stimulation in the absence of extracellular Ca^{2+}. Although desensitized cells cannot respond to a second IgE signal, they can still respond to some other secretory agonists. This suggests that the secretory machinery is intact, but that early receptor-induced transduction or translational mechanisms become downregulated. Unfortunately, relatively little is known about the biochemical events involved in desensitization.

Other Issues Pertinent to Mast Cell/Basophil Activation

Putative Mediators of Glucocorticoid Effects

Since glucocorticoids dramatically reduce allergic inflammation and their ability to bind to an intracellular receptor and alter transcription of a family of genes is well known, their role in IgE-receptor mediated activation of mast cells and basophils remains controversial. *In vivo* experimental models have demonstrated a reduced anaphylactic activity as the result of prior therapy with glucocorticoids, but *in vitro* studies have been less convincing.

The dependence of glucocorticoid effects on new protein synthesis in better characterized models led for the search for an anti-inflammatory protein that might mediate this effect. A series of similar proteins which bind both Ca^{2+} and phospholipid, and possessed inhibitory activity toward PLA_2 were described (lipocortin, macrocortin, lipomodulin). Although appealing, the widely held view that new lipid mediator synthesis and perhaps exocytosis in the mast cell was regulated by these proteins has been severely undermined. Specifically, lipocortin has been shown to block phospholipases *in vitro*, not as the result of enzyme inhibition, but rather because, at the high concentrations used to demonstrate inhibition, it binds available phospholipid substrate and does not allow the phospholipid access to the enzyme – a situation that could not occur *in vivo* at physiologically realistic levels of lipocortin.

Sodium Cromoglycate

Sodium cromoglycate is a widely used anti-allergic drug the principal action of which was initially thought to be the 'stabilization' of mast cells and the prevention of exocytosis. Although more recent studies demonstrate inhibitory effects of the drug on a

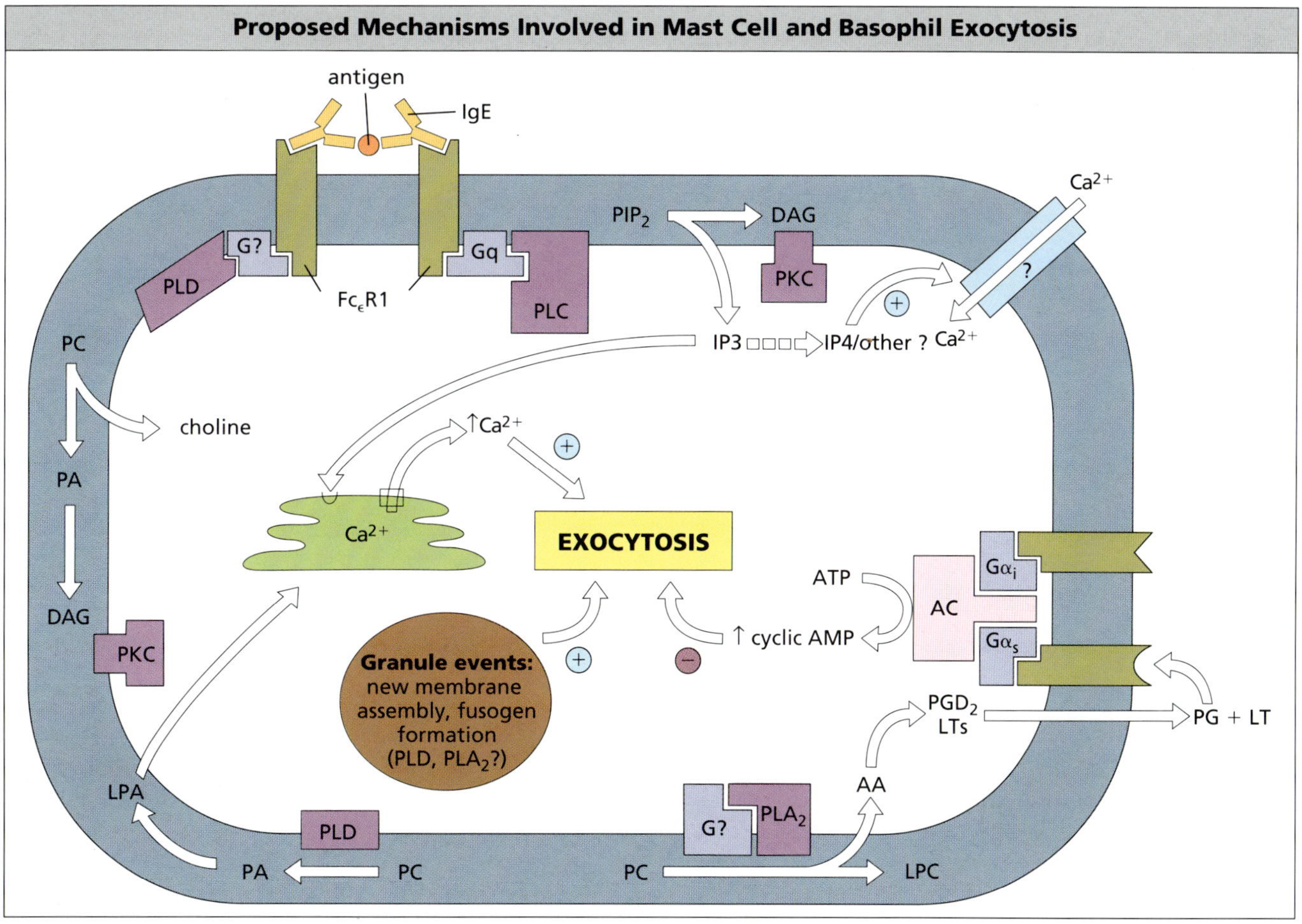

Fig. 4.15 Proposed mechanisms involved in mast cell and basophil exocytosis.

number of cells using a variety of different experimental inflammatory parameters, work by one group of investigators has associated inhibition of mast cell exocytosis to a partially characterized cromoglycate-binding protein of 60 kDa associated with the plasma membrane of RBL-2H3 cells. Although a role for this binding protein in Ca^{2+} influx has been proposed, confirmation of these data are lacking in this or any other mast cell models.

Future Directions

A synthesis of the biochemical mechanisms involved in mast cell activation is shown schematically in Fig. 4.15, but many of these mechanisms are controversial and the subject of considerable investigative attention. Challenging studies are seeking to identify both the intracellular portions of the IgE receptor that contribute to signal transduction and the membrane proteins that translate $Fc_{\epsilon}R1$ cross-linking into a biochemical signal. The role of lipid second messengers mechanisms of their genesis is rapidly envolving. Although desensitization is not well understood, characterizing its biochemical mechanism may be of considerable importance in an effort to develop pharmacological agents able to downregulate $Fc_{\epsilon}R1$ mediated activation of mast cells.

Further Reading

Freissmuth M, Casey MJ, Gilman AG. G proteins control diverse pathway of transmembrane signalling. *FASEBJ* 1989; **3**:2125–2131.

Ishizaka K, Ishizaka T. Allergy. In: Paul WE, ed. *Fundamental Immunology, Second Ed.* New York: Raven Press, 1989:867–888.

Kennerly DA. Mechanisms of 1,2-diacylglycerol formation during receptor-mediated cellular activation. *Advances in Regulation of Cell Growth* 1989;**1**:27–57.

Oliver JM, Seagrave JC, Stump RF, Pfeiffer JR, Deanin GG. (1988) Signal Transduction in RBL–2H3 Cells. In: Becker EL, ed. *Progress in Allergy.* Basel: Karger, 1988:**42**:185–245.

Waite M, ed. The Phospholipases In: *Handbook of Lipid Research*. New York: Plenum Press, 1987: **5**.

Chapter 5

Mast Cell and Basophil Functions

Introduction

Mast cells are the primary initiating cells of immediate hypersensitivity reactions. By binding IgE with high affinity and responding to allergen challenge with the rapid secretion of a wide array of mediators, mast cells can induce fast and dramatic changes in their local environment. Particular examples are the immediate bronchoconstrictor response that follows bronchial allergen challenge; rhinorrhoea and nasal blockage following nasal allergen challenge; and the weal-and-flare response following the intradermal injection of allergen into an atopic subject. An appreciation of the biology of the mast cell is therefore fundamental to the understanding of the mechanism of allergic diseases.

Mast Cell Heterogeneity

Mast cells are tissue cells which are distributed widely throughout mammalian tissues. They are present at both mucosal and serosal surfaces, in lymphoid tissues and connective tissues, and are associated with nerves, blood vessels and tumours. The tissue disposition of mast cells distinguishes them from basophils, which are essentially blood leucocytes and invade tissues only during inflammatory events.

Although mast cells share many characteristics, it has been known since the pioneering experiments of Maximov in 1906 that they do not represent an homogenous population. Extremes of mast cell heterogeneity may be illustrated by comparison of the mast cell in the bronchial or nasal mucosa with that in the skin. In the bronchial or nasal mucosa, the mast cell is situated at the interface with the external environment and is one of the first cells to interact with inhaled allergens. Evidence that this cell participates in allergic responses comes from the presence of mast cell-derived mediators in lavage fluid after allergen provocation. In contrast, the skin mast cell is located in the dermis, well away from the external environment. This cell is found in association with nerves and blood vessels and may play a role in angiogenesis. However, it may also participate in immediate allergic responses, as observed by the production of a weal that is largely histamine-mediated at the site of intradermal injection of allergen. As will be seen, the local environment of these two mast cells has helped them to develop into cells with distinct phenotypes and functions including sensitivity to non-immunological activation and modulation by drugs of their mediator secretion.

Historically, the classification of rodent mast cell subtypes has been based on phenotypical differences between cells found at connective tissue sites, particularly the skin and peritoneal cavity, and at mucosal sites, particularly the intestinal mucosa. Clearly there are large phenotypical differences between these cells, including their size, histamine content and their proteoglycan and neutral protease composition, the latter determining their staining characteristics (Fig. 5.1). Furthermore, these subtypes show differences in function which appear to parallel, in the majority of cases, their differences in phenotype.

Human mast cells are quite different from those of rodents and, consequently, extrapolation across the species can be dangerous. However, there do appear to be separate human phenotypes associated with mucosal and connective tissue sites which may be differentiated by their neutral protease content. In the intestinal mucosa, the majority of the mast cells contain only one neutral protease, tryptase, and are thus designated MC_T. In the skin, the majority of mast cells contain chymase and carboxypeptidase in addition to tryptase and are hence designated MC_{TC}. It is becoming apparent that there are major differences in the maturation processes for these two phenotypes and, moreover, that phenotype alone cannot explain many of the complexities of mast cell heterogeneity, particularly in functional characteristics. For example, mast cells recovered from the airways by bronchoalveolar lavage (BAL) are phenotypically similar to those dispersed from lung tissue, but are smaller, contain less histamine, and are more sensitive to IgE-dependent stimuli and to modulation of histamine release by sodium cromoglycate. To take a second example, skin mast cells secrete histamine in response to substance P, while those of the intestinal submucosa do not, although both are predominantly of the MC_{TC} phenotype. These examples suggest that the environment is likely to superimpose functional differences on local mast cells, regardless of their major phenotype.

Development of Mast Cells

Studies in mice have suggested that mast cell precursors originate in the bone marrow and are carried by

Comparison of Rat Mast Cell Sub-Types		
	Mast cell source	
	peritoneal cavity	intestinal mucosa
alternative names	connective tissue mast cell (CTMC) typical mast cell	mucosal mast cell (MMC) atypical mast cell
size	10–20 μm	5–10 μm
formaldehyde fixation	resistant	sensitive
staining	safranin O	alcian blue
T-cell dependence in development	no	yes
protease content	chymase (RMCP I)	chymase (RMCP II)
proteoglycans m.w.	heparin 750–1000 kDa	chondroitin sulphate di-B 100–150 kDa
histamine 5-hydroxytryptamine	10–20 pg/cell 1–2 pg/cell	~1 pg/cell <0.5 pg/cell
prostaglandin D_2 leukotriene C_4	+ –	+ ++
activated by IgE-dependent compound 48/80 substance P	 yes yes yes	 yes no no
inhibited by sodium cromoglycate	yes	no

Fig. 5.1 Comparison of rat mast cell sub-types.

the blood to their final tissue of deposition, where they mature into recognizable mast cells under the influences of local cytokines. Rodent studies suggest that division and commitment of progenitor cells in the bone marrow is stimulated by the presence of IL-4 and IgE complexes. The role of stem cell factor (SCF) from stromal cells in this stage of mast cell precursor proliferation is not yet established.

Elegant studies performed by Kitamura and colleagues in Japan have demonstrated the obligate requirement for SCF and its receptor, the so-called c-kit proto-oncogene ligand (Fig. 5.2). While such experiments indicate the basic necessities for mast cell development in the tissues, they do not explain the heterogeneous nature of mast cells at different tissue sites. Clues to this come from parasitology, where increased T-lymphocyte numbers and mast cell proliferation are observed in the intestinal mucosa following nematode infestation. These mast cells have the morphological and immunocytochemical characteristics of rodent mucosal mast cells. Tissue culture experiments support the view that T-lymphocyte-derived

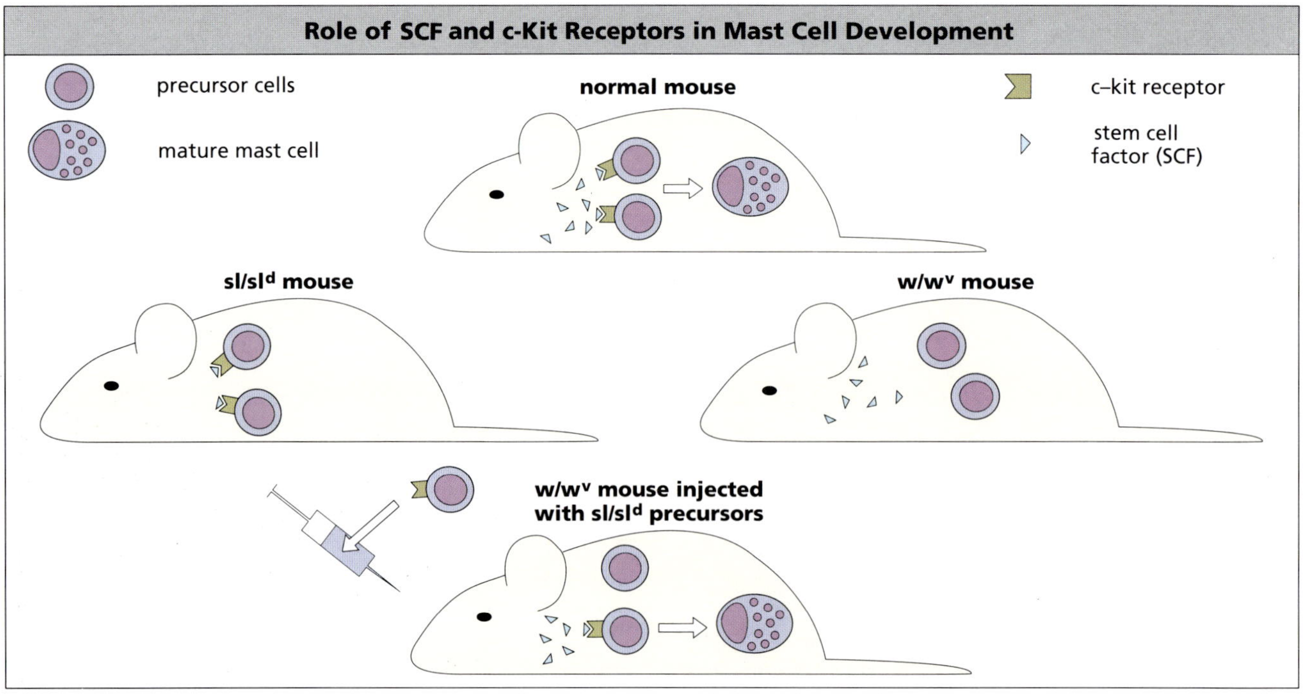

Fig. 5.2 The role of SCF and c-kit receptors in mast cell development. In normal mice, stem cell factor (SCF) produced by stromal cells interacts with c-kit receptors on progenitor cells, and stimulates them to grow into mature mast cells. Sl/sl^d mice are deficient in SCF and w/w^v mice precursors do not bear c-kit receptors. Neither mouse has mature mast cells. Injection of sl/sl^d precursors into w/w^v mice leads to mast cell maturation.

cytokines are responsible for this directed maturation. One is the glycoprotein IL-3, which promotes the proliferation and maturation of murine mast cell progenitor cells. The other is IL-4, a lymphokine which cannot support mast cell proliferation when used in isolation but augments the effects of IL-3 and may be involved in maturation of mast cells of the mucosal phenotype.

In rodent studies, when immature IL-3-dependent bone marrow derived mast cells, which have the characteristics of mucosal mast cells, are co-cultured with 3T3 fibroblasts, they change their phenotype into that of connective tissue mast cells. More recently, SCF has been shown to provoke the same phenotype shift in immobilized immature murine mast cells. Interestingly, the continued presence of IL-3 prevents the switch, indicating the dominance of the mucosal mast cell pathway in uncommitted mast cell precursors. While these experiments may suggest that mast cells have the ability to switch phenotypes readily, the weight of evidence would suggest that this may occur only with uncommitted progenitors as used in these experiments. The presence of committed murine mast cell precursor cells has been demonstrated by their separation through density gradient centrifugation and subsequent culture of the precursor subsets. These data allow us to assemble a flow chart for mast cell development (Fig. 5.3).

Attempts to culture human mast cells using the same methods as used for rodent cells have thus far been disappointing. Prolonged culture of bone marrow or cord blood cells in the presence of IL-3 and IL-4 has led to the production of basophils as the predominant metachromatic cell. It should be pointed out at this stage that basophils stain with myelocytic markers expressed by most granulocytes, while mast cells share membrane surface antigens with monocytes and macrophages, indicating that mast cells and basophils do not come from the same progenitor cells (see Fig. 5.3).

Evidence that the human MC_T are dependent on T-cell products for their development comes from two types of *in vivo* investigation. Firstly, there is a predominance of MC_T in areas of inflammation in which there is heavy T-cell infiltration. Such observations have been made in the joints, the skin and the eye. Secondly, in cases of AIDS or combined immunodeficiency syndrome where T-lymphocyte function is severely compromised, gastrointestinal biopsies have shown an almost complete absence of MC_T. In these subjects, MC_{TC} numbers were normal, making it unlikely that MC_{TC} are derived from MC_T or that switching of mature phenotypes occurs. Experiments in which mast cells cultured from human cord blood were over 80 per cent MC_{TC}, irrespective of the presence of IL-3 in the culture medium, suggest that a committed precursor exists, at least for MC_{TC}.

From these studies, it appears that the primary commitment of a precursor is to a phenotype which may be characterized by its profile of neutral protease production. As a consequence, the more subtle functional differences between mast cells of an apparently identical phenotype seem to result from the influence of the local environment during maturation.

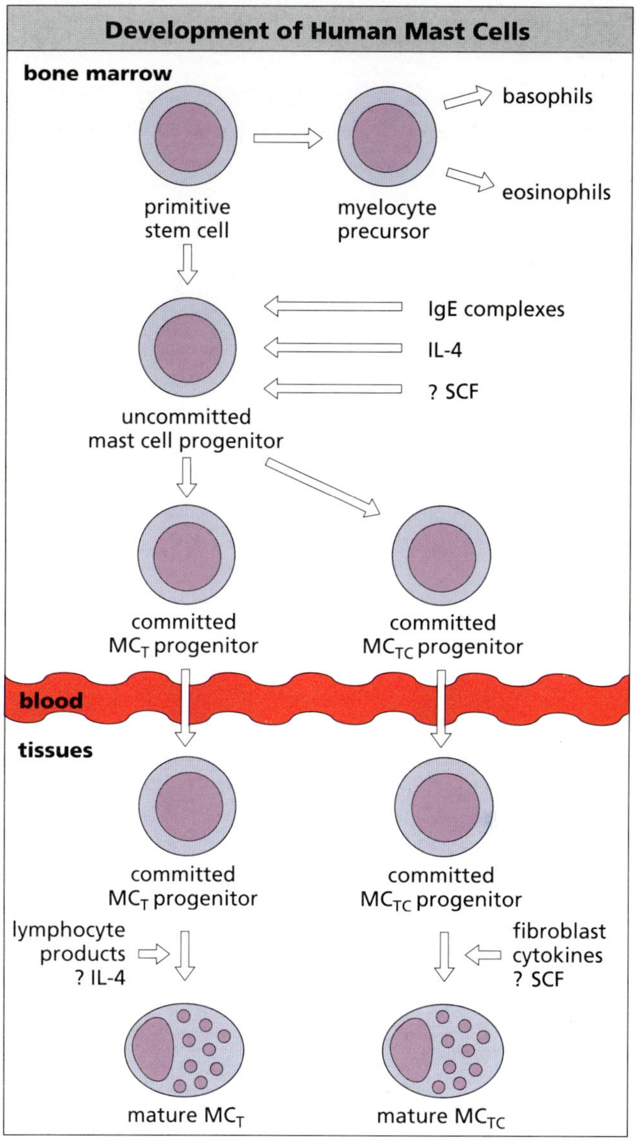

Fig. 5.3 Development of human mast cells. Stem cell division and development into progenitors with various degrees of commitment takes place in the bone marrow. Committed precursors are released into the blood and migrate into the tissues where they develop into mature mast cells, determined by the presence of cytokines.

Histological Appearance

The histological appearance of mast cells and basophils has fascinated scientists ever since the innovative experiments of Paul Ehrlich in the 1870s, which showed them to stain metachromatically with analine dyes. Indeed dyes such as toluidine blue are used routinely today to visualize mast cells and basophils (Fig. 5.4). This histochemical reaction, in which the basic dye interacts with the acidic proteoglycans of the mast cell or basophil, has several drawbacks. Firstly, it does not distinguish between mast cells and basophils, differentiation of which relies on other morphological characteristics. Secondly, staining conditions have to be carefully controlled and even then true metachromasia may be difficult to interpret, leading to inaccurate estimation of mast cell numbers. Finally, fixation with formaldehyde may prevent some mast cells from being

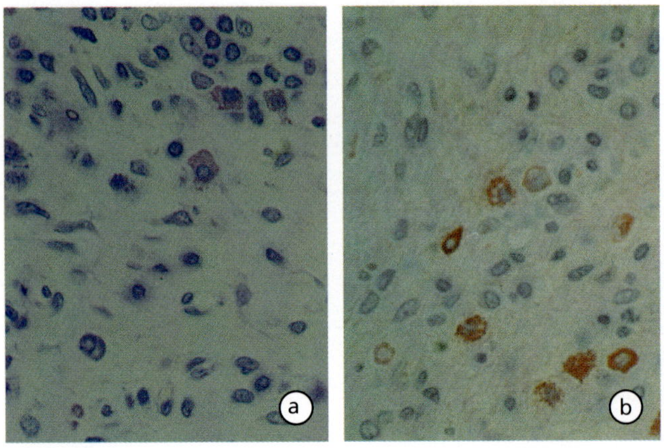

Fig. 5.4 Mast cells in human bronchial biopsy stained (a) with acidic toluidine blue – note the reddish metachromasia of the mast cell granules – and (b) with anti-mast cell tryptase (AAI monoclonal antibody) (With acknowledgements to S Wilson and PH Howarth.)

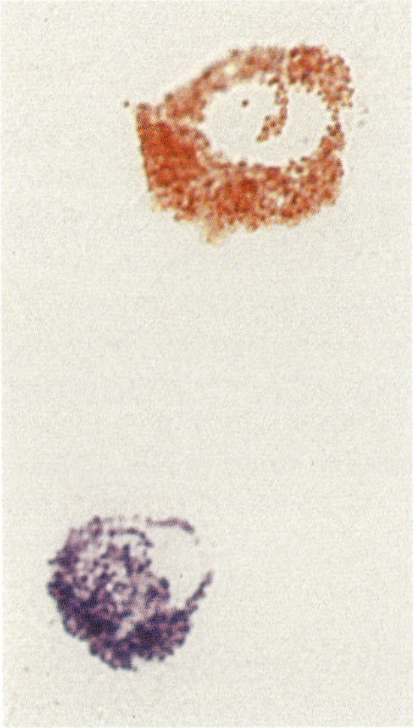

Fig. 5.5 Immunocytochemical identification of human MC_T and MC_{TC}. A cytospin preparation of human mast cells was incubated with anti-chymase antibody and the MC_{TC} stained brown by immunoperoxidase. The subsequent addition of anti-tryptase antibody followed by the development of immunoalkaline phosphatase stains the MC_T blue. The anti-tryptase antibody does not bind to the tryptase of the MC_{TC} because of interference by the primary peroxidase stain. (Reproduced with permission from Drs A-M Irani and LB Schwartz.)

stained. Today mast cells are best visualized for light microscopy by the use of immunocytochemistry, using antibodies to either the granular neutral protease, tryptase, which is present in all mast cells (see Fig. 5.4), or the c-kit receptor on the mast cell surface.

While sensitivity to formaldehyde fixation may be a problem when trying to estimate total mast cell numbers in a tissue, it has been used as an indication of mast cell heterogeneity in rodents (see Fig. 5.1). The granular proteoglycan of rat connective tissue mast cells is comprised mainly of the highly charged heparin, whose affinity for alcian blue dye is unaffected by formaldehyde fixation. In contrast, the condroitin di-B proteoglycan of the mucosal mast cell is less highly charged and its ability to stain with alcian blue is blocked by formaldehyde. Thus, comparisons of numbers of alcian blue positive cells observed after formaldehyde fixation with those observed after fixation in Carnoy's fixative (a milder chloroform-based fixative) have been used to assess the relative proportions of the two mast cell subpopulations in a tissue. Attempts have been made to use these techniques to distinguish human mast cell subpopulations. While some differences in staining have been reported, the finding that all mast cells contain at least 65 per cent heparin suggests that any differences in staining characteristics would be small and influenced by the state of solubilization of the granule matrix.

Immunocytochemistry is a far more discerning way to distinguish mast cell phenotypes. Monoclonal antibodies to rat mast cell chymases allow the ready separation of connective tissue mast cells, which contain rat mast cell protease I (RMCP I), from mucosal mast cells, which contain RMCP II. Human mast cell phenotypes may be separated by use of monoclonal antibodies to human mast cell tryptase and either chymase or carboxypeptidase. Using adjacent sections, the anti-tryptase antibody will stain both MC_T and MC_{TC} while the chymase or carboxypeptidase antibody will stain only MC_{TC}. Alternatively a double-staining technique developed by Schwartz may be used (Fig. 5.5). Basophils do not stain using these techniques as they contain only minute amounts of tryptase, less than 1 per cent of that contained in an MC_T, and are devoid of chymase. The use of protease immunocytochemistry allows a study of distribution throughout different tissues of the major human mast cell phenotypes (Fig. 5.6). Two observations may readily be made from this figure. Firstly, MC_T predominate at mucosal surfaces, while MC_{TC} predominate in connective tissues, and, secondly, a mixture of MC_T and MC_{TC} is found in all tissues. Thus, it is likely that different microenvironmental conditions within a tissue will determine the mast cell phenotype at the local level, either by influencing the deposition of precursors or mast cell maturation. This hypothesis is strengthened by the observations that disease processes may influence the proliferation of a particular mast cell phenotype. For example, increased numbers of MC_T have been found in the nasal mucosa of seasonal rhinitic patients in season, in acutely inflamed lesions of atopic dermatitis and in the conjunctiva in vernal conjunctivitis. Conversely increased MC_{TC}

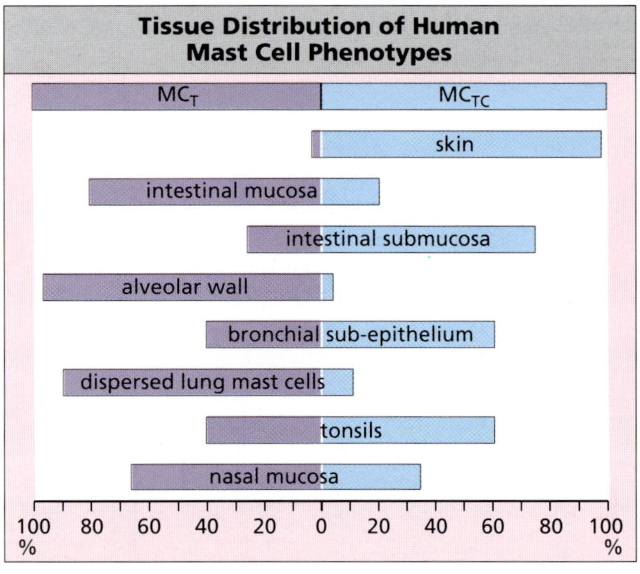

Fig. 5.6 Tissue distribution of human mast cell phenotypes. (Based on data from normal tissue studies by Drs A-M Irani and LB Schwartz.)

numbers are found in the skin in systemic mastocytosis and in the lung associated with fibrotic disease.

Human mast cells and basophils may also be distinguished by transmission electron microscopy. Fig. 5.7 shows a typical human basophil which is characterized by a multilobed nucleus and by the presence of relatively few granules which are larger and often more electron-dense than those of mast cells. Mast cells, by contrast, are larger and contain a monolobed nucleus which is often eccentric. The cytoplasm is packed with granules which appear more electron-dense in MC_{TC} than in MC_T (see Fig. 5.7). In their natural tissue environment, mast cells have a variable shape which has been described as polyhedral, fusiform, ovoid or even rectangular. When isolated for detailed examination, they are rounded and usually measure 6–13 μm in diameter. Detailed tomography suggests that the mean diameter of the human skin mast cell (MC_{TC}) is approximately 10 μm whereas that of the lung mast cell (MC_T) is approximately 9 μm. Thus the great size diversity of the two rodent mast cell subtypes (see Fig. 5.1) does not appear to extend to man. Mast cells recovered by BAL are smaller and less granular, which suggests a partially degranulated cell.

Detailed ultrastructural examination of the secretory granules show them to contain the distinct crystalline structures which characterize the human mast cell (Fig. 5.8). Electron microscopic studies of human lung mast cells, which are likely to be the MC_T phenotype, reveal three types of crystalline structure, scrolls, gratings and lattices. Estimates of the basic periodicity of the crystalline structures have been put at 6.0–7.5 nm, which suggests a common basic unit, probably the heparin-tryptase complex.

Similar studies in human skin mast cells, presumably of the MC_{TC} phenotype, have shown them to be more electron dense. The basic crystalline structures are still seen, indicative of the tryptase content of these cells, but they are overlaid with amorphous material, which suggests that chymase and carboxypeptidase are not crystallized with heparin in the same way as tryptase.

Mast Cell Mediators

The mast cell has the capacity to generate a wide variety of preformed and newly generated inflammatory mediators which are capable of inducing both immediate and long-term effects on their target organs. For practical purposes, the discussion of mast cell mediators has been divided into three sections, primary effector mediators, inducers of chronic inflammation, and proteoglycans and enzymes.

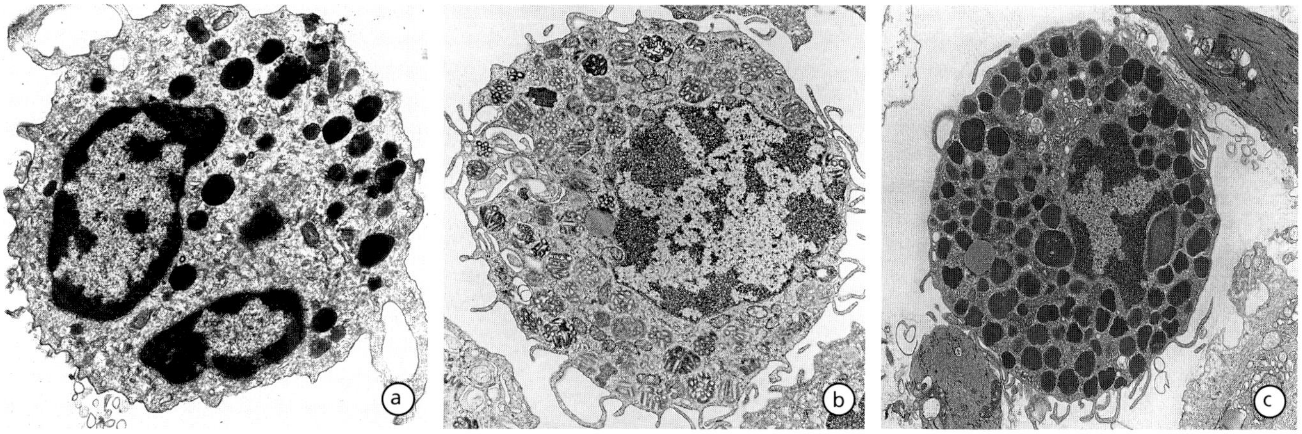

Fig. 5.7 EM of (a) human circulating basophil, (b) human lung mast cell and (c) human skin mast cell.

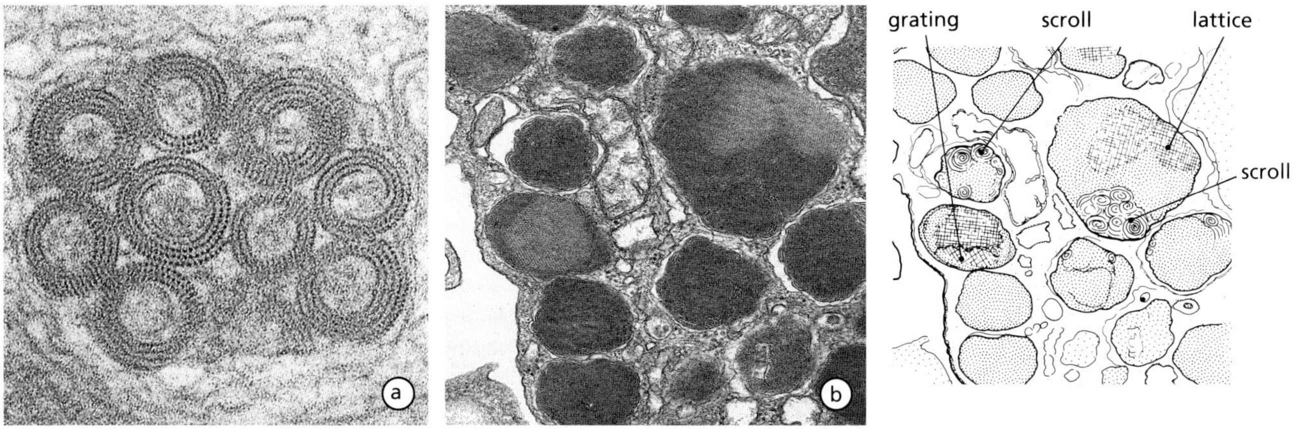

Fig. 5.8 Crystalline structures of human mast cell granules (a) Scrolls seen in a human lung mast cell (MC_T), (b) scrolls, gratings and lattices seen in a human skin mast cell (MC_{TC}). Note increased density and amorphous material content in the skin mast cell.

Primary Effector Mediators

The term primary effector mediators has been used to group those mast cell-derived, pharmacologically active substances which are involved in the production of the symptoms of immediate hypersensitivity or allergic reactions. These include histamine, prostaglandin D_2 and leukotrienes.

5-Hydroxytryptamine (serotonin) is found in many rodent mast cells, particularly connective tissue mast cells. It is not synthesized by the cells but is taken up from extracellular sources by an active uptake process in the cell membrane similar to that found in the human platelet. Human mast cells do not appear to have this uptake process and hence contain no 5-hydroxytryptamine.

Histamine

Histamine is a primary amine synthesized from histidine in the Golgi apparatus, from where it is transported to the granule for storage in ionic association with the acidic residues of the glycosaminoglycans (GAG) side chains of heparin. The histamine content of mast cells dispersed from lung and skin is similar at 2–5 pg/cell while that of the smaller mast cell recovered by BAL is around 1 pg/cell. Taking into consideration the mean mast cell density of the lung and skin, approximately 5×10^3 mast cells/mm^3, the enormous histamine storage capacity of these tissues of 10–12 μg/g is apparent.

Following mast cell activation, the solubilization of the granular contents and the breakdown of the granules and cytoplasmic membranes lead to the rapid dissociation of histamine from the granule matrix by exchange with sodium ions in the extracellular environment. Extracellular histamine has a wide variety of biological effects which are mediated through its interaction with specific H_1-, H_2- or H_3-receptors (see Chapter 15, Fig. 15.7). In asthma, histamine is implicated in bronchoconstriction, vasodilatation, oedema caused by leakage of plasma proteins from post-capillary venules, stimulation of bronchoconstrictor reflexes and mucus secretion. In rhinitis, histamine is responsible largely for the rhinorrhoea but plays a smaller role in nasal blockage. In the skin, the ability of histamine to induce oedema, vasodilatation and axon reflexes provides it with a pivotal role in the weal-and-flare response and implicate it strongly in urticaria.

In the extracellular environment and in the circulation, histamine has a half-life of less than one minute because of its rapid metabolism to inactive products by histamine-N-methyl histamine (70 per cent) and diamine oxidase, alternatively named histaminase (30 per cent). Normal levels of circulating histamine are 0.05–0.2 ng/ml which suggests a continuous low level of release of histamine into the circulation. When levels reach around 1 ng/ml, the typical systemic effects of histamine, namely flushing, headache and hypotension, are observed. Although a good marker of systemic anaphylaxis, the measurement of circulating histamine as a quantitative indicator of a local allergic response, e.g. asthma provocation, is unreliable because of its rapid systemic metabolism.

Prostaglandins

Immunological activation of mast cells results not only in degranulation but also in the liberation of arachidonic acid from phospholipids in the cell membrane, as described in Chapter 4. Further metabolism of this 20-carbon fatty acid may proceed along either of two independent pathways, the cyclo-oxygenase pathway towards prostaglandins and the lipoxygenase pathway towards leukotrienes.

The enzymes which comprise the cyclo-oxygenase complex are a ubiquitous group of membrane-associated enzymes which have the capacity to initiate the oxidation of arachidonate into the hydroperoxy derivative, PGG_2, which is then reduced to the hydroxy derivative PGH_2. The route of further metabolism of these unstable intermediates to stable prostanoids is cell specific. In the mast cell, the most abundant, if not the only, prostanoid formed is prostaglandin D_2 (PGD_2). Maximal generation of PGD_2 following immunological activation of isolated human mast cells is 100–150 p/mol/10^6 cells, some thirty to forty times less than the amount of histamine released.

Once released into the extracellular environment, PGD_2 is rapidly metabolized by 11-ketoreductase to a product similar to $PGF_{2\alpha}$, with the exception that the hydroxyl groups of the cyclopentane ring are in an α, β configuration rather than in a coplanar α-geometry. This compound, 9α, 11β-PGF_2, has biological activity similar to that of PGD_2 and is only slowly metabolized by reduction to 13,14-dihydro-15-keto-9α,11β-PGF_2. Because of its extended life, measurement of 9α, 11β-PGF_2 in the circulation represents a far more reliable determinant of mast cell degranulation than does measurement of the parent, PGD_2.

In systems tested so far, the biological activities of PGD_2 and 9α,11β-PGF_2 are essentially similar. In the lung, they act as bronchoconstrictor agents with a potency some thirty times greater than that of histamine. Most of the activity is due to a direct effect on bronchial smooth muscle, while a smaller amount is reflex-mediated. Interestingly, the direct effects on bronchial smooth muscle induced by $PGD_{2\alpha}$, 9α, 11β-PGF_2, PGF and thromboxane A_2 (TXA_2) all appear to be mediated through the same receptor, termed the TP_1-receptor on account of its affinity for TXA_2. Finally, it has been suggested that PGD_2 contributes to nasal blockage in rhinitis, while in the skin it has vasodilator properties.

Leukotrienes

The second arm of the arachidonate metabolism pathway is the so-called lipoxygenase pathway which has the capacity to generate a wide variety of leukotriene and hydroxyeicosatetraenoate (HETE) products. Despite this potential diversity, individual cell products are limited and may even be stimulus-specific. In the mast cell, the only lipoxygenase product identified is LTC_4. This sulphidopeptide leukotriene is synthesized by the action of 5-lipoxygenase on arachidonic acid, followed by conjugation of the LTA_4 intermediate with glutathione under the influence of LTC-synthase, a unique glutathione-S-transferase enzyme. Activated human mast cells produce 6–20 pmol LTC/10^6 cells, some 300–800 times less than the amount of histamine generated under similar conditions. Extracellular enzyme –mediated elimination of glutamate and glycine leads to the formation of LTD_4 and LTE_4 respectively. Together, LTC_4, LTD_4 and LTE_4 comprise the complex previously known as slow-reacting substance of anaphylaxis (SRS-A), so named because of its ability to cause a slow contraction of guinea pig small intestine.

Leukotrienes C_4 and D_4 are rapidly metabolized by a variety of pathways to either LTE_4 or inactive metabolites. Together with their renowned ability to adhere non-specifically to both biological surfaces and laboratory plasticware, this makes them notoriously difficult to assay in biological fluids after *in vivo* generation. However, LTE_4 may have an extended biological half-life and its concentration in the urine has been used recently as an approximate measure of its generation during allergic reactions.

Biologically, LTC_4 and LTD_4 are highly potent bronchoconstrictor agents which apparently act at different receptors on the surface of the bronchial smooth muscle cell. Leukotrienes provoke increased permeability of post-capillary venules, which is demonstrable as a prolonged weal response to intradermal injection. Sulphidopeptide leukotrienes are also potent vasoconstrictors in both the pulmonary and coronary vascular beds, the latter being of potential importance in systemic anaphylaxis.

Platelet activating factor (PAF)
A further lipid-derived mediator, PAF, may play a role in the acquisition of bronchial hyperresponsiveness. The biology of PAF is described in Chapter 8. Mast cell ability to synthesize PAF has been known for some time, and recent experiments suggest that they may release it extracellularly. Thus PAF may eventually be added to the ever-growing list of mast cell-derived mediators.

Role of primary mediators in acute allergic responses
The functional participation of mast cell mediators during an allergic or pseudo-allergic response will be determined by two factors:

- the array and relative concentrations of the mediators released from the mast cell;
- the relative sensitivity of the target tissues to each mediator.

With the knowledge that mast cells release histamine, PGD_2 and LTC_4 in approximate molar ratios of 1000:25:2 during allergic stimulation, it is possible to predict responses (Fig. 5.9). As histamine is more effective as an inducer of vascular leakage than PGD_2 or LTC_4, conditions in which this response is dominant are sensitive to antihistamine therapy. Examples are allergen-induced skin wealing and rhinorrhoea. In contrast, the effectiveness of histamine, PGD_2 and LTC_4 in causing bronchoconstriction are approximately the inverse of the amounts released. As a consequence all will play a role in an immediate bronchoconstrictor response to allergen provocation.

Inducers of Chronic Inflammation
Mast cell activation *in vivo* has long been associated with the influx into the microenvironment of inflammatory cells, initially neutrophils then eosinophils. Furthermore, allergic reactions stimulate the further production of allergen-specific IgE from B-lymphocytes. However, in such reactions *in vivo*, many cells are activated, either primarily or secondarily, and so the provenance of the pro-inflammatory factors is difficult to define.

Of the mediators discussed so far, the sulphidopeptide leukotrienes increase adherence of leucocytes to vasculature endothelium, while PAF is a potent chemoattractant for both neutrophils and eosinophils. Moreover, a number of peptides, varying from tetramers to oligopeptides, have been proposed as mast cell-derived neutrophil and eosinophil chemoattractants. However, the only two to have been structurally characterized, the eosinophil chemotactic tetrapeptides Val-Gly-Ser-Gln and Ala-Gly-Ser-Gln, are likely to be merely degradation products of larger molecules.

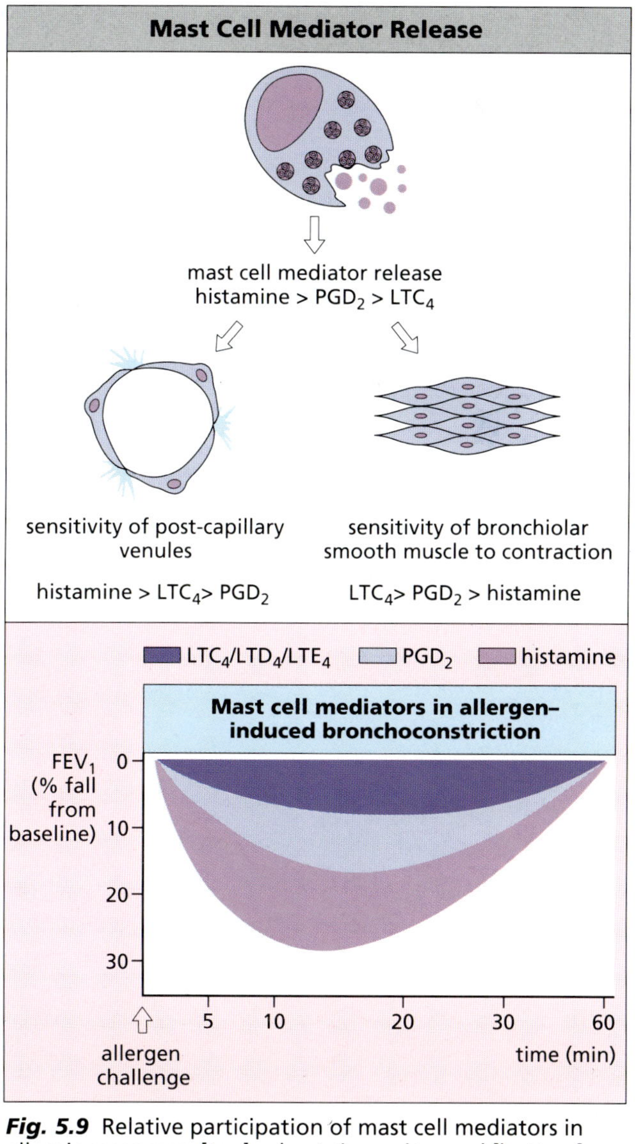

Fig. 5.9 Relative participation of mast cell mediators in allergic responses: [top] role at tissue sites and [bottom] participation of histamine, PGD_2 and leukotrienes in an early asthmatic response provoked by allergen.

Of possible greater significance is the localization of the cytokines IL-3, IL-4, IL-5, IL-6 and TNF_{α} to mast cells. As described in Chapter 3, this group of cytokines, previously associated only with TH_2 lymphocytes, upregulates allergic inflammation. In particular, they induce the switch of B-cell immunoglobulin synthesis to IgE (IL-4), support basophil and mast cell differentiation and development (IL-3 and IL-4), increase endothelial cell VCAM expression (IL-4) and stimulate eosinophil proliferation, migration and activation (IL-5).

Most mast cell studies have been performed by probing cytosolic mRNA of mouse cell lines and rat mast cells for cytokine message. However, cytokine studies are now being extended into human mast cells with evidence of TNF_{α} production by skin mast cell coming from mRNA probing and cell proliferation assays for product. More recently immunocytochemical staining has localized preformed IL-4, IL-5, IL-6 and TNF_{α} to human lung, skin and nasal mast cells (Fig. 5.10). The IgE-dependent generation of these cytokines to provide a rapid and localized trigger to T-cell activation and eosinophil migration presents an attractive hypothesis to explain the initiation of allergic inflammation.

Proteoglycans and Enzymes

Proteoglycans

Proteoglycans comprise the major structural unit of the mast cell granule. They are large molecules which contain a long protein core of repeating serine and glycine units, to which highly sulphated glycosaminoglycan (GAG) side chains are attached by xylose-galactose-galactose-glucuronic acid links. These links are unique to proteoglycans. It is the nature and degree of sulphation of the GAG side chains which determine the molecular species of proteoglycans, i.e. heparin or chondroitin, and the length of the protein core which determines the molecular weight. Other mast cell mediators are packaged in an inactive but readily released form in ionic combination with the GAGs: histamine is found in association with the carboxylic acid residues of glucuronic and iduronic acids while tryptase, and possibly other proteases, associate largely with the highly sulphate glycosamines (Fig. 5.11). The crystalline appearance of human mast cell granules suggests that there may be up to three consistent types of protein–proteoglycans association, which correlate with the scroll, lattice and grating patterns seen under the electron microscope.

In rat connective tissue mast cells, the major proteoglycan is a 750 kDa heparin, which equates to up to 140 repeating GAG units. Rat mucosal mast cells contain the less highly sulphated chondroitin-di-B. These differences account for the variety in patterns of metachromatic staining described earlier. Proteoglycans from mast cells from both human lung and skin appear to comprise approximately 65 per cent heparin and 35 per cent chondroitin sulphate. At approximately 60 kDa, which equates to approximately 30 repeating units, human mast cell heparin is smaller than that of the rat. Basophils contain chondroitin sulphate.

During mast cell degranulation, the cationic mediators dissociate from heparin by ionic exchange, initially with Ca^{2+} then with Na^{+}. Those mediators with isoelectric points close to neutrality, e.g. histamine and acid hydrolases, dissociate rapidly while the process is slower with the more highly charged neutral proteases.

Neutral proteases

The disposition of tryptase, chymase and carboxypeptidase in the granules of human mast cells has already been described. The relative concentrations of these three enzymes in MC_{TC} and MC_{TC} are shown in Fig. 5.12.

Human mast cell tryptase is a unique enzyme in that it is a 134 kDa tetramer stored in close association with the sulphate groups of heparin and chondroitin sulphate. The component monomers have molecular weights of 31–35 kDa and are all recognized by a series of monoclonal antibodies directed to different epitopes. This suggests that the monomers

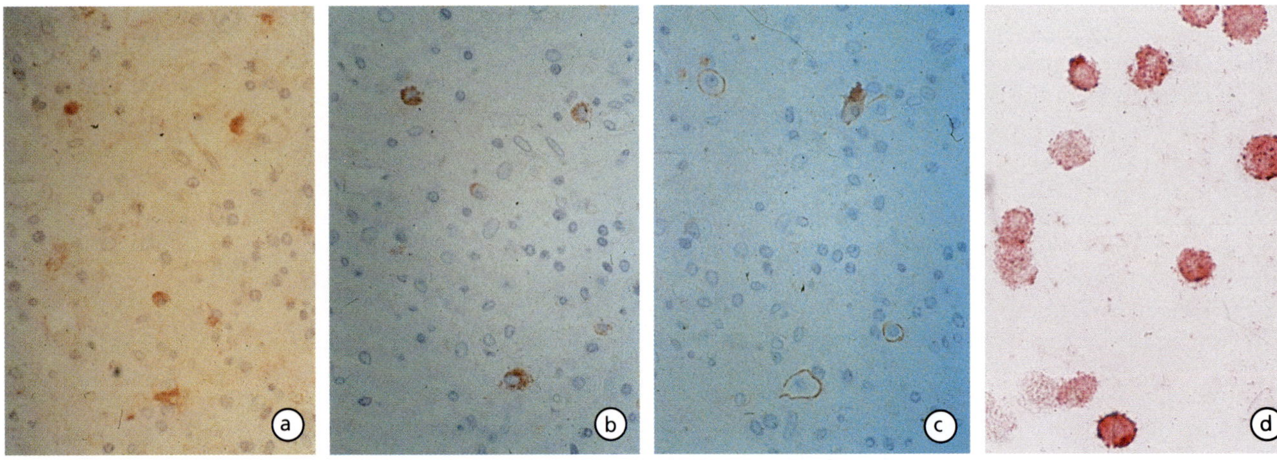

Fig. 5.10 Immunocytochemical localization of IL-4 to human mast cells. (a,b,c) Biopsy of human rhinitic nasal mucosa. Sequential 2μm sections were stained (from left to right) with monoclonal antibodies 3H4 to IL-4, AAl to mast cell tryptase and 409 to IL-4. (With acknowledgements to Dr P Bradding.) (d) Dispersed skin mast cells stained using antibody 3H4 to IL-4. (With acknowledgements to Drs C Heusser and Y Okayama.)

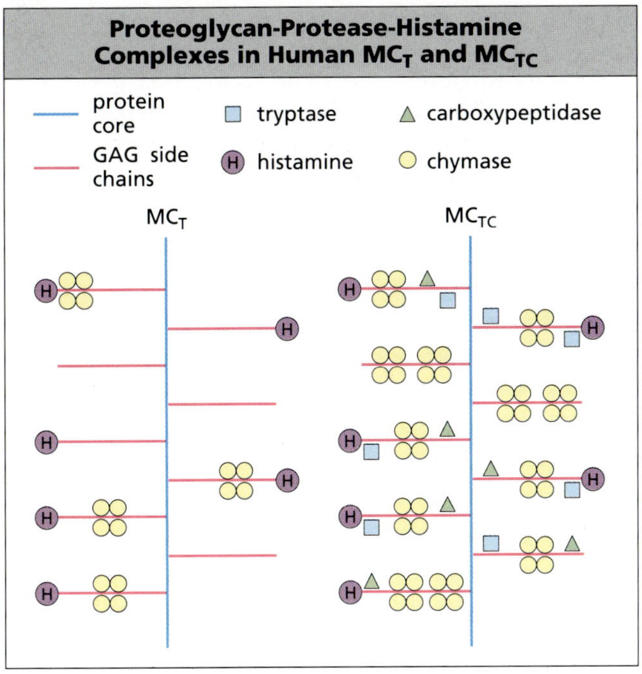

Fig. 5.11 Diagrammatic representation of proteoglycan–protease–histamine complexes in human MC$_T$ and MC$_{TC}$ mast cells. The proteoglycan comprises a protein core with GAG side chains. Tryptase, chymase, carboxypeptidase and histamine associate ionically with the GAGs.

Distribution of Neutral Proteases in Human Mast Cells

Protease	Cellular content (pg/cell)	
	MC$_T$	MC$_{TC}$
tryptase	10.0	35.0
chymase	–	4.5
carboxypeptidase	–	10.0

Fig. 5.12 Distribution of neutral proteases in human mast cells. (Data from studies by LB Schwartz, NM Schechter and SM Goldstein.)

are structurally very similar, differing possibly only in the addition of non-protein residues. Once released from the granular matrix, tryptase assumes the trypsin-like activity from which it was named. While no clear biological function has been demonstrated, the actions of tryptase include a rapid inactivation of fibrinogen, a weak activity like that of kallikrein, cleavage of the C3a fraction and activation of types I–V collagenases. Metabolism of the bronchodilator neuropeptide VIP, but not of the bronchoconstrictor neuropeptide substance P, suggests that mast cell tryptase may produce an imbalance in these peptides within the lung, thus favouring bronchoconstriction. Furthermore, experiments in the dog suggest that tryptase may increase bronchial hyperresponsiveness.

The functional control of tryptase, which is activated immediately on reaching the neutral pH of the extracellular environment, is particularly novel. Unlike other, trypsin-like enzymes, there are no known anti-proteases for tryptase. Since this enzyme is only active as a tetramer, it is instead regulated by the presence of heparin or other similarly charged proteoglycan which is stablizes this form. Thus, the enzyme is active in a high-proteoglycan concentration close to the mast cell but, on diffusion away from this environment, it dissociates into its monomeric form and becomes inactive.

Human mast cell chymase is an N-glycosylated 30 kDa monomeric chymotrypsin-like enzyme. Within the mast cell granule, it is bound ionically to heparin but not to chondroitin sulphate. Unlike tryptase, chymase is readily inhibited in the extracellular environment by α_1-antichymotrypsin, α_1-proteinase inhibitor and α_2-macroglobulin. Like tryptase, little is known about its biological role. The evidence that it converts angiotensin I to angiotensin II and degrades bradykinin and many neuropeptides suggests a role for chymase in the local control of blood flow. Chymase has also been shown to separate the epidermis from the dermis, thereby incriminating it in skin blistering such as bullous pemphigoid and bullous mastocytosis.

Human mast cell carboxypeptidase was definitively recognized only in 1987 and thus represents the most recently found of the human mast cell neutral proteases. Structurally it is a 34.5 kDa monomer with unique substrate characteristics which slightly resemble that of pancreatic carboxypeptidase B. Like this latter enzyme, mast cell carboxypeptidase appears to be a zinc metallo-exopeptidase. Few studies have yet been made on its biological function.

Acid hydrolases

In addition to mast cell-specific neutral proteases, the mast cell is also a source of acid hydrolases which are present too in the lysosimal granules of other inflammatory cells. These include β-hexosaminidase, β-glucuronidase and β-galactosidase.

Mast Cell Activation

Mast cells and basophils are characterized by the presence within the cell membrane of high affinity receptors for IgE. These receptors, termed $Fc_\epsilon R1$, comprise dimeric α, β and γ sub-units which, between them, traverse the 5 nm thickness of the cell membrane. The α-sub-units have a unique affinity for the fourth domain of the Fc_ϵ chain of IgE which it binds with an affinity of approximately 1 x 10^9/M. Cross-linkage of IgE by the interaction of allergen with specific determinants on the Fab portion of the molecule brings the receptors into juxtaposition and initiates mast cell activation. In the laboratory, IgE receptor cross-linkage may be induced artificially by the use of anti-IgE antibodies or antibodies to the $Fc_\epsilon R1$ receptor.

Immunological stimulation of human mast cells leads to the exocytosis of the preformed granule-associated products and the generation of newly synthesized eicosanoids. Morphologically, mast cell degranulation proceeds by compound exocytosis which is characterized by solubilization of the granule contents seen as granule swelling, fusion of the granular and plasma membrane and exteriorization of the granule contents (Fig. 5.13). The details of the biochemistry which relates to these events is contained in Chapter 4.

Mast cells may also be activated by non-immunological stimuli. It has recently been demonstrated that human skin mast cells, in contrast to those of the lung, adenoid, tonsil or large intestine, release histamine in response to substance P, VIP, somatostatin, compound 48/80, morphine, and the complement anaphylatoxins C5a and C3a (Fig. 5.14). Interestingly, this reactivity does not parallel protease phenotyping, and both mixed intestinal and tonsillar mast cell populations contain large numbers of MC_{TC} mast cells which appear unresponsive to neuropeptide stimulation (see Fig. 5.6).

Examination of the characteristics of IgE-dependent and neuropeptide-induced mediator release from human skin mast cells shows marked differences. IgE-dependent activation leads to a relatively slow (5-minute) degranulation and generation of PGD_2 and LTC_4. In contrast, neuropeptide stimulation leads to rapid (15-second) release of preformed mediators without the generation of either PGD_2 or LTC_4. When viewed under the electron microscope, the morphology of degranulation produced by immunological and non-immunological stimulation appears identical. However, biochemical processes which lead to mediator release appear to be different (Fig. 5.15). The ability of the skin mast cell to respond to non-immunological stimulation by release of its preformed histamine, proteoglycans and proteolytic enzymes only extends its possible biological function from allergy into control of local inflammation, blood flow regulation or angiogenesis.

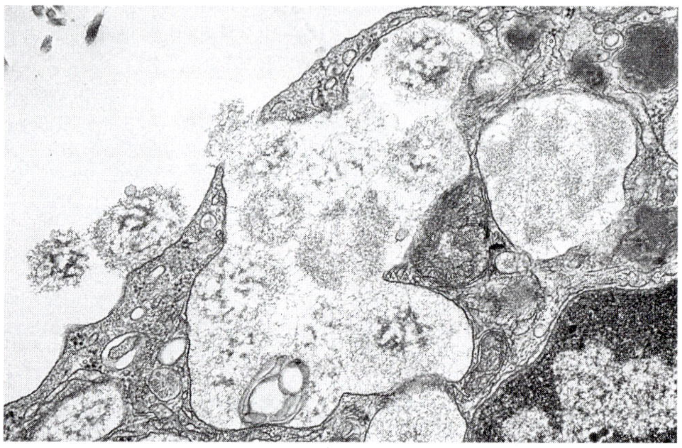

Fig. 5.13 EM of compound exocytosis stimulated in an isolated human skin mast cell by IgE-dependent activation. Granules swell as they move towards the cell membrane. Following membrane fusion, the granular contents are exposed to the extracellular environment where ion exchange and passive diffusion occur to release the contents, so causing compound exocytosis.

Histamine Release Induced from Human Mast Cell Sub-Populations by Anti-IgE and Substance P

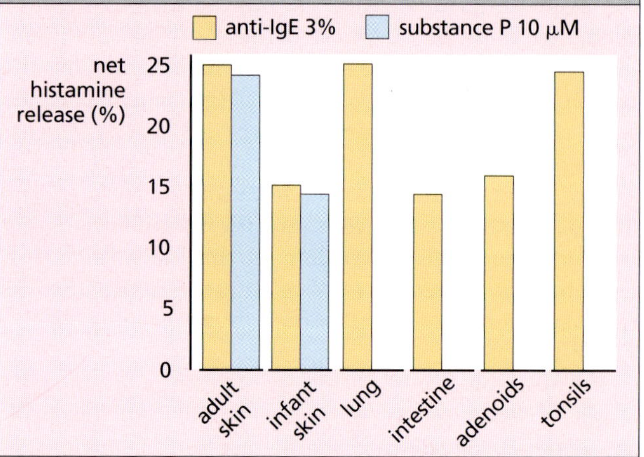

Fig. 5.14 Histamine release induced from human mast cell sub-populations by anti-IgE and substance P.

Modulation of Mast Cell Mediator Release

The central role of the mast cell in the initiation of allergic responses makes it an ideal target for anti-allergic drug therapy. As a consequence, mast cell models, particularly those of the rat peritoneal mast cell *in vitro* and the rat cutaneous mast cell *in vivo*, have been widely used for the screening of potential drugs. However, it has now been recognized that there are considerable differences in mast cell populations, both between species and between tissues in a single species and in response to drug modulation.

Mast Cell Activation by Anti-IgE and Substance P

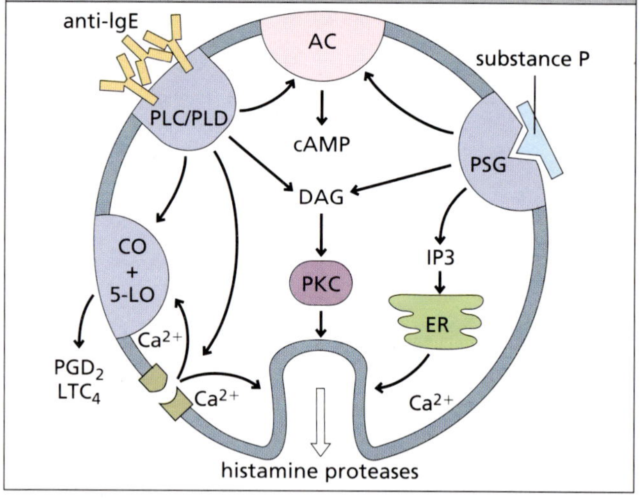

Fig. 5.15 Mast cell activation by anti-IgE and substance P. IgE-dependent activation is initiated through phospholipases C and/or D (PLC/PLD) which generate diacyglycerol (DAG), which in turn stimulates protein kinase C (PKC), an enzyme critical for the degranulation process. Influx of calcium from the extracellular medium by opening of calcium channels is also stimulated. Membrane-associated cyclooxygenase (CO) and 5-lipoxygenase (5-LO) are stimulated to generate PGD_2 and LTC_4. In contrast, substance P–induced activation is initiated through a pertussis-sensitive G-protein (PSG), and through the generation of DAG and IP3 which stimulate PKC and mobilize intracellular calcium from the endoplasmic reticulum (ER) and the inner surface of the membrane respectively. No PGD_2 or LTC_4 synthesis occurs with this stimulus. Both stimuli activate adenylate cyclase (AC) to elevate intracellular cyclic AMP.

Sodium cromoglycate, introduced initially as a mast cell stabilizer, exhibits marked heterogeneity. In the rat, it is a potent inhibitor of mediator release from connective tissue mast cells, while not inhibiting mucosal mast cells. In guinea pigs and mice, it is essentially ineffective. Its activity in human mast cells is shown in Fig. 5.16. When examined in human lung mast cells, high concentrations are needed to produce only modest inhibition of histamine release (Fig. 5.17). Furthermore those cells show rapid tachyphylaxis to the inhibitory effects of sodium cromoglycate.

Mast cells recovered from the airway lumen by BAL, which are of the same protease phenotype as those dispersed from lung tissue, have a strikingly different response to sodium cromoglycate. These cells are more potently inhibited and there is no obvious sign of tachyphylaxis. Similar results are found with mast cells dispersed from the large intestine. Unlike mast cells of rat skin, human skin mast cells are totally unresponsive to sodium cromoglycate. These results indicate that mast cell responsiveness cannot be predicted from a knowledge of its protease phenotype and confirm that extrapolations may not be made from one species to another. β-Adrenoceptor stimulants which interact with cell surface β_2-receptors to elevate intracellular cyclic AMP levels are both more potent and more effective inhibitors of mast cell histamine release than sodium cromoglycate (see Fig. 5.17). Moreover, while they are poor inhibitors of rat mast cell or human basophil histamine release, they are equally effective in all human mast cell populations. Finally, they are more effective inhibitors of eicosanoid synthesis than of degranulation, which suggest that this pathway is more susceptible to drug modulation (Fig. 5.18).

At concentrations which would not cause toxicity *in vivo*, other drugs used in the treatment of allergic diseases, including corticocosteroids, histamine H_1-antagonists and theophylline, have negligible effect on mast cell mediator release.

The Role of Mast Cells in Allergic Disease

The mast cell has long been regarded as central to the initiation and mediation of the early phase of allergic inflammation and may also be responsible for the initiation of chronic allergic inflammation. The mechanisms by which mast cell activation may achieve those ends are summarized in Fig. 5.19.

Mast cell-derived histamine, PGD_2 and LTC_4 together produce the symptoms of the early response

Effect of Sodium Cromoglycate Against Human Mast Cell Sub-Populations

Tissue	Inhibitory Effects	Tachyphylaxis	Mast Cell Phenotype
lung			
dispersed mast cells	+	yes	$MC_T \gg MC_{TC}$
BAL mast cells	+++	no	$MC_T \gg MC_{TC}$
intestine	+++	no	$MC_T \simeq MC_{TC}$
tonsil	++	yes	$MC_T \simeq MC_{TC}$
skin	–	–	$MC_T \ll MC_{TC}$

Fig. 5.16 Effect of sodium cromoglycate on human mast cell populations.

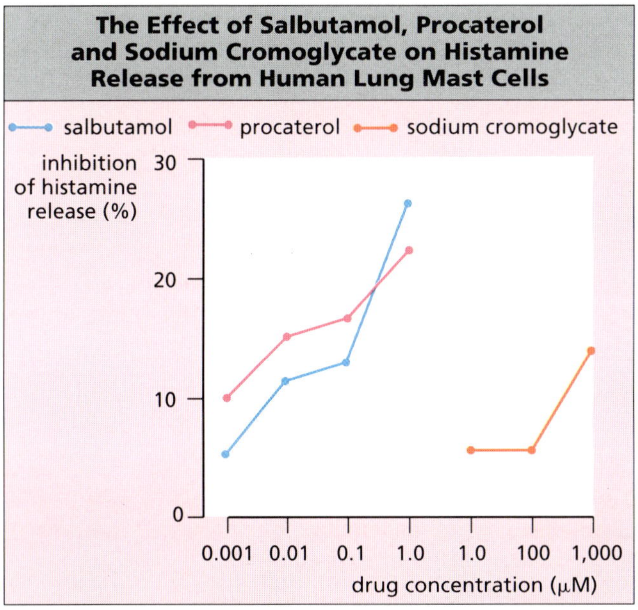

Fig. 5.17 The effect of salbutamol, procaterol and sodium cromoglycate on histamine release from human lung mast cells initiated by 3% anti-IgE.

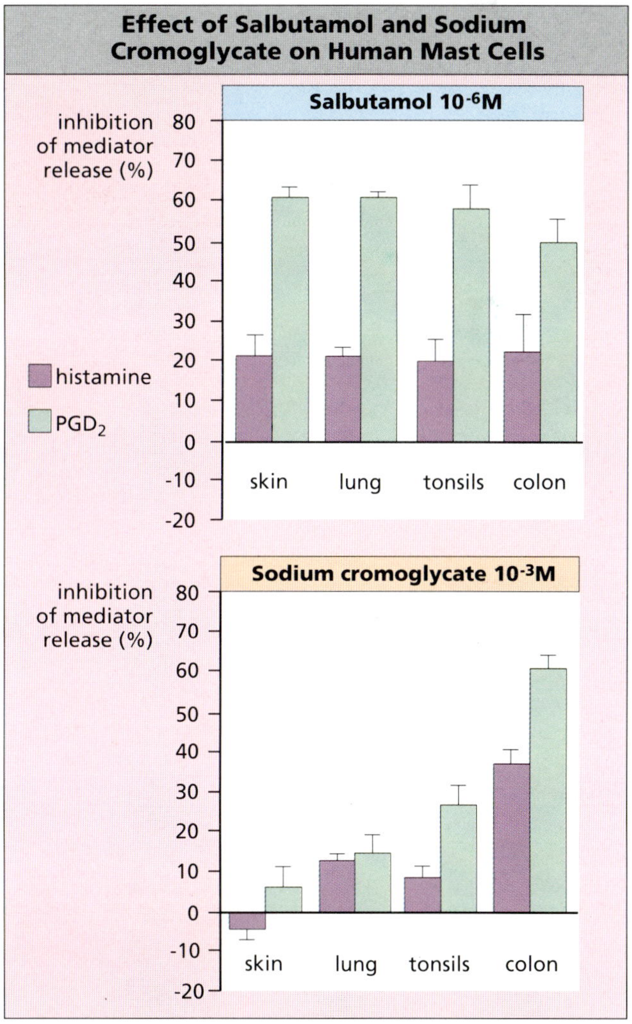

Fig. 5.18 Effect of salbutamol and sodium cromoglycate on histamine and PGD_2 release from human mast cells.

to allergen challenge. Their action may be supplemented by the generation of kinins by tryptase and of TAME-esterases by mast cells and by neuropeptide release following nerve stimulation. In the lungs these mediators induce bronchoconstriction, oedema in the airway walls and the secretion of mucus. These events are all characteristic of an acute asthmatic episode. In the nose, mast cell mediators induce rhinorrhoea, blockage and sneezing by actions on both the vasculature and sensory nerve endings. In the skin, local vasodilatation and oedema are responsible for the weal that follows allergen injection, while the flare is propagated by axon reflex-mediated vasodilatation, stimulated primarily by histamine.

The role of the mast cell in the initiation of chronic allergic inflammation is less well established. However, recent observations that mast cells contain IL-3, IL-4, IL-5, IL-6 and TNF_{α} and that they may release these preformed products as a rapid local pulse suggest a major role in the initiation of chronic inflammation. The concomitant generation of LTC_4, PAF, chemotactic factors and cytokines would initiate leucocyte adhesion, migration and priming. Once at the site of challenge, mediator release from these migratory cells would then be induced by interaction with allergen or high local concentrations of cytokines. IL-4 would also act as a stimulus for the prolonged *de novo* synthesis of IL-3, IL-4, IL-5, IL-10 and GM-CSF by TH_2 lymphocytes, necessary to induce IgE-production from B cells and to support the chronic allergic inflammatory response.

The mast cell can, therefore, be regarded as a primary initiating cell for both the early allergic response and for chronic allergic inflammation.

Role of the Mast Cell in Acute and Chronic Allergic Inflammation

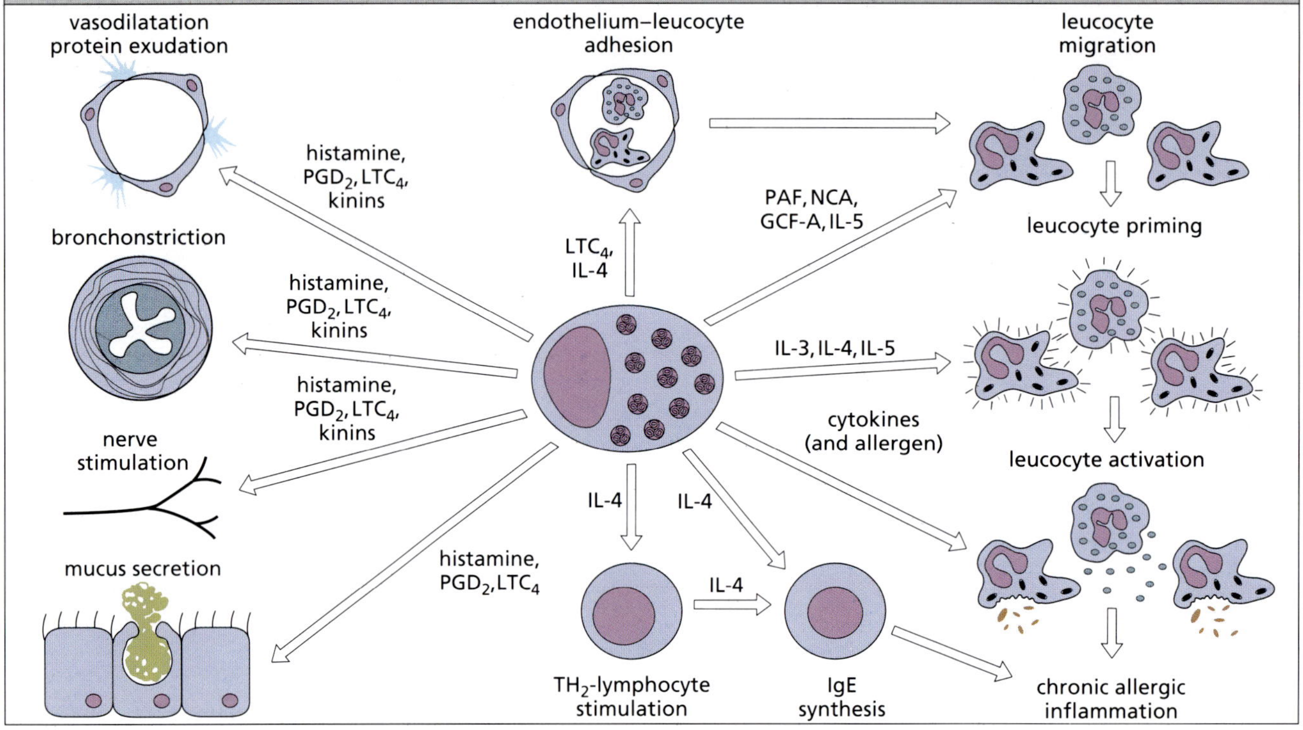

Fig. 5.19 The role of the mast cell in acute and chronic allergic inflammation.

Further Reading

Caulfield JP, El-Lati SG, Thomas G, Church MK. Dissociated human foreskin mast cells degranulate in response to anti-IgE and substance P. *Lab Invest* 1990; **63**: 502–510.

Church MK, El-Lati SG, Caulfield JP. Neuropeptide-induced secretion from human skin mast cells. *Int Arch Allergy Appl Immunol* 1991;**94**:310–318.

Galli SJ, Austen KF, eds. *Mast Cell and Basophil Differentiation and Function in Health Disease*. New York: Raven Press, 1989.

Galli SJ, Lichtenstein LM. Biology of mast cells and basophils. In: *Allergy: Principles and Practice*, Middleton E et al, eds. St. Louis: Mosby, 1988, pp. 106–134.

Holgate ST, ed. *Mast Cells, Mediators and Disease*. Dortrecht: Kluwer, 1988.

Holgate ST, Robinson C, Church MK, Mediators of immediate hypersensitivity. In: *Allergy: Principles and Practice,* Middleton E et al, eds. St Louis: Mosby, 1988, pp 135–163.

Schwartz LB, ed. Neutral Proteases of Mast Cells. *Monographs in Allergy*. Basel: Karger, Vol. 27, 1990.

Chapter 6

Eosinophils

Introduction

In 1879, Ehrlich studied aniline dyes as stains for peripheral blood smears and observed that a certain leucocyte type with cytoplasmic granules avidly bound acidic dyes. Thus, he developed a staining procedure to identify eosinophils; he was also the first to associate their proliferation with disease. Because the cell's granules had a marked affinity for the reddish-orange coloured eosin (Eos was the goddess of dawn in Greek mythology), he coined the term 'eosinophil'. Ehrlich's staining procedure was soon widely adopted. By the early years of the twentieth century, eosinophilia had become a hallmark of parasitic and allergic diseases.

Although we still do not fully understand many aspects of eosinophil function, they are certainly active participants in important physiological and pathophysiological events. Eosinophils kill many species of helminths and other parasites and probably play a role in defence against infection; they also probably play a role in inflammatory responses in the lung, skin, and heart. To do this, eosinophils elaborate inflammatory mediators that initiate tissue damage in these organs. The following discussion will review findings that support such conclusions.

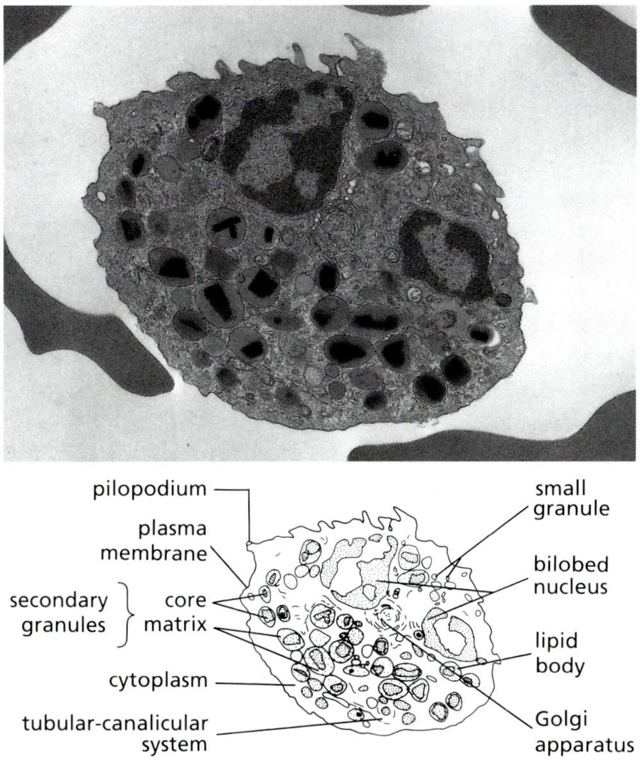

Fig. 6.1 A typical human eosinophil, showing two parts of the bilobed nucleus and several intact secondary granules; the granules show the opaque core and lucent matrix. (×14,000). (Courtesy of Dr H Kita.)

Structure and Contents

Morphology

Eosinophils share some structural similarities with other granulocytes, but the mature human eosinophil is slightly larger than the neutrophil, and is usually round or ovoid with a bilobed nucleus. The distinctive feature of mammalian eosinophils is the presence of characteristic secondary granules (Fig. 6.1). Two other types of granules have been described in eosinophils: the so-called small granules, which reportedly contain acid phosphatase and arylsulfatase; and the primary granules, which are round, uniformly electron dense, and are characteristically seen in eosinophilic promyelocytes.

Cellular Constituents (Fig. 6.2)

Excluding the secondary granules, the major components of the eosinophil include:

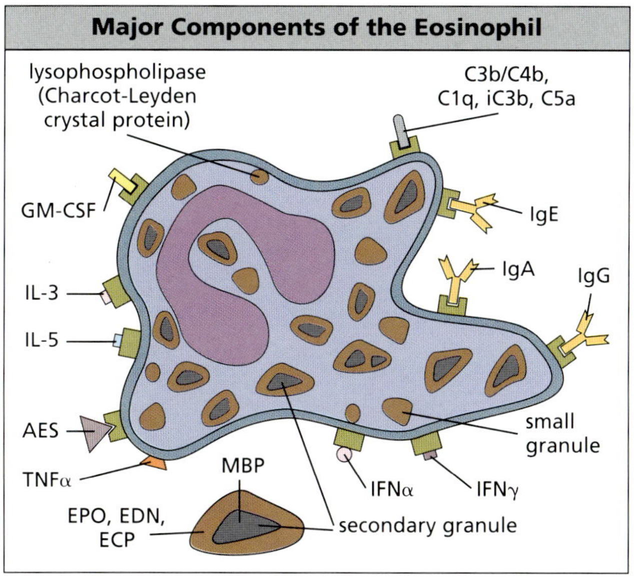

Fig. 6.2 Diagrammatic representation of an eosinophil, showing major internal structures and surface receptors. Adapted from Gleich GJ. Current understanding of eosinophil function. *Hospital Practice* 1988; **23**:137.

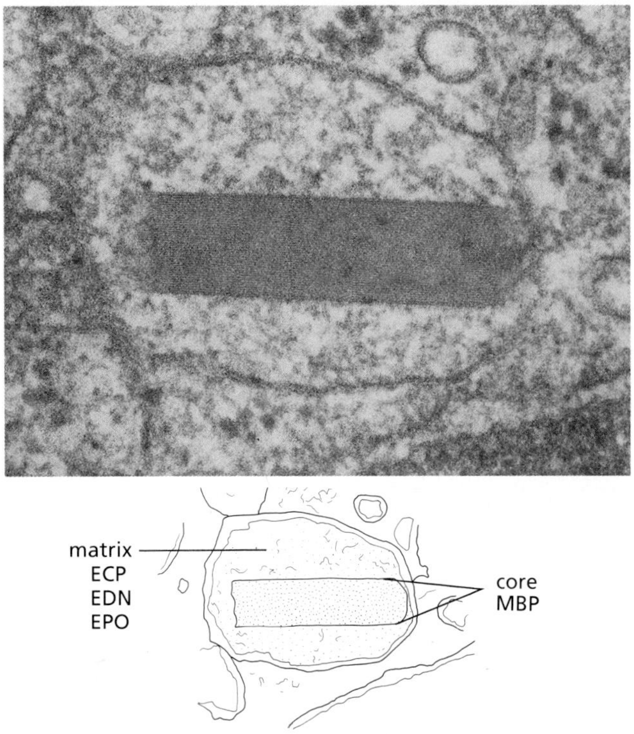

Fig. 6.3 A rat eosinophil secondary granule. The crystalline core is MBP and the remaining constituents are in the surrounding matrix. Note the linear arrays in the cystralloid core (×160,000). (Courtesy of Dr E deHarven).

- receptors for immunoglobulins, growth factors, and complement components on the cell membrane surface;
- Charcot–Leyden crystal (CLC) protein (lysophospholipase) within the cell membrane and in primary granules;
- arylsulfatase B, eosinophil collagenase, and other enzymes, including those able to generate PAF, LTC_4, and substance P; and
- antigenic determinants recognized by antiserum to eosinophils.

These constituents play many roles in eosinophil function. For example, the ability of the eosinophil to kill parasites and other targets has been linked to immune effectors, including IgG, IgA, secretory IgA, IgE, and complement fragments, and to the existence of receptors for these molecules. Likewise, various haematopoietic growth factors influencing eosinophil differentiation such as IL-3, IL-5, and GM-CSF, as well as TNF-α, IFN-α, and IFN-γ stimulate mature eosinophils. The distinctive hexagonal, bipyramidal CLC, the crystallized form of lysophospholipase, was observed in 1872 in sputum from patients with asthma. Moreover, the protein that crystallizes *in vitro* to give CLCs is lysophospholipase and is found in both eosinophils and basophils in comparable quantities. Other enzymes associated with the eosinophil include arylsulfatase B, and eosinophil collagenase which degrades types I and III collagen, the two major connective tissue components of human parenchyma. An enzyme reaction produces PAF, an ether-linked phospholipid that has numerous potent biological activities. Eosinophils produce LTC_4 and substance P; both have potent activities on blood vessels and smooth muscles. Finally, certain membrane proteins are the antigens recognized by anti-eosinophil sera. Specific antisera and murine monoclonal antibodies to human eosinophils have been produced.

Secondary Granule Proteins

As expected from the avidity of secondary granules for the acidic dye eosin, these granules contain basic substances; in fact, four distinctive cationic proteins are associated with the granules. Fig. 6.3 shows the localization of the different granule constituents, and Fig. 6.4 summarizes the features of these proteins.

Major Basic Protein (MBP)

By electron microscopy, the secondary granule core reveals a crystalline lattice structure, suggesting it is made up of a single substance (Fig. 6.3). The crystalloid core is major basic protein (MBP), and the remaining components are in the surrounding matrix. Latest data on human MBP indicate a single polypeptide chain of 117 amino acid residues (about 16 per cent arginine) and an isoelectric point (pI) of 10.9. The recently determined cDNA for MBP reveals that MBP is translated as a 25.2 kDa preproprotein, with the 9.9 kDa pro-portion being rich in glutamic and aspartic acids and having a pI of 3.9. The calculated pI for proMBP is 6.2, which suggests that MBP is translated as a non-toxic precursor, masking the toxic effects of mature MBP and protecting the eosinophil as the protein is processed through the endoplasmic reticulum to the granule core.

Because in the guinea pig MBP accounts for one quarter of the eosinophil's protein content, it seemed reasonable to hypothesize that MBP had much to do with the cell's functions. The earliest studies found that MBP is toxic to schistosomula (larvae) of the intestinal parasite *Schistosoma mansoni*. Further studies showed that MBP's toxic effects extended to a variety of parasites, including *Brugia malayi* and *B. pahangi*, the bloodstream trypomastigote stage of the protozoan *Trypanosoma cruzi*, newborn larvae of *Trichinella spiralis*, and juvenile *Fasciola hepatica*. MBP is also toxic to certain bacteria *in vitro*, including *Escherichia coli* and *Staphylococcus aureus*.

Another early finding was the *in vitro* dose-related toxicity of MBP for murine tumour cells and human tracheal and intestinal epithelial cells, lymph node cells, and skin cells. Subsequently, MBP concentrations in blood from patients with eosinophilia and sputum from patients with asthma all had MBP levels equal to or greater than those causing cell damage *in vitro*.

As circumstantial evidence for MBP's toxicity in asthma, an immunofluorescence technique found intense staining for MBP in lung tissue specimens from patients with asthma in association with damage to bronchial epithelium. In addition, incubation of human peripheral blood leucocytes with MBP causes concentration-dependent histamine release. The release process is calcium-, temperature-, and energy-dependent, and it is not cytotoxic. Also, MBP is a unique and strong platelet agonist, and it is able to activate neutrophils. Altogether, these findings

Some Properties of Human Eosinophil Secondary Granule Proteins and Their Encoding cDNA and Gene

Protein	Physical properties		Molecular biology		Biological activities
MBP	Site Molecular weight Isoelectric point Plasma levels (ng/ml)	granule core 13.8 kDa 10.9 186	**cDNA** ~900 nt (prepro-MBP)	**Gene** 3.3 kb 5 introns 6 exons	potent helminthotoxin and cytotoxin histamine release from basophils and rat mast cells neutralizes heparin bactericidal increases bronchial reactivity to methacholine in primates unique, strong platelet agonist provokes bronchospasm in primates
ECP	Site Molecular weight Isoelectric point Plasma levels (ng/ml)	granule matrix 18–21 kDa 10.8 17	**cDNA** ~725 nt (preECP)	**Gene** ~1.2 kb 1 introns in UTR	potent helminthotoxin potent neurotoxin inhibits cultures of peripheral blood lymphocytes histamine release from rat mast cells weak RNase activity bactericidal
EDN	Site Molecular weight Isoelectric point Plasma levels (ng/ml)	granule matrix 18–19 kDa 8.9 20	**cDNA** ~725 nt (preEDN)	**Gene** ~1.2 kb 11 introns 12 exons	potent neurotoxin inhibits cultures of peripheral blood lymphocytes potent RNase activity weak helminthotoxin
EPO	Site Molecular weight Isoelectric point Plasma levels (ng/ml)	granule matrix 66 kDa 10.8 26	**cDNA** ~2500 nt (2106 nt ORF)	**Gene** ~12 kb 1 introns 12 exons	in the presence of H_2O_2+halide: kills micro-organisms and tumour cells releases histamine from rat mast cells inactivates leukotrienes in the absence of H_2O_2+halide: kills Brugia microfilariae damages respiratory epithelium promotes bronchospasm in primates

Fig. 6.4 Properties of human eosinophil secondary granule proteins. The cDNAs were used to calculate the isoelectric points of the proteins. Adapted from Haman KJ, Gleich GJ. Eosinophil structure and function: roles in host defence and pathogenesis in disease. In Sorg C, ed. *Local Immunity*, **6**: Natural Resistance to Infection, 60–88. Stuttgart: Gustav Fischer Verlag, 1990.

indicated that the eosinophil might be an effector cell for tissue damage in bronchial asthma and that MBP might be a prime mediator of such damage.

Eosinophil Cationic Protein (ECP)

The core of the secondary granule is surrounded by a matrix which contains three well-characterized cationic proteins (Fig. 6.3). ECP is one of these; ECP and MBP have different properties and are distinct molecules (Fig. 6.4). The cDNA sequence for ECP codes for a preproprotein of 160 amino acids and a protein of 133 amino acids. Despite its highly basic nature, there is no evidence for a proECP analogous to that of MBP. The nucleotide sequence of ECP is similar to that of eosinophil-derived neurotoxin (EDN), rat pancreatic RNase, and human angiogenin,which are members of the RNase gene superfamily. ECP is a weak ribonuclease.

ECP has several activities: it is a potent toxin for schistosomula of *S. mansoni,* and is eight to 10 times as active as MBP, though not as abundant in granules. ECP is also toxic *in vitro* for newborn larvae of *T. spiralis* and microfilariae of *B. pahangi* and *B. malayi*. The guinea pig is exquisitely sensitive to neurotoxic activity produced by extracts of eosinophils, and ECP is a potent neurotoxin. Culture of human peripheral blood lymphocytes in the presence of ECP shows a dose-dependent inhibition of proliferation induced by phytohaemagglutinin and by a one-way mixed lymphocyte reaction. Finally, ECP damages certain target cell membranes by causing pore formation.

Eosinophil-Derived Neurotoxin (EDN)

Another cationic protein in the granule matrix is EDN, which is indistinguishable from the previously reported eosinophil protein X. As noted above, eosinophils contain a powerful neurotoxin capable of severely damaging myelinated neurons in experimental animals. Using the Gordon phenomena (a neurotoxic reaction in rabbits) as an endpoint, EDN was purified from eosinophil granules. Initially, the partial N-terminal sequence, and later the complete amino acid sequence of EDN deduced from the cDNA, showed marked amino acid sequence homology to ECP. EDN, however, has about 100 times more RNase activity than ECP, but is a relatively weak helminthotoxin. Comparison of amino acid sequences shows that EDN possesses fewer strongly basic amino acids, resulting in a much lower pI. Because cationic charge may be an important determinant of cytotoxicity, these characteristics may explain EDN's relative lack of helminthotoxic potency.

Eosinophil Peroxidase (EPO)

The third cationic protein in the granule matrix is EPO, which differs from neutrophil or monocyte myeloperoxidase in its absorption spectra and haem prosthetic groups. It consists of two subunits (a heavy chain of 53 011 Da and a light chain of 12 712 Da) in a 1:1 stoichiometry. Comparison of the EPO nucleotide sequence to that of other peroxidases, such as myeloperoxidase and thyroid peroxidase, indicates the existence of a multigene peroxidase family. In the

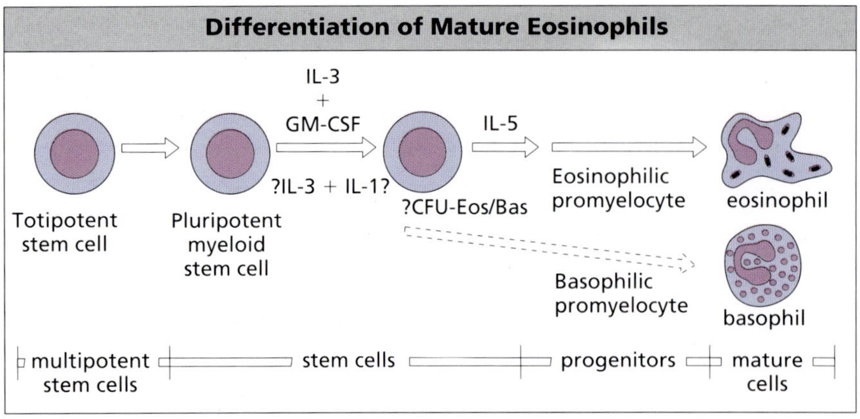

Fig. 6.5 Bone marrow differentiation from totipotent haematopoietic stem cell to mature eosinophils. Adapted from Slifman, NR , Adolphson, CR, Gleich G.J. Eosinophils: biochemical and cellular aspects. In: Middleton EJ, Reed CE, Ellis EF, Adkinson NF Jr., Yunginger JW, eds. *Allergy: Principles and Practice*, 3rd Ed., Vol. 1, 179–205, St Louis: C.V. Mosby Co, 1988.

presence of H_2O_2, purified EPO is able to oxidize halides to form highly reactive hypohalous acids. EPO prefers Br^- to Cl^- in these reactions. Because eosinophils generate H_2O_2 and have an active halogenation capability, the killing of micro-organisms by the EPO+H_2O_2+halide system has been tested. The results show that EPO+H_2O_2+halide not only kills many micro-organisms, including *E. coli*, schistosomula, microfilariae of *B. pahangi* and *B. malayi*, trypanosoma, toxoplasma, and mycobacteria, but also kills mast cells and tumour cells.

Furthermore, EPO at lower concentrations and when supplemented by H_2O_2+halide induces rat mast cell degranulation and histamine release. EPO also binds to microbes such as *S. aureus*, *T. cruzi* and *Toxoplasma gondii*, which potentiates the killing of these organisms by mononuclear phagocytes. Similarly, tumour cells adsorb EPO, which potentiates their lysis by H_2O_2. Incubation of LTC_4 or LTD_4 with EPO+H_2O_2+halide rapidly decreases their biological activity on smooth muscle, and EPO+H_2O_2+halide decreases the chemotactic activity of LTB_4. Thus, the EPO+H_2O_2+halide system is able to mediate the destruction of numerous organisms, and may regulate the concentrations of several leukotrienes during inflammation and immediate hypersensitivity.

Ontogeny of Eosinophils

Eosinopoiesis

Eosinophils are produced in the bone marrow under the influence of differentiation factors, including IL-l, IL3, IL-5, and GM-CSF. Fig. 6.5 illustrates the currently accepted model of eosinophil differentiation, based on the concept of a totipotent haematopoietic stem cell giving rise to pluripotent stem cells which in turn give rise to stem cells committed to one or two lines of differentiation. Because, under clonal conditions, eosinophil-type colonies contain both eosinophils and basophils, these cells may derive from a common precursor. For murine eosinophils, IL-1 and IL-3 appear to act synergistically by increasing the number of eosinophil colony-forming cells, whereas IL-5 acts later in eosinophil differentiation by causing the generation of mature eosinophils from precursor cells. For human eosinophil production, IL-5, IL-3, and GM-CSF are active. Once eosinophil differentiation has begun, the cell undergoes characteristic morphogical changes until it is functionally mature.

Life Cycle, Kinetics and Distribution

Eosinophils are formed in the bone marrow, and are present in the peripheral blood as they travel to their final site of deposition in the tissues. Thus, the life cycle of the eosinophil may be divided into marrow, blood, and tissue phases.

The bone marrow transit time in humans is about 4.3 days. In peripheral blood the eosinophil has a half-life of less than one day; it then migrates into the tissues, probably by diapedesis at endothelial intercellular junctions. Consequently, changes in

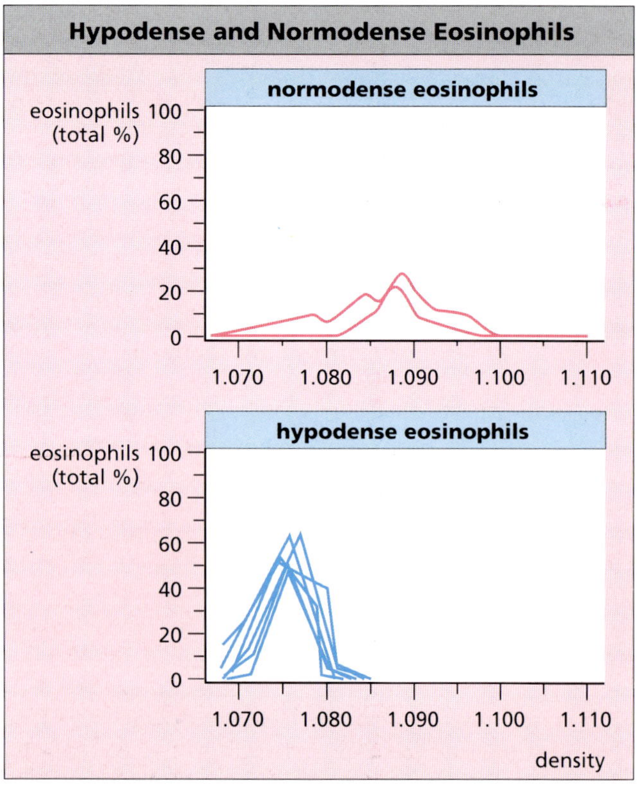

Fig. 6.6 Comparison of buoyant densities of normodense and hypodense eosinophils. The hypodense eosinophil contains similar numbers of granules as normodense eosinophils, but the individual granules are smaller. Adapted from Peters MS, Gleich GJ, Dunnette SL, Fukuda T. Ultrastructural study of eosinophils from patients with the hypereosinophilic syndrome: A morphological basis of hypodense eosinophils. *Blood* 1988; **71**: 780.

vascular permeability may greatly affect the ability of eosinophils to infiltrate tissues and may also contribute to the pathogenesis of clinical syndromes. The tissue life span of eosinophils has not been well studied: it is probably in the range of two to five days, depending partly on the tissue studied. In rats, the ratio of tissue to blood eosinophils is between 200:1 and 300:1; in humans, the ratio is about 100:1. In rats, eosinophils tend to dwell in tissues whose epithelial surfaces are exposed to the external environment, at the 'first line of defence' where mast cells also tend to reside. In humans, the gut appears to be the most heavily populated site; normally few eosinophils are present in human lung, and none in human skin. In disease states, however, many organs may be infiltrated by eosinophils, and the kinetics of eosinophil production may be altered.

Hypodense Eosinophils

Several studies have shown that patients with eosinophilia-associated diseases, such as the hypereosinophilic syndrome, parasitism, asthma, allergic diseases, and neoplasia, have two populations of peripheral eosinophils that may be distinguished on the basis of their density (Fig. 6.6). The light density or hypodense eosinophils have a peak density of 1.075–1.077; the normodense eosinophils have a peak density of 1.088. In peripheral blood of normal persons, less than 10 per cent of the eosinophils are hypodense. But patients with eosinophilia-associated diseases have a much higher proportion of circulating hypodense eosinophils, and their numbers are positively correlated with the degree of eosinophilia.

Hypodense eosinophils may be 'activated' cells:

- hypodense eosinophils appear to be more metabolically active than normodense eosinophils, with increased oxygen consumption and increased ability to generate superoxide anion;
- hypodense eosinophils show increased production and/or releasability of LTC_4 after incubation with IgG-coated beads or calcium ionophore A23187;
- hypodense eosinophils show potent cytotoxic activity for antibody-coated targets, and have greater numbers of IgG_{Fc}, IgE_{Fc}, and complement receptors. Moreover, IgE-dependent cytotoxicity for the schistosomula of *S. mansoni* appears to be restricted to hypodense eosinophils, and they are more active parasite killers.

Whether hypodense eosinophils originate from the bone marrow or are derived in the blood and tissues from normodense cells remains controversial (Fig. 6.7). The smaller granule size in hypodense eosinophils may be because of maturation or piecemeal degranulation. Hypodense eosinophils may be partially degranulated by a prior activation step; e.g. incubation of normodense cells with IL-5 causes release of granule proteins into the culture medium.

Production of Mediators and Toxic Oxygen Metabolites

In addition to the toxic cationic proteins, eosinophils secrete the lipid mediators, PAF and LTC_4, and the superoxide ion, $\dot{O}_2^-$ (see Fig. 6.8).

Platelet Activating Factor (PAF)

Although named because of its biological effects on platelets (see chapter 8), PAF is the most potent known chemotactic factor for eosinophils, and under certain conditions may be an eosinophil activating factor. PAF also causes aggregation and stimulation of neutrophils, activation of macrophages, increased vascular permeability of skin, contraction of guinea pig lung parenchyma strips, and an anaphylactoid reaction after injection into rabbits. PAF is produced by

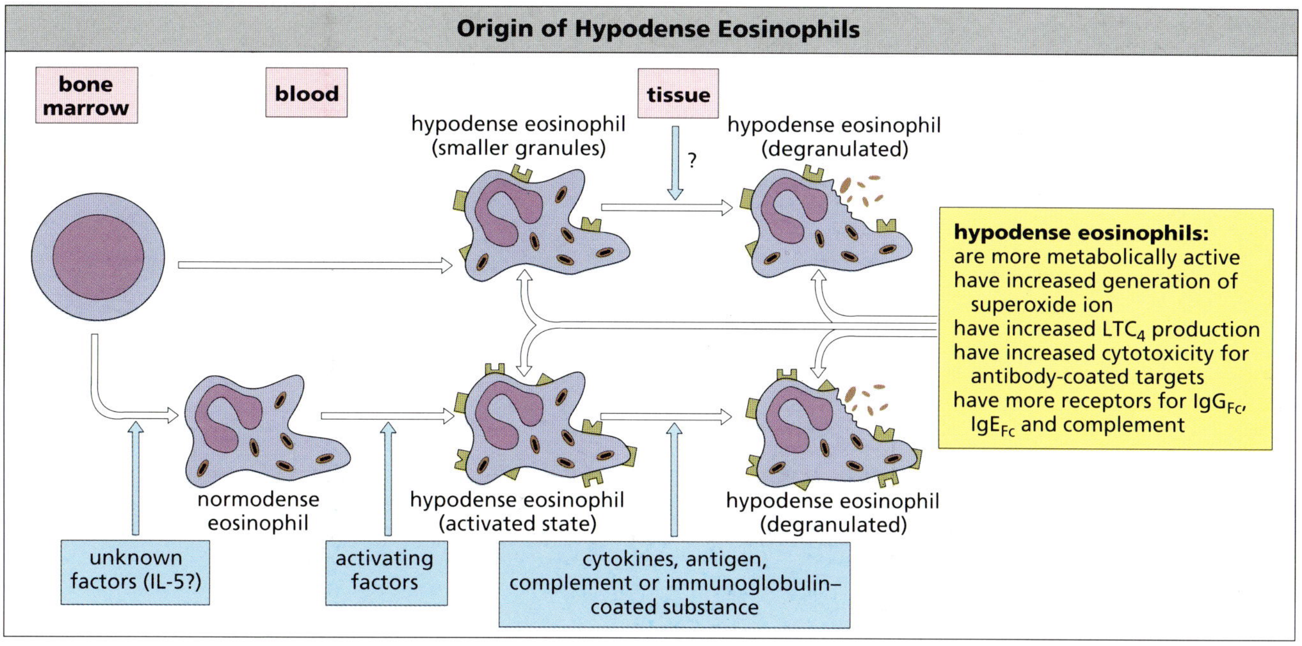

Fig. 6.7 Current hypotheses regarding the origin of hypodense eosinophils. The properties of hypodense eosinophils are well studied; however, the mechanism(s) for producing hypodense eosinophils are less well defined.

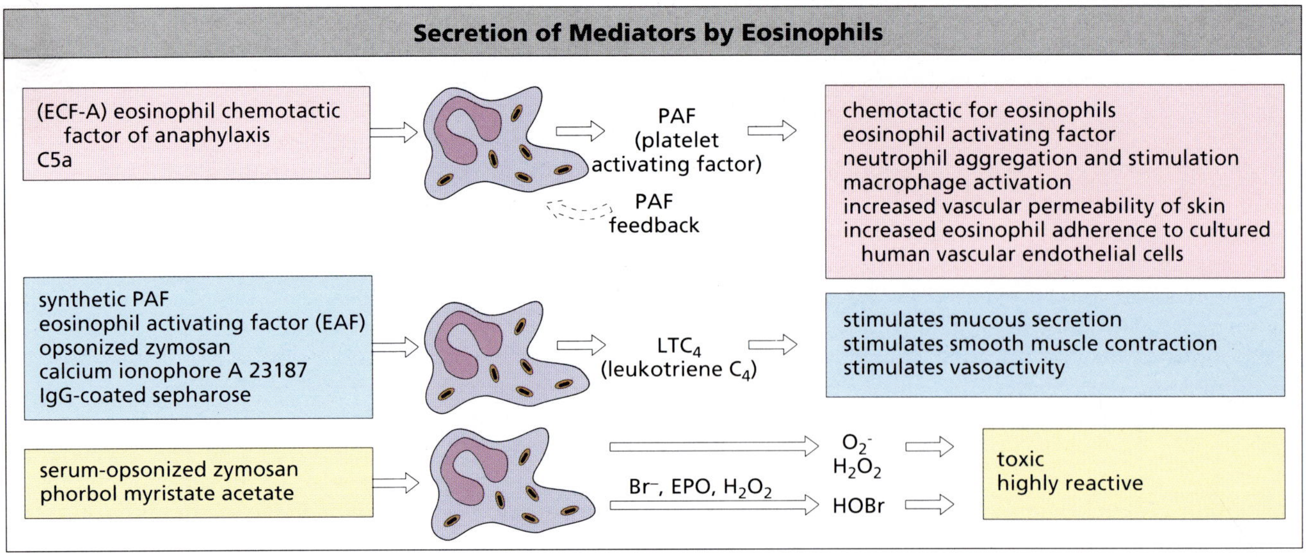

Fig. 6.8 Secretion of mediators and toxic oxygen metabolites by eosinophils.

stimulated eosinophils, platelets, neutrophils, macrophages, monocytes, basophils and endothelial cells. Secretion of PAF from eosinophils is stimulated by several naturally occurring eosinophilotactic substances, such as eosinophil chemotactic factor of anaphylaxis (ECF-A) and C5a. Therefore, PAF is probably a mediator in the inflammatory and hypersensitivity diseases in which eosinophils participate. Whether PAF is able to stimulate or suppress its own production and secretion from eosinophils is still being debated.

Leukotrienes

Resting blood eosinophils do not synthesize leukotrienes, but early experiments showed that eosinophils stimulated by the calcium ionophore A23187 or opsonized zymosan do produce appreciable amounts of LTC_4 (previously called the slow-reacting substance of anaphylaxis, or SRS-A). LTC_4 is a potent mediator, producing smooth muscle contraction, mucous secretion, and changes in vascular permeability. Other stimuli causing eosinophils to secrete LTC_4 include: IgG-coated sepharose beads, synthetic PAF (PAF-acether), and eosinophil activating factor (EAF). Eosinophils produce more LTC_4 when the EPO+H_2O_2+halide system is inhibited, which suggests a mechanism for self-modulation of eosinophil LTC_4 production. In contrast to eosinophils, neutrophils elaborate predominantly LTB_4, a potent neutrophil chemotactic factor, but a weaker eosinophil chemotactic factor.

Superoxide, Hydrogen Peroxide and Hypobromous Acid (HOBr)

In response to *in vitro* stimulation by phorbol myristate acetate (PMA) or serum-opsonized zymosan particles, eosinophils generate two potentially toxic oxygen metabolites, the superoxide radical anion, O_2^-, and H_2O_2. The presence of H_2O_2 may then give rise to

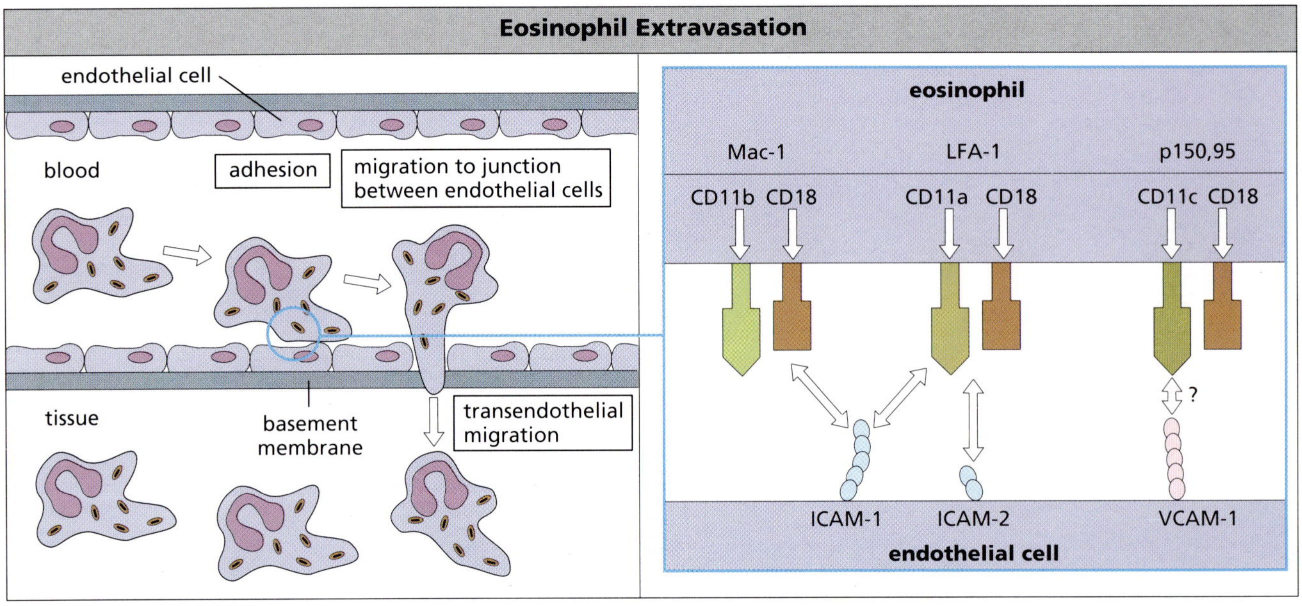

Fig. 6.9 Eosinophil extravasation and a model for adhesion molecules and receptors on endothelial cells. [left] the three steps involved in extravasation; [right] the integrin family of adhesion receptors on eosinophils are shown Adapted from Springer TA. Adhesion receptors of the immune system. *Nature* 1990; **346**: 425.

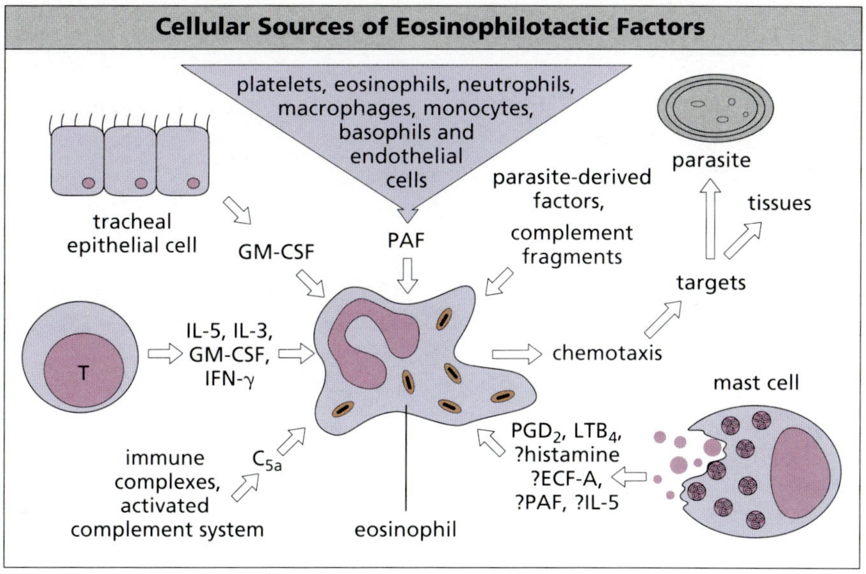

Fig. 6.10 The cellular sources of eosinophilotactic factors.

the potentially cytotoxic hypohalous acids such as HOBr:

$$H_2O_2 + Br^- + H^+ \xrightarrow{EPO} HOBr + H_20$$

Although Cl^- and I^- are also oxidized by EPO+H_2O_2, Br^- seems the likely reactant *in vivo* because the physiological concentrations are sufficiently high and because EPO prefers Br^- to Cl^- and I^-. Superoxide production is higher in hypodense than in normodense eosinophils. EAF and IL-1 also influence superoxide production.

Eosinophil Accumulation

Adhesion Molecules (Fig. 6.9)
Currently there is intense research into the adhesive interactions of cells with other cells and with the extracellular matrix. To act effectively, leucocytes must both circulate as non-adherent cells in blood and migrate as adherent cells through tissues. Three families of adhesion receptors facilitate these interactions:
(1) the immunoglobulin superfamily – includes the antigen-specific receptors of T and B lymphocytes and the intercellular cell adhesion molecule-1 (ICAM-1), expressed on the surface of vascular endothelial cells, and the vascular-cell adhesion molecule-1 (VCAM-1);
(2) the integrin family – important in dynamic regulation of adhesion and migration. Eosinophils express the lymphocyte function related antigen (LFA-1), macrophage antigen-1 (Mac-1), and p150,95; and
(3) the selectins – known to be prominent in lymphocyte and neutrophil interaction with vascular endothelium.

Many of the adhesion molecules have several functions; indeed, some are used as receptors by viruses.

Eosinophil Chemotactic Factors
Eosinophils are motile cells, and can respond to stimuli by chemokinesis (non-directional movement) and chemotaxis (directed migration to a site across a stimulus concentration gradient). Several chemotactic factors are implicated in the modulation of the influx and accumulation of eosinophils in tissues or sites of inflammation. *In vitro* studies have ascribed eosinophilotactic activity to many compounds (Fig. 6.10). However, as noted by CJF Spry (1988), the isolation of chemotactic factors that are specific *in vivo* for eosinophils remains elusive. For example, PAF is also chemotactic for neutrophils. Recent studies have shown the importance of LTB_4 (in guinea pigs), PGD_2 (in isolated dog trachea), IL-5, and GM-CSF.

Activation

Activation of eosinophils can be described as the augmentation of the effector properties of eosinophils. Many of the substances which are chemotactic for eosinophils or which enhance eosinophil survival also activate eosinophils as judged by surface receptor expression and enhanced function, such as respiratory burst, production of inflammatory mediators, and cytotoxicity. Cytokines produced by many cells, especially those of the immune system, are involved in eosinophil activation. The earliest studies to discover activated eosinophils utilized eosinophils from patients with eosinophilia and from parasitized individuals. These eosinophils had structural and functional differences compared to eosinophils from normal individuals. Fig. 6.11 shows various eosinophil activating factors and their sources.

In addition to these endogenous factors, parasites, e.g. schistosomula of *S. mansoni*, produce exogenous eosinophil activating factors. In one study the parasite-derived factor enhanced the cytotoxic capabilities of eosinophils more than neutrophils, suggesting a mechanism to explain why eosinophils are more toxic than neutrophils for schistosomula.

Relationship to Other Cells

Eosinophils and Endothelial Cells (Fig. 6.12)
The first study, in 1987, documented extended viability, lowered density, enhanced parasite killing activity, and enhanced LTC_4 production by peripheral blood eosinophils after coculture with bovine

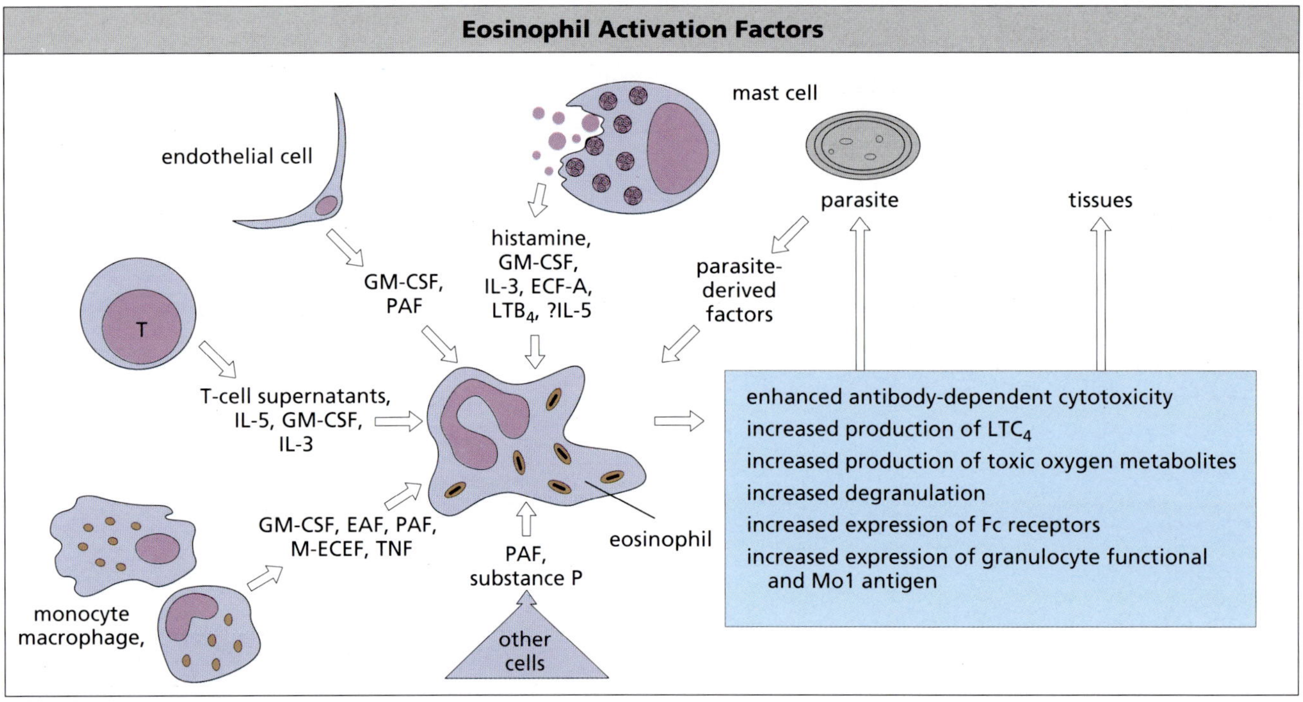

Fig. 6.11 The cellular sources and effects of eosinophil activating factors.

endothelial cells. Eosinophils cultured with either conditioned medium from cultures of bovine endothelial cells or human umbilical vein endothelial cells showed similar increased survival and activation. Not all the soluble factors secreted by endothelial cells have been identified. It is known that endothelial cells secrete growth factors; for example, TNF and IL-1 stimulate endothelial cells to produce GM-CSF. In a later study using human endothelial cell-conditioned medium, eosinophil survival was enhanced, but other cell types were unaffected. When endothelial cells were stimulated with IL-1, the resulting cell-conditioned medium caused increased eosinophil survival; conversely, endothelial cells stimulated with PAF showed no enhancement of eosinophil survival. TNF and IL-1 enhance endothelial cells' adhesive capacity for eosinophils and also for neutrophils, basophils and monocytes. These findings

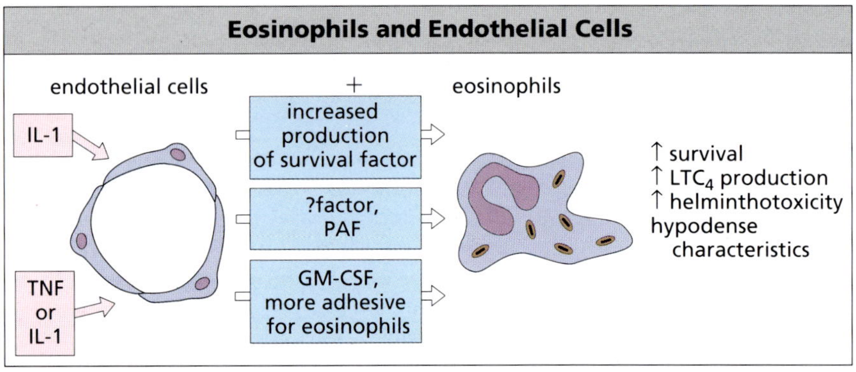

Fig. 6.12 Influence of endothelial cells on eosinophils.

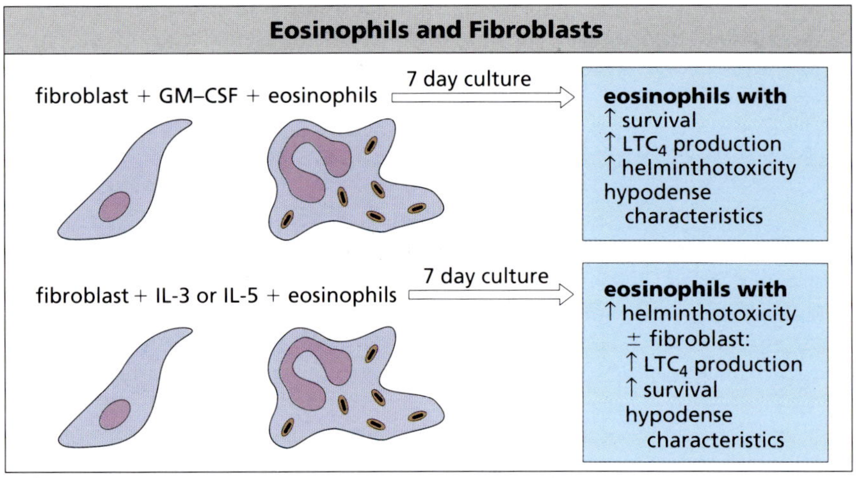

Fig. 6.13 Influence of fibroblasts on eosinophils.

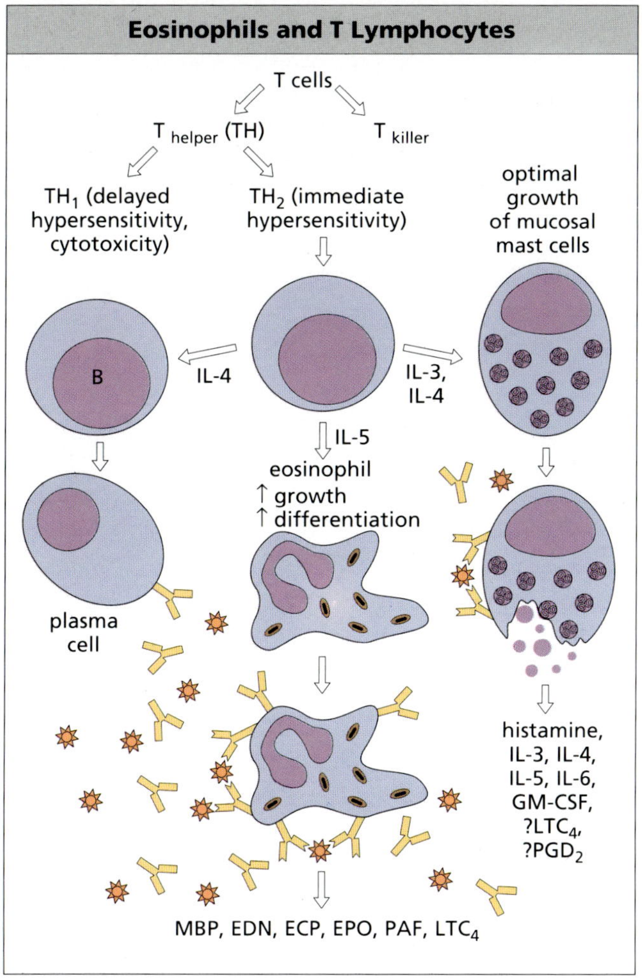

Fig. 6.14 B cells, eosinophils, and mucosal mast cells are involved in the TH_2 immediate hypersensitivity response. Antigen-specific IgG, IgA, and IgE antibodies on eosinophils and IgE mast cells can be bridged by antigen and allow release of toxic inflammatory mediators. Adapted from Coffman RL. T-helper heterogeneity and immune response patterns *Hospital Practice* 1989; **24**: 101.

have given rise to the hypothesis that the abundance of eosinophils during inflammation may result from non-selective recruitment of leucocytes combined with the release of local factors by endothelial cells that promote the survival of eosinophils but not of other cells.

Eosinophils and 3T3 Fibroblasts (Fig. 6.13)
Coculture studies with 3T3 fibroblasts were prompted by research showing enhanced survival of mast cells cocultured with 3T3 fibroblasts. Normodense human eosinophils cultured for seven days with GM-CSF and 3T3 fibroblasts survived longer than eosinophils cultured with either GM-CSF or fibroblasts alone; as well, they were hypodense and showed enhanced LTC_4 production and helminthotoxicity.

Another study investigated the culture of IL-3 and 3T3 fibroblasts with peripheral blood eosinophils. IL-3 enhanced the helminthotoxicity of freshly isolated eosinophils, but after seven days of culture, both IL-3 and 3T3 fibroblasts were necessary for helminthotoxicity. IL-3 was sufficient for extended viability, LTC_4 production and formation of hypodense eosinophils. Almost identical results have been shown with IL-5.

Eosinophils and T Lymphocytes (Fig. 6.14)
The two types of helper T (TH) cells are distinguished by the cytokines they synthesize. In general, the TH_1 subset regulates delayed-type hypersensitivity and cytotoxic reactions and TH_2 subset regulates immediate hypersensitivity or allergic reactions. By secretion of IL-4 and synergy with IL-5, the TH_2 cells stimulate B cells to produce IgA, IgG and IgE. TH_2 cells also secrete IL-5, a potent stimulator of eosinophil growth and differentiation. The immunoglobulin receptors on an increased population of eosinophils encounter an increased concentration of antibodies, and when the antibodies are bridged by appropriate antigens, toxic

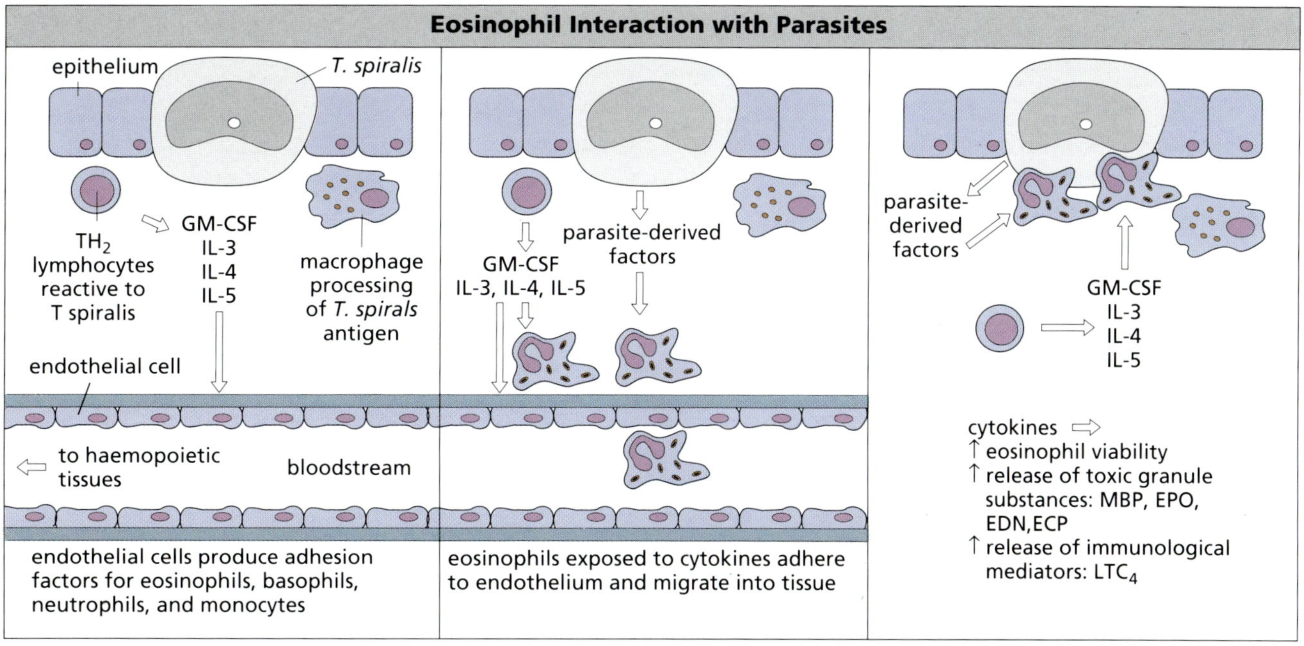

Fig. 6.15 [left] cytokines play a role in the development of eosinophilia; [middle] cytokines influence the migration of eosinophils to the tissue; this is the next stage in the development of the lesion; [right] cytokines influence the functions of the mature eosinophils in the lesion. Adapted from Silberstein DS, Austen KF, Owen WF Jr. Hemopoietins for eosinophils. In: *Hematology/Oncology Clinics of North America* 1989; **3**, 3: 525–526.

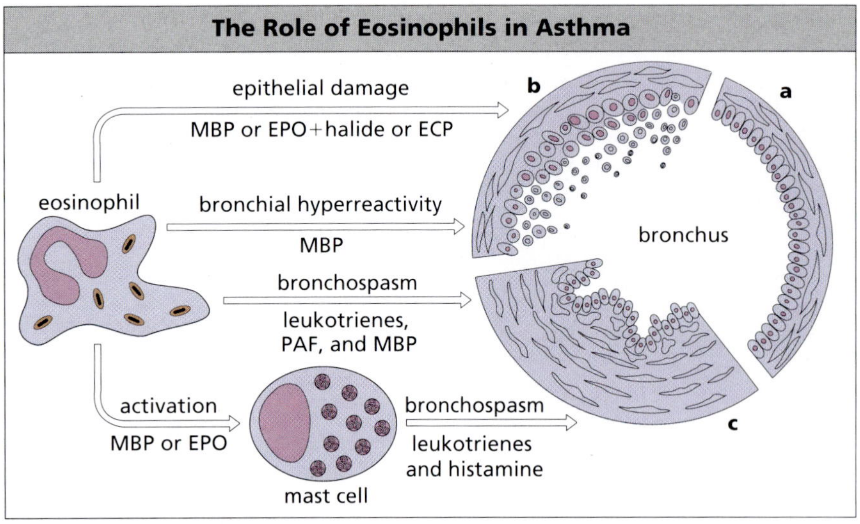

Fig. 6.16 (a) normal bronchus; (b) bronchus damaged by MBP, ECP or EPO showing epithelial desquamation; (c) smooth muscle hypertrophy, constriction, and oedema of the lamina propria, resulting in a reduction in the calibre of the airway.

granule contents and other mediators of inflammatory reactions are released. TH_2 secretion of IL-3 and IL-4 also enhances the growth of mast cells. Subsequently, the high-affinity IgE receptors on mast cells are bridged by allergen, releasing inflammatory mediators and cytokines capable of a 'feedback' effect on the immediate hypersensitivity reaction.

Model of Eosinophil Interaction with Parasites. Fig. 6.15 shows a possible scheme for the eosinophil response to a *T. spiralis* infection. The larva in the epithelium releases its soluble antigens into the tissues; these are processed by macrophages and stimulate TH_2 lymphocytes. The TH_2 cells secrete cytokines which stimulate eosinophil production and trigger endothelial cells' adhesion mechanisms for eosinophils, neutrophils and monocytes. The eosinophils move towards the parasite under the influence of the cytokines GM-CSF, IL-3, and IL-5, and possibly factors produced by the parasite itself. At the lesion the eosinophils, which have enhanced viability, degranulate and release their toxic granule constituents and immunological mediators.

Role of Eosinophils in Allergic Diseases

Lung

Infiltration of eosinophils into the bronchial wall and lumen and the resulting damage to the respiratory epithelium are two prominent pathological features of asthma. The pathogenesis of these features involves several steps, including enhanced eosinopoiesis, recruitment to the lungs, activation and release of putative effector molecules such as MBP (Fig. 6.16). Fig. 6.17 shows a tenfold increase in airway responsiveness two hours after 1 mg of MBP was instilled into the lung. PAF and leukotrienes may also act as contractile agonists for smooth muscle. PAF may also contribute to bronchial hyperresponsiveness in asthma by its ability to stimulate eosinophil degranulation. MBP or EPO+halide+H_2O_2 may induce mediator release from lung mast cells which in turn could contribute to smooth muscle contraction or hyperreactivity.

These results suggest a model system for asthma as a chronic late-phase response in the lung. Fig. 6.18 summarizes this, and shows the immediate allergic reaction initiated by allergen bridging mast cell IgE.

Skin

The relevant skin diseases are atopic dermatitis, chronic urticaria, episodic angioedema associated

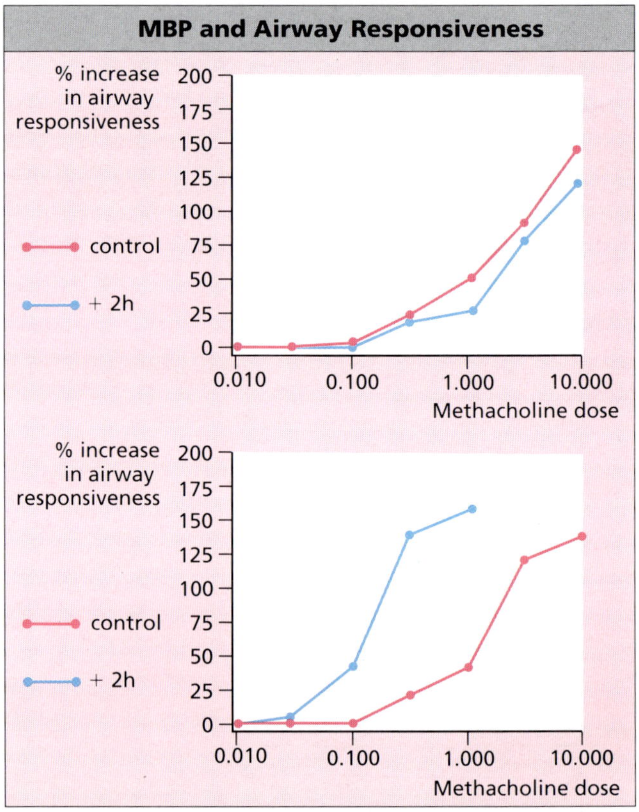

Fig. 6.17 An *in vivo* experiment with MBP in primate lung. Two hours after intratracheal instillation of [top] column buffer and [bottom] MBP (1.0mg), there was a tenfold increase in airway responsiveness to methacholine by MBP, as indicated by a shift to the left in dose-response curves (see Chapter 14). Column buffer, EPO, ECP, and EDN did not increase the airway responsiveness. Adapted from Gundel R, Letts LG, Gleich GJ. Human eosinophil major basic protein induces airway constriction and airway hyperresponsiveness in primates. *J Clin Investigation* 1991; **87**:1470.

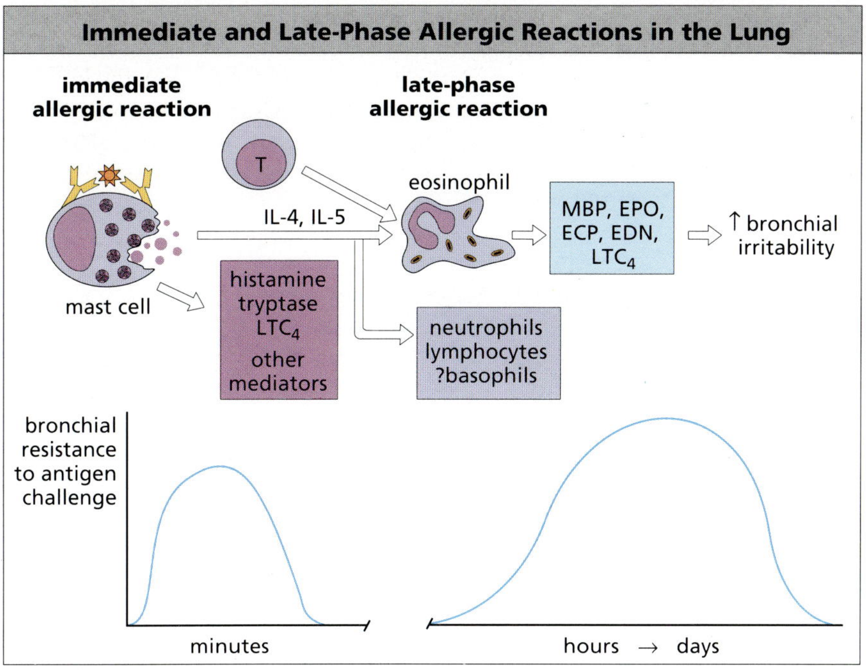

Fig. 6.18 [top] The cells and mediators prominent in the immediate and late-phase reaction. Mast cells are important in the immediate response; eosinophils in the late response; [bottom] the increased bronchial irritability during the late-phase reaction.

with eosinophilia, Well's syndrome, and recurrent facial oedema associated with eosinophilia.

Atopic dermatitis is frequently associated with increased serum IgE and peripheral blood eosinophilia, but eosinophils are not prevalent in the skin lesions. Immunofluorescence studies, however, show extensive extracellular MBP staining, indicative of eosinophil infiltration and degranulation.

The remaining four skin diseases manifest both oedema and extracellular deposition of MBP. In

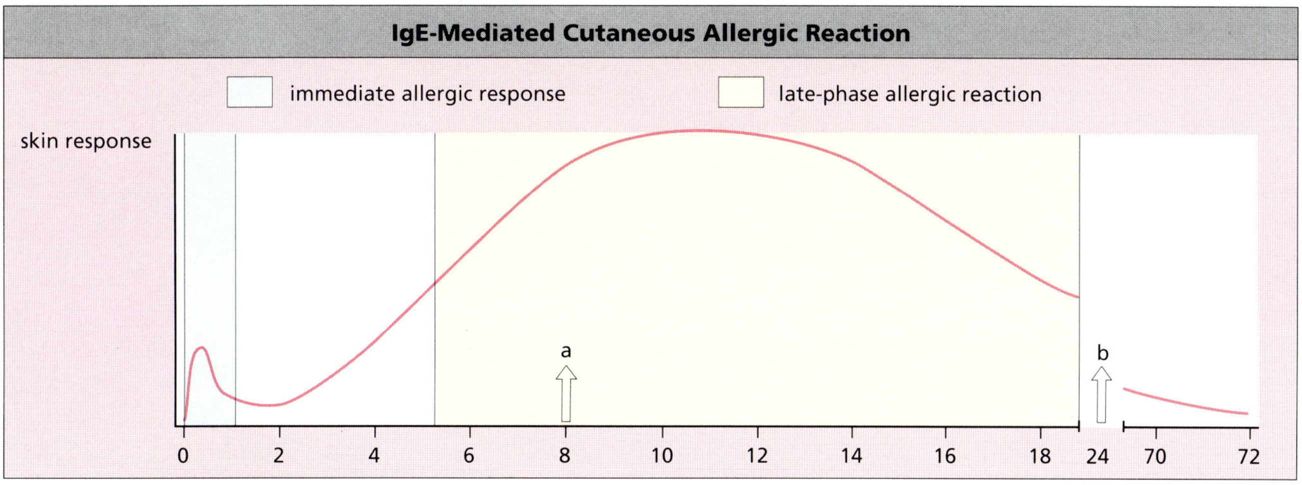

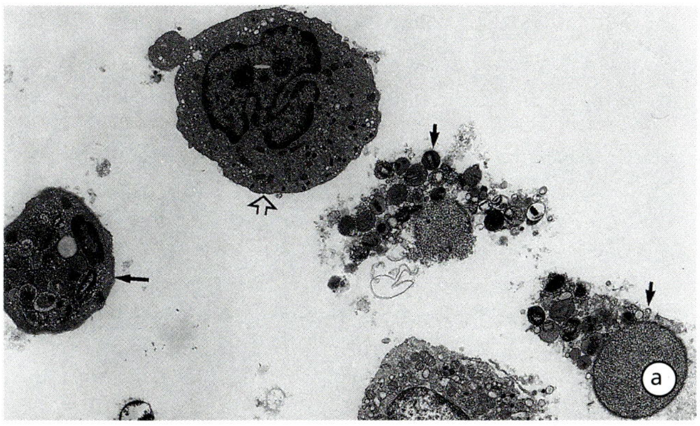

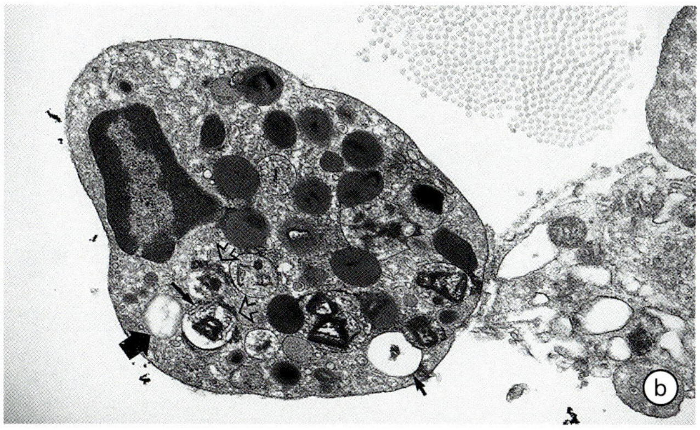

Fig. 6.19 Immediate weal-and-flare and late-phase cutaneous reactions. [top] Immediate weal-and-flare reaction peaks at 10–20 mins; few eosinophils seen. By 1–3 hr extensive extracellular MBP, EDN, and neutrophil elastase deposition. At 3–4 hr, late-phase reaction apparent with erythema, warmth, oedema, pruritus, and tenderness over a larger area. Late-phase reaction skin response, maximal at 6–12 hr, gradually subsides by 24–72 hours. [bottom] The cells involved in immediate and late-phase reactions: (a) at 8 hr – degranulated eosinophil without membranes (short dark arrow), eosinophil with lucent granules (long dark arrow) and intact neutrophil (open arrow); (b) at 24 hr – the eosinophil is intact, but some cores dissolved. (EMs provided by Dr KM Leiferman.)

chronic urticaria, MBP and ECP skin deposits are seen in the virtual absence of intact tissue eosinophils. Episodic angioedema associated with eosinophilia is characterized by recurrent attacks of fever, urticaria, and angioedema of the face, neck, trunk, and extremities. Blood eosinophils in episodic angioedema display morphological abnormalities, including granular changes, which suggest activation. In skin biopsies, diffusely infiltrating dermal eosinophils show marked abnormalities, suggesting degranulation; mast cells also appear to degranulate. On immunofluorescence, the biopsies show intense extracellular MBP staining. Patients with eosinophilia and recurrent facial oedema also have extracellular dermal MBP and elevated serum MBP. Well's syndrome is an eosinophilic cellulitis with oedematous and infiltrative plaques in the dermis, and characteristic eosinophilic deposits called 'flame figures' which show intense MBP staining.

The IgE-mediated cutaneous late-phase reaction has been compared to the late-phase response in asthma. Fig. 6.19 shows the skin response versus time in a typical weal-and-flare cutaneous reaction. The cutaneous late-phase reaction is dependent on IgE: IgE depletion abolishes both the immediate and late-phase reaction, and neither eosinophil nor neutrophil accumulation and degranulation occur.

Other Organs

Other organs with documented involvement of eosinophils in allergic disorders include the eye, the upper airway, and the paranasal sinuses. An early study found elevated levels of MBP and CLC protein in tears from patients with vernal keratoconjunctivitis; the MBP levels seemed to correlate with the severity of the disease. In a second study, biopsy specimens of conjunctiva from other patients with vernal keratoconjunctivitis and patients with giant papillary conjunctivitis showed MBP deposition, but specimens from normal controls showed no MBP deposition. In a third study that tested MBP levels in soft contact lenses, ten patients wearing contact lenses had giant papillary conjunctivitis, but only one of the 10 with an atopic history had MBP elevated on the lenses.

When seasonal allergic rhinitis patients had a nasal challenge with antigen, MBP, ECP, and EDN were found to be elevated in the nasal lavage during the late response several hours after challenge. In biopsy specimens of paranasal sinus tissue from chronic sinusitis patients with chronic asthma and/or allergic rhinitis, the tissues were extensively infiltrated with eosinophils. A direct association was seen between extracellular MBP deposition and mucosal damage.

Conclusions

The eosinophil is essentially a tissue inflammatory cell which matures in the bone marrow and is transported by the blood to its tissue of deposition. Migration and deposition in tissues may be influenced by cytokines, especially IL-5. The activated eosinophil may release its preformed mediators, MBP, ECP, EDN, and EPO, and generate LTC_4, PAF, and superoxide anions. Eosinophil-derived products probably play a major role in parasite killing and in the later inflammatory stages of asthma, rhinitis, conjunctivits, and cutaneous allergies.

Further Reading

Coffman RL. T-helper heterogeneity and immune response patterns. *Hospital Practice* 1989; **24**: 101.

Gleich GJ. Current understanding of eosinophil function. *Hospital Practice* 1988; **23**: 137.

Gleich GJ, Adolphson CR. The eosinophilic leukocyte: Structure and function. *Advances in Immunol* 1986; **39**: 177.

Hamann KJ, White S.R, Gundel RH, Gleich GJ. Interactions between respiratory epithelium and eosinophil granule proteins in asthma: The eosinophil hypothesis. In: Farmer SG, Hay DWP, eds: *The Airway Epithelium: Structure and Function in Health and Disease*. New York: Marcell Dekker Inc. In press.

Gundel RH, Letts LG, Gleich GJ. Human eosinophil major basic protein induces airway constriction and airway hyperresponsiveness in primates. *J Clin Invest* 1991; **87**: 1470.

Lamas AM, Marcotte GV, Schleimer RP. Human endothelial cells prolong eosinophil survival. Regulation by cytokines and glucocorticoids. *J Immun* 1989; **142**: 3978.

Leiferman KM, Fujisawa T, Gray BH, Gleich GJ. Extracellular deposition of eosinophil and neutrophil granule proteins in the IgE-mediated cutaneous late phase reaction. *Laboratory Investigation* 1990; **62**: 579.

Slifman NR, Adolphson CR, Gleich GJ. Eosinophils: Biochemical and cellular aspects. In Middleton E Jr, Reed CE, Ellis EF, Adkinson NF Jr, Yunginger JW, eds. *Allergy: Principles and Practice*, 3rd Ed, Vol 1. St. Louis: CV Mosby Co, 1988.

Springer TA. Adhesion receptors of the immune system. *Nature* 1990; **346**: 425.

Spry CJF. Eosinophils. A Comprehensive Review and Guide to the Scientific and Medical Literature. Oxford: Oxford University Press, 1988.

Weller PF. The immunobiology of eosinophils. *New England J Med* 1991; **324**: 1110

Chapter 7

Mononuclear Phagocytes and Dendritic Cells

Mononuclear Phagocytes

Cells of the macrophage/monocyte lineage are ubiquitous in the human body. Although there is great heterogeneity in morphology and function, which is probably determined by local tissue factors, the cells originate from the same bone marrow stem cell. Tissue macrophages are closely allied to dendritic cells and are strategically located at mucosal surfaces. Cells of the macrophage/monocyte lineage perform their role in host defence by non-specific endocytosis, by acting as accessory cells to lymphocytes in specific immunity, by releasing pro-inflammatory mediators for granulocytes, and by the secretion of over 100 bio-active substances with inflammatory and hormonal activities (Fig. 7.1).

Structure and Development of the Macrophage/MonocyteLineage

The mononuclear phagocyte system is a diffuse network of cells which arises in the bone marrow from the pluripotential stem cell. Under the control of glycoproteins, called colony stimulating factors, the stem cell develops into a committed cell for the mononuclear granulocyte lineage and then subsequently develops into a monoblast. Monoblasts are approximately 10 to 20 μm in diameter, have a half-life of 12 hours, and undergo one division in order to become promonocytes (see Figs 7.2 and 7.3). They are weakly phagocytic and demonstrate adherence to glass and plastic surfaces.

Promonocytes

Promonocytes are also 10 to 20 μm in diameter. They have a basophilic cytoplasm and have a high nuclear to cytoplasmic ratio. They are weakly phagocytic and adhere to glass plates. There is some peroxidase activity and they can synthesize DNA. Promonocytes undergo two divisions and develop into monocytes. During inflammation, promonocytes proliferate and are released into the circulation.

Functions of the Mononuclear Phagocyte System
1. non-specific endocytosis
2. inducible accessory cells for antigen presentation
3. secretion of bio-active substances
4. pro-inflammatory activity

Fig. 7.1 Mechanisms by which cells of the mononuclear phagocyte system perform their role.

Monocytes

Monocytes are approximately 10 to 18 μm in diameter, exist mainly in the circulation and have a bilobed nucleus. They contain approximately 30 azurophilic granules located near the Golgi complex and they have a reduced nuclear to cytoplasmic ratio. Their half-life within the circulation is approximately 10

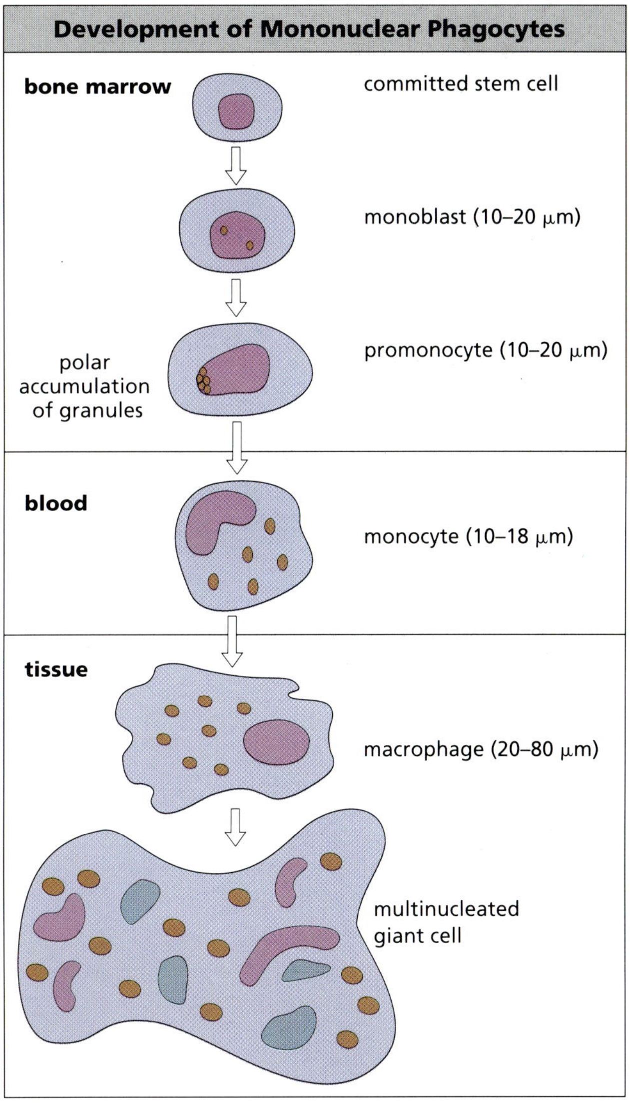

Fig. 7.2 Development of cells of the macrophage/ monocyte lineage from the stage of committed stem cell.

hours, after which they migrate to the extravascular pool. There is no evidence of a marginating pool of monocytes such as there is with neutrophils. As monocytes mature, they contain increased quantities of lysosomes and have increasing phagocytic activity. They are heterogeneous with regard to cell density, size, morphology and surface antigen expression. In the absence of local inflammation, this migration into the extravascular space occurs in a random fashion. The basal production rate of monocytes is about seven million cells per hour per day, and this is increased during inflammation to about 28 million cells per hour per day.

Macrophages

Circulating blood monocytes migrate into the tissues to form tissue macrophages, where they can exist in three forms (Fig. 7.3):

(1) cells which line serous cavities such as alveolar spaces, and exist in connective tissue as histiocytes;
(2) fixed-tissue macrophages, for example the Kupffer cells in the liver and the osteoclasts of bone. Fixed-tissue macrophages do not mount a respiratory 'burst' when activated. This mechanism may be important in protecting the host tissues from damage during endocytosis;
(3) activated macrophages, responding to a local inflammatory insult. When macrophages are activated they increase their size, express more surface antigen, and have augmented secretory and pro-inflammatory activities. It is interesting that patients who have received bone marrow transplantation develop the same karyotype as the donor in their alveolar macrophages and Kupffer cells at approximately two months, indicating that these cells are repopulated by cells of marrow origin.

Cells of the Mononuclear Phagocyte System in Normal and Inflamed Tissue

Cells	Localization
committed stem cells	bone marrow
monoblasts	bone marrow
promonocytes	bone marrow
monocytes	bone marrow (one day) blood (three days)
macrophages	tissues
free, normal state	
histiocytes	connective tissues
alveolar macrophages	lung
pleural/peritoneal	serous cavities
fixed, normal state	
Kupffer cells	liver
osteoclasts	bone
microglial cells	central nervous system
synovial A cells	joints
mesangial cells	kidney
fixed-tissue macrophages	spleen, lymph nodes, bone marrow
inflammation	
exudative macrophages	any inflamed tissue
activated macrophages	any inflamed tissue
elicited macrophages	any inflamed tissue
multinucleated giant cells	any inflamed tissue

Fig. 7.3 Sites of cells of the mononuclear phagocyte system.

Replication of cells of the monocyte/macrophage lineage

Replication of the macrophage lineage is under the control of specific growth factors produced by fibroblasts and lymphocytes. Colony stimulating factor-1 (CSF-1) is a glycoprotein with a molecular weight of 60 kDa and is lineage-specific for mononuclear phagocytes. Cells of this lineage also respond to factors which affect other haemopoietic lineages, e.g. granulocyte macrophage colony stimulating factor (GM-CSF) and granulocyte colony stimulating factor (G-CSF), which affect myeloid and mononuclear cell lineages; and interleukin-3 (IL-3), which affects myeloid, erythroid and lymphoid lineages. A soluble factor (probably interferon-gamma, [IFN-γ]) promotes formation of giant cells when added to cultured macrophages.

As cells of the monocyte/macrophage lineage mature, they lose their capacity to proliferate. Multinucleated giant cells and epithelioid cells in chronic inflammation represent fusion of macrophages caused by the failure of cytokinesis during mitosis. Monocytes and macrophages appear in these lesions before giant cells and are thus thought to be their precursors (Fig. 7.4).

Changes in Cellular Functional Characteristics with Maturation of Mononuclear Phagocytes

Property	promonocyte	monocyte	immature macrophage	mature macrophage *
proliferation	++++	+++	++	0
azurophilic granules	+++	++	±	0
lysosomes	+	++	++++	++++
glass adherence	+	++	+++	+++
endocytosis	±	+	+++	++++
Fc receptors	+	++	+++	+++
lymphocyte interactions	?	++	++++	++++
non-specific esterase	+++	+++	+++	+++
lysosomal secretion	?	++	++	++

* (similar in function to multinucleated giant cells)

Fig. 7.4 Properties of cells of the mononuclear phagocyte system.

Functions of Mononuclear Phagocytes

Secretory products of mononuclear phagocytes
Cells of the mononuclear phagocyte system congregate in most subacute or chronic inflammatory reactions. One of their responses is the secretion of approximately 100 bio-active substances. These substances include polypeptide hormones, e.g. (IL-1) and tumour necrosis factor (TNF); complement components; components of the coagulation pathways; bio-active lipids, e.g. the leukotrienes, prostanoids, and platelet activating factor; reactive oxygen intermediates and a host of other substances (Fig. 7.5).

A single macrophage product can have diverse activities, and a single activity can reflect the action of many macrophage products. Few products arise solely from macrophages. Cellular secretion is under complex control and varies with the state of maturation of the mononuclear phagocyte. Lysosome and complement components are secreted in all phases of activation. The secretion of other substances, for example arachidonic acid metabolites, acid hydrolases, and neutral proteases, is triggered and regulated by engagement of specific receptors, by endocytosis, or by exposure to membrane active drugs, such as tumour promoters, ionophores and endotoxins. Local tissue pH and local oxygen tension are also important in the regulation of secretion.

Surface Receptors (Fig. 7.6).
Cells of the mononuclear phagocyte system exhibit a wide range of surface antigen receptors. These receptors can be broadly divided into those with 'immune' and 'non-immune' functions. The expression of immune receptors greatly increases with maturation of the cell.

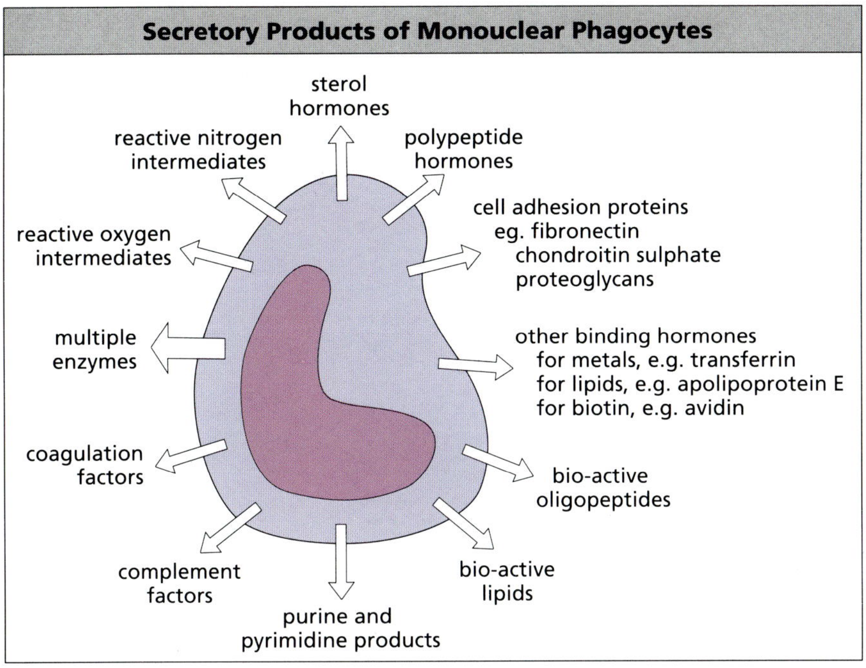

Fig. 7.5 Mononuclear phagocytes congregate in areas of inflammation, and secrete approximately 100 bio-active substances.

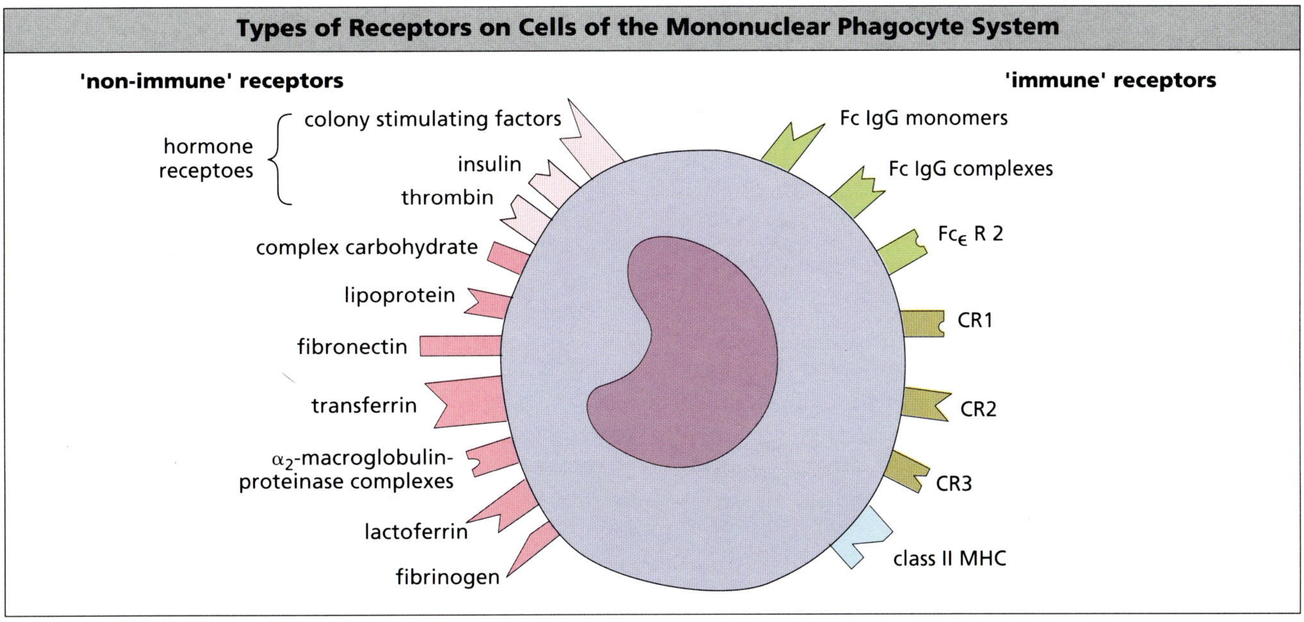

Fig. 7.6 Receptors on cells of the mononuclear phagocyte system.

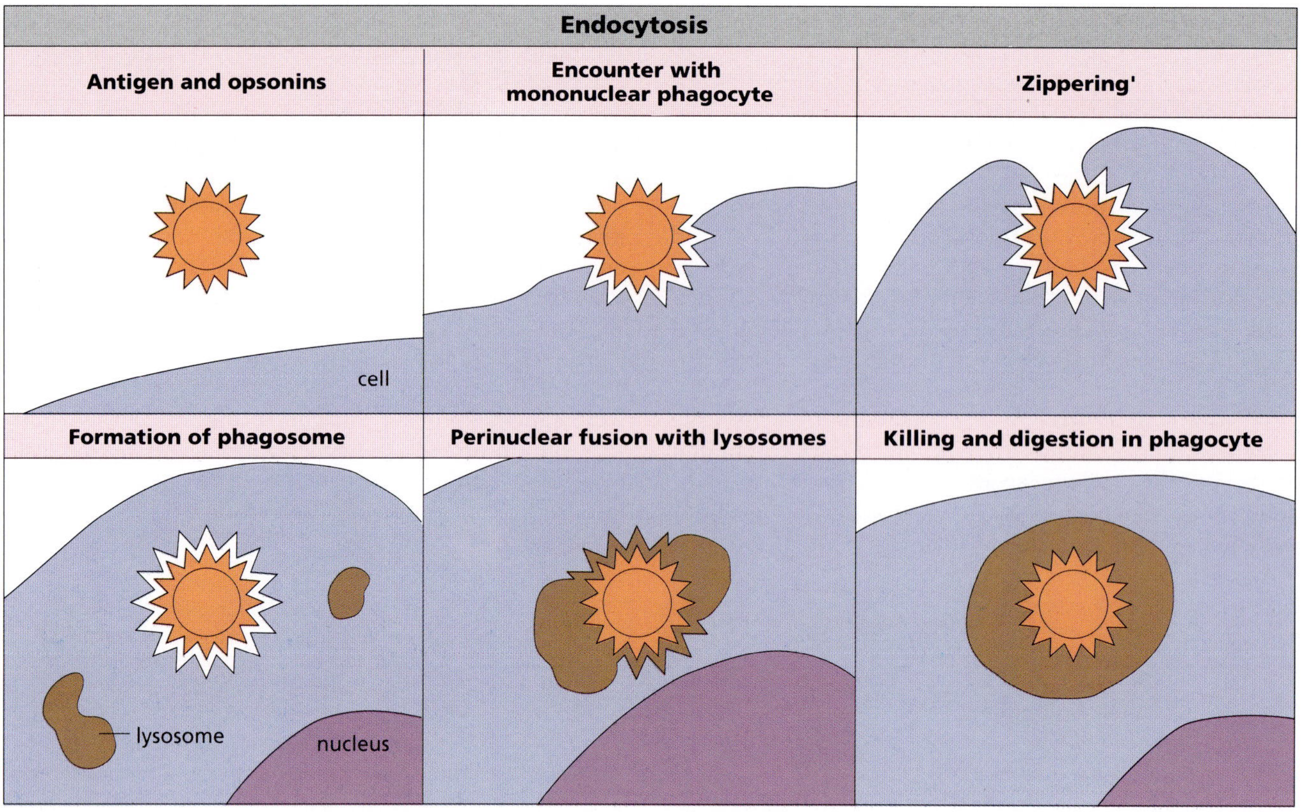

Fig. 7.7 Phagocytosis of an opsonized particle by a mononuclear phagocyte.

These receptors include those for the constant component of IgG monomers and IgG complexes; low-affinity receptors for the constant component of IgE ($Fc_{\epsilon}R2$), the expression of which is enhanced in allergic diseases such as bronchial asthma; and receptors for the complement components C3b, C3bi and C3d, which are also increased in allergic disease. All cells of the mononuclear phagocyte system bear class II histocompatibility (MHC) antigens which facilitate antigen presentation. However, antigen presentation in these cells is inducible and therefore not inherent, as it is in cells of the dendritic network.

There are many stimuli which increase receptor expression on monocuclear phagocytes. These stimuli include antigens, endotoxins, soluble factors such as the complement and coagulation components, and lymphokines produced by T cells.

In addition to immune receptors, the cells of the mononuclear phagocyte system exhibit a wide variety of other receptors indicating their diverse role in homeostasis.

Endocytosis

The most prominent function of mononuclear phagocytes is phagocytosis of opsonized particles (Fig. 7.7). Typical opsonins include IgG and the complement component C3b.

In order for ingestion to occur, the particulate antigen is circumferentially surrounded by the membrane of the cell during a process called sequential 'zippering' between opsonins and receptors. Once zippering is completed, a membrane-bound vesicle, which is distinct from the plasma membrane, is formed. This is called a phagosome. The phagosome

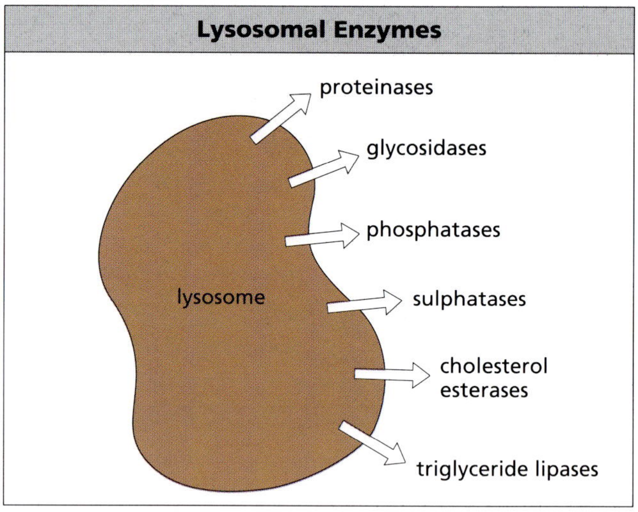

Fig. 7.8 Hydrolytic enzymes in lysosomes of mononuclear phagocytes.

then fuses with primary and secondary lysosomes in the cytoplasm of the phagocyte to form granules called phagolysosomes. Subsequent killing and acid digestion occur in these granules. This fusion occurs in the perinuclear area, to which the phagosomes have been guided by microtubules in an energy-requiring process. There are more than 40 hydrolytic enzymes present within lysosomes, which are located mainly in the perinuclear area where this process is completed (Fig. 7.8).

In free-tissue macrophages, e.g. alveolar macrophages, the killing process is augmented by a respiratory 'burst' which produces oxygen radicals (see Fig. 7.12).

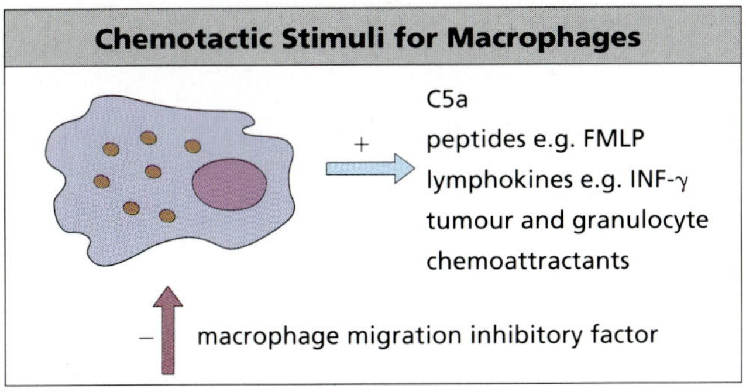

Fig. 7.9 Substances which cause chemotaxis of macrophages to sites of inflammation.

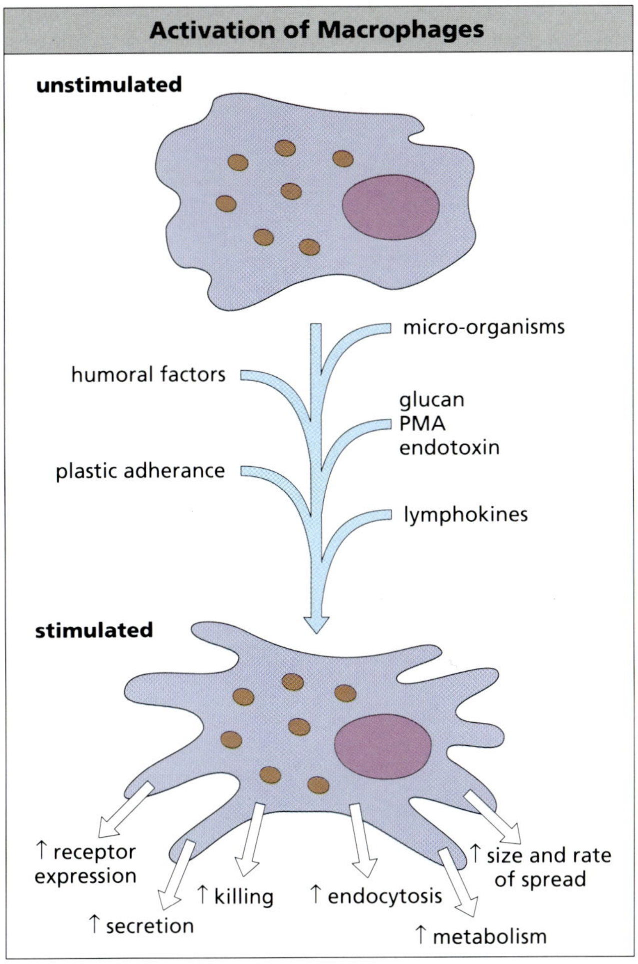

Fig. 7.10 Activation of macrophages causes them to undergo a wide variety of morphological, functional, and metabolic changes.

Chemotaxis

Chemotaxis occurs when cells move along a concentration gradient, and it is necessary in order to recruit cells from the circulating pool to sites of inflammation. Macrophages can be recruited and localized to sites of inflammation by various substances (Fig. 7.9):
(1) C5a, which is released indirectly by immune complexes and by bacteria via the alternative or classical pathways, or else directly by proteolytic enzymes themselves;
(2) peptides such as N-formyl-methionyl-leucyl-phenylalanine;
(3) lymphokines;

Properties of Activated Inflammatory Macrophages
Non-specific inflammatory events
↑ size and ruffling of plasmalemma ↑ rate of spread ↑ adherence to glass ↑ rate and extent of phagocytosis ↑ secretion ↑ cellular ATP ↑ O_2 consumption ↑ antigen presentation ↑ surface receptor expression
Lymphokine-mediated events
↑ H_2O_2 receptors ↑ microbicidal activity ↑ tumour cytostasis and killing ↑ chemotaxis

Fig. 7.11 Properties of activated inflammatory macrophages: some of the changes are non-specific changes and occur irrespective of the inciting agent; others are specific lymphokine-mediated events.

(4) chemoattractants from granulocytes and tumour cells;
(5) macrophage migration inhibition factor (MIF) and some proteolytic enzymes which prevent the random migration of macrophages away from sites of active inflammation.

Macrophages also release numerous chemotactic factors for other cells. These include leukotriene B_4, platelet activating factor, TNF, C5a, and a 10 kDa molecule which has yet to be characterized fully.

Activation of macrophages

Activation of macrophages enhances their activity to kill facultative intracellular micro-organisms and tumour cells. Macrophages can be activated directly by stimuli such as endotoxins, or indirectly by lymphokines. Activation can also occur with products of activated complement components or with IFN-γ. This activation is not specific for the primary inciting agent and indeed activated macrophages show an enhanced cytotoxicty for unrelated organisms. There are many causes of macrophage activation (Fig. 7.10):
(1) opsonized micro-organisms;
(2) opsonized tumour antigens;
(3) lymphokines, e.g. IFN-γ and GM-CSF;
(4) hormonal factors, e.g components of the complement or coagulation systems;
(5) glucan or phorbol diesters;
(6) agents which release cytokines such as TNF, which in turn may lead to auto-activation of the same macrophage.

When macrophages are activated, a wide range of morphological, functional and metabolic changes occur (Figs 7.10 and 7.11). There is an increase in size, with more pronounced ruffling of the plasma membrane, increased adherence and rate of spread on glass and plastic surfaces, increased rate and extent of phagocytic activity, and enhanced secretion. The metabolic changes include an increase in consumption of cellular ATP and oxygen. Receptor expression is enhanced, as is antigen presentation.

These events are mostly non-specific and occur irrespective of the inciting agent. Specific lymphokine-mediated events include increased microbicidal and tumoricidal activity, and increased production of the hydrogen peroxide radical (see Fig. 7.11).

Macrophage activation is a complex phenomenon. Mononuclear phagocytes are very heterogeneous, and cells taken from different sites differ in their responsiveness. These differences are most likely due to environmental and maturational influences.

Metabolism of macrophages

Macrophages process many antigenic stimuli by endocytosis and subsequent acid digestion in the phagolysosome system. This process is usually accompanied by an increase in oxygen consumption. This is associated with increased oxidation of glucose by the hexose-monophosphate shunt. This respiratory burst, however, is not dependent on endocytosis, and may occur alone when macrophages are stimulated by immune complexes, ionophores or certain tumour promoters. The respiratory burst can help degrade ingested micro-organisms or, by releasing reactive oxygen species into the extracellular milieu, can lead to tissue damage and inflammation.

During activation of macrophages, a membrane-associated oxidase (pyridine-nucleotide-dependent oxidase, or PNDO) converts oxygen to the superoxide radical (Fig. 7.12).

$$0_2 \longrightarrow 0_2^{\cdot}\text{(superoxide)}$$

Either spontaneously, or via an enzyme called dismutase, hydrogen peroxide is formed:

$$0_2^{\cdot} + 0_2^{\cdot} + 2H \longrightarrow H_2O_2 + O_2\text{(hydrogen peroxide)}$$

Superoxide and hydrogen peroxide then interact to yield the hydroxyl radical and singlet oxygen. Hydrogen peroxide reacts with and is inactivated by GSH peroxidase, with subsequent oxidation of reduced GSH (glutathione). Reduced GSH is regenerated by GSH reductase and this is accompanied by oxidation of reduced NADPH derived from the activated hexose-monophosphate shunt.

Products of this respiratory burst are microbicidal and can cause tissue inflammation. The macrophage is protected by its stores of GSH peroxidase and catalase. These reactive oxygen species are used most effectively in association with granule-derived peroxidases, especially myeloperoxidase.These granule-derived peroxidases catalyse hydrogen-peroxide-mediated oxygenation of halide ions to hypohalides:

$$\text{Halide anion} + H_2O_2 \longrightarrow \text{Halide radicals}$$

One product of this reaction, namely hypochloride, is extremely microbicidal, especially when it reacts with either ammonia or amines to form chloramines.

Endocytosis therefore may or may not be associated with a respiratory burst by activation of a membrane-bound oxidase. Both processes work together for enhanced microbicidal and inflammatory activity, especially when hypohalide ions are formed. Fixed-tissue macrophages do not exhibit the respiratory burst.

Antigen processing and presentation

Cells of the mononuclear phagocyte system are a major determinant of innate immunity because of their strategic location near portals of entry to the body. They are responsible for endocytosis of most particulate matter entering via these routes. They

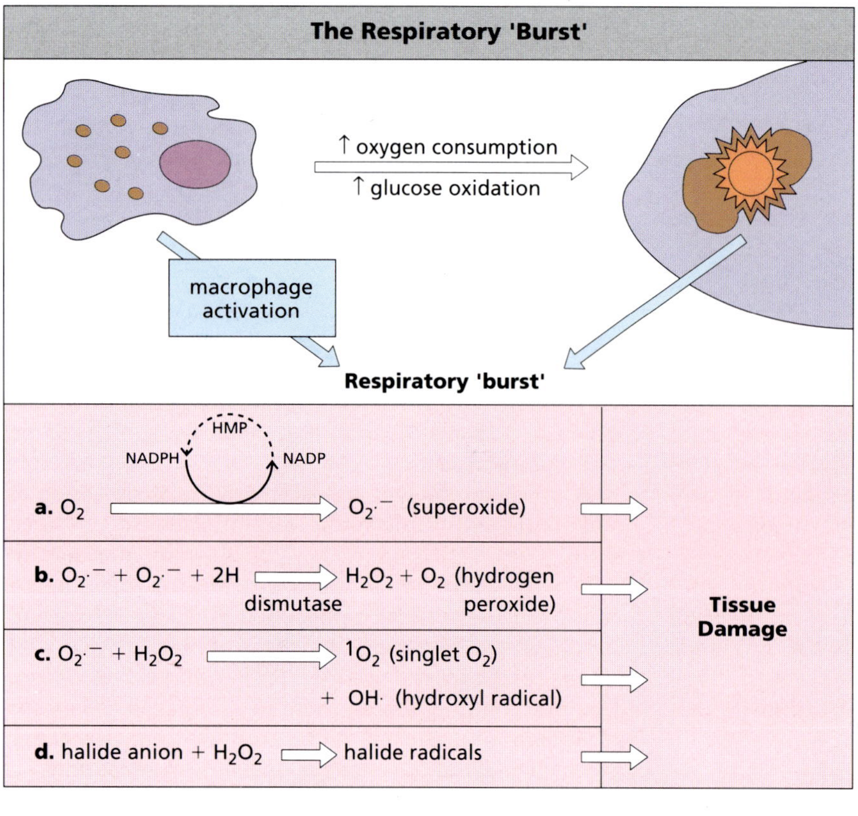

Fig. 7.12 The respiratory burst, which usually accompanies endocytosis and acid digestion of opsonized particles in the phagolysosome system. It may also occur without endocytosis, for example when macrophages are stimulated by immune complexes, ionophores, or certain tumour promotors.

can be activated to become antigen-presenting cells, bearing characteristic class II MHC receptors which enable interaction with T lymphocytes.

Antigens opsonized with immunoglobulin and complement interact with cells of the mononuclear phagocyte system. The antigen is processed intracellularly to become approximately eight to 24 amino acids in size. The processed antigen is then presented to T lymphocytes in association with class II MHC antigen on the surface of the phagocyte. The T cell then produces cytokines which, in addition to other functions, serve to activate resting macrophages for enhanced microbicidal, tumoricidal and secretory roles. One of the main lymphokines secreted by T cells is INF-γ.

The function of antigen processing and presentation is in the most part inducible in cells of the mononuclear phagocyte system, whereas in the closely allied dendritic cell network it is more constitutive. Activated macrophages can also augment or diminish non-specifically the proliferation of lymphocytes by producing other cytokines (e.g. IL-1).

Macrophages therefore are inherently involved in all aspects of immunity, from non-specific innate immunity to complex cell-mediated immunity involving both T and B cells. They are also immune effector cells by virtue of the products they secrete when activated. It is important to note that class II MHC antigen expression on mononuclear phagocytes can be augmented by certain cytokines (such as INF-γ produced from T cells) once an antigen is recognized, and also by 'auto-activation' by TNF which is produced by the macrophages themselves (Fig. 7.13).

Role of the Mononuclear Phagocyte System in Allergic Diseases

Mononuclear phagocytic cells in the lungs include alveolar macrophages, interstitial macrophages, circulating blood monocytes and airway macrophages. (Fig. 7.14).

There is now abundant evidence that macrophages are inherent airway cells and do not arrive there purely via the mucociliary escalator from the distal alveoli. The number of macrophages in the bronchial mucosa of asthmatic patients, as identified with the HAM 56 pan-macrophage marker, is significantly increased as compared to normals. Many of these cells express phenotypic characteristics of blood

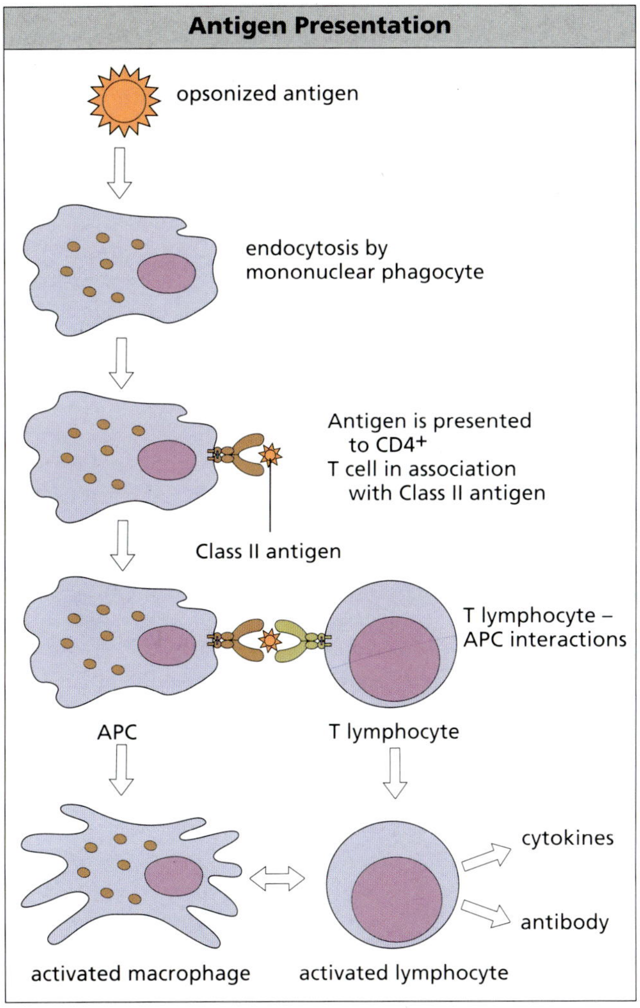

Fig. 7.13 Cells of the mononuclear phagocyte system are located near portals of entry to the body, and are responsible for endocytosis of foreign matter entering via these routes. Once activated, they become antigen-presenting cells bearing class II MHC receptors which enable interaction with T lymphocytes.

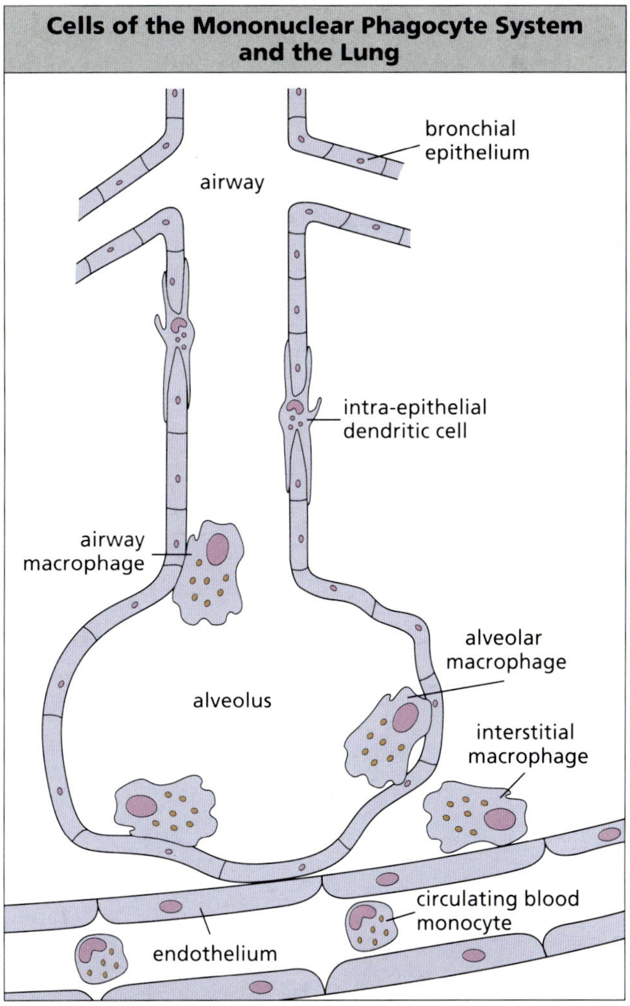

Fig. 7.14 Macrophages are inherent airway cells, and their numbers in the bronchial mucosa are significantly increased in patients with asthma.

monocytes. HLA class II antigen is expressed on the infiltrating cells and on airway epithelial cells in patients with asthma. There is also a significant difference in the numbers of primed T cells, which included T memory cells, staining positive with UCHL1 monoclonal antibody between asthmatic and normal subjects. Viable macrophages have recently been shown to reside directly on top of the epithelium at the air-surface interface of human airways. By isolated segmental bronchoalveolar lavage of the large airways it is now known that macrophages are the predominant white cell at this site in normals and in subjects with mild asthma.

Lung macrophages are relatively long-lived phagocytes, surviving more than one month. Most of these cells arise from the bone marrow rather than by proliferation of locally resident cells.

It now seems probable that the cells of the monocuclear phagocyte system are involved in the pathogenetic process of asthma (Fig. 7.15).

In 1975, IgE receptors ($Fc_{\epsilon}R$) on macrophages were first described by implicating the role of IgE antibodies in macrophage-dependent cytotoxic damage to parasites. It is now believed that the $Fc_{\epsilon}R$ expressed on the surface of macrophages is identical to that on T and B lymphocytes. This receptor is referred to as $Fc_{\epsilon}R2$ and differs in both structure and function from the $Fc_{\epsilon}R1$ on mast cells and basophils. The most important functional difference is that the $Fc_{\epsilon}R2$ on macrophages is a lower affinity receptor and has the potential to be activated preferentially by IgE immune complexes. Approximately 5 to 10 per cent of peripheral blood mononuclear cells and lung macrophages from normal non-atopic humans bear $Fc_{\epsilon}R2$. This number increases in atopic subjects to approximately 20 per cent in mildly atopic asthmatic subjects. Patients with severe asthma and atopic eczema who have been treated with corticosteroid have a substantially lower percentage of $Fc_{\epsilon}R2$-positive peripheral blood monocytes. Thus monocytes and macrophages of asthmatic patients appear to have enhanced expression of $Fc_{\epsilon}R2$ which can be modulated by corticosteroid treatments.

Mononuclear phagocytes derived from asthmatic subjects exhibit other functional abnormalities. They show increased complement receptor expression compared with those of normal subjects, and also greater enhancement of receptor expression following stimulation with casein. The numbers of peripheral blood monocytes which form rosettes with complement-coated red blood cells are significantly increased in asthmatic patients after allergen bronchoprovocation, but not after histamine-induced bronchoconstriction. The respiratory burst of cultured macrophages obtained from subjects with asthma is increased as compared with that observed in macrophages from normal subjects. Analysis of bronchoalveloar lavage (BAL) fluid from patients with asthma following antigen challenge reveals increased amounts of β-glucuronidase, whereas macrophage intracellular levels of β-glucuronidase are decreased as compared to the levels found in BAL fluid from non-atopic control subjects. This suggests that macrophage secretory progress may be activated by allergen. It has also been shown that the total numbers of mononuclear phagocytes present in BAL fluid are increased at 48 and 96 hours after antigen challenge. The macrophages stain positively for peroxidase, suggesting that a population of monocytes had entered the lung from the local vascular compartment.

Mononuclear phagocytes may participate in airways inflammation by the release of factors which can modulate the function of other cells. Thus macrophages release numerous chemotaxins which include leukotriene B_4 (LTB_4) platelet-activating factor (PAF), TNF, C5a, platelet-derived growth factor, and a 10 kDa molecule that has yet to be characterized fully. Furthermore, macrophages secrete a 6 kDa glycoprotein which increases the bactericidal activity of neutrophils. Peripheral blood mononuclear cells also secrete a range of pro-inflammatory cytokines with granulocyte activating properties including IL-1, TNF, colony stimulating factors, and histamine releasing factors. They also secrete a range of heat-stable factors of heterogenous size and charge, which prime eosinophils and neutrophils for increased leukotriene generation following subsequent stimulation, and factors which prime eosinophils for enhanced cytotoxicity against *Schistosoma mansoni*; one of these factors is eosinophil cytotoxicity enhancing factor. Lung macrophages are also able to modulate the generation of leukotriene by eosinophils. Howell *et al* identified an activity secreted by asthmatic lung macrophages which augmented eosinophil generation of both LTC_4 and PAF. Partial purification obtained the major activity in substantial purity and, based on its neutralization by specific antibody, it was characterized as GM-CSF. GM-CSF stimulates

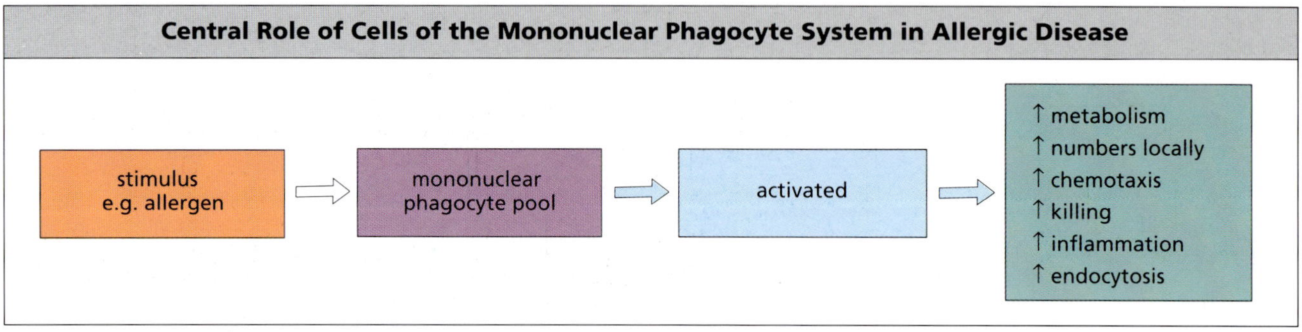

Fig. 7.15 Cells of the mononuclear phagocyte system are now thought to be involved in the pathogenesis of allergic disease.

the proliferation and differentiation of normal granulocytes and monocytes from stem cells, primes granulocytes for enhanced generation of LTC_4 and PAF, induces histamine release from basophils and enhances eosinophil survival in culture. In addition, GM-CSF activates macrophages to become tumoricidal, to express class II antigen, and to release PGE_2; it also stimulates neutrophils and macrophages to secrete other cytokines such as IL-1, TNF, G-CSF, and M-CSF.

The enhanced generation of a granulocyte activating factor by monocytes derived from asthmatic subjects which is capable of increasing the capacity of human neutrophils to produce LTB_4 and eosinophils to produce LTC_4 following subsequent stimulation has recently been demonstrated. Incubation of monocytes from corticosteroid-sensitive asthmatic subjects (those who show over 30 per cent improvement in FEV_1 after two weeks' treatment with 40 mg prednisolone per day) with 10^{-8} M hydrocortisone inhibited the production of the enhancing activity, whereas in corticosteroid-resistant asthmatic subjects (those who show less than 15 per cent improvement in FEV_1 after two weeks' treatment with 40 mg prednisolone per day), hydrocortisone concentration up to 10^{-4} M did not suppress the release of the enhancing activity. The molecule has been purified to homogeneity and is a peptide of 3 kDa molecular weight.

Macrophage/lymphocyte interaction is apparent in asthma. There are elevated numbers of T lymphocytes in BAL fluid from asthmatic subjects after localized allergen challenge and in the submucosa from biopsies obtained from asthmatic subjects. Furthermore, peripheral blood T cells appear to be activated in acute asthma. Macrophages initiate lymphocyte responses to antigen/allergen through the elaboration of IL-1, which stimulates T-cell IL-2 receptor expression and IL-2 secretion. T cells, under the influence of IL-2, differentiate to secrete additional lymphokines including IL-4, one of whose functions is to enhance the expression of $Fc_\epsilon R2$ on peripheral blood mono-nuclear cells cultured *in vitro*. Alveolar macrophages derived from asthmatic subjects *in vitro* show enhanced generation of LTB_4 in response to an IgG stimulus when primed with a lymphocyte product, INF-γ. These data suggest that macrophage-lymphocyte interaction is important in atopic disease states.

Macrophages, in common with lymphocytes and platelets, produce a number of histamine releasing factors (HRFs). HRFs are an incompletely characterized group of molecules with molecular weights of between 15 and 30 kDa, and they are distinct from other cytokines produced from macrophages which may in themselves cause histamine release. HRFs all cause histamine release from basophils and mast cells via an interaction with cell-surface-bound IgE. There is now abundant evidence that HRF/ mast cell/basophil interaction is implicated in allergic disease states.

Macrophage products can influence bronchial smooth muscle function through the elaboration of mediators which can stimulate contraction or which can alter the contractile state. Thromboxane A_2 (TXA_2) is a potent smooth muscle constrictor produced form arachidonic acid via the cyclo-oxygenase pathway and is generated in large quantities by alveolar macrophages. It is elevated in BAL fluid in patients with asthma. PGE_2 is a potent bronchodilator *in vivo* and *in vitro* and is released in large quantities by alveolar macrophages. Workers have measured the ratio of bronchoconstricting prostanoids to bronchodilating prostanoids and found that asthmatic subjects generate greater amounts of bronchoconstricting prostanoids than do controls, and suggesting that the asthmatic state may be related to the ratio of these mediators in the lungs of these patients.

Dendritic Cells

Dendritic cells have a characteristic morphology (Fig. 7.16) and are found in the following areas:

- the epidermis and dermis, e.g. the Langherhans' cells which constitute about 2 per cent of all epidermal cells.
- the paracortical areas of lymph nodes, i.e. interdigitating cells.
- the B-cell germinal centres of the spleen, i.e. follicular dendritic cells.
- the thymus, where they may be important in recognition of self antigens.
- the bronchial epithelium (interdigitating cells) where they are four to eight times more potent than alveolar macrophages as antigen-presenting cells.

Their secretion of IL-1 and TNF is much less when compared to peripheral blood monocytes and alveolar macrophages. They are related functionally to fixed-tissue macrophages, although their origin is different. It has emerged that they are derived from the bone-marrow and are continually repopulated from a mobile pool of precursor cells. They express a wide

Dendritic Cell

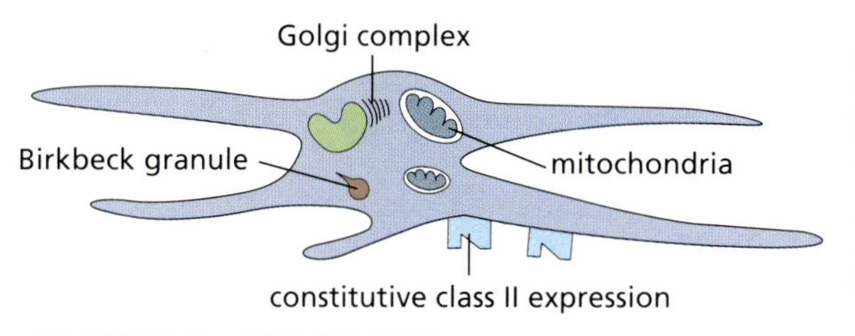

Characteristics of dendritic cells

1. distinctive morphology
2. Birkbeck granule in cytoplasm
3. located at sites of maximum antigen encounter
4. constitutive antigen presentation
5. non-phagocytic
6. high class II expression

Fig. 7.16 Dendritic cells are morphologically distinct, and play a key role in enhancing immunogenicity.

variety of surface markers of the monocyte/macrophage lineage, including MHC class II antigen.

Morphologically they are distinctive. They contain a lobulated or indented nucleus, a clear cytoplasm with rough endoplasmic reticulum, a well-defined Golgi complex, numerous mitochondria and they are devoid of tonofilaments. Their most characteristic ultrastructural feature is the presence of distinctive cytoplasmic granules (Birkbeck granules), the function of which is unclear. These granules usually appear in thin sections as rods with a central zipper-like striation, but can sometimes be seen as 'tennis racket'-like structures with an expansion at one end.

In contrast to other white cells, dendritic cells do not phagocytose and kill micro-organisms, or exhibit a respiratory burst, and unlike lymphocytes, dendritic cells do not secrete cytokines or immunoglobulins. However, when dendritic cells are mixed together with lymphocytes, they act as powerful accessory cells for lymphocyte growth and differentiation. Antigens gain access to the spleen or lymph nodes via the blood and lymph respectively. There is long-standing evidence that sensitization to transplantation and contact antigens in the skin require intact afferent lymphatics. Dendritic cells are present in afferent (but not efferent) lymph and they have been noted in afferent lymph following the application of transplant or contact allergen. If antigen is applied to the skin, one can identify antigen-bearing dendritic cells draining the lymph nodes between eight and 48 hours later, suggesting that Langherhans' cells in the epidermis bind the antigen and carry it to the lymph node.

The thesis is thus emerging that dendritic cells are specialized to pick up antigens and to take them to the T-cell areas of the spleen or lymph nodes via the blood or lymph respectively, where clones of antigen-specific T cells can be selected from the recirculating pool. Later, enlarged T cells leave the lymphoid organ in large numbers in the efferent lymph, thereby gaining access to the blood steam via the thoracic duct. These sensitized cells can leave the blood and accumulate in an antigen-non-specific way in any inflammatory site.

The dendritic cell network therefore plays a key role in enhancing immunogenicity. Dendritic cells pick up antigen in the tissues and move it to lymphoid organs for interaction with T-lymphocytes. Dendritic cells enhance binding of specific T lymphocytes and promote the induction of lymphokines and growth factors required for lymphoblastic proliferation of clonally specific T cells.

Further Reading

Johnson RB. Monocytes and macrophages; Current concepts. *New Eng J Med*; **318**:12:747–753

Johnson RB Jnr, Zucker-Franklyn D. Monocytes and macrophages. In: Zucker-Franklyn D, Greaves MF, Grossi CE, Marmont AM, eds. *Atlas of blood cells; function and pathology*, 2nd Ed. Philadelphia: Lea and Febiger.

Nathan CF. Secretory produces of macrophages. *J Clin Invest* 1987; **79**:319–326.

Werb Z. *Phagocytic cells:* Chemotaxis and effector functions of macrophages and granulocytes. In: Stipes DP, Stokes JD, Wells JV, eds. *Basic and Clin Immun*, 6th Ed. Norwark, Connecticut: Appleton and Lange.

Howell CJ, Pujol JL, Crea AEG, et al. Identification of an alveolar macrophage derived activity in bronchial asthma which enhances leukotriene C4 generation by human eosinophils stimulated by ionophore as granulocyte macrophage colony-stimulating factor (GM-CSF). *Am Rev Resp Dis* 1987; 1340–1347.

Cohn ZA. The activation of mononuclear phagocytes: fact, fancy and future. *J Immunol* 1978; **121**:813–6.

Unanue ER, Allen PM. The basis for the immunoregulatory role of macrophages and other accessory cells. *Science* 1987; **236**:551–7.

Chapter 8

Platelets

Introduction

The platelet is the smallest blood element and, being devoid of a nucleus, it is often considered not to be a true cell type. Classically, platelets have been thought to be produced in bone marrow as products of budding of the large precursor cell line, the megakaryocyte, although recently this view has been challenged. Recent mathematical, experimental and clinical evidence has suggested that blood platelets may in fact be produced as fragmentation products of megakaryocytes in the pulmonary vasculature.

Although the production of platelets remains controversial, the appearance of platelets in the circulation is not disputed and their presence within the vascular system is viewed as providing a mechanism for repairing damaged areas of the vasculature. The evidence that platelets are active participants in physiological homeostatic mechanisms, and that they are central to the development of pathological conditions such as thrombosis and related cardiovascular disorders, is considerable. However, it is now apparent that platelets can also behave as effector cells in allergic inflammatory responses, and that they have many properties which make them analogous to blood leucocytes. When observed under the electron microscope (Fig. 8.1), unstimulated platelets have a characteristic discoid appearance and contain a variety of granular structures connected via an open canicular network. Three granule types have been described: dense bodies, alpha granules, and lysosomes (Fig. 8.2), and these granules contain a range of biologically active substances.

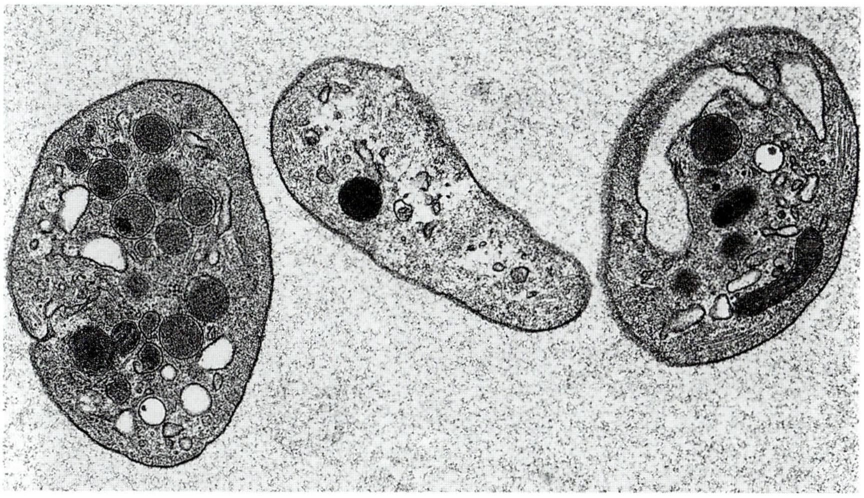

Fig. 8.1 An electron micrograph of a human platelet. (×30,000). (Courtesy of Dr CM Lees, Ciba-Geigy Research Centre, Horsham, West Sussex.)

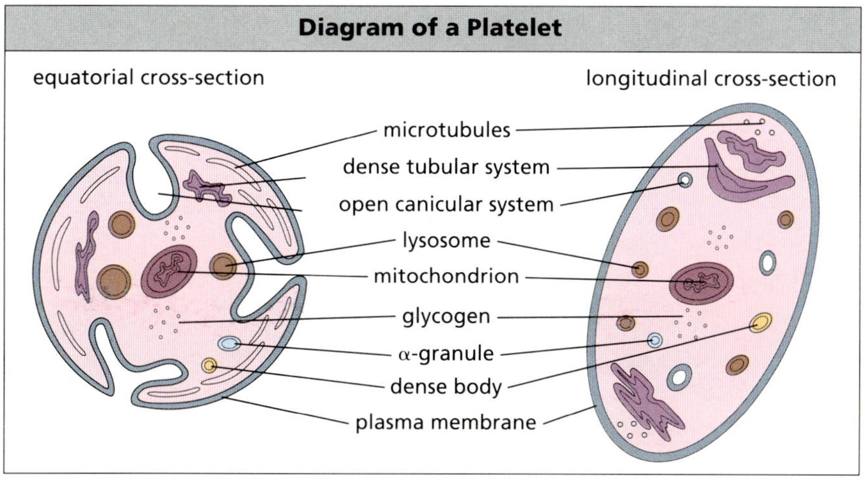

Fig. 8.2 A schematic representation of a human platelet showing both the longtitudinal and equatorial cross-sections.

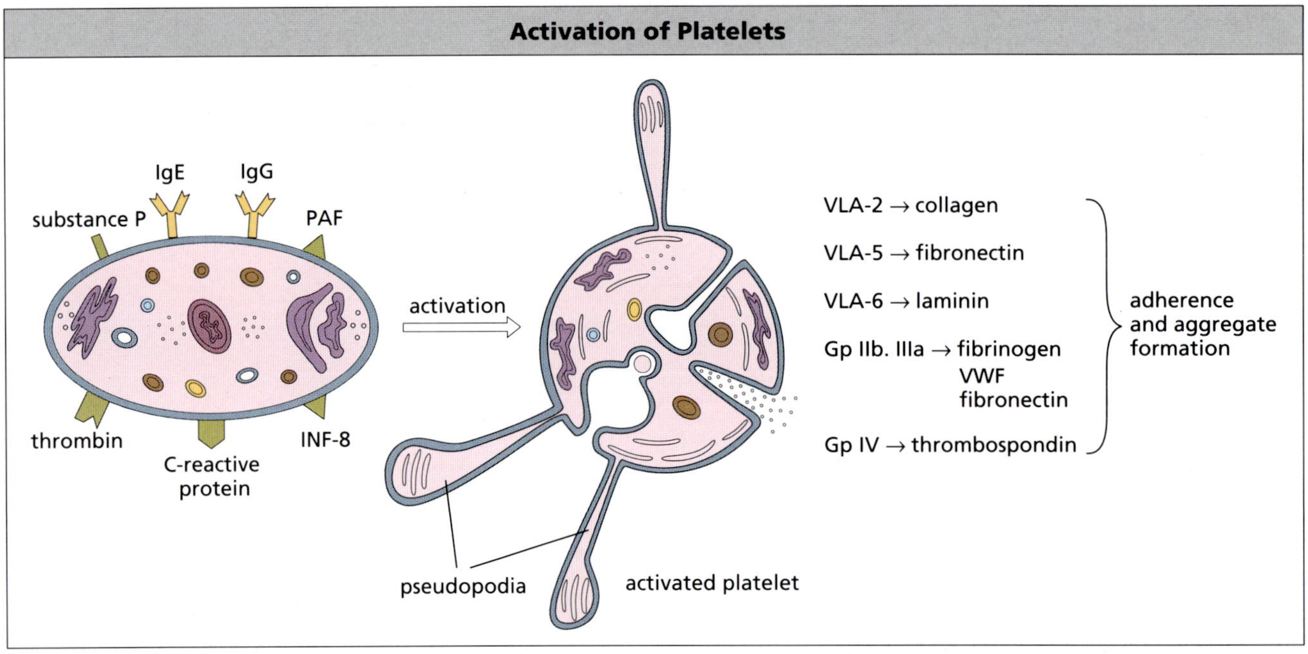

Fig. 8.3 Diagrammatic representation of receptors present on human platelets for endogenous agonists and the major classes of adhesive molecules expressed following platelet activation.

Surface Receptors on Platelets

Human platelets have been shown to possess a range of receptors on their surface. These receptors can be stimulated by a variety of circulating agonists, which cause them to change shape and to form pseudopodia (Fig. 8.3). In particular, the fibrinogen receptor protein Gp II_bIII_a is exposed, and thus enables the binding of circulating fibrinogen which in turn allows platelet to platelet interactions to occur and platelet aggregates to form. Aggregation of platelets is also associated with release of both alpha- and dense-granule contents, some of which lead to further platelet stimulation (eg ADP, 5-HT) (Fig. 8.4). Upon stimulation, platelets also release a variety of biologically active molecules from membrane phospholipids, such as cyclooxygenase and lipoxygenase metabolites of arachidonic acid, and the ether-linked phospholipid, platelet activating factor (PAF) (Fig. 8.4). Some of the platelet-derived mediators are also capable of activating and recruiting leucocytes. Also of interest is the observation that platelets can interact with leucocytes such as neutrophils in the synthesis of novel mediators of arachidonic acid metabolism that neither platelets nor neutrophils can synthesise alone. The significance of such observations to the pathology of allergic inflammatory responses is not yet known. However, since platelets and neutrophils are often observed in close proximity to one another in tissues obtained from inflammatory lesions, this may be indirect evidence that the cells are co-operating to produce novel mediators.

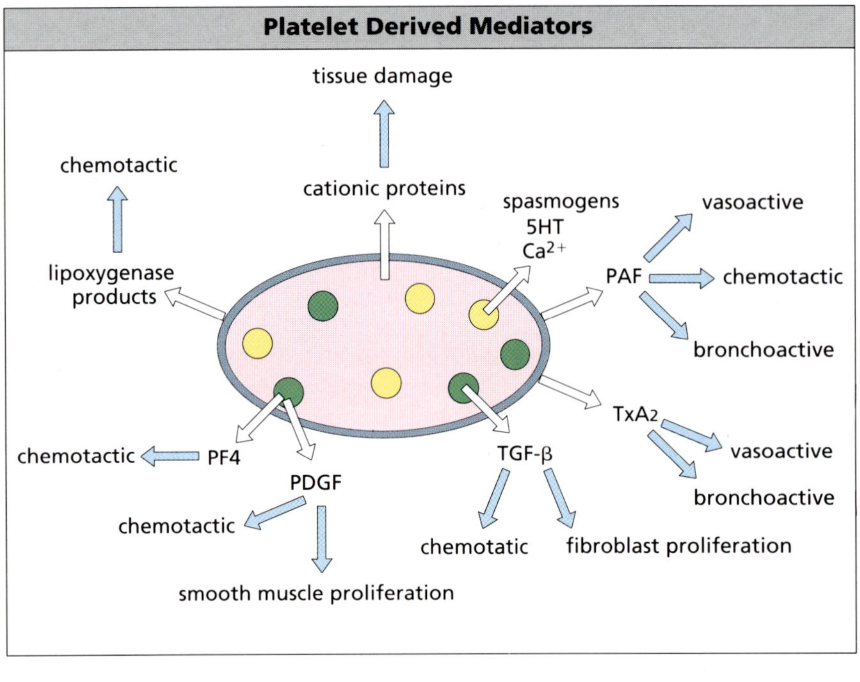

Fig. 8.4 Diagrammatic representation of inflammatory mediators derived from platelets.

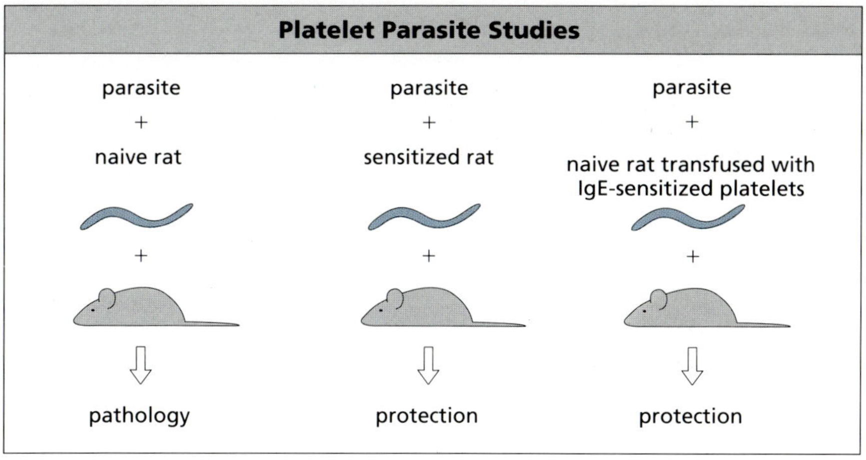

Fig. 8.5 Diagrammatic representation of experiments performed to demonstrate the recruitment of IgE sensitized platelets in the expulsion of parasitic infections.

Platelets as Inflammatory Cells

Many experts view platelets as participants in a non-allergic defence mechanism, particularly against bacterial invasion, while others suggest that circulating platelets offer host defence against parasite invasion. However, these views have not gained widespread acceptance largely because of the prominent role of the platelet in thrombosis and haemostasis. Nonetheless, the participation of platelets in defence mechanisms is exemplified by the knowledge that in certain lower organisms such as caterpillars, the response to a foreign body is characterized by the adhesion of haemocytes (primitive leucocytes) to the surface of the foreign body, with the subsequent aggregation of further haemocytes to form a capsule. This capsule is remarkably similar to the gross morphology of a platelet plug, suggesting that the primary haemostasis in higher mammals is a phylogenetic vestige retained from the behaviour of primitive leucocytes. It would not be surprising, therefore, if other properties of the haemocyte have been retained by mammalian platelets in relation to the defence of the host organism.

Platelets have been shown to undergo chemotaxis and phagocytosis, and to initiate vascular permeability. In addition, platelets release a range of mediators relevant to the inflammatory process. Platelets are known to release bactericidal products such as β-lysin, mediators chemotactic for neutrophils including 12-HETE and platelet derived growth factor (PDGF), mediators of tissue damage (eg oxygen free radical species), vasoactive agents, and a variety of spasmogens (Fig. 8.4).

Platelets have also been demonstrated to possess both IgE and IgG receptors. In the case of the IgE-dependent activation of platelets, a very strong case has been presented recently for these having a fundamental physiological role in aiding the removal of parasitic infections. The passive transfer to naive rats of platelets bearing IgE antibodies against *Schistosomula* can protect the recipient animals from a subsequent challenge with this parasite (Fig. 8.5). The IgE receptors found on platelets, being of the IgE $FC_{\epsilon}R$ II type, are of relatively low affinity compared with the IgE receptors found on mast cells and basophils, but they are comparable to similar receptors found on other inflammatory cell types such as alveolar macrophages and eosinophils.

In animals, IgE-dependent activation of platelets has been shown to release cytotoxic free radicals in sufficient quantities to kill parasites *in vitro*. IgE receptors have also been demonstrated on a proportion of human platelets, and this proportion increases in subjects with known allergic disease. Activation of these receptors by an appropriate antigenic stimulus induces the release of oxygen free radical species but does not cause the classical platelet aggregation and secretion of mediators as described above. IgE-dependent platelet activation may, therefore, represent a novel form of platelet activation distinct from the classical platelet aggregation and secretion of mediators which has been so well characterized (see Fig. 8.6). This distinction is exemplified by the recent observation that anti-allergic drugs such as sodium cromoglycate and nedocromil sodium inhibit IgE-dependent release of free radicals from platelets whilst having no effect on classical platelet aggregation. The mechanisms of this inhibition are unknown, but recently PAF antagonists have been demonstrated to inhibit IgE-dependent free radical generation by eosinophils; this raises the possibility that if similar mechanisms operate in platelets, the production of PAF may play a key role in the generation of free radicals in inflammatory cells.

Other endogenous stimuli may also stimulate the release of oxygen free radicals from platelets. These include the neuropeptide substance P, C-reactive protein, and lymphokines such as interferon-γ and tumour necrosis factor. This suggests that the generation of free radicals by platelets may be stimulated by non-immunological mechanisms as well as by IgE-mediated allergic responses. Furthermore, another lymphokine, termed platelet activating suppressive lymphokine (PASL), has recently been described: this is capable of down-regulating the inflammatory activity of platelets.

Platelets obtained from individuals with aspirin-sensitive asthma also release cytotoxic free radicals following incubation *in vitro* with aspirin or related non-steroidal anti-inflammatory drugs (NSAID). In addition, platelets from these subjects also exhibit abnormal metabolism of hydrogen peroxide. No other blood element from these individuals has been

The Production and Function of Platelets

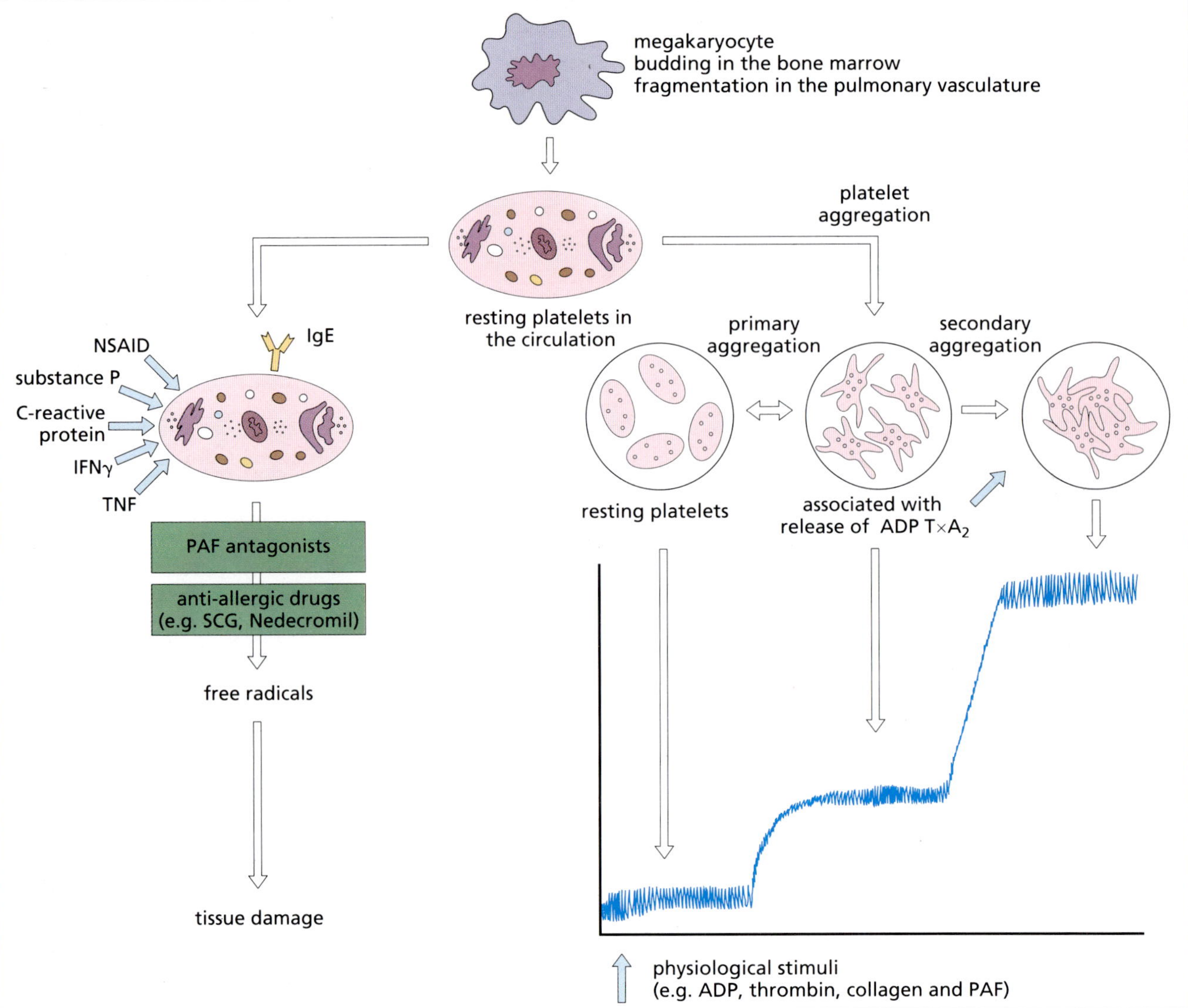

Fig. 8.6 Production and function of platelets. Platelets are produced from megakaryocytes, either by budding in the bone marrow or by physical fragmentation within the pulmonary vasculature. It is now apparent that platelets within the vasculature can undergo different forms of platelet activation.

demonstrated to show such abnormalities, neither do platelets from patients with other types of asthma. This observation has considerable significance in that it represents the first true cellular abnormality in aspirin-sensitive individuals, a finding which may open up new diagnostic possibilities for the early detection of this subset of asthmatics.

Platelets in Asthma

In Vitro Observations

Platelets from asthmatic patients have been repeatedly demonstrated to behave abnormally *in vitro* (Fig. 8.7). Often this abnormality has been demonstrated as an impairment of the second wave of platelet aggregation that would normally occur when platelets are challenged in a Born aggregometer with agonists such as ADP, adrenaline, or thrombin. A similar abnormality of platelet function has also been shown in various pathological conditions where platelets are partially refractory to stimulation *in vitro*, suggesting that platelets are over-stimulated in asthmatic patients.

***In Vitro* Platelet Aggregation in Asthma**
abnormal second phase aggregation to ADP, adrenaline and collagen.
reduced release of 5-HT, PF4
reduced intraplatelet nucleotides
increased resting cytoplasmic Ca^{2+}, IP3
reduced uptake of 5-HT
abnormal lipoxygenase activity
increased oxygen free radical formation

Fig. 8.7 Some of the platelet abnormalities in asthmatics that have been detected *in vitro*.

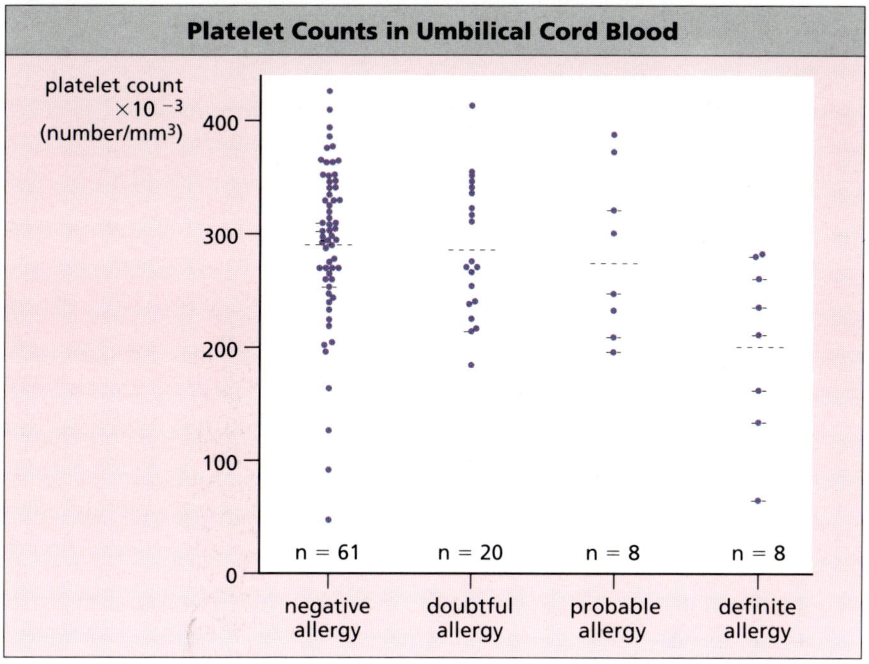

Fig. 8.8 Platelet count in umbilical cord blood of infants followed up at 18 months of age for atopic symptoms. The lowest platelet counts were found in cord blood from those infants who developed definite atopy. (Data modified from Magnusson CGM and De Weck AL, *Allergy*, 1989, **44**, 143-151.)

Evidence for the involvement of humoral elements in bringing about this abnormality derives by the observation that the responsiveness of platelets from asthmatics can be partially restored after incubation with plasma from normal subjects. Conversely, platelets from normal subjects develop altered responsiveness *in vitro* following incubation with plasma from asthmatic patients.

The incidence of abnormal platelet responsiveness is higher among patients having high serum IgE titres, suggesting a possible relationship with the allergic process. This is of potential importance in the light of recent observations made in neonates that umbilical cord IgE levels correlate with the degree of thrombocytopaenia at birth (Fig. 8.8).

Furthermore, the extent of neonatal thrombocytopaenia has been considered to be a useful parameter for predicting newborns at risk of developing allergic disease in later life. It has been suggested that a low platelet count at birth represents ongoing intra-uterine sensitization, although precisely what platelets are doing at this stage of the disease can only be speculative at this time.

***In Vivo* Platelet Abnormalities in Asthma**
increased plasma levels of PF4/TXB_2
increased circulating platelet aggregates
thrombocytopaenia
prolonged bleeding time
reduced platelet survival time
reduced platelet regeneration time
abnormal megakaryocytes at autopsy
increased platelets in BAL fluid
platelet aggregates within microvasculature

Fig. 8.9 Some of the platelet abnormalities that have been detected *in vivo* in asthmatics.

There have also been studies indicating that platelets from asthmatic subjects have an abnormal lipoxygnase pathway, reduced intraplatelet nucleotide levels and increased resting inositol triphosphate (IP_3) levels. However other investigators, albeit using classical *in vitro* tests normally reserved for detecting abnormalities of platelet function in the context of thrombosis and haemostasis, have failed to find significant abnormalities *in vitro* in platelets from asthmatics; this suggests that these discrepancies may relate to differences in methodology. Because platelet activation in allergy may induce oxygen free radical release in the absence of classical aggregation or degranulation, it may be necessary to develop new tests to study these aspects of platelet function.

In Vivo Observations

A number of clinical observations have suggested that platelet activation is a feature of both provoked and spontaneous attacks of asthma (Fig. 8.9). A wide range of techniques have been used to demonstrate platelet activation as a feature of asthma (Fig. 8.10). In 1955, Storck and his colleagues reported that thrombycytopaenia occurred in allergic subjects following allergen challenge. This has recently been confirmed by other investigators.

Markers of Platelet Activation
release of PF4
release of β-TG
β-TG : PF4 ratio
plasma and urinary TXB_2
circulating platelet microaggregates
survival time of ^{111}indium radiolabelled platelets

Fig. 8.10 Summary of some of the recognised markers of platelet activation *in vivo*.

The appearance of the platelet-specific proteins, β-thromboglobulin and platelet factor 4 (PF4) in the systemic circulation of asthmatics following antigen or excercise-induced bronchoconstriction has also been demonstrated. In one study, the release of PF4 was shown to parallel bronchoconstriction following allergen provocation, although similar changes in platelets were not observed when the patients underwent comparable bronchoconstriction induced by inhalation of methacholine. Again there are a number of studies which have not confirmed these *in vivo* findings of platelet activation, although it must be noted that in some, there was an elevation of specific platelet markers which did not attain statistical significance due to intersubject variation.

Platelet aggregates have been observed in the microvasculature of the lungs of asthmatic subjects during late-onset airways obstruction following allergen provocation (Fig. 8.11). Platelet-derived markers have also been demonstrated in bronchoalveolar lavage (BAL) fluid, as have platelets themselves. Furthermore, platelets have been observed undergoing diapedesis in ashtmatics (Fig. 8.12) and on epithelial surfaces of symptomatic asthmatics (Fig. 8.13) suggesting that like leucocytes, platelets migrate into inflamed tissues. In experimental animals, platelets have been observed to undergo diapedesis into the lung with subsequent apposition on to airway smooth muscle.

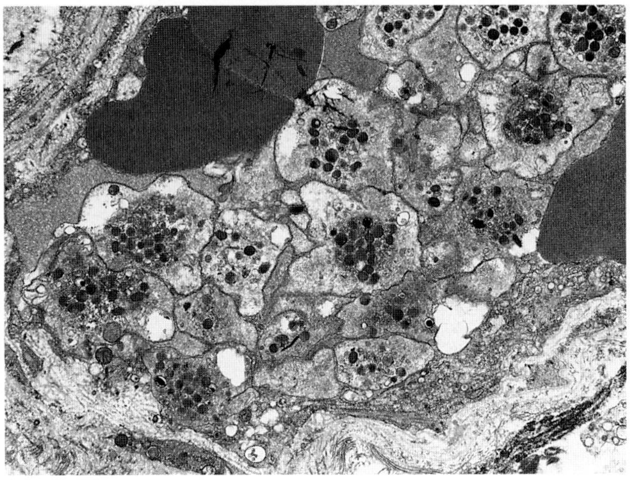

Fig. 8.11 Intravascular platelet aggregates in the lamina propria of the bronchus in a subject with mild asthma. (× 17,000). (Reproduced from Beasley R *et al, Am Rev Respir Dis* 1989; **139**: 806–17 with permission.)

Other clinical observations also support the role of platelet activation in asthma (Fig. 8.9). Shortened platelet survival time has been reported to be a feature of allergy and platelet regeneration time is shortened in asthmatics with acute symptoms. Both of these parameters have been suggested to be useful indices of *in vivo* platelet activation leading to accelerated platelet consumption. Shortened platelet survival time can be corrected by treatment of asthmatics with glucocorticosteroids or ketotifen. There have been negative studies in this regard, although in one study investigations were only reported for three subjects, and in another platelet survival time was shown not to be altered in allergic asthmatics as a result of a single allergen challenge. Support for the theory of accelerated platelet consumption in asthmatics comes from the report that allergic subjects have a mild haemostatic defect in that they have a prolonged bleeding time.

Studies at autopsy of asthmatics who died of status asthmaticus have also revealed large numbers of megakaryocytes in the lungs. Normal lungs contain only the occasional megakaryocyte. Given that the lung has been suggested to be the organ responsible for the fragmentation of megakaryocytes into platelets, this observation may have implications in furthering our understanding of platelet abnormalities in asthma and other pulmonary diseases.

The precise mechanisms by which platelets are activated in asthma and their contribution to the pathophysiological changes which characterize this disease have not yet been determined. However, in

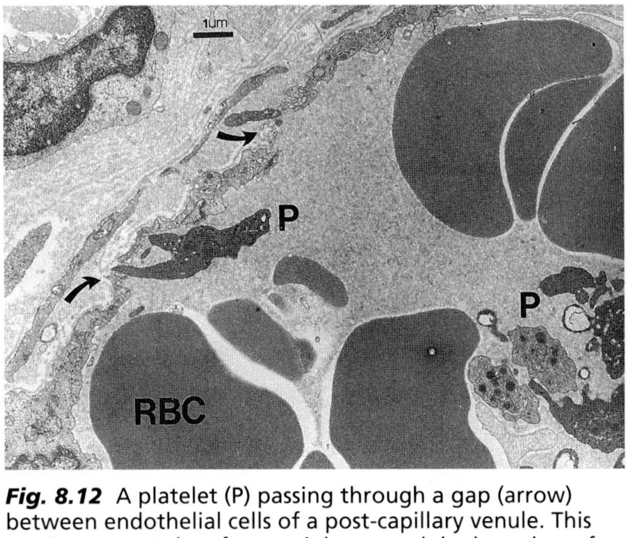

Fig. 8.12 A platelet (P) passing through a gap (arrow) between endothelial cells of a post-capillary venule. This specimen was taken from a right upper lobe bronchus of a subject with mild, non-atopic asthma. (× 13,000).(Courtesy of Drs A. and L. Laitinen.)

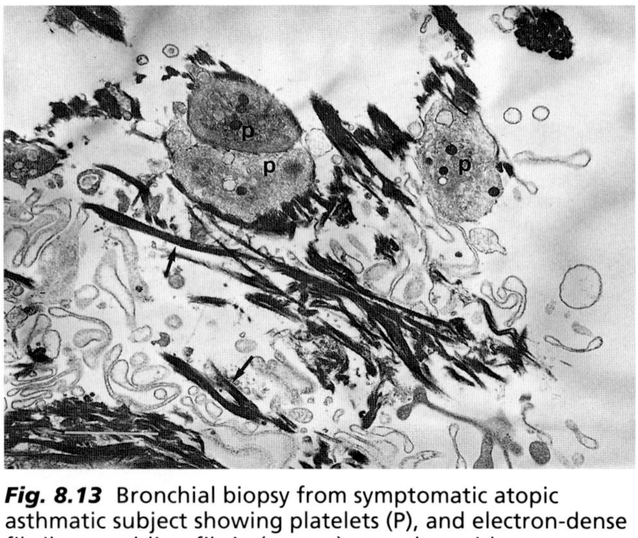

Fig. 8.13 Bronchial biopsy from symptomatic atopic asthmatic subject showing platelets (P), and electron-dense fibrils resembling fibrin (arrows), together with membranous debris at the luminal edge from where surface epithelium was lost. Glutaraldehyde and osmium tetroxide. (Scale bar = 2μm). (Courtesy of Dr PK Jefferey.

experimental animals, selective platelet depletion with specific anti-serum reduces the ability of allergen to induce an eosinophil infiltrate into the lungs of sensitized animals. The mechanisms by which platelets may be involved in eosinophil recruitment involve chemoattractant factors such as PF4 and lipoxygenase metabolites of arachidonic acid metabolism, and the generation of platelet-derived histamine releasing factor (PDHF) which has been shown to elicit an eosinophil infiltrate into the lungs of rabbits. As eosinophil products (See Chapter 6) have been implicated in the tissue damage observed in the lung in asthma, and as asthma considered to be an inappropriate parasite-killing response, these results suggest that platelets may have a beneficial role in recruiting eosinophils into tissues in order to expel parasites (Fig. 8.14).

Platelets have also been shown to be necessary for the induction of bronchial hyperresponsiveness induced by allergen in experimental animals. It is therefore of interest that both platelet-derived histamine releasing factor (a peptide) and platelet-derived hyperreactivity factor (a lipid) can induce bronchial hyperreactivity (Fig. 8.15). It is not yet apparent whether these substances require the presence of eosinophils or whether they interact directly with the smooth muscle of airways. The generation of platelet-derived hyperreactvity factor occurs in response to stimulation of both human and guinea pig platelets by PAF, but it is not released following stimulation of platelets with classical agonists such as thrombin or collagen.

Such results suggest that, like IgE-dependent activation of platelets, release of this potentially important substnance is unrelated to classical aggregation and secretion. This is supported by the finding that sodium cromoglycate can inhibit the generation of these materials even though it does not inhibit platelet aggregation.

The knowledge of whether PAF is involved in the pathogenesis of asthma must await the outcome of controlled clinical studies with selective antagonists but it is of interest that one such drug, BN 52063, has been shown to inhibit the platelet activation

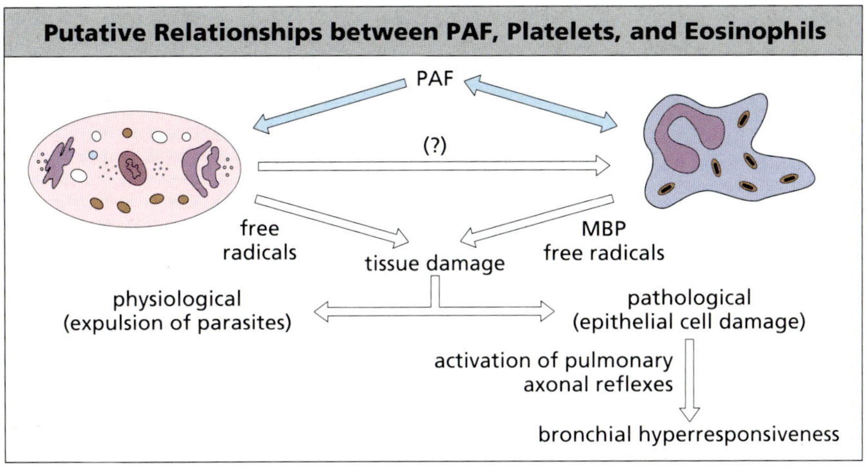

Fig. 8.14 Schematic representation of the possible relationship between PAF release from inflammatory cells, the activation of platelet and eosinophils, with release of cytotoxic materials and the subsequent induction of tissue damage. Physiologically, this cascade is involved in the removal of parasitic infections, but it may also contribute to the tissue damage underlying the bronchial hyperresponsiveness characterizing asthma when activated inappropriately.

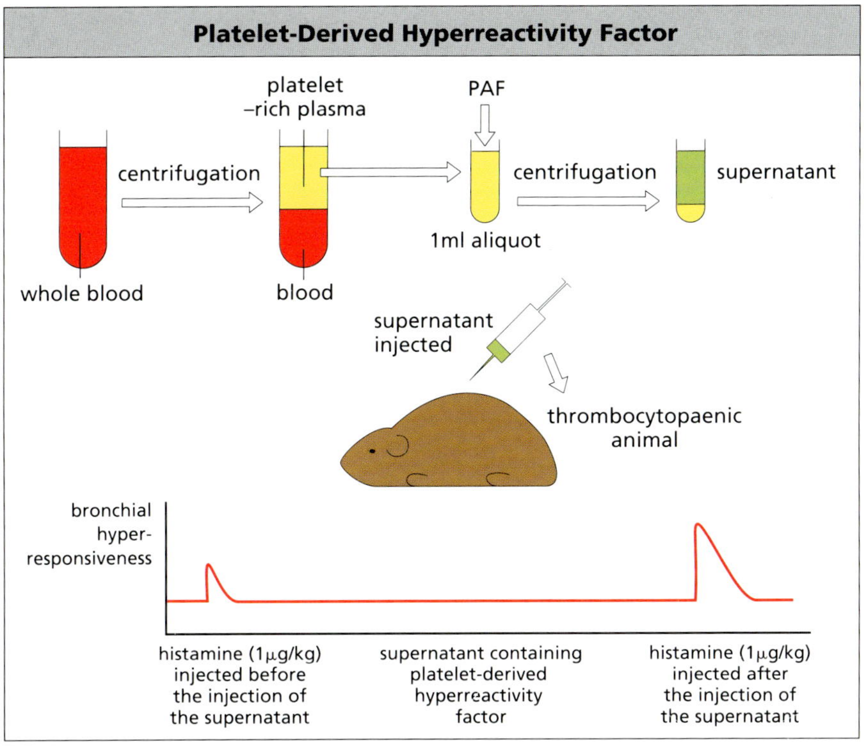

Fig. 8.15 Generation of platelet-derived hyperreactivity factor from human platelets by PAF. Administration of this material to thrombocytopaenic animals results in increased airways responsiveness to intravenous histamine and other spasmogens.

associated with excercise-induced bronchoconstriction in asthmatics (Fig. 8.16).

Exposure of asthmatics to inhaled PAF also results in platelet activation within the circulation, assessed as increased expression of platelet-associated von Willebrand factor, but it does not result in overt aggregation and secretion since neither thrombocytopaenia nor release of PF4 into plasma have been detected following exposure of people to PAF.

Conclusion

It is clear that platelets can behave as effector cells in allergic inflammatory conditions and may provide a vital role in the defence of the body against parasitic infections. Inappropriate activation of platelets to behave as inflammatory cells may be involved in the pathophysiology of allergic diseases by recruiting eosinophils and thereby contributing to the acute increase in bronchial hyperresponsiveness associated with this disease. Furthermore, the realization that platelets can release transforming growth factor beta (TGF-β), known to be capable of stimulating fibroblast proliferation, and PDGF, a known smooth muscle mitogen, suggests that platelets may also be involved in initiating and perpetuating the structural changes underlying sub-epithelial fibrosis and smooth muscle proliferation which may contribute to chronic airways hyperreponsiveness (Fig. 8.17).

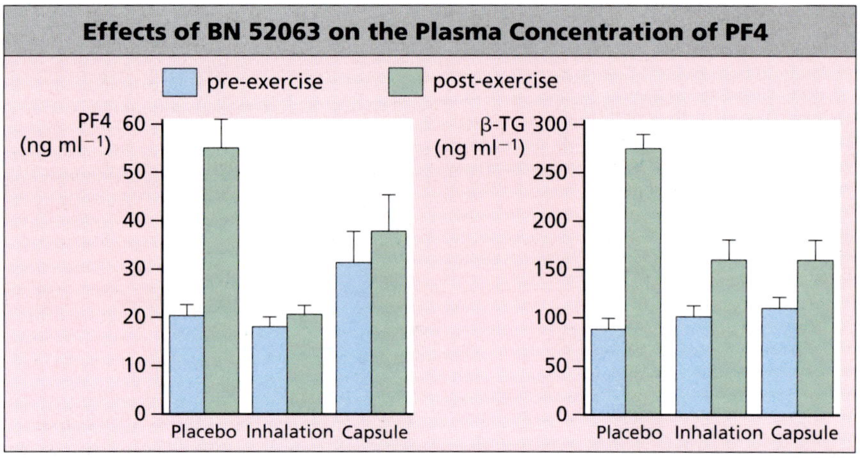

Fig. 8.16 Effects of BN 52063 on the plasma concentrations of PF4 [left] and β-TG [right] before and five minutes after the exercise challenge. Note the significant inhibition of increase in protein levels after pretreatment with BN 52063. (Printed with permission from Wilkens et al. Platelet activation and exercise induced asthma, *Br J Clin Pharmacol*, 1990, **29**.

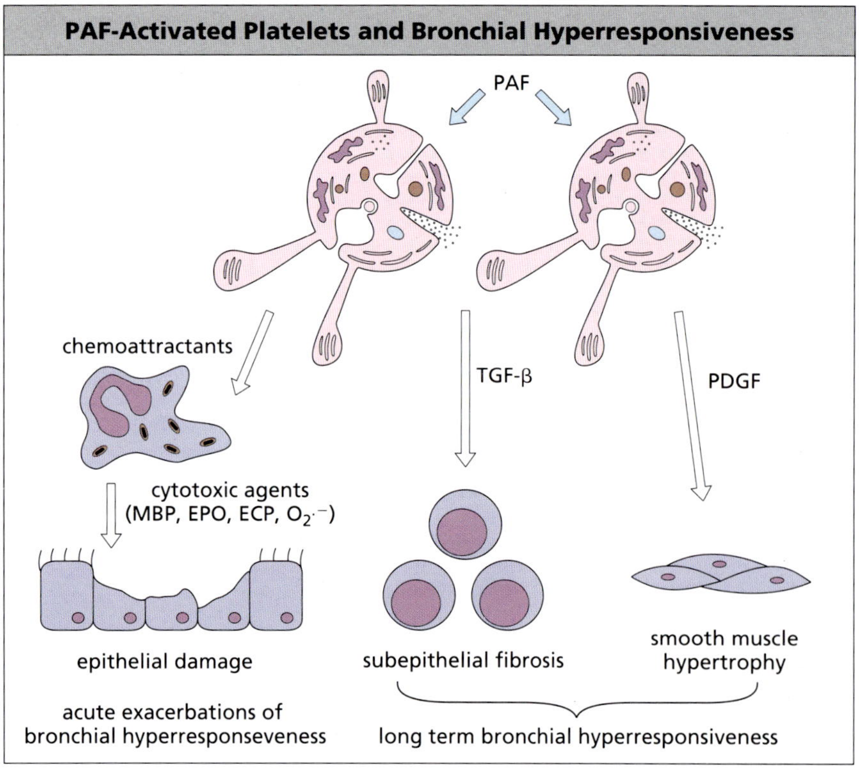

Fig. 8.17 Schematic representation of the relationship between PAF activated platelets and the induction of acute exacerbations of bronchial responsiveness via recruitment of eosinophils, as well as long term bronchial hyperresponsiveness as a result of inducing repair processes in the airways.

Further Reading

Page CP. The platelet as an inflammatory cell. *Immunopharmacol* 1989;**17**:51-59.

Joseph M. Platelets in Allergy. In: *The Platelet in Health and Disease* Ed: Page CR. Oxford: Blackwell Scientific, 1991.

Chapter 9

Lymphocytes, Allergy and Asthma

Introduction

The most important function of the lymphocyte is to recognize and respond directly to exogenous antigens. Other inflammatory cells recognize antigen through non-specific surface binding of immunoglobulin. T lymphocytes also have the capacity to influence the production, lifespan and activation of granulocytes as well as other cell types. It is likely that they play a role in the regulation of all inflammatory responses. B lymphocytes secrete immunoglobulin (Ig), and are responsible for the exaggerated IgE response characteristic of atopy. This chapter is concerned with the immunobiology of T and B lymphocytes, and the importance of these cells in allergic inflammation.

T Lymphocytes

Functional Divisions of T Lymphocytes

T lymphocytes form the majority of lymphocytes in the peripheral blood and are widely distributed throughout the body in lymphoid organs including the spleen and thymus, and at mucosal surfaces.

In addition to receptors for antigen, T lymphocytes express many other surface molecules or markers. T lymphocytes may be divided into broad functional subsets based on the expression of various surface markers, whereas other markers are present on all T lymphocytes (Fig. 9.1). The markers have been internationally standardized using monoclonal antibodies and catalogued using clusters of differentiation (CD) numbers. All mature post-thymic T lymphocytes express (amongst others) the markers CD2 and CD3. CD3 consists of a group of four polypeptide chains (γ, δ, ϵ, and ζ), which are closely associated with the antigen receptors on the surface of the T lymphocyte (Fig. 9.2). It is this group of molecules which conveys the activation signal to the T lymphocyte following binding of specific antigen to the receptor. The CD2 molecule is concerned with binding to LFA-3, an adhesion molecule found on T lymphocytes, as well as other cell types.

The first major functional division of T lymphocytes arises from the nature of the antigen receptor itself. The majority of T lymphocytes possess an antigen receptor composed of two covalently linked polypeptide chains called α and β, whereas a minority use two distinct chains called γ and δ (different from those in the CD3 molecule). The properties of these cells are discussed below.

CD3 $T_{\alpha\beta}$ lymphocytes may be further divided into two major functional subsets according to whether they express the markers CD4 or CD8 (Fig. 9.1).

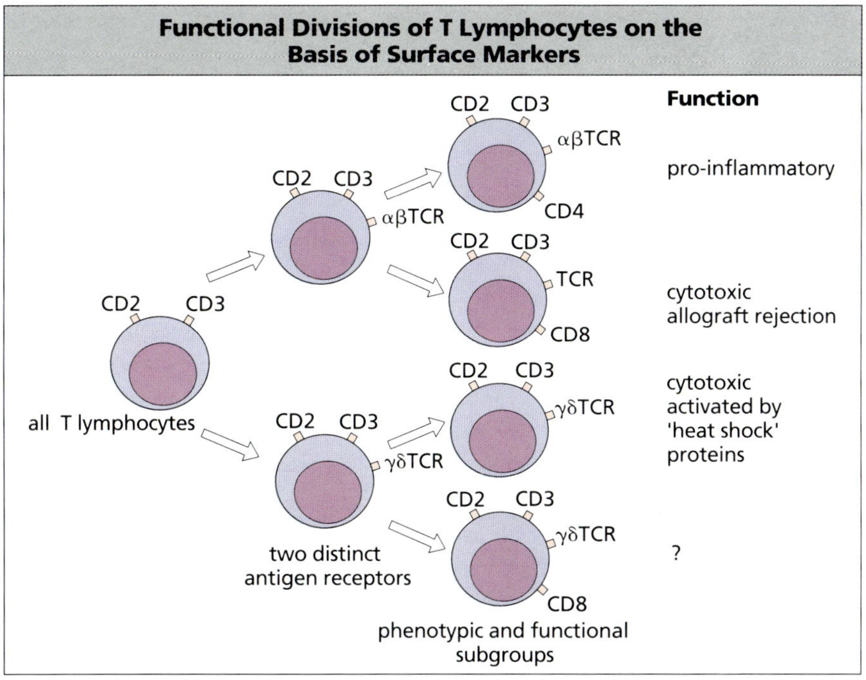

Fig. 9.1 The major functional subdivisions of T lymphocytes. All T lymphocytes are characterized by expression of the surface markers CD2 and CD3. The expression of $\alpha\beta$ or $\gamma\delta$ receptors delineates two major T-lymphocyte groups. $T_{\alpha\beta}$ cells may be divided into two further subgroups according to their expression of CD4 or CD8.

CD4+ T lymphocytes are traditionally called helper cells because one of their functions is to interact with B lymphocytes to produce antibody (although it is now clear that these cells have many other pro-inflammatory functions as well). For this reason they are referred to in this chapter as pro-inflammatory cells. CD8+ T lymphocytes have the ability directly to recognize and kill malignant or virally-infected cells. In addition, they kill cells bearing non-self histocompatibility antigens and are therefore largely responsible for the rejection of allografts.

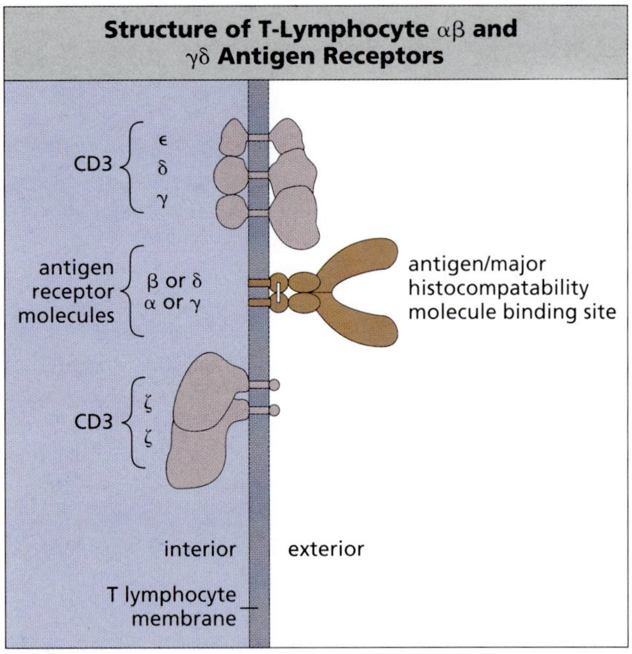

Fig. 9.2 Basic structure of T-lymphocyte αβ or γδ antigen receptors. The two receptor polypeptides are lined on the cell surface by disulphide bridges. The fine structure of the polypeptides varies between cells, thus determining their antigen specificity. Very little of the receptor lies within the cell cytoplasm, so that when the receptors are presented with antigen, the activation signal is transmitted by the CD3 molecules γ,δ,ε, and ζ which are closely associated with the antigen receptor molecules on the cell surface, and which traverse the cell membrane.

Most CD3 $T_{\gamma\delta}$ lymphocytes express neither CD4 nor CD8, although a small subset of these cells (particularly in the gut epithelium) are CD8+. There is insufficient knowledge of their function at present to ascertain whether the CD8+ cells form a functional subgroup.

Ontogeny of T Lymphocytes

T lymphocytes derive their name from the fact that they are largely dependent on the presence of the thymus for normal development. Hairless or 'nude' mice, which lack a thymus, develop few $T_{\alpha\beta}$ lymphocytes with limited antigen specificity. Some $T_{\gamma\delta}$ cells may also be found, raising the possibility that some T lymphocytes may develop extra-thymically. T-lymphocyte development occurs early in fetal life (Fig. 9.3). In man, primitive thymocytes begin to colonize the thymus around weeks 7–8 of fetal development. The earliest thymocytes express the marker CD7. These cells retain the capacity to develop, depending on environmental conditions, into erythroid or myeloid cells as well as lymphoid cells. During weeks 8–9 of gestation, thymocytes begin to express cytoplasmic CD3 and surface CD2. By 9.5 weeks, T-lymphocyte antigen-receptor molecules appear in thymocytes, first $T_{\gamma\delta}$ cells and then $T_{\alpha\beta}$ cells at 10 weeks. These lineages develop independently. When antigen receptor molecules appear, surface CD3 can

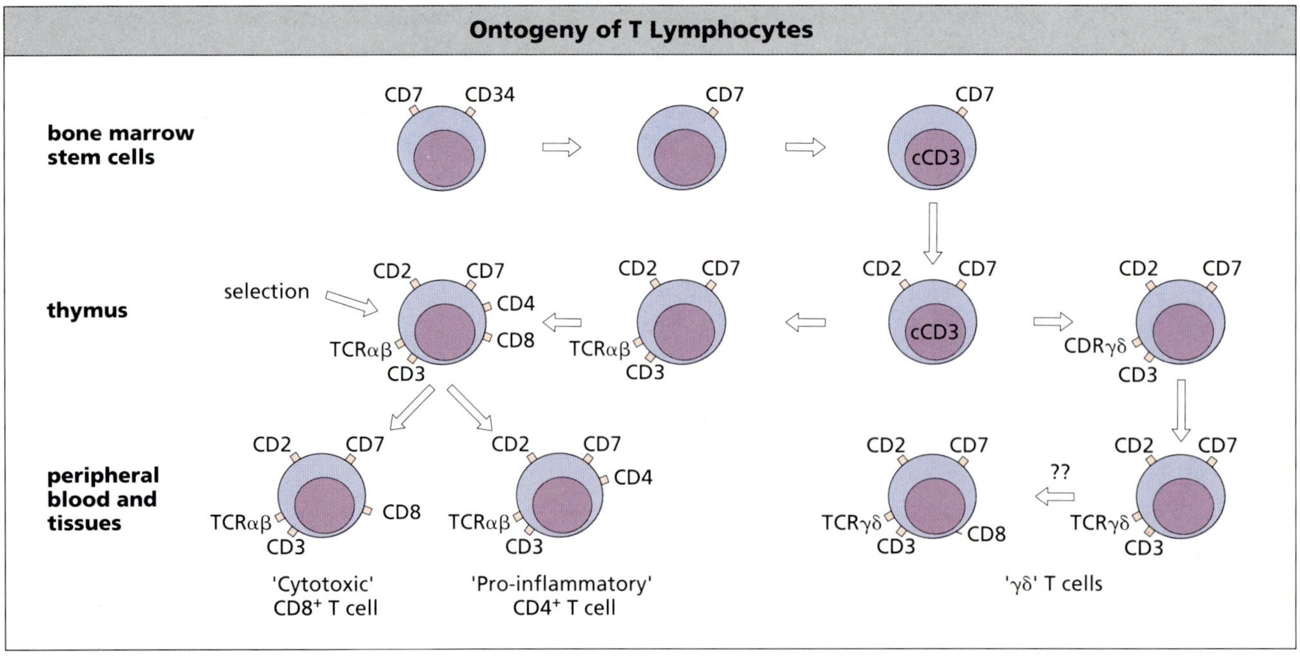

Fig. 9.3 T-lymphocyte ontogeny. Thymocyte precursors arrive in the primitive thymus around week 7 of fetal development. During thymic development, the thymocytes randomly rearrange and express either αβ or γδ receptor genes. Cells with receptors which happen to recognize self antigens (i.e. the majority) are then eliminated, whereas those cells recognizing foreign antigens proliferate and reach the exterior. $T_{\alpha\beta}$ cells are selected at the double positive stage, when they express both CD4 and CD8. Those cells which recognize antigen presented on MHC class I molecules retain CD8 and lose CD4, whereas those recognizing antigen presented by MHC class II molecules retain CD4 and lose CD8.
(C = cytoplasmic molecule not yet expressed on cell surface.)

be expressed. $T_{\alpha\beta}$ cells initially express both CD4 and CD8, then expression of one of these is lost, resulting in a cell of the mature phenotype.

During development in the thymus the T-lymphocyte antigen repertoire is defined and many of those cells recognizing self antigens are eliminated (see below). It is probable that local humoral influences as well as physical interactions with thymic stromal cells play an important part in this process.

The T-Lymphocyte Antigen Receptor and its Repertoire

The structure of the T-lymphocyte antigen receptor has only recently been defined. As previously stated, the receptor is composed of a pair of polypeptide chains, α and β or γ and δ, which are usually linked by disulphide bridges and whose fine structure determines antigenic specificity (see below). T lymphocytes do not recognize antigenic molecules in isolation; they do so only in association with major histocompatibility (MHC) molecules (Fig. 9.4). $CD4^+$ T lymphocytes recognize antigens in association with MHC class II molecules (found principally on the surface of antigen-presenting cells, e.g. monocytes, macrophages, B lymphocytes and dendritic cells), whereas $CD8^+$ cells recognize antigen in association with MHC class I molecules (found on all body cells). This is reflected in the role of $CD8^+$ cytotoxic T lymphocytes, which recognize any host cells expressing foreign antigen as a result of infection or malignant transformation, whereas $CD4^+$ pro-inflammatory T lymphocytes need only recognize foreign antigen presented by antigen-presenting cells.

This system of antigen recognition involves a series of events as follows:

(1) Coding of the T-lymphocyte receptor polypeptide chains (α/β or γ/δ) by T-lymphocyte receptor genes.
(2) Positive selection in the thymus for T-lymphocyte clones which recognize foreign antigens in association with self MHC antigens.
(3) Elimination of T-lymphocyte clones recognizing self antigens.
(4) Expansion of useful clones in the periphery (this takes place largely after they are exposed to specific antigen).

The Nature of the Antigen Recognized by T Lymphocytes

Recent experiments have revealed some other fundamental characteristics of T-lymphocyte antigen recognition:

- Antigens require processing by 'antigen-presenting' cells before they can be recognized by T lymphocytes. This processing involves cleavage of the antigens into short polypeptide fragments.
- T lymphocytes recognize small peptides (derived from the foreign-protein antigens) typically 10–20 amino acid residues in length. Synthetic oligopeptides are equally effective in activating sensitized T lymphocytes.
- Unlike B lymphocytes, T lymphocytes cannot bind to antigen directly but rely on accessory 'antigen-presenting' cells to present them with antigen-derived oligopeptide fragments. This may have evolved as a guidance system allowing T lymphocytes to recognize small quantities of antigen. Thus, T lymphocytes recognize the *amino acid sequences* of peptides derived from antigenic proteins. This should be contrasted with antibodies, which recognize the *three-dimensional structures* of antigenic proteins – this relies on the proteins being intact.

In a manner similar to that seen for immunoglobulins, the genes encoding the T-lymphocyte receptor polypeptides are arranged in segments which are brought together by enzymatic splicing as the T lymphocyte develops; once a gene is productively rearranged it is expressed, and further development ceases. The genes encoding the α and γ chains comprise three segments: variable (V), joining (J) and

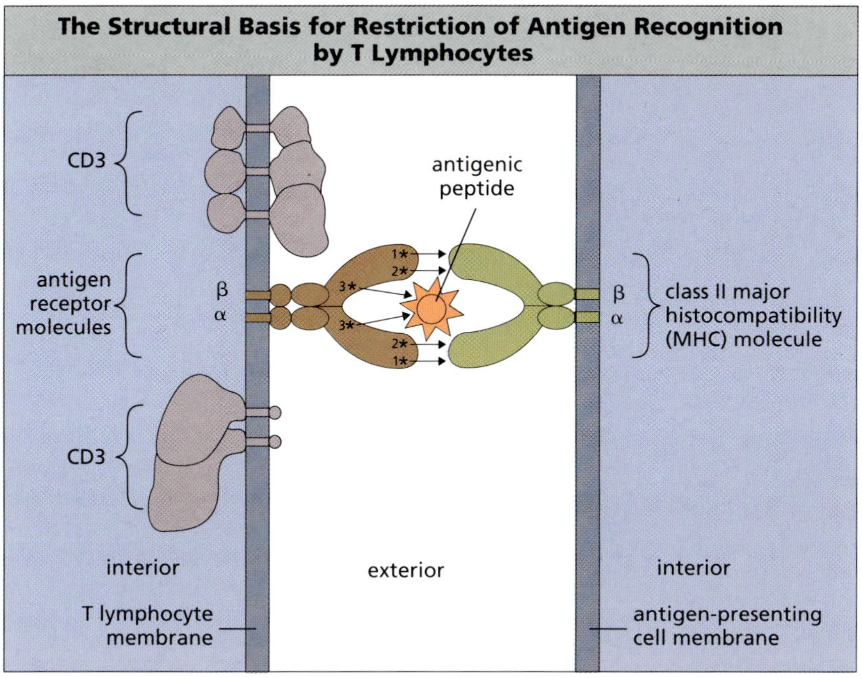

Fig. 9.4 The structural basis for restriction of antigen recognition by T lymphocytes. T lymphocytes can recognize antigen-derived peptides only when presented by self MHC class I ($CD8^+$ cytotoxic cells) or MHC class II ($CD4^+$ pro-inflammatory cells) molecules, as T lymphocytes require contact both with the antigenic peptide and with the class I/II molecule for activation. The hypervariable regions of the T-lymphocyte antigen-receptor molecules, CDR1–3, are shown as numbered asterisks in the figure. CDR1 and CDR2 contact the histocompatibility molecule, whereas CDR3 contacts the antigenic peptide. The hypervariable regions are created by the mechanisms shown in Figs 9.5 and 9.6.

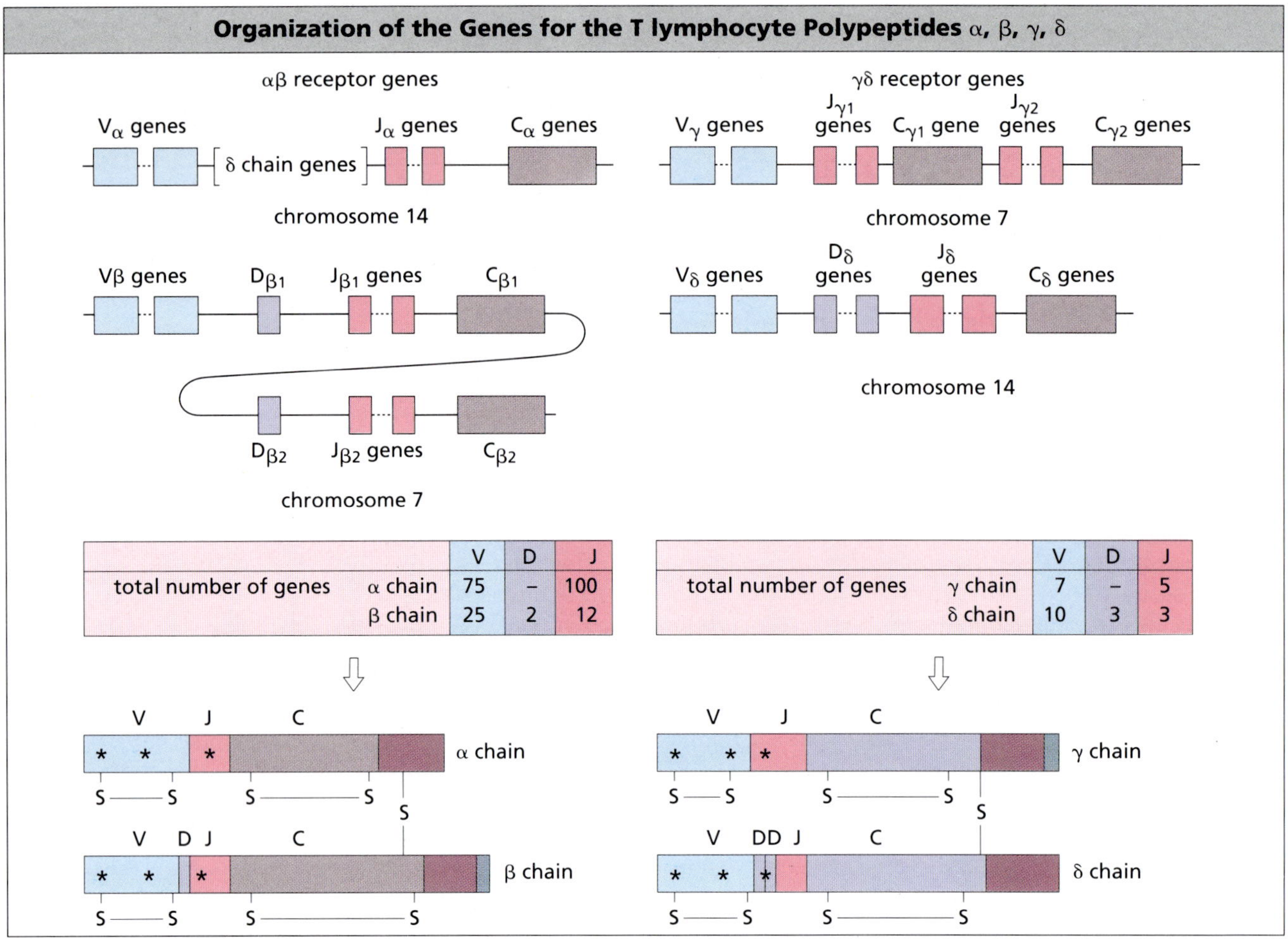

Fig. 9.5 The organisation of the genes for the T-lymphocyte receptor polypeptides α, β, γ and δ. The genes are arranged in order on various chromosomes as shown in the figure. Note that the δ chain genes lie entirely within the α chain genes. Each complete chain is encoded by three (α and γ chains) or four (β and δ chains) gene segments. During thymocyte development, particular segments are brought together by enzymatic looping out of the intervening DNA. The hypervariable regions on each of the chains (marked by asterisks which correspond to those in Fig. 9.4) are created by variations in the structure of the V segment genes and also by the variable structure and joining of the V, D and J segment genes (Fig. 9.6). —S—S— shows the positions of intra- and inter-chain disulphide bridges. Shaded regions on chains correspond to the hydrophobic transmembrane regions.

Generation of T Lymphocyte Antigen Receptor Diversity	
αβ receptor	γδ receptor
variable use of V-region genes	
75 V_α genes 25 V_β genes	7 V_γ genes 10 V_δ genes
variable ues of D-region genes	
2 D_β genes used singly but read in all frames	2–3 D_δ genes often used in tandem and read in all frames
variable ues of J-region genes	
100 J_α genes 12 J_β genes	5 J_γ genes 3 J_δ genes
'N-region addition' (addition or removal of one or a few extra DNA bases at the joining regions)	
V–J region (α chain) V–D regions (β chain)	V–J region (γ chain) V–D_1, D_1–D_2, D_2–D_3 regions (δ chain)

Fig. 9.6 Mechanisms of variability in T-lymphocyte antigen receptor chain structure. The total numbers of possible chains created by the variable use of V, D and J segments and N-region addition far exceed the total number of T lymphocytes in the body.

constant (C). The β and δ chain genes possess an additional diversity (D) segment. During development, V(D)JC sequences are brought together to form genes encoding the complete receptor polypeptide (Fig. 9.5). Variability in receptor specificity is brought about by the mechanisms listed in Fig. 9.6. By analogy with immunoglobulins, most of the variability between the V-region genes is confined to two 'hypervariable' regions, CDR1 and CDR2. A third 'hypervariable' region, CDR3, is formed by the V(D)J junctional region. The combinatorial possibilities for these various gene segments are very large (at least 10^{16} for αβ receptors – far greater than the total number of T lymphocytes in the entire body). It should be remembered that T-lymphocyte receptor development takes place early in fetal life as described above; therefore, the entire acquisition of the T-lymphocyte receptor repertoire and elimination of anti-self receptors occur independently of exposure to foreign antigens. This is in contrast to immunoglobulin genes, which mutate somatically during B-lymphocyte proliferation after exposure to antigen, so that their antigen specificity may be further enhanced.

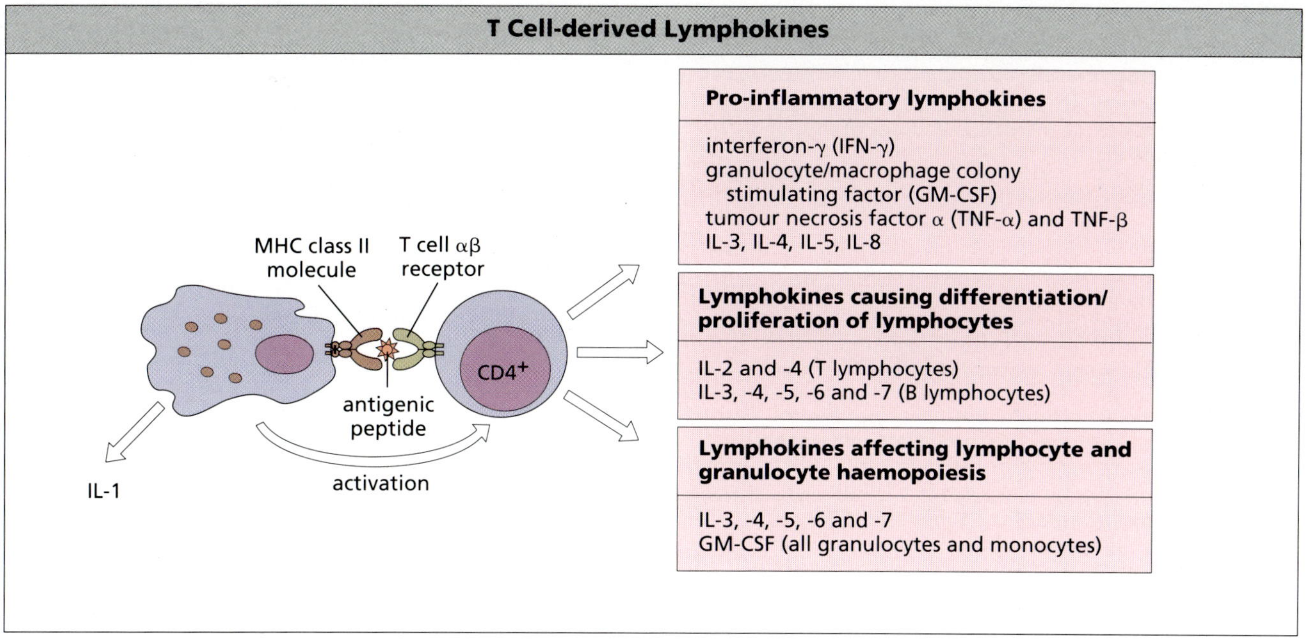

Fig. 9.7 Pro-inflammatory spectrum of $CD4^+$ T-lymphocyte derived lymphokines. This list is not meant to be exhaustive but does emphasize the importance of lymphokines in: (1) attracting granulocytes to sites of inflammation and activating them *in situ*; (2) influencing the amount and class of antibody responses; and (3) regulating the production of granulocytes and lymphocytes in the bone marrow.

Recently, the structural basis for the three-way interaction between the T-lymphocyte receptor, the MHC molecule, and the antigenic peptide has been elucidated. Of great interest is the interaction of the MHC molecule with the T-lymphocyte 'hypervariable' regions (CDR1-3 described above). One computer model suggests that the antigenic peptide sits in a trough between the class I molecule and T-lymphocyte receptor, in contact with CDR3, whilst the other two 'hypervariable' regions, CDR1 and CDR2, are in direct contact with the HLA molecule (Fig. 9.4). This provides a structural basis for the restriction of T-lymphocyte antigen recognition by MHC molecules.

The CD4 and CD8 molecules also play an important part in the recognition of foreign peptides by T lymphocytes, and indeed can bind directly to MHC molecules. The suggestion is that these molecules may act as associative recognition elements, binding to non-polymorphic parts of the MHC class I and II molecules. Their importance for the triggering of T lymphocytes probably depends on the affinity of the T-lymphocyte receptor for its ligand; the lower the affinity of the T-lymphocyte receptor for a particular peptide, the more significant the contribution of the CD4/8 molecule.

T lymphocytes therefore acquire their antigen specificities randomly, depending on the particular combinations of T-lymphocyte receptor-gene segments which they express. The thymus is then responsible for the positive selection of those T lymphocytes with reactivity against foreign antigenic peptides and the elimination of those reacting with self peptides. Although the sequence of events by which this selection process occurs is not well understood, it has been shown in many experiments that the introduction of a foreign antigen into the thymus during thymocyte development results in elimination of T lymphocytes recognizing this antigen. Again the CD4 and CD8 molecules seem to influence this process: T lymphocytes with low binding affinities for self antigens may be spared in the thymus if they also express low levels of CD4 or CD8. This would suggest that T-lymphocyte turnover in the thymus is large, as indeed it is. In the mouse, $CD4^+8^+$ (double-positive) thymocytes have an average lifespan of 3 days and are renewed at a rate of $5x10^7$ cells per day. On the other hand, $CD4^+$ or $CD8^+$ (single-positive) cells which are derived from these double-positive cells are produced at a much lower rate of $lx10^6$ cells per day. Thus the vast majority (98 per cent) of $CD4^+8^+$ cells die intrathymically. There is now good evidence to suggest that the cells which die are anti-self, and only 'useful' cells which recognize foreign antigens are rescued from death.

Functional Properties of T Lymphocytes

$CD4^+$ pro-inflammatory $T_{\alpha\beta}$ lymphocytes

Although $T_{\alpha\beta}$ lymphocytes have traditionally been called helper cells because they can help B lymphocytes to make antibody, it is now clear that these cells, after activation by specific antigenic peptides, secrete many proteins called lymphokines which, by their effects on other cells, have the potential to orchestrate inflammatory responses irrespective of whether or not antibody production is part of the response. Lymphokines have the capacity to augment the turnover and increase the activity of every cell in the granulocyte series, as well as exerting effects on macrophages and other cells not of the haemopoietic series. A list of the more common lymphokines derived from $CD4^+$ T lymphocytes is shown in Fig. 9.7. The general properties of lymphokines which are relevant to the genesis of inflammation are listed in

General Pro-inflammatory Functions of Lymphokines
increasing the production of granulocytes from precursor cells both in the bone marrow and locally at sites of inflammation
prolonging the survival of specific granulocytes, thereby causing their accumulation in tissues
direct chemotaxis of specific granulocytes to sites of inflammation
priming of specific granulocytes for an enhanced response to physiological activating stimuli
influencing the activation of B lymphocytes and the classes of antibodies which they produce in immune responses

Fig. 9.8 Mechanisms by which CD4⁺ T-lymphocyte-derived lymphokines may influence the types and numbers of inflammatory cells appearing during the course of an immune response, as well as whether the response is predominantly cell-mediated or antibody-mediated.

Fig. 9.8. Further details of the properties of the various lymphokines may be found in Chapter 3.

To consider some examples of these properties relevant to allergic inflammation, interleukin-5 (IL-5) has been shown specifically to increase the production of eosinophils from precursors in the bone marrow, to prolong the life of eosinophils *in vitro* from several days to several weeks, and to prime eosinophils for an enhanced response to physiological activating stimuli such as opsonized helminthic larvae. IL-3 exerts a similar series of effects on mast cells and their precursors. IL-4 enhances the production of IgE by B lymphocytes, whereas interferon-γ (IFN-γ) inhibits this process; therefore T-lymphocyte products are likely to be intimately involved in the allergen-specific IgE response which characterizes atopy. It is easy to see how secretion of specific lymphokines may be responsible for the predominance of particular granulocytes in inflammatory situations, e.g. the predominant eosinophil infiltration seen at sites of allergic inflammation.

In the mouse, some evidence exists for distinct functional subsets of CD4⁺ T lymphocytes. This is based on the differing profiles of lymphokine secretion of individual T-lymphocyte clones after activation *in vitro* (Fig. 9.9). TH_1 cells are more efficient at participating in delayed-type hypersensitivity reactions, whereas TH_2 cells preferentially help B lymphocytes to produce all classes of immunoglobulins, including IgE. No similar functional dichotomy has so far been described in man.

Two Functional Types of CD4⁺ T Lymphocytes in the Mouse

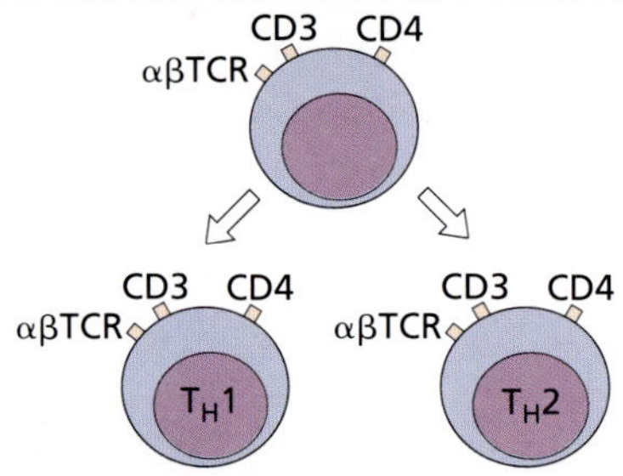

	T_H1	T_H2
Lymphokine synthesis		
IL-2	+	–
IL-3	+	+
IL-4	–	+
IL-5	–	+
interferon γ	+	–
GM-CSF	+	+
TNF-β (lymphotoxin)	+	–
Help for B lymphocytes		
IgG, IgA, IgM	+	+++
IgE	–	+
Delayed-type hypersensitivity	+	–

Fig. 9.9 Two functional types of CD4⁺ T lymphocyte in the mouse. As a result of their different basic profiles of lymphokine synthesis, TH_1 cells appear to be better equipped to participate in cell-mediated immune responses, whereas TH_2 cells tend to promote an antibody response (including the synthesis of IgE).

CD8⁺ cytotoxic $T_{\alpha\beta}$ lymphocytes

Killing of cells infected by viruses and intracellular bacteria and of malignant cells is usually effected by CD8⁺ T lymphocytes which recognize antigenic peptides on the surface of such cells (derived from viral or bacterial proteins or novel cellular proteins expressed as a result of malignant transformation) in association with MHC class I molecules. CD8⁺ cytotoxic cells tend to spare innocent bystander cells, suggesting that contact-specific activation is more important for killing than secretion of soluble factors. Furthermore, cytotoxic T lymphocytes can detach and lyse new targets.

Cytotoxic T lymphocytes in culture produce proteins called perforins. Electron microscopy shows that aggregates of perforins form tubules which effectively 'punch holes' in the target cell membrane. In addition, it has been noted that target cells killed by cytotoxic T lymphocytes undergo nuclear shrinkage and fragmentation of their DNA, processes characteristic of programmed cell death or apoptosis. This raises the possibility that cytotoxic T lymphocytes kill target cells by switching on a pre-programmed cell-death mechanism, which may be of particular relevance to the elimination of viruses. If initiation of this process requires specific cellular contact, this might explain how bystander cells are spared.

$T_{\gamma\delta}$ lymphocytes

Little is known as yet about the function of these T lymphocytes, but their abundance at mucosal surfaces suggests that they might have a role to play in mucosal inflammation. They possess relatively few V- and J-region genes to encode their antigen receptors; furthermore, at least in the mouse, one particular V_γ gene is preferentially used at any given site (e.g. cells expressing $V_{\gamma 7}$ are predominant in the intestinal mucosa whereas $v_{\gamma 5}$ cells predominate in the skin). This might suggest that these cells have a limited antigenic repertoire; on the other hand, since most of the variability in the γ and δ chain-encoding genes

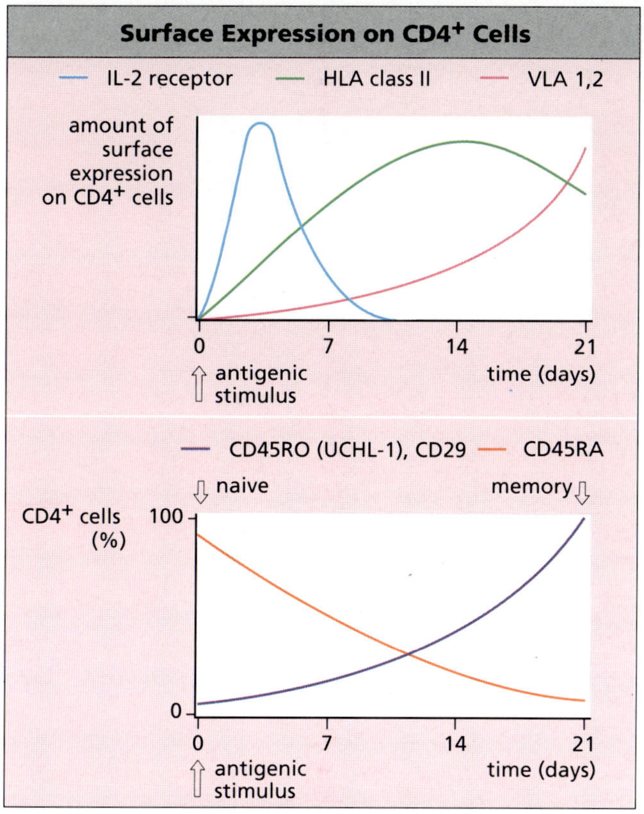

Fig. 9.10 [top] Expression of activation markers on the surface of T lymphocytes after they have been presented with specific antigen. These markers can be used to identify activated T lymphocytes in tissues and body fluids. [bottom] Reciprocal expression of CD45RA and CD45RO on T lymphocytes. Naive cells, which have never been exposed to antigen, express high levels of CD45RA which is progressively lost after activation. At the same time, the expression of CD45RO as well as CD29 are progressively increased. The functional significance of these changes is not known, but they do provide useful clues as to whether or not the T lymphocytes arriving at a given site have been previously exposed to antigen.

arises from the V(D)J joining region (Figs 9.5, 9.6), the repertoire might still be considerable.

Cytotoxicity, which need not be restricted to MHC class I molecules, is one property of these cells. They can also be activated by heat-shock proteins, a range of highly conserved proteins secreted by a wide variety of cells in response to physical, chemical or immunological insults. Similar proteins can also be found in bacteria, especially mycobacteria. Because of their possible limited antigenic repertoire and their sensitivity to heat-shock proteins, the suggestion has been made that $T_{\gamma\delta}$ lymphocytes may serve as 'sentinels' at mucosal surfaces, being activated (through heat-shock proteins) in response to any form of mucosal injury. At the present time this remains speculative. It will be important in the future to define better the phenotypic and functional characteristics $T_{\gamma\delta}$ lymphocytes if (as is likely) they are present at sites of allergic mucosal inflammation.

Other T-Lymphocyte Surface Molecules

T lymphocytes express many other surface molecules in addition to the αβ or γδ antigen receptor, CD2, CD3, and CD4 or CD8. The account of other molecules given below is not exhaustive, but rather is meant simply to highlight some other molecules whose functional significance is at least partly understood. Expression of such molecules by T lymphocytes at sites of inflammation can be detected by staining with specific antibodies, providing clues as to their functional properties and degree of activation.

Activation molecules

Some molecules appear or increase in number on the surface of T lymphocytes after activation by specific antigen (Fig. 9.10 [top]). Expression of these molecules by T lymphocytes at sites of inflammation implies that they have been activated and are secreting lymphokines. The receptor for IL-2 (a lymphokine produced by activated T cells which is essential for their own continued proliferation) appears on the surface of T lymphocytes about 24 hours after activation. In the absence of further antigenic exposure, it persists for several days and then declines. MHC class II molecules appear on the surface of T lymphocytes soon after activation by antigen. Their function on T lymphocytes, which do not present antigen, is unknown but they are useful markers of cellular activation. The VLA family of molecules is concerned with binding of cells to tissue matrix substances such as laminin, collagen and fibronectin. T lymphocytes begin to express VLA-l and VLA-2 after two to three weeks of chronic stimulation *in vitro*. The appearance of these molecules might be related to the need for T lymphocytes to adhere to tissues at sites of chronic inflammation.

Many other molecules are increased in numbers on the surface of T lymphocytes after activation; these molecules include the cellular receptors for transferrin and corticosteroids.

Naive and memory T lymphocytes

The CD45R surface molecule is found on both $CD4^+$ and $CD8^+$ T lymphocytes and can be found in a number of structural forms, including two called CD45RA and CD45RO. These forms are produced by differential splicing of the mRNA transcript of the CD45R gene. CD45RA and CD45RO are expressed on T lymphocytes in a reciprocal fashion: CD45RA 'high' cells are CD45RO 'low', and vice versa. CD45RO 'high' cells are also CD29 'high', whereas CD45RA 'high' cells are CD29 'low'. These changes reflect different maturational stages of T lymphocytes rather than distinct lineages (Fig. 9.10 [bottom]). Activation of CD45RA 'high' cells results in down-regulation of this marker and up-regulation of CD45RO and CD29 on the same cells. These changes do not revert when the activating antigen is removed, in contrast to some of the activation markers described previously. CD29, CD45RO 'high' T lymphocytes show enhanced help for immunoglobulin production, enhanced responses to recall antigens, and greater cytotoxicity in comparison to CD45RA 'high' cells. Furthermore, CD29 'high' cells constitute 40 per cent of adult peripheral blood T lymphocytes but less than 5 per cent of the T lymphocytes in neonatal umbilical-cord blood. For these reasons CD45RO, CD29 'high' cells are thought

Antibody Molecule

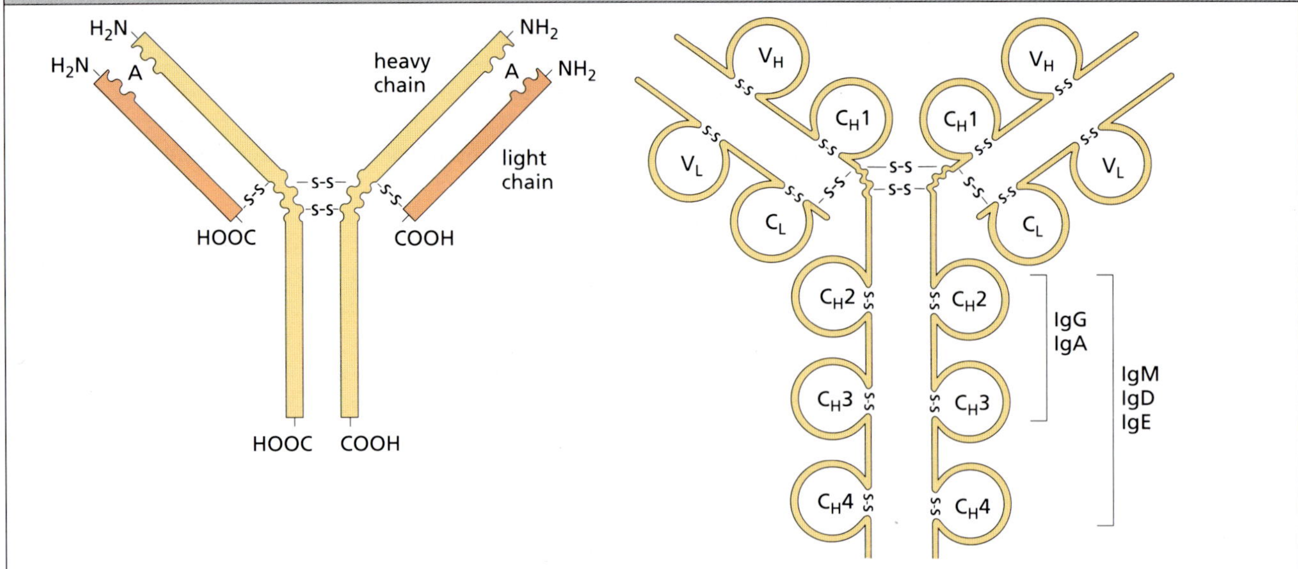

Fig. 9.11 [left] Schematic representation of an antibody molecule. The molecule is symmetrical, with two heavy and light polypeptide chains held together by disulphide bridges. There are two identical antigen binding sites formed by the variable ends of the heavy and light chains. [right] The heavy and light chains are pulled by intra-chain disulphide bridges into partly homologous domains as shown.

to be memory cells which have previously been activated by exposure to specific antigen. Arrival of such cells at sites of experimental antigen challenge implies specific recruitment of T cells which have previously been exposed to the initiating antigen.

Adhesion molecules
The presence of VLA molecules on activated T lymphocytes has already been mentioned. In addition, T lymphocytes express LFA-1, which binds to a molecule called ICAM-1, an adhesion molecule found on vascular endothelial cells. Activated T lymphocytes also express LFA-3, the ligand for CD2 (which is also expressed on all T lymphocytes). Thus, T lymphocytes have the capacity to adhere to endothelial surfaces and to each other.

Of great interest is the recent demonstration of T-lymphocyte tissue-specific homing receptors. Migration of T lymphocytes into tissues takes place at specialized post-capillary vascular sites called high endothelial venules (HEV), which are found in all lymphoid organs except the spleen. *In vivo*, T lymphocytes bind preferentially to HEV. They have also been described in various chronic inflammatory lesions, such as tuberculin reactions in the skin. In man, a monoclonal antibody (Hermes-3) binds to endothelial cells and inhibits adhesion of T lymphocytes to HEV in Peyer's patches in the gut, but not in other lymphoid tissues. Antibodies against the more ubiquitous adhesion molecules such as ICAM-1 also partly inhibit this adhesion, so that the two groups of molecules may function in concert, with molecules such as that recognized by Hermes-3 conferring tissue specificity. These observations imply that subgroups of T lymphocytes, perhaps with specific functions, may accumulate preferentially in specific tissues.

B Lymphocytes

Functional Spectrum of B Lymphocytes
B lymphocytes are responsible for the synthesis of specific antibodies on exposure to antigen. Each individual B lymphocyte secretes a single antibody of uniform structure, and thus of uniform antigen specificity. This same antibody is also expressed on the B-lymphocyte cell surface, and it is through this surface-bound antibody that the cell recognizes specific antigen. Antibodies form an indispensable part of the immune response, called the humoral response because it is concerned partly (but not exclusively) with the neutralization of antigens in solution.

Antibodies are large molecules composed of four polypeptide chains, two light and two heavy chains, joined by disulphide bridges. The three-dimensional structure of antibodies is necessary to enable them to bind to antigen. Antibodies recognize the shape of antigens, in contrast to T lymphocytes which, as we have seen, recognize small oligopeptides derived from the native antigen.

The Structure and Functions of Antibodies
Antibodies are symmetrical molecules with two antigen-binding sites (Fig. 9.11 [left]). They are required to bind to and neutralize a potentially limitless number of environmental antigens, and this is reflected in the wide variability of antibody structure. Most of this variability lies in the 100 amino-terminal amino acid residues of the heavy and light chains of the antibody – called the variable (V) regions – whilst the carboxy-terminal ends are relatively uniform or constant (C) in structure. The C regions of the heavy chains can be grouped according to overall structure into classes or isotypes (called μ, δ, γ1–4, α1, 2 and ϵ), corresponding to the classes of antibody

Properties of Antibodies
Properties of antigen binding (variable) region
binding and neutralization of soluble antigens
forms B lymphocyte receptor for antigen
Properties of class-specific (Fc) region
fixation of complement (IgG1-3, IgM)
activation of monocytes and granulocytes through their Fc receptors (IgG, IgE, ?IgA)
indirect killing of cells and organisms by complement activation by activation of granulocytes by antibody-dependent cell cytotoxicity by other effects, e.g. immobilisation of organisms
crossing of the placenta (IgG1, 3, 4)
concentration in secretions (IgA)
immediate-type hypersensitivity (IgE)

Fig. 9.12 General properties of antibodies. These can be divided into: (1) the properties of the variable region, the function of which is to bind antigen; and (2) the properties of the constant regions of the molecules which depend on the antibody class.

seen in the circulation and on the B-lymphocyte surface (IgM, IgD, IgG1–4, IgA1,2 and IgE). The light chain C regions have two basic alternative structures – κ and λ. The C regions are composed of partly homologous repeating sequences: heavy chains have three (IgG, IgA) or four (IgM, IgD, IgE) such sequences (C_H1–4), whilst light chains have only one (C_L1). These sequences are fashioned by intra-chain disulphide bridges into 'domains' (Fig. 9.11 [right]). The heavy chains are glycosylated, usually at the CH2 domain. The significance of this is unknown. In addition to this basic four chain structure, IgM exists in the serum as a polymer of 5 four-chain molecules linked by disulphide bonds. IgA exists mostly as a monomer in the circulation, but is also found at high concentrations in the secretions at most mucosal surfaces, where it exists as a dimer, the two four-chain molecules being joined by a third small polypeptide called the J chain. In addition, secretory IgA is associated with a fourth secretory (S) protein, which is essential for its transport across epithelial surfaces.

The variable regions of immunoglobulins are concerned with binding and neutralization of antigens, whereas the structure of their constant (Fc) regions confer class-specific properties (Fig. 9.12). Eosinophils and neutrophils have receptors for the Fc portions of IgG, whilst mast cells, basophils, eosinophils and B lymphocytes themselves (see below) have Fc receptors for IgE. Granulocytes may be activated non-specifically through these receptors if their bound antibody is cross-linked by antigen. Thus, mast cells and eosinophils may be activated by exposure to allergens only in the presence of allergen-specific IgE. This of course is the basis of immediate hypersensitivity.

B-Lymphocyte Differentiation

Rearrangement of immunoglobulin genes in a pluripotential stem cell in the bone marrow commits the cell to the B-lymphocyte lineage. Of the two sets of immunoglobulin genes in the cell (one on each chromosome), only one set is rearranged and expressed, a phenomenon called allelic exclusion. This means that B lymphocytes from a single stem cell express identical antibody molecules. Little is known about early B-lymphocyte differentiation in the bone marrow, but it is likely that it is under the control of local environmental and growth factors. As with T lymphocytes in the thymus, only a small percentage of the B lymphocytes in the bone marrow ever survive to leave it; this may reflect a process whereby cells making anti-self antibodies are removed. Mature circulating B lymphocytes, which have not yet encountered specific antigen, are known as virgin B cells. These cells express surface IgM and IgD only. Activation by specific antigen is followed by proliferation and somatic mutation of the immunoglobulin gene (see below), so that the antigen-binding affinity of the antibody produced by the cells increases as they divide. The class (isotype) of the antibody may also change (see below), in which case the cell surface immunoglobulin isotype changes correspondingly. Some activated B lymphocytes are transformed into short-lived plasma cells secreting large amounts of antibody (up to 2000 molecules per second) whilst others become memory cells which respond more promptly when they re-encounter antigen. These cells always switch their antibody isotype away from IgD and IgM. Primary immune responses (the first encounter with a particular antigen) are characterized by the production of IgM by virgin B lymphocytes, then other immunoglobulin classes as the cells proliferate and switch isotype. Secondary immune responses may involve IgG, IgA, IgE or any combination of these three.

B lymphocytes cannot, in most cases, proliferate in response to antigen alone, but require help (in the form of cell contact and lymphokines) from $CD4^+$ pro-inflammatory T lymphocytes. This necessitates processing of the antigen by B lymphocytes into oligopeptide fragments and presentation to T lymphocytes in association with MHC class II molecules on the B-lymphocyte surface (see Fig. 9.13). B lymphocytes therefore function as antigen-presenting cells. The exact site where this T-lymphocyte/B-lymphocyte/antigen interaction occurs is unknown; many believe that it does not occur at sites of inflammation but at local lymph nodes, where activated B lymphocytes proliferate in the germinal centres of the lymph node follicles and are in intimate contact with T lymphocytes and macrophages.

Antibody Diversity

B lymphocytes can make many more antibody molecules than there are genes in the entire human genome. By analogy with T lymphocytes, this is achieved by the variable combination of gene segments which encode the immunoglobulin heavy and light chains. In addition, the V-region genes of both

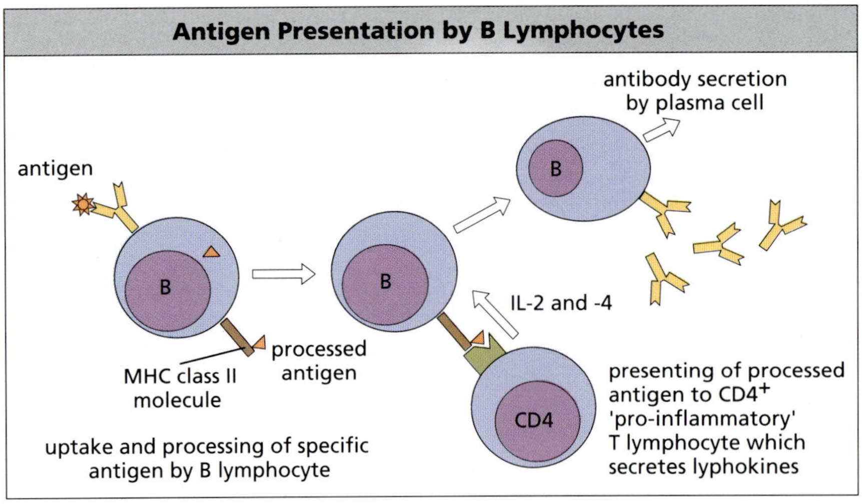

Fig. 9.13 Before they can proliferate in response to antigen, B lymphocytes have to process the antigen by cleaving it into small fragments, and present these fragments to T lymphocytes bound to MHC class II molecules. Lymphokines from the activated T lymphocytes then allow proliferation to take place. Thus T lymphocytes can influence the extent of antibody responses as well as the predominant antibody class which is secreted.

heavy and light chains have a high mutation rate during proliferation of the B lymphocyte on exposure to antigen, a phenomenon called somatic hypermutation, which is not seen in T lymphocytes. This mechanism is responsible for the increased affinity of antibody produced during the course of an immune response.

The genes encoding the heavy chains and the κ and λ light chains are arranged in three separate clusters on different chromosomes (Fig. 9.14). The V-region cluster for the heavy chains comprises multiple V, D, and J segments (as with T lymphocytes) which can be joined to any of the C-region segment genes. A separate C-region gene encodes each antibody class. The V-region V segments can be divided into families of between 4 and 100 genes, with over 75 per cent sequence homology within a family. The V segments contain three hypervariable regions, which form the sites on the antibody-variable regions which actually bind to the antigen. The light chain clusters have V, J, and C segments but no D segment. The κ cluster has hundreds of V segments, five J segments and a single C segment. The exact numbers of λ genes are not precisely known. During B-lymphocyte development, V/(D)/J/C segments are brought together to form a single gene encoding one heavy or one light chain. Expression of one functional heavy and light chain gene switches off further gene

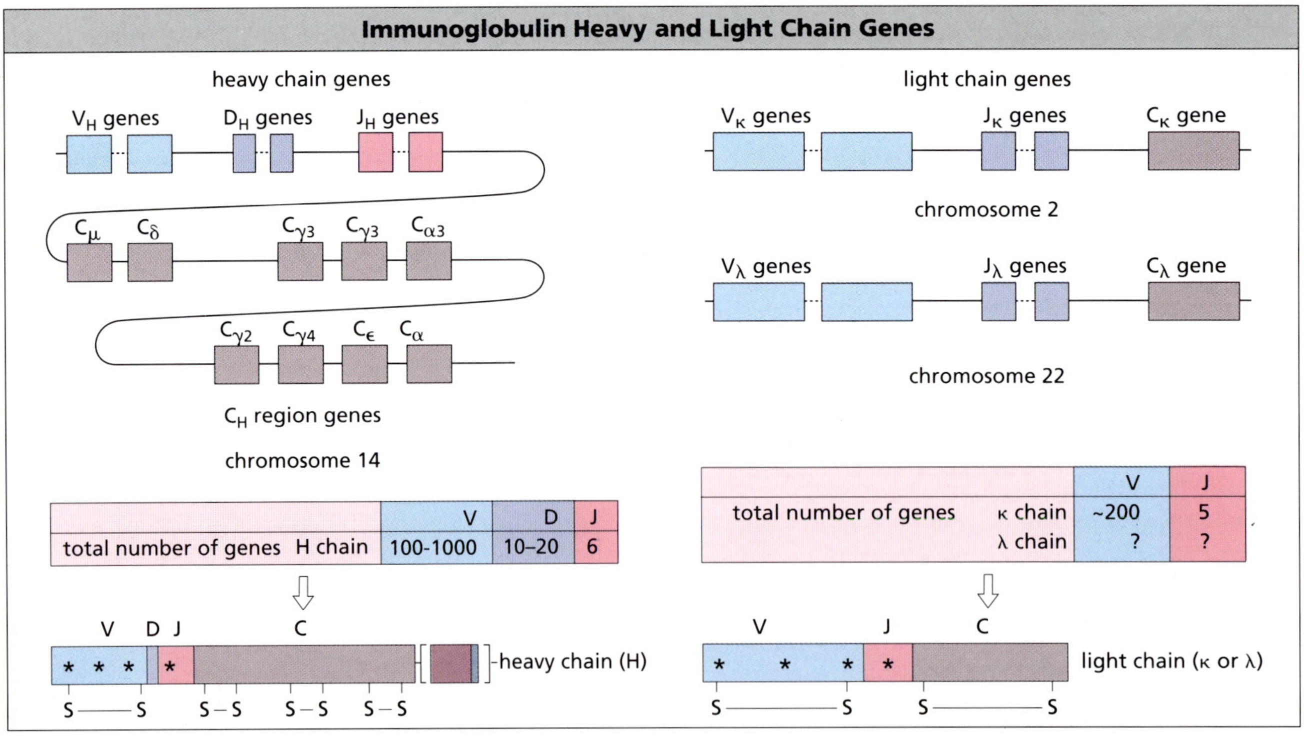

		V	D	J
total number of genes	H chain	100-1000	10–20	6

		V	J
total number of genes	κ chain	~200	5
	λ chain	?	?

Fig. 9.14 Organization of the immunoglobulin heavy and light chain genes. One V, (D), J and C segment are brought together in each B lymphocyte to form the genes for the heavy and light chains. There is a separate gene for each C_H region (which determines the class of the antibody). In any cell, only one of the two sets of immunoglobulin genes (one on each chromosome) is rearranged. The hypervariable regions (marked by asterisks) on the chains form the antigen binding site and arise through the use of variable V, D and J genes; as well, there is further variability induced at the junctional regions (Fig. 9.15). The heavy chain genes encode a terminal hydrophobic portion (shaded) which is responsible for membrane binding of the immunoglobulin. If the immunoglobulin is to be secreted, this portion is cleaved off during mRNA processing.

Generation of Antibody Diversity	
variable use of V, D and J region genes	
heavy chains	light chains
100-1000 V_H genes	>100 V_K unknown numbers of V_λ
10-20 D_H genes	none
6 J_H genes	5J_K genes unknown numbers of J_λ
random association of heavy and light chains	
junctional diversity (the precise DNA base at which V, D and J segments joins may vary)	
N-region diversity (addition or removal of one of a few nucleotides between gene segments)	
heavy chains	light chains
V-D, D-J	none
somatic hypermutation (further mutation of the V-region gene hypervariable regions after exposure to antigen)	

Fig. 9.15 Generation of antibody diversity. These mechanisms are similar to those used by T lymphocytes to generate diverse antigen-binding specificities, with the important exception that T-lymphocyte variable region genes cannot mutate somatically after exposure to specific antigen. As with T-lymphocyte receptors, the possible numbers of combinations of segments are enormous, far exceeding the total number of B lymphocytes in the body.

rearrangement, thus effecting allelic exclusion. In the case of the heavy chain, IgM- and IgD- C- region segments are expressed first. As a result of exposure of the B lymphocyte to antigen, the same V(D)J segments may be joined to different C segments (Fig. 9.14), thus changing the class of the antibody without altering its antigen specificity (class switching). Whether an immunoglobulin is membrane-bound or secreted depends on the carboxy-terminal amino acid sequence of the heavy chain C segments. There are two forms, hydrophobic (causing membrane retention) and hydrophilic (allowing secretion). Variation here operates at the level of splicing of the mRNA after the gene has been transcribed. Antibody diversity is therefore created by the mechanisms shown in Fig. 9.15.

B-Lymphocyte Activation

Antibody production requires exposure of B lymphocytes to specific antigen and contact with CD4⁺ T lymphocytes. Lymphokines (most of them derived from activated CD4⁺ T lymphocytes) and other soluble factors are also important. One useful classification of these factors is those involved in 'priming', 'progression' and 'proliferation' (Fig. 9.16).

(1) Priming refers to an enhanced response of B lymphocytes to subsequent antigen exposure, not accompanied by entry of the cells into the proliferative cycle. IL-4 and IgE can prime B lymphocytes, IgE acting through surface CD23, the IgE Fc receptor. Antibodies to a variety of other surface molecules (Fig. 9.16) can also prime B lymphocytes. The function of these is not yet known, though some will almost certainly prove to be receptors for molecules such as IL-4.

(2) Progression refers to entry of cells into the proliferative cycle but without actual cell division. This is accompanied by a number of cell surface changes (Fig. 9.16). IL-1, the complement fragment C3d and the B-lymphocyte growth factor $BCGF_{low}$ enhance progression, whereas IFN-γ and immune complexes inhibit it (the latter possibly by negative feedback on

Control of B Lymphocyte Activation

priming	progression	proliferation
resting	exposed to antigen	

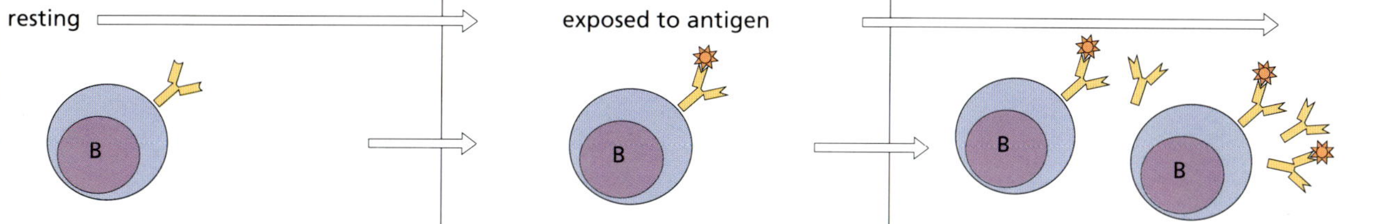

cell is 'primed' for enhanced response to antigen but not committed to division	cell begins to replicate DNA and progress towards replication	cell divides progressively with secretion of antibody
Enhanced by		
IL-4 IgE (via CD23, the Fc receptor) antibodies to the surface molecules CD20, CD21, CD22 and CDw40	IL-1 complement fragment C3d $BCGF_{low}$ (acts on CD23)	IL-2 interferon-γ IL-5 IL-6 soluble form of CD23
Cell surface changes		
↑ CD23	↓ IgD ↓ CD23 (with release of soluble form) ↑ MHC class II molecules	appearance of IL-2 receptor

Fig. 9.16 Control of B-lymphocyte activation, which can be thought of as occurring in three stages as shown. Proliferation is influenced by a complex array of lymphokines and other growth factors. Note the interesting role of IgE and $BCGF_{low}$, which both act on the CD23 IgE F_c receptor. Binding of $BCGF_{low}$ to CD23 causes cleavage and secretion of the latter. This soluble CD23 molecule can further enhance B-lymphocyte proliferation.

Fc receptors). $BCGF_{low}$ also acts on the CD23 molecule, which on activation is cleaved to a soluble molecule of lower molecular weight which itself enhances B-lymphocyte proliferation.

(3) Proliferation refers to actual B-lymphocyte division and is enhanced by a number of lymphokines (Fig. 9.16).

In addition to promoting B-lymphocyte proliferation non-specifically, some lymphokines derived from $CD4^+$ pro-inflammatory T lymphocytes can influence the production of particular antibody isotypes. For instance, IL-4 increases synthesis of IgG1 and IgE, but reduces synthesis of IgG2 and IgG3. IFN-γ inhibits IgE secretion. IL-5 can enhance IgA secretion, which may be important in mucosal inflammation. IgE antibody itself may play an interesting role, since this antibody can prime resting B lymphocytes, but may also block the action of $BCGF_{low}$ by its binding to CD23.

T and B Lymphocytes in Allergic Inflammation and Asthma

Asthma and allergic rhinitis are characterized by mucosal inflammation, which in turn is believed to be responsible for many of the pathophysiological features of these diseases. $CD4^+$ T lymphocytes, as well as eosinophils and mast cells, are particularly abundant at such sites of mucosal inflammation. $CD4^+$ T lymphocytes can respond directly to antigens encountered at mucosal surfaces and, by the secretion of lymphokines, bring about the accumulation and activation of specific granulocytes. The direct activation of T lymphocytes by antigen and their subsequent direct effects on granulocytes form one major possible mechanism for the genesis of allergic inflammation, which is independent of the presence or absence of IgE (Fig. 9.17).

B lymphocytes in atopic subjects secrete IgE in response to airborne allergens and other antigens. The control of this process is evidently very complex, but is in part influenced by products of $CD4^+$ T lymphocytes. In atopic subjects, allergen-specific IgE bound to granulocyte Fc receptors may activate these cells directly on exposure to allergens, with release of inflammatory mediators. This forms a second major possible mechanism for the genesis of allergic inflammation which depends on the presence of allergen-specific IgE (Fig. 9.17).

It will be important in the future to delineate the relative importance of these two parallel mechanisms in the pathogenesis of allergic inflammation and asthma. Whereas direct degranulation of mast cells

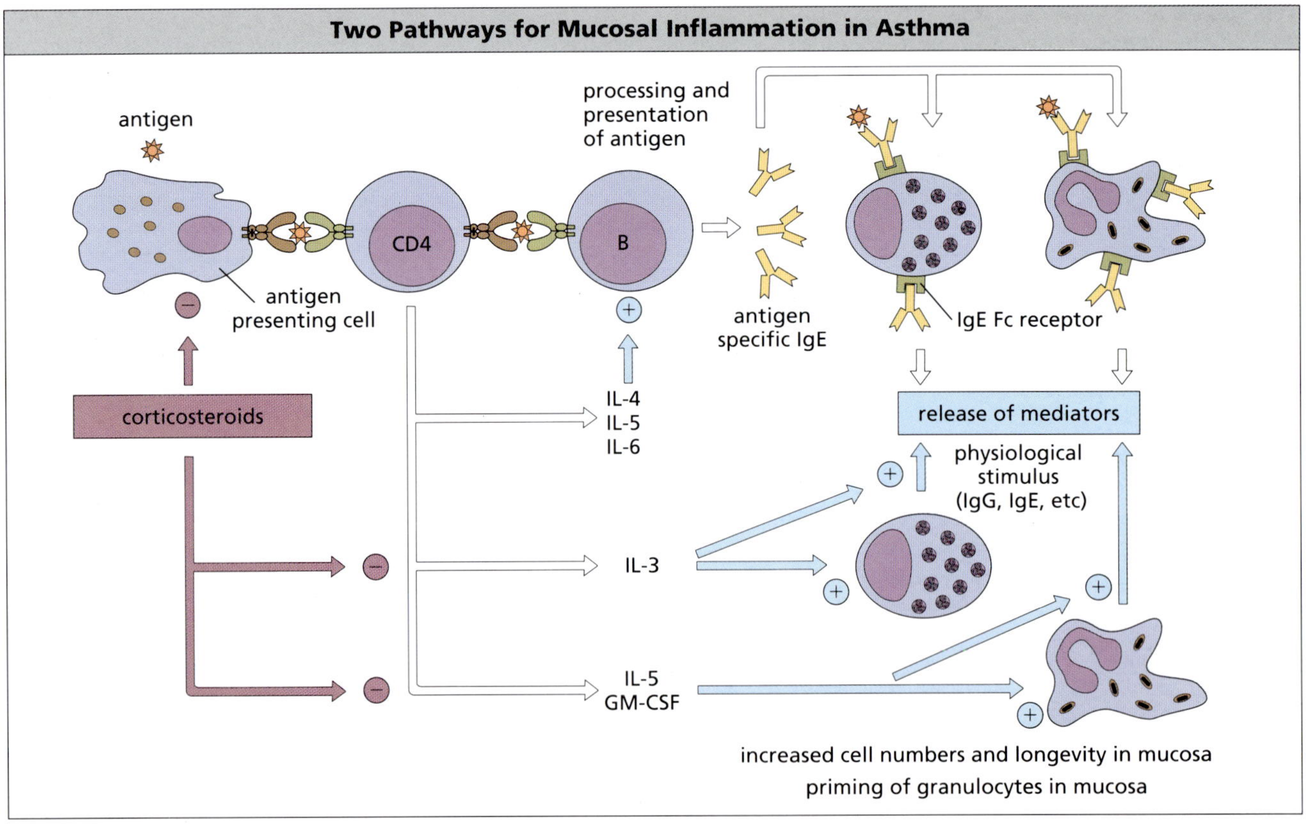

Fig. 9.17 Two pathways for antigen-mediated bronchial mucosal inflammation in asthma.
[upper pathway] Antigens may also activate granulocytes (such as mast cells and eosinophils) directly if the latter possess surface-bound antigen-specific IgE which is cross-linked after antigen exposure. This mechanism is not obviously applicable to non-atopic subjects.
[lower pathway] Antigens (including airborne allergens) may activate T lymphocytes directly, leading to release of lymphokines which subsequently activate granulocytes such as eosinophils. This mechanism need not involve antigen-specific IgE.
The lower mechanism (which is inhibited by corticosteroids) may be more important in chronic disease, whilst the upper (which is partly inhibited by granulocyte-stabilizing drugs such as nedocromil and cromoglycate, but not by corticosteroids) might be responsible for acute exacerbations of symptoms following exposure of atopic subjects to allergens.
+ = stimulatory effect; − = inhibitory effect.

and eosinophils on exposure to allergens may be important in producing acute exacerbations of rhinitis and asthma in atopic patients, inflammation orchestrated by activated T lymphocytes may be more important in chronic disease. A predominant role for activated $CD4^+$ T lymphocytes provides a unifying hypothesis for the pathogenesis of asthma in both atopic and non-atopic individuals. Corticosteroids, the mainstay of prophylactic therapy for both asthma and allergic rhinitis, are extremely inhibitory to T lymphocytes but have little effect on granulocyte function. Corticosteroids may therefore ameliorate allergic inflammation by inhibiting lymphokine production by T lymphocytes, rather than by a direct effect on granulocytes.

Since T lymphocytes may be able to accumulate specifically in different tissues, it will be important in future studies to characterize the properties of cells actually at the sites of allergic inflammatory responses in terms of their antigen specificities and profiles of lymphokine production. Only then will it be possible to appreciate fully their role in allergic diseases and asthma. With regard to B-lymphocyte function, a better understanding of the regulation of IgE secretion in atopic subjects may lead to new approaches to the therapy of these diseases.

Further Reading

Allison JP, Lanier LL. The structure, function and serology of the T cell antigen receptor complex. *Ann Rev Immunol* 1987; **5**:503–40.

Claverle J-M, Drochnika Chalufour A, Bougaeleret L. Implications of a F_{ab} like structure for the T cell receptor. *Immunol Today* 1989; **10**:10–14.

Janeway CA, Jones B, Hayday A. Specificity and function of cells bearing Fγδ receptors. *Immunol Today* 1988; **9**:73–76.

Kronenberg M, Sul G, Hood KE, Shastri N. The molecular genetics of the T cell antigen recognition. *Ann Rev Immunol* 1986; **4**:529–91.

Marrack P, Kappler, J. The antigen-specific major histocompatibility complex-restricted receptor on T cells. *Adv Immunol* 1986; **38**:1–30.

Mosmann TR, Coffman RL. Th1 and Th2 cells: different patterns of lymphokine secretion lead to different functional properties. *Ann Rev Immunol* 1989; **7**:145–73

Romagnani S, Del Prete G, Maggi C, Parronchi P, Tiri A, Macchia D, Giudizi MG, Almengogna F, Ricci M. Role of Interleukins in induction and regulation of human IgE synthesis. *Clin Immunol Immunopathol* 1989; **50**:513–518.

Sanders ME, Makgoba MW, Shaw S. Human naive and memory cells: reinterpretation of helper-inducer and suppressor-inducer subsets. *Immunol Today* 1989; **9**:195–98.

Schleimer RP, Claman HN, Oronsky A, eds. Anti-inflammatory steroid action: basic and clinical aspects. London: Academic Press, 1989.

Chapter 10

Neutrophils

Introduction

Neutrophilic polymorphonuclear leucocytes, or 'neutrophils', are white blood cells of the myeloid series. They are produced in the bone marrow and normally circulate with a short half-life before their removal, mainly by the spleen. Neutrophils are essential for host defence against infection and have functions ideally suited to this role. They are exquisitely responsive to signals generated in infected or injured tissues, which induce them to migrate rapidly through tissues to the site of perturbation. They are the first cells to arrive and are immediately effective in the killing of bacteria. A pivotal role in the inflammatory response is suggested by their involvement in the generation of inflammatory oedema, and the dependence of monocyte migration upon the initial accumulation of neutrophils. The beneficial effects of neutrophils in host defence were first recognized a century ago, by Metchnikoff in his description of phagocytes digesting bacteria. A variety of diseases, characterized by a common susceptibility to infection, have now been linked to specific defects in neutrophil structure and function.

More recently it has become apparent that neutrophils are widely involved in diseases that are responsible for many illnesses and premature deaths. It seems that the neutrophil-mediated processes which protect the host can also cause these inflammatory diseases. For example, the proteolytic enzymes and reactive oxygen species which enable the neutrophil to move rapidly through tissues and to kill bacteria have also been implicated in many inflammatory diseases. The development of safe and rational strategies for the treatment of inflammatory diseases will require a deeper understanding of this central paradox, which is likely to be achieved only by a detailed dissection of the cellular and molecular biology of neutrophil behaviour in inflammation.

Some neutrophil-mediated injury to local tissues is likely to be inevitable, even in the 'beneficial inflammation' associated with the eradication of bacteria. However, it is generally considered that potentially injurious neutrophil processes tend to be effectively counter-balanced by tissue defences, thus minimizing injury. It is possible, nevertheless, that loss of control of neutrophil behaviour may lead to chronic inflammation. The neutrophil is often perceived as an immutable, end-stage cell which digests its way through tissues, killing bacteria before finally disintegrating. However, it is now clear that neutrophil behaviour may be modulated by environmental influences, and that its interactions with other cells are both subtle and complex.

Structure, Origin and Physiological Behaviour

Morphology

Neutrophils are easily recognized on giemsa- or Wright-stained cytological preparations by their distinctive nuclei and pinkish cytoplasm (Fig. 10.1). On electron microscopy, the cells have a mean diameter of about 7μm, a multilobed nucleus and a large number of granules. When the cell is stained for

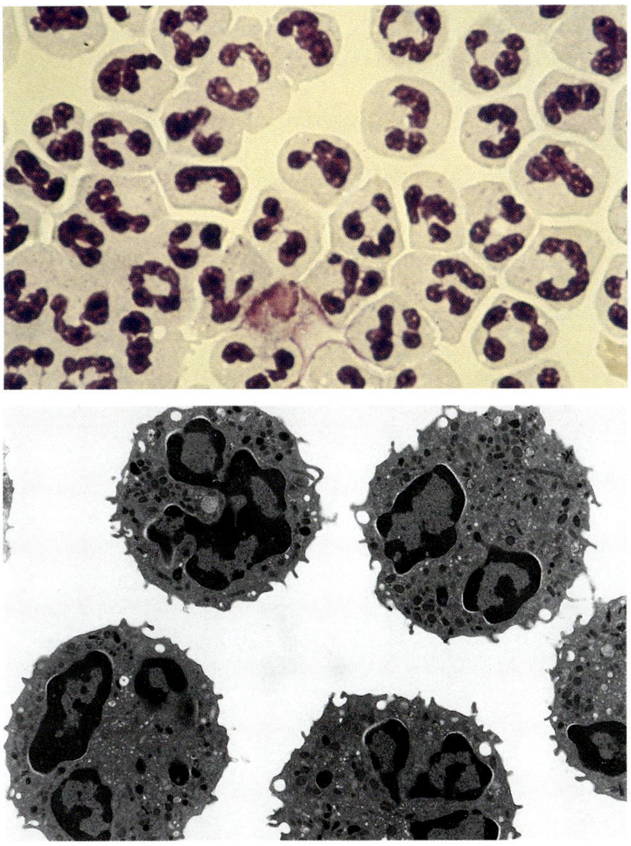

Fig. 10.1 [above] Light microscopy of a cytospin preparation of purified human neutrophils, stained with Wright's modified giemsa. Note the slightly pink cytoplasm and lobulated nucleus with loosely granular chromatin (oil immersion X 1000). [below] EM of human neutrophils. Note the large numbers of cytoplasmic granules (X 12,000). (Courtesy of Jan Henson.)

peroxidase, the granules appear heterogeneous, with larger 'azurophil' (or 'primary') granules, which are peroxidase positive, and the 'specific' (or 'secondary') granules, which are peroxidase negative. Other subcellular structures, such as Golgi apparatus and mitochondria are scarce, although human neutrophils do contain some smooth endoplasmic reticulum. The neutrophil membrane is of prime importance, since it contains both the receptors which detect inflammatory mediators and the molecules involved in transduction of external signals into cellular responses. Finally, there is an intimate arrangement between the cell membrane and the cytoskeletal framework of the cell, which resides mainly in the submembrane region and is responsible for complex motility functions such as polarization, spreading, chemotaxis and phagocytosis.

Granule Contents

The compartmentalization of antimicrobial agents within granules provides an opportunity for selective and controlled delivery to the target particle within the phagolysosome. Granules may also provide a mechanism for exocytosis of protein receptors at the leading front of the migrating cell. Neutrophil granules contain a variety of proteins, many of which are highly cationic and enzymatically active (Fig. 10.2). By contrast with monocyte-macrophage cells, the synthesis and assembly of granules in the short-lived neutrophil occurs only during the promyelocyte/myelocyte stage of granulocytopoiesis: granule products cannot be reconstituted once released.

A number of granule proteins have been implicated in bacterial killing, for example, myeloperoxidase, which is intimately involved in the generation of toxic reactive oxygen species in the phagolysosome.

Constituents of Human Neutrophil Granules

	Azurophil granules	Specific granules
Microbicidal enzymes	lysozyme myeloperoxidase	lysozyme
Neutral proteinases	elastase collagenases cathepsin G	collagenase
Acid hydrolases	phosphatases lipases sulphatases histonase cathepsin D β glycerophosphatase esterase neuraminidase 5' nucleotidase	phosphatases
Others	bactericidal/permeability inducing protein defensins cationic proteins glycosaminoglycans chondroitin sulphate heparin sulphate	lactoferrin VIT B_{12} binding protein C3bi receptor cytochrome B flavoproteins

Fig. 10.2 Typical constituents of human neutrophil granules.

Others appear capable of killing bacteria *in vitro* without the requirement of oxygen. For example, collaborative effects of various granule constituents have been examined only recently, and it is clear that some agents previously thought, from *in vivo* studies, to have little antibacterial activity may have major roles in concert with other factors. Certain granule proteins do have clear antibacterial effects *in vitro*.

Bactericidal/Permeability-inducing Protein

Bactericidal/permeability-inducing protein (BPI) accounts for virtually all neutrophil activity against certain susceptible organisms, principally Gram-negative bacteria, and in particular *Escherichia coli*. Such activity is abolished by specific anti-BPI antibodies, and purified BPI causes lesions in target bacteria which are indistinguishable from those induced by intact neutrophils. BPI is tightly bound within neutrophil azurophil granules; its antibacterial activity appears to be restricted to the intracellular environment, where it is likely to be mediated primarily through a combination of electrostatic and hydrophobic interactions with the outer membrane of the bacterium, and secondarily by hydrolysis of bacterial phospholipids.

Defensins are cationic peptides (e.g. HNP-1, HNP-2 and HNP-3) whose antibacterial effects correlate with their charge, which is determined by the arginine content. Defensins kill a variety of Gram-positive organisms, fungi and viruses *in vitro*. Unlike BPI, defensins appear in the extracellular medium upon neutrophil degranulation and they are potentially toxic to mammalian cells. The mechanisms of their toxicity are uncertain. Cathepsin E is a neutral proteinase derived from azurophil granules, whose antibacterial activity does not appear to depend on enzymic action. Lactoferrin is an Fe-binding glycoprotein which is only found in specific granules. Its antibacterial action is related in part to competition with Fe-requiring bacteria for an essential growth factor. Lysozyme is a highly cationic protein with a very specific disruptive effect on bacteria which contain susceptible cell wall peptidoglycans. However, very few organisms of relevance to human disease have cell wall components susceptible to cleavage by lysozyme, which raises questions about the role of this widely distributed granule enzyme. The physiological functions of many granule contents of the neutrophil are poorly understood.

Neutrophil Ontogeny, Maturation and Circulation

More than half of the work of the bone marrow is dedicated to the production of neutrophils. However, because mature neutrophils have a short half-life in the blood, there are comparatively few circulating at any given time. *In vitro* studies with colonies of marrow cells have shown that progenitor cells give rise to cells which are committed to a single lineage of myeloblasts, which then divide further through a promyelocyte stage to metamyelocytes. These are essentially end-cells because they do not divide further. They enter a large bone marrow pool where they mature through 'band' forms into fully mature segmented neutrophils (Fig. 10.3).

Constitutive granulocytopoiesis is under the control of growth factors, such as IL-3 which is non-specific and GM-CSF and G-CSF which are lineage specific. It is now becoming clear that the interaction between stem cells and stromal cells in the bone marrow, including endothelial cells, epithelial cells and fibroblasts, is of profound importance. Stromal cells, by a combination of the production of soluble mediators and complex cell contact interactions appear to exert critical controls on stem cells. Furthermore, stromal cell release of growth factors is profoundly sensitive to external agents, such as IL-1 and TNF which are released from inflamed sites, thus providing a highly sensitive inducible component (see Fig. 10.3), which rapidly mobilizes more cells when required. Factors which exert negative influences on granulocytopoiesis, e.g. TGF_{β}, have also been identified. Thus the molecular mechanisms of the background constitutive production of neutrophils and the enormous potential for inducible amplification are now becoming clearer.

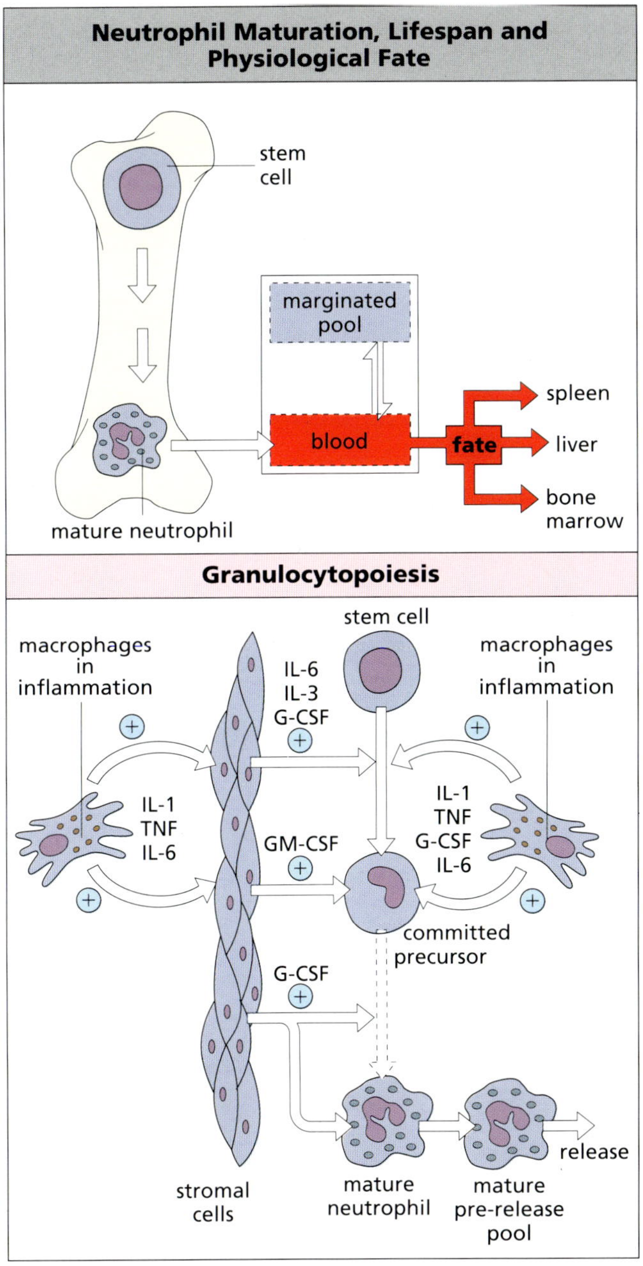

Neutrophil Circulation and Physiological Fate

Mature neutrophils exist in the blood compartment with a half-life of about 6 hours. About half of the neutrophils in the vascular compartment at a given time do not circulate. This physiological retention of neutrophils by the lung may allow the rapid release of a pool of neutrophils in stress or injury, and the presence of large numbers of neutrophils may increase the lungs' defences against inevitable exposure to inhaled micro-organisms or toxins.

The physiological fate of neutrophils has received little formal study. It was thought until quite recently that the oral cavity or the gut provided a 'sump' for effete neutrophils. However, the availability of methods to label mature blood neutrophils without greatly influencing their behaviour *in vivo* has shown that neutrophils meet their fate mainly in the spleen and, to a lesser extent, the liver and bone marrow (Fig. 10.3). It is likely that mononuclear phagocytes of these organs play an important role.

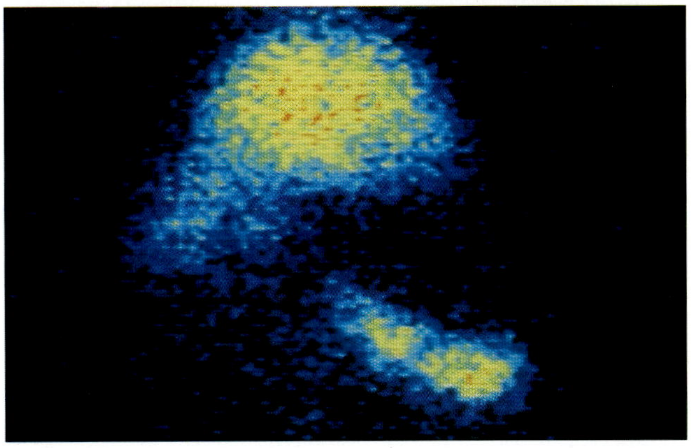

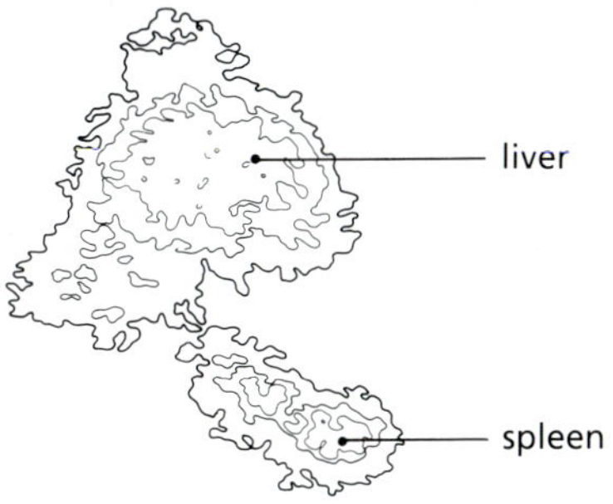

Fig. 10.3 Neutrophils are released from bone marrow into the bloodstream where the circulating pool is in dynamic equilibrium with the marginated pool [left]. Maturation in the bone marrow occurs constitutively under the influence of cytokines released by stromal cells in the marrow. During inflammation, a variety of agents released from the inflamed site are carried in the bloodstream to the bone marrow where marked amplification of granulocytopoiesis is induced. Neutrophils meet their fate physiologically in the spleen, liver and bone marrow. This is illustrated by a gamma camera scintigram of a rabbit taken after intravenous injection of a pulse of ^{111}indium-labelled neutrophils [above]. By 24 hours (6 half-lives), no labelled cells were circulating, and the scintigram shows that generally they remain localized in the spleen and liver.

The Neutrophil in Inflammation

External gamma camera scinitigraphy can be used to monitor the movement of radiolabelled neutrophils to inflamed sites both in experimental models and in human disease (Fig. 10.4). Changes in neutrophil behaviour which are set in motion by tissue injury or infection are illustrated in Fig. 10.5. For the purpose of discussion, these events are considered separately, although many are likely to occur simultaneously *in situ*.

Chemotactic Factors and Their Receptors

When injected into tissues, many inflammatory agents lead to neutrophil migration (Fig. 10.6). However, the numbers of true chemotactic factors, i.e. agents which cause directed migration via ligation of specific neutrophil receptors, is likely to be quite restricted. True chemotaxins include C5a and certain chemotactic bacterial products, exemplified by the synthetic analogue Fmet-leu-phe (fMLP). Recent data suggest that chemotactic cytokines, such as IL-8, also act via specific neutrophil receptors. It is likely that agents which themselves are not chemotactic *in vitro*, eg. TNF, IL-1, PAF, exert neutrophil-attracting effects *in vivo* by inducing the release of specific chemotaxins from other cells in the microenvironment. They may also induce the expression on local microvascular endothelial cells of adhesive molecules which influence neutrophil adhesion and transmigration.

Chemotaxins take effect by binding to specific receptors. FMLP and C5a receptors have now been cloned and are identified as members of the G-protein-linked/rhodopsin receptor superfamily. Chemo-attractant receptors are mobile and may be swept back from the leading edge of the cell and internalized, then recycled. Activation of neutrophils rapidly increases the number of receptors on the neutrophil surface, indicating the presence of a reserve population of chemoattractant receptors which may be contained within specific granules.

Neutrophil Activation

Neutrophil chemotactic responses are likely to be mediated through common mechanisms which cause rapid formation of inositol phosphates, diacylglycerol and a marked increase in free intracellular calcium – $[Ca^{2+}]_{ic}$ (Fig. 10.7). Modulating effects of guanosine triphosphate (GTP) and the inhibitory effects of certain bacterial toxins indicate a role for a guanine nucleotide-binding protein (G-protein) which may be unique to the neutrophil (Gc). Stimulation of the G-protein receptor complex activates phospholipase C which hydrolyzes phosphatidyl inositol (4,5)-bisphosphate into inositol trisphosphate (IP3) and 1,2-diacylglycerol (DAG). The IP3 causes rapid release of Ca^{2+} from intracellular stores, followed by a slower influx from the extracellular environment. DAG activates protein kinase C (PKC) to promote protein phosphorylation processes critical to cell locomotion and degranulation. It is also intimately associated with membrane-associated NADPH oxidase which converts 0_2 to 0_2^-.

Although the same general pathways are activated by many chemotaxins, there are finer levels of control for individual agents and for specific neutrophil functions, such as degranulation, superoxide production and motility. For example, LTB_4 is a good chemotaxin

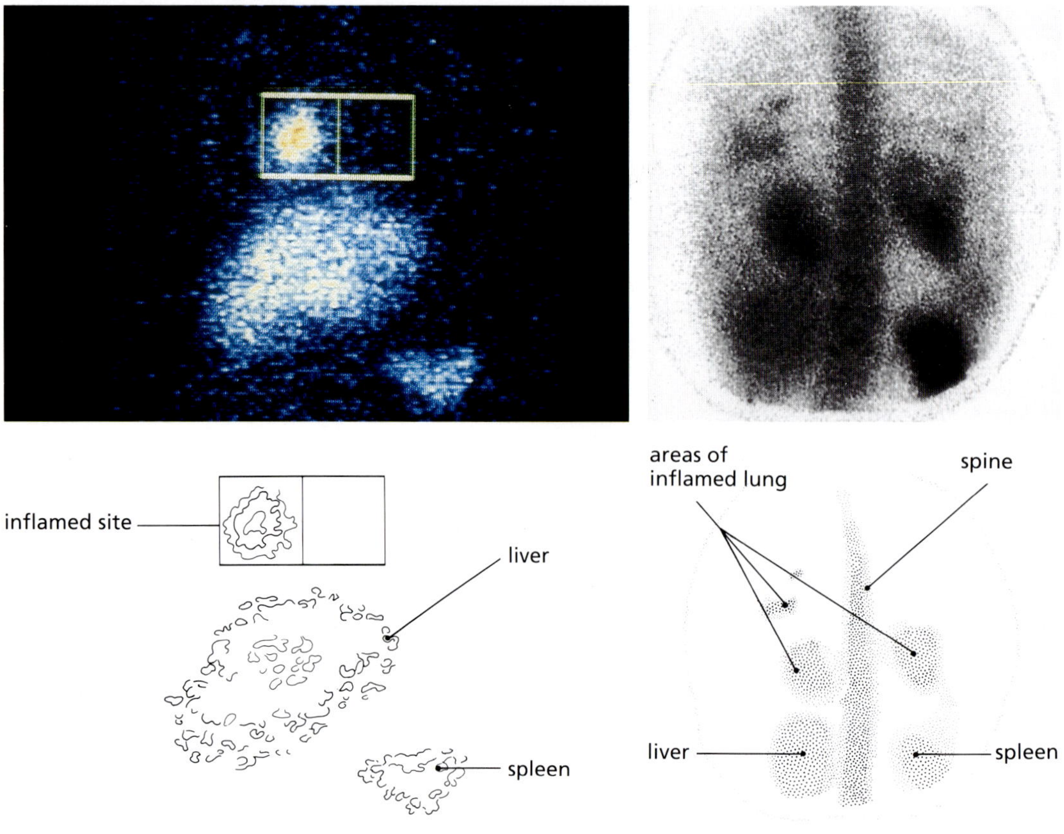

Fig. 10.4 [left] Neutrophil migration to an inflamed site in rabbit lung, illustrated by a gamma camera scintigram, taken 24 hours after intravenous injection of ^{111}indium-labelled neutrophils into a subject with streptococcal right upper lobe pneumonia. [right] Neutrophil migration to multiple areas of lung inflammation and infection in a patient with bronchiectasis. (Courtesy of Professor JP Lavender.)

but a poor secretagogue. This may be related to the observation that, unlike other chemotaxins, LTB_4 stimulation does not cause the later rise in $[Ca^{2+}]_{ic}$.

Neutrophils crawl and wriggle, rather than swim, to the inflamed site. The protrusive and retractive movements of the cell membrane necessary for this are likely to be mediated by subplasmalemmal filaments of the cytoskeleton linked to the membrane. One of the earliest events in the stimulated neutrophil is a change of neutrophil shape from the

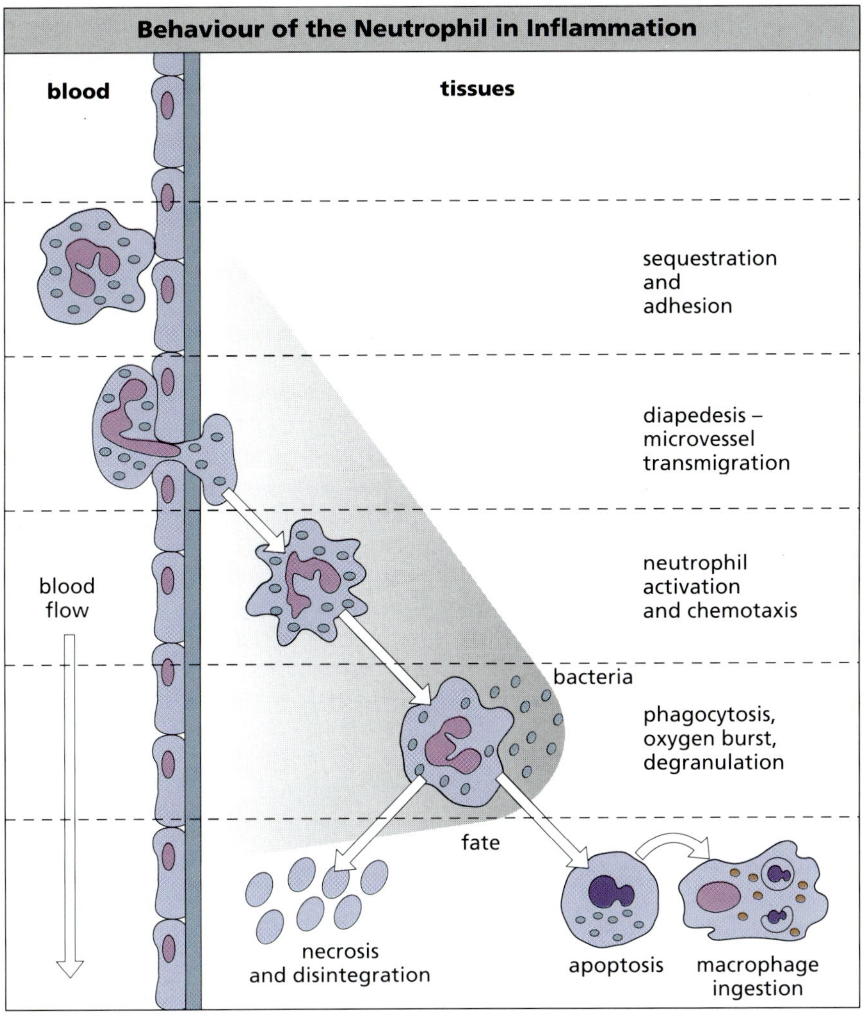

Fig. 10.5 Neutrophil behaviour in inflammation.

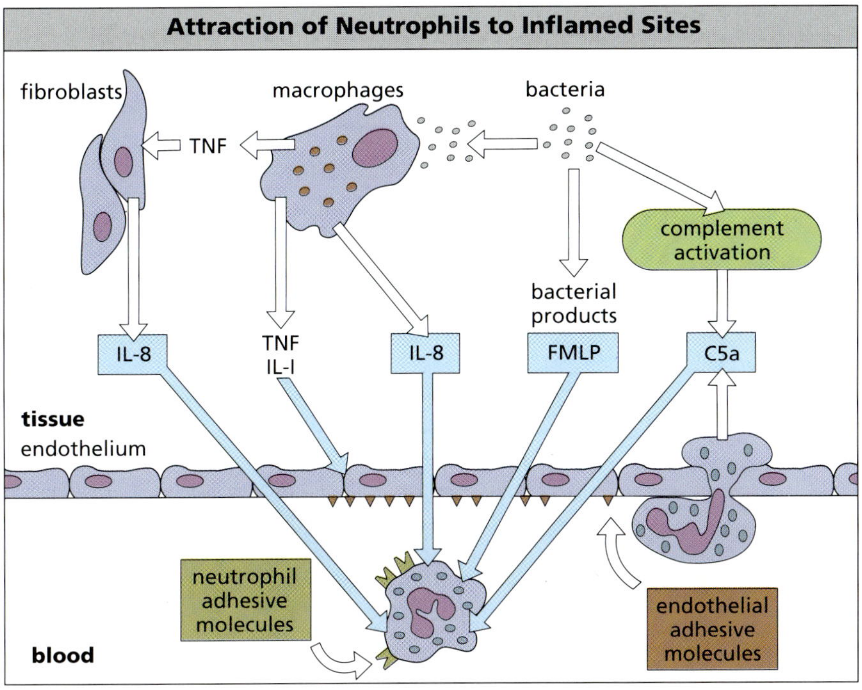

Fig. 10.6 The generation of chemotaxins (IL-8, C5a and bacterial factors, e.g. FMLP) which activate neutrophils and attract them to the inflamed site. Macrophages also produce IL-1 and TNF which act on endothelial cells to express adhesion molecules and on fibroblasts in a paracrine fashion to release more IL-8.

normally spherical cell to a polarized form (Fig. 10.8). This is associated with a reduction in cell deformability and in the mechanical changes which are the prelude to directed locomotion and phagocytosis, in which actin polymerization plays a prominent role. When the neutrophil is in a resting state, about half of its actin complement is insoluble and forms a branching network under the cell membrane which extends into and controls the formation of pseudopodia and other conformational changes. The network is composed of actin monomers (G-actin) which are polymerized to form actin-filaments (F-actin) which in turn are cross-linked into a web by another protein, actin-binding protein (ABP). The remaining 50 per cent of actin is maintained in a soluble form by agents which inhibit polymerization, providing the opportunity for considerable amplification of the actin framework upon activation (see Fig. 10.8). Profilin appears to sequester G-actin whereas gelsolin binds to the end of actin, preventing polymerization. Gelsolin has an additional inhibitory effect by cleaving binding sites between actin filaments, further restraining the formation of an insoluble actin web. These proteins are controlled in turn by second messengers generated during activation. For example, the affinity of profilin for actin is reduced by inositol phosphates. Gelsolin is under dual control: Ca^{2+} promotes its effects in cleaving actin filaments and blocking monomer addition, whereas inositol phosphates inhibit these effects.

Once formed, the actin web can be induced to contract by myosin which is activated locally by the action of a Ca^{2+}-calmodulin-dependent myosin light chain kinase. Although the control mechanisms are poorly understood, the mechanical responses critical for most neutrophil functions are centrally linked to early events in signal transduction. How gel-sol changes and membrane conformational changes are regulated locally in the very precise fashion required for such complex events as phagocytosis and degranulation is as yet poorly understood.

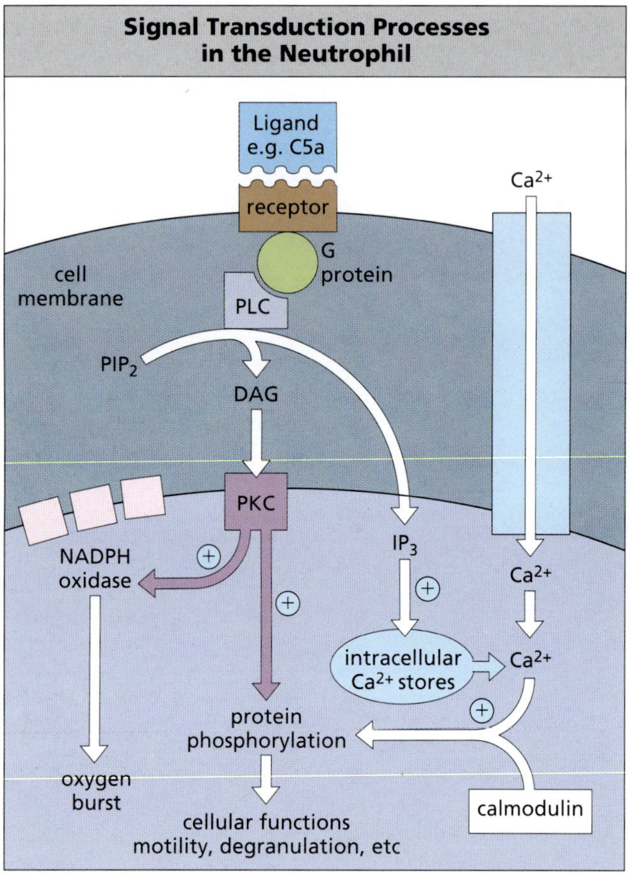

Fig. 10.7 Major pathways of signal transduction in the neutrophil.

Neutrophil Migration

Adhesion

The identification of a group of patients with defective surface adhesion proteins drew attention to the role of a group of surface glycoproteins in neutrophil adhesion to endothelial cells and their subsequent migration from blood into extravascular tissues. In these patients, the common β chain of a small group of transmembrane heterodimeric glycoproteins – the CD11/18 complex – is defective. The complex is formed of three members – CD11a/CD18 (LFA-1), CD11b/CD18 (CR3) and CD11c/CD18 (p150,95) representing a subfamily of transmembrane heterodimeric adhesive proteins, the integrins, many of

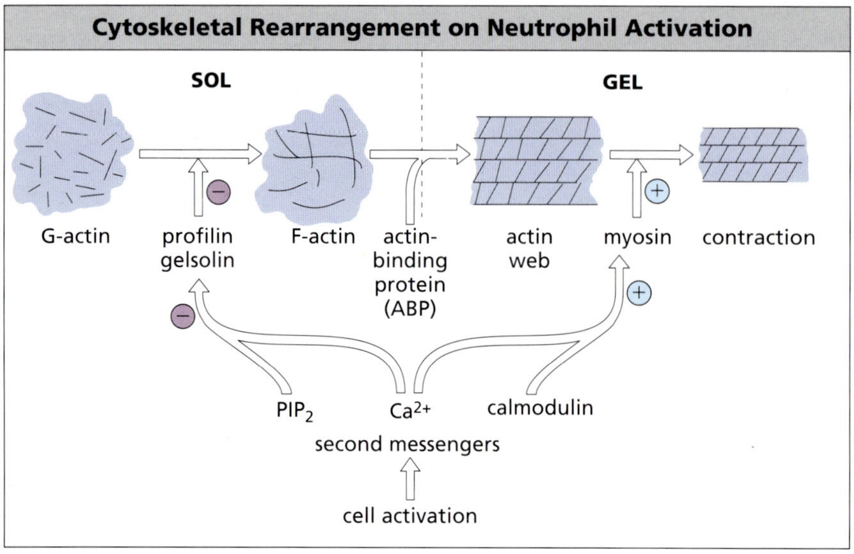

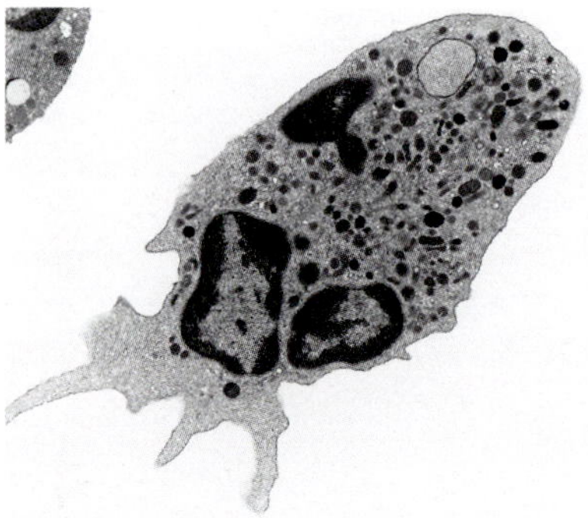

Fig. 10.8 [left] Major skeletal events during neutrophil activation and polarization. [above] EM of neutrophil polarized by exposure to fMLP. (Courtesy of Jan Henson).

which are involved in important cellular recognition processes. Leukocyte adhesion molecule deficiency (LAD) patients suffer from a variety of recurrent infections and from skin ulcers to which neutrophils fail to migrate (Fig. 10.9). Neutrophils from the blood of these patients also fail to show stimulated adhesiveness to endothelial cells *in vitro*. Monoclonal antibodies raised against the neutrophil surface have demonstrated other important molecules and suggest an adhesive/transmigration role for L-selectin, a member of the selectin family of adhesive molecules that are characterized by a structure which includes a lectin domain and an EGF-like domain.

A variety of adhesive receptors have now been identified on the surface of endothelial cells stimulated by endotoxic lipopolysaccharide or by cytokines, some of which represent ligands for neutrophil surface adhesive receptors (Fig. 10.10). ICAM-1 and ICAM-2 are members of the immunoglobulin supergene family, whereas ELAM-1 and GMP-140 are selectins. The exact temporal and physical relationships between neutrophil and endothelial surface adhesive proteins is yet to be established. Endothelial cells are sensitive to cytokines like IL-1, which induces ELAM-1 expression over several hours. It is likely that chemotactic factors, such as C5a, exert their early effects mainly upon the neutrophil surface where they may rapidly induce not only upregulation of adhesive molecules but also promotion of activated states of expressed integrins by enhancing the affin-

Clinical Features
delayed umbilical cord separation
destructive skin ulceration
poor wound healing with dystrophic scars
repeated septicaemia
neutrophilia and prolonged neutrophil lifespan

Fig. 10.9 Leukocyte adhesion deficiency (LAD). [left] Clinical features of patients defective in the leukocyte adhesion molecule complex CD11/18. [below left] The appearance of the elbow with dystrophic scars and an active area of necrotic ulceration. [below] Histology of an area of pneumonia at necropsy of the same patient, showing large numbers of neutrophils in microvessels but not in tissues. (Reproduced with permission, *Clin Exp Immunol*, 1991; **84**: 223–231).

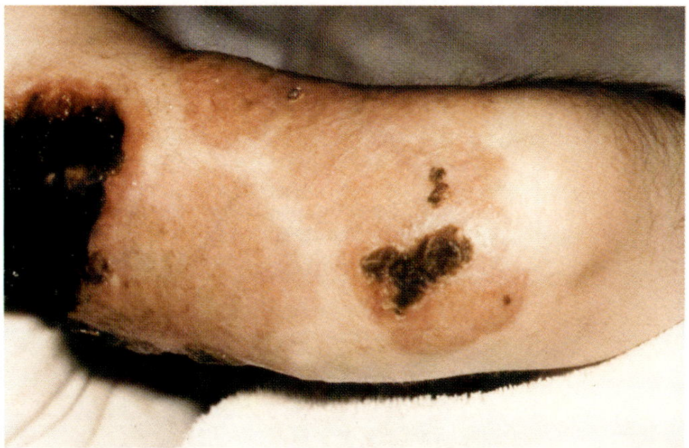

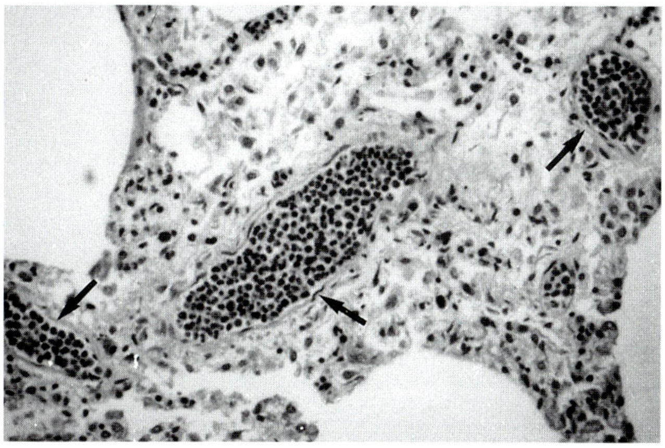

Cell type	Workshop cluster designation	Common nomenclature	Ligand(s)
Integrins			
neutrophil	CD11a/CD18	LFA-1	ICAM-1, ICAM-2, ICAM-3 (immunoglobulin superfamily)
neutrophil	CD11b/CD18	CR3 (Mac-1)	C3bi ICAM-1 fibrinogen
neutrophil	CD11c/CD18	p150,95	C3bi? endothelial ligand fibrinogen
Selectins			
neutrophil	W/D	L-selectin (mel 14 mouse)	endothelial CHO
endothelial	—	GMP-140 PADGEM	sialated Lewis X antigen (CD15 on neutrophil)
endothelial		ELAM-1	sialated Lewis X antigen (CD15 on neutrophil)
Others			
neutrophil	CD44	HCAM?	hyaluronate receptor

Table title: **Adhesive Molecules and Ligands Relevant to Neutrophil/Endothelial Interactions**

Fig. 10.10 A variety of adhesive molecules are important, in neutrophil/endothelial interactions leading to adhesion and transmigration.

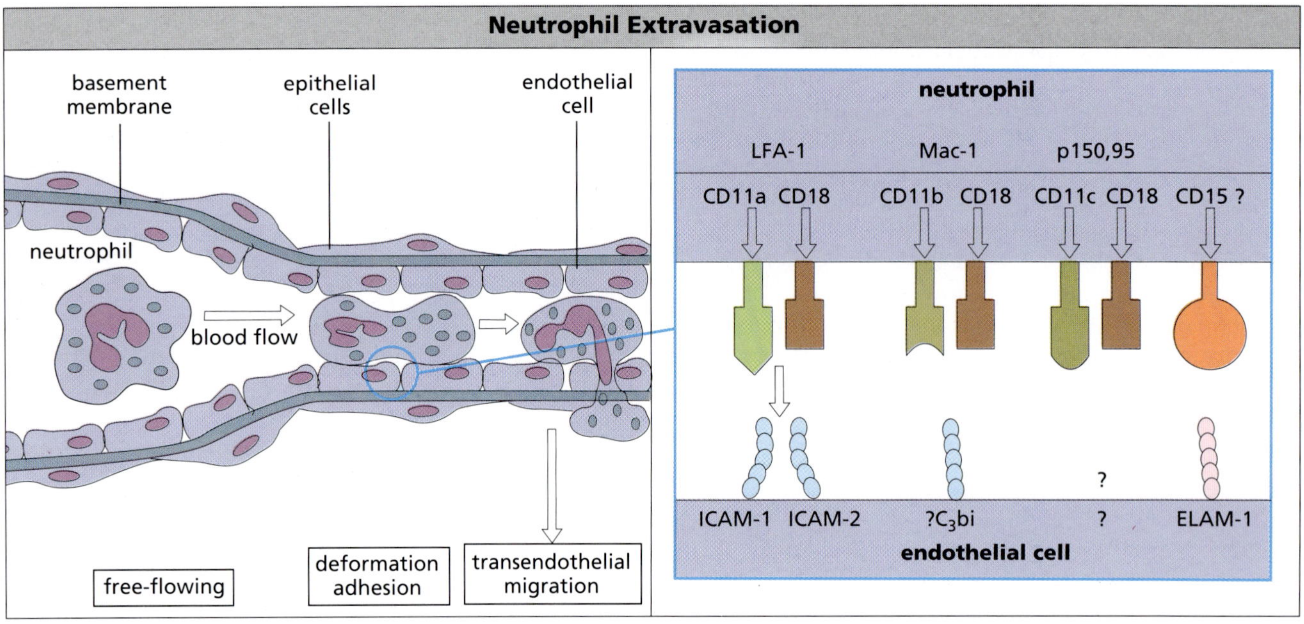

Fig.10.11 Sequestration, adhesion and transmigration of neutrophils in pulmonary capillaries.

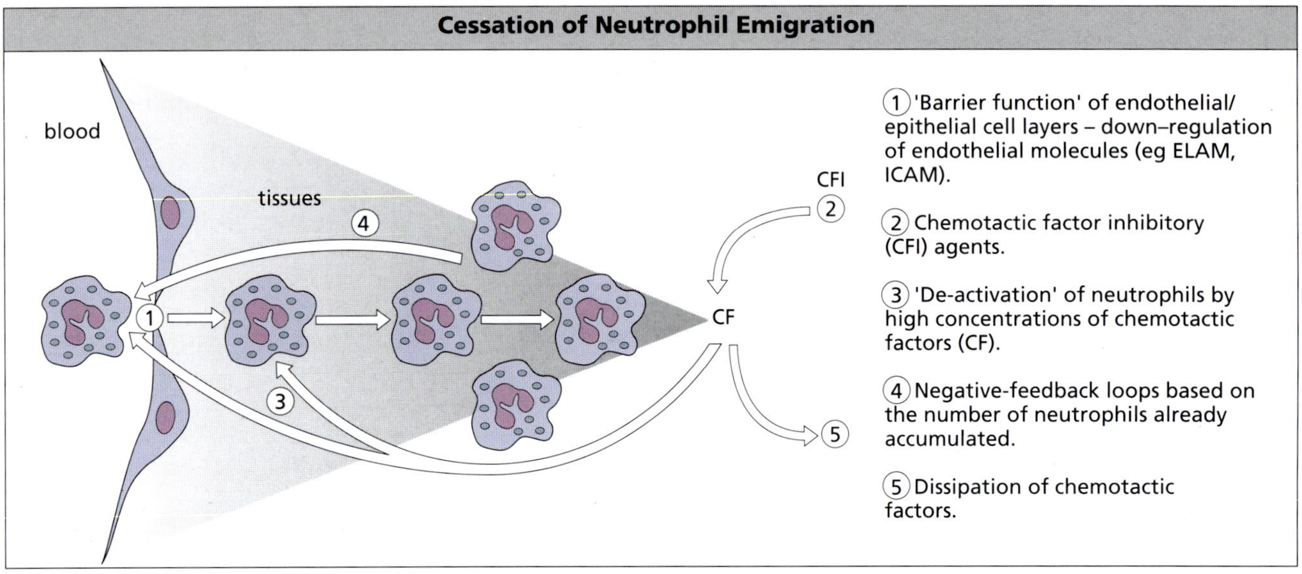

Fig. 10.12 Neutrophil locomotion to the inflamed site and possible mechanisms for cessation of migration.

ity of their individual dimers. 'On-off' switching mechanisms of adhesive molecules are presently being addressed experimentally: their elucidation will be of profound importance in our understanding of attachment/detachment processes which must occur both during the transient adhesion events observed as marginated neutrophils 'roll' along the endothelium of post-capillary venules and during the process of capillary transmigration *en route* to the inflamed site. Other factors are also involved in the sequestration of neutrophils in specialized vascular beds, such as the pulmonary microcirculation (Fig. 10.11). Although low levels of expression of adhesive molecules by neutrophils and pulmonary microvascular endothelial cells may contribute, neutrophil margination and demargination in response to exercise does not appear to be dependent on the neutrophil CD11/18 complex, and recent evidence suggests that neutrophil deformability and other physical properties may be more important.

Since the mean diameter of neutrophils is about 7μm while that of the pulmonary capillary is about 5.5μm, neutrophils are normally required to deform and 'squeeze' through pulmonary capillaries. A number of inflammatory mediators have been shown to greatly reduce neutrophil deformability, thus retarding neutrophil transit through pulmonary microvessels. Moreover, unlike other vascular beds, it appears that neutrophil migration to inflamed sites in the lung occurs mainly through capillaries rather than through post-capillary venules. Thus it seems likely that factors influencing neutrophil rheology could have major amplication effects in neutrophil sequestration which occurs early in the evolution of acute inflammation, at least in the lung.

The study of the effects of anti-CD11/18 antibodies in inflammatory models in rabbits has produced some interesting results. Anti-CD18 MoAbs block neutrophil migration into skin sites of *Streptococcus pneumoniae* infection but not to lung sites of infection,

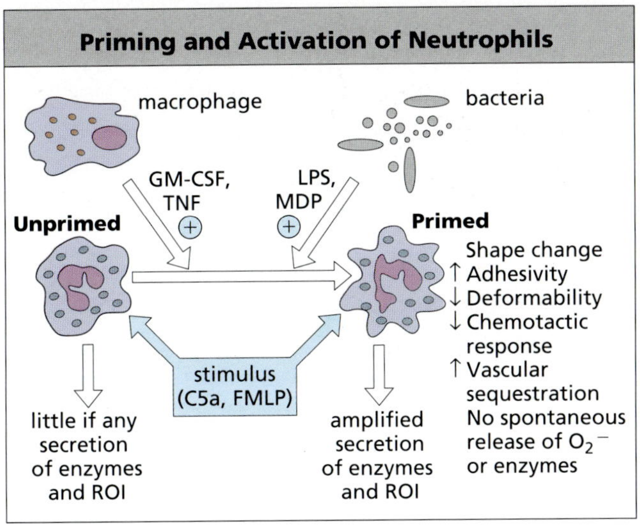

Fig. 10.13 Neutrophil states in tissues – priming (enhanced state of readiness) and activation (triggering).

whereas neutrophil migration in response to *E. coli* endotoxin is blocked both in the lung and in the skin. This suggests that CD11/18-dependent and independent processes may govern neutrophil migration in the lung in response to different stimuli. The possibility of stimulus-specific neutrophil responses raises exciting possibilities for incisive approaches in the future design of novel and specific anti-inflammatory strategies.

Transmigration
Since Addison's classical light microscopical observations in 1843, it has been recognized that emigrating neutrophils squeeze between endothelial cells by a process of diapedesis. Florey's more detailed electron microscopical studies indicated that this does not necessarily cause endothelial injury, indeed there is recent evidence that endothelial cells may actually assist neutrophil transit. The further passage of neutrophils through the basement membrane inevitably requires degradation of matrix proteins, but it is likely that this is normally tightly controlled and that gaps are rapidly re-formed by mechanisms which may again involve the endothelial cell. In the hypothetical example of neutrophil migration to an inflammatory focus in a lung airspace (see Fig. 10.11), the neutrophil must then traverse the epithelial cell layer, which, unlike endothelial cells, is formed by 'tight' intercellular junctions. Neutrophils can migrate between epithelial cells *in vitro* without causing injury or loss of electrical resistance of the epithelial monolayer. The mechanisms whereby the tight junctions are broached and re-sealed are obscure.

Although neutrophils can traverse cellular 'barriers' without necessarily causing major disruption, even in acute 'beneficial' inflammation which resolves spontaneously, there is often evidence of some endothelial and epithelial injury. Therefore, this stage of inflammation is likely to represent a point where any interference with local control mechanisms could amplify inflammatory tissue injury considerably, and it is interesting that many inflammatory diseases are characterized by evidence of excessive endothelial and epithelial injury and persistent microvascular leakiness.

Chemotaxis
After penetration of the cellular 'barriers', neutrophils undergo directed migration, or chemotaxis, towards the inflammatory focus. Chemotaxis does not require new protein synthesis, but the details of energy supply, sensing mechanisms and local motor mechanisms remain obscure. Sustained chemotaxis is likely to occur in part through sweeping back occupied receptors which are internalized, recycled and re-presented at the leading edge.

It is important to understand how neutrophil migration ceases both in terms of the events which lead to cessation of chemotaxis in a single cell and the environmental changes at the inflamed site whereby populations of neutrophils are no longer attracted. Deactivation of individual cells is likely to occur by a combination of several mechanisms, but factors leading to cessation of influx are poorly understood (Fig. 10.12). Nevertheless, it is clear that neutrophil influx ceases remarkably early in the evolution of acute inflammation and the elucidation of the mechanisms responsible is likely to be important in the understanding of inflammatory diseases, many of which are characterized by persistant accumulation of inflammatory cells.

The States of the Neutrophil

The presence of neutrophils in tissues is not in itself synonymous with injury. Neutrophils have been shown to synthesize a variety of proteins, including the Fc receptor and protein components of CR1 and CR3 as well as stress proteins, in response to environmental changes. Neutrophil function can also be modulated or primed by a more rapid mechanism which does not require protein synthesis. Low concentrations of a variety of inflammatory agents (Fig. 10.13), which are not themselves effective secretagogues, can markedly enhance the subsequent responses of neutrophils to secretagogues such as C5a. Priming agents appear to exert population effects whereby primed cells are recruited to form a pool of cells which are in an enhanced 'state of readiness'. The molecular mechanisms of priming are poorly understood as yet, but $[Ca^{2+}]_{ic}$ is likely to play a central role. A variety of neutrophil functions other than degranulation and 0_2^- release are modulated by priming (see Fig. 10.12) and these may also have bearing in some disease states.

Phagocytosis, Degranulation and the Respiratory Burst

Bacteria and other foreign particles are phagocytosed most effectively when coated with an opsonizing IgG or with opsonic components of C3 (see Fig. 10.14). Particles coated with IgG are recognized by the Fc receptors (FcR) of the neutrophil. It is now accepted that there is a small group of FcRs which form a subgroup of the immunoglobulin supergene family. The specific roles of FcR1, FcR2 and FcR3 are presently being dissected. Particles coated with opsonizing complement components of C3, such as C3b and C3bi, are recognized by complement receptors (C3Rs) type 1 (CR1) and type 3 (CR3), respectively, on the neutrophil surface. CR1 is a glycosylated protein which has four allelic forms, and CR3 is a cation-dependent member (CD11b/CD18) of the integrin family which also plays an important role in adhesion of stimulated neutrophils to endothelial cells.

Receptor function is greatly upregulated by inflammatory mediators such as C5a, probably from a combination of newly expressed receptors and their transformation into an activated state. Activation of CR1 and CR3 also confers the capacity for internalization as well as binding. Receptor activation is independent of protein synthesis and may be mediated through PKC activation and phosphorylation of proteins. Ligation of FcR or activated C3R promotes pseudopod protrusion and the early motility events required for phagocytic vesicle formation. However, unlike Fc-mediated phagocytosis, which causes release of 0_2^-, H_2O_2, and a variety of eicosanoids, C3R (either CR1 or CR3) -mediated phagocytosis does not, suggesting that it may play an important role in clearance of debris during the resolution phase of inflammation.

Engulfment of particles is accompanied by movement of granules, or lysosomes, to the site of phagosome formation, where they fuse with the phagosome into which they discharge their contents. It appears that specific and azurophil granules may be under different control mechanisms, specific granules being the first to accumulate and degranulate. Some external secretion of granule enzymes occurs inevitably as a consequence of this process but how significant this is quantitatively, and what its mechanisms and purposes are is uncertain. Mobilization and translocation of granules to the phagolysosome are likely to be effected by cytosolic or cytoskeletal contractile proteins and appear to be triggered by the rapid rise in $[Ca^{2+}]_{ic}$ which occurs during neutrophil activation. Like the release of (0_2^-) from stimulated neutrophils, the degree of chemotactic superoxide anion peptide-stimulated secretion of granule enzymes may be greatly enhanced by a variety of agents, such as bacterial lipopolysaccharide (LPS), which are poor secretagogues in their own right. Excessive external secretion of potentially toxic neutrophil products may well lead to circumstances that favour inflammatory diseases.

A variety of reactive oxygen intermediates (ROI) are also generated in response to phagocytosis. It is likely that all of the associated events occur within the membrane of the neutrophil. The presumed progenitor of the ROI, (0_2^-) is formed in the plasma and phagosomal membrane by transfer on to oxygen of an electron from an electron transport chain driven by NADPH oxidase (Fig. 10.15). Many ROIs are potentially highly toxic, but are also so labile that is is difficult to be sure of their relevance *in vivo*. There is, however, good evidence that ROI are important in bacterial killing and, in particular, the H_2O_2-MPO-Halide system described by Klebanoff represents a highly effective bactericidal mechanism. The respiratory burst may also have an important role in acidifying the phagolysosome microenvironment, facilitating

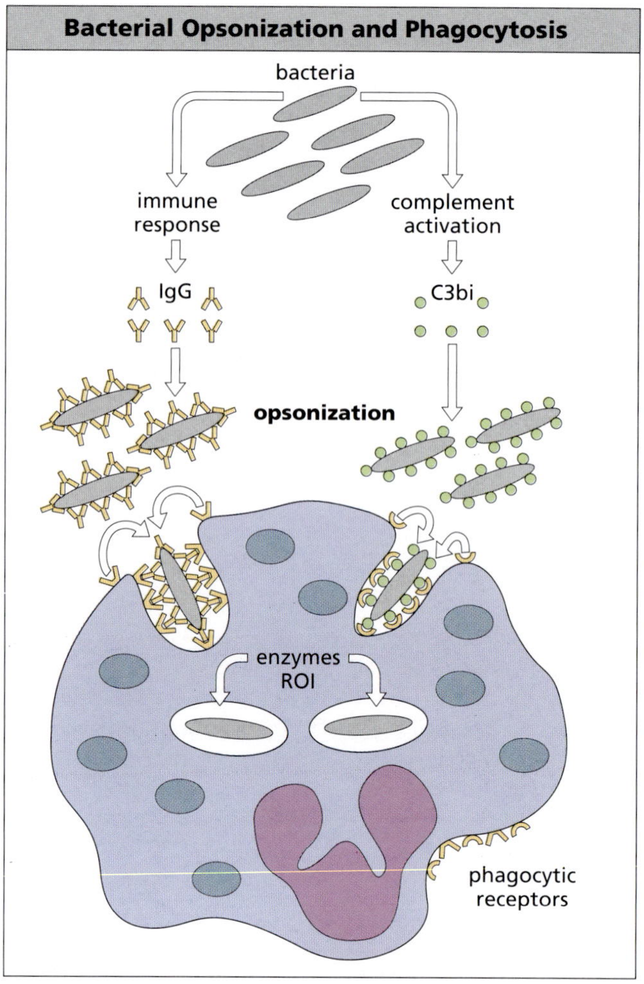

Phagocytic Receptors		
Integrin		
CD11b/CD18	CR3	binds <C3bi-coated particles
CD11c/CD18	p150,95	binds <C3bi-coated particles
Immunoglobulin		
CD16	FcR3	low affinity receptor for IgG
CD32	FcR2	low affinity receptor for IgG
CD64	FcR1	high affinity receptor for IgG

Fig. 10.14 Phagocytosis. Phagocytes engulf particles opsonized by complement or antibody, using surface receptors in a 'zipper-like' mechanism proposed by Wright and Silverstein. This results in information of a phagosome with which lysosomes fuse, releasing their enzymic contents into the newly-formed phagolysosome.

the action of some of the important degradative acid hydrolases from the azurophil granules.

Neutrophil Fate in Inflammation

Neutrophils contain a large number of agents with the capacity to injure human tissues, and yet their fate at inflamed sites has received little formal study. Although it is widely assumed that extravasated neutrophils disintegrate before being removed by phagocytes, this would inevitably result in the disgorgement into the local environment of large amounts of histotoxic neutrophil contents. However, Metchnikoff's classical observations a century ago

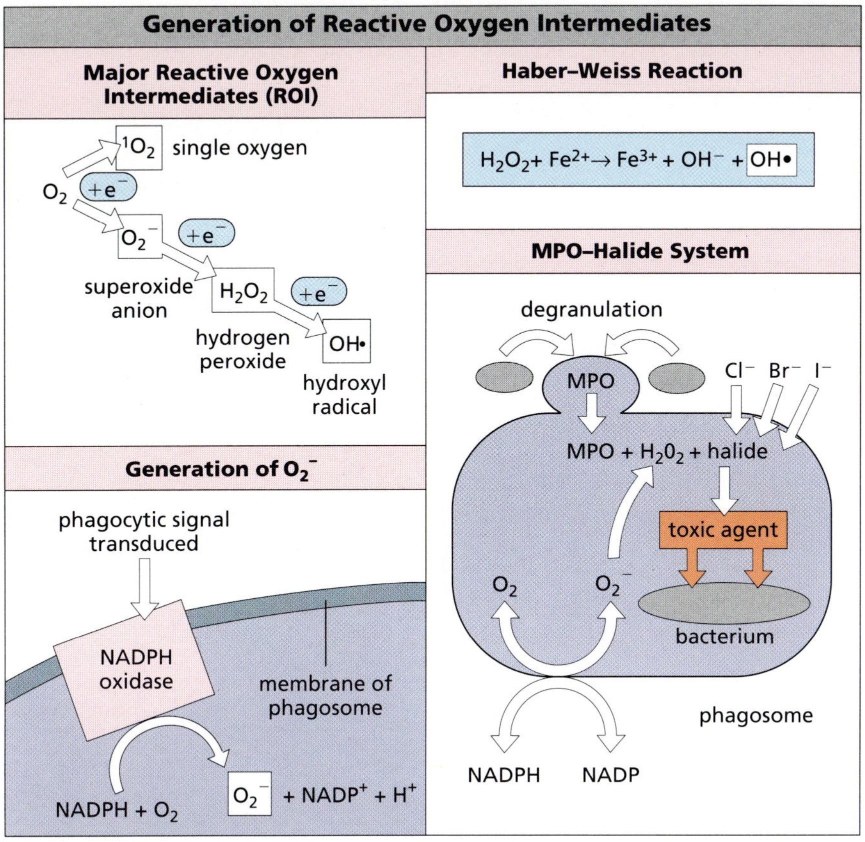

Fig. 10.15 The oxygen burst and the formation of reactive oxygen intermediates (ROI). O_2^- is produced by NADPH oxidase and further intermediates by the Haber-Weiss reaction or myelorepoxidase-halide system (after Klebanoff).

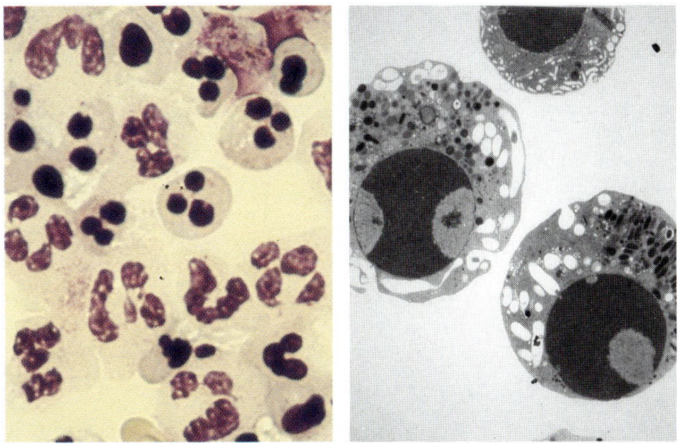

Fig. 10.16 Aged neutrophils with features of apoptosis (programmed cell death): [left] light microscopy demonstrates a subpopulation of cells with nuclear chromatin condensation and cytoplasmic vacuolation (X 1000); [right] electron microscopy demonstrates the chromatin changes, prominent nucleolus and dilatation of the endoplasmic reticulum characteristic of apoptosis.

suggested an alternative fate. He pricked tadpole tail fins with a rose thorn and then observed the cellular events that occurred during the evolution and resolution of inflammation. Rather than neutrophil disintegration, he observed the uptake of apparently intact effete neutrophils by local macrophages. Neutrophils have been described within macrophages in human tissues, but the possible importance of these observations as an injury-limiting mechanism for neutrophil removal has not really been appreciated. In support of this hypothesis, it has been shown in Edinburgh that ageing neutrophils (Fig. 10.16) derived from blood or from inflamed human tissues undergo 'apoptosis' (programmed cell death), a process associated with endogenous endonuclease activation which leads to macrophage recognition and phagocytosis of the intact senescent cell (Fig. 10.17). Programmed cell death occurs in other situations, such as thymus involution and embryological remodelling, where there is no evidence of tissue injury or inflammation (which, in the developing embryo could presumably have catastrophic consequences). Such analogies have interesting implications for the control of inflammation, and the observation that macrophages rapidly degrade apoptotic neutrophils without being stimulated to release pro-inflammatory mediators lends further credence to a role for this process in the limitation of tissue injury and termination of inflammation.

Summary and Future Prospects

In 'beneficial inflammation', neutrophil-associated events are tightly controlled so that inflammatory tissue injury is limited and inflammation ceases promptly:

- neutrophil migration is rapid;
- contact time between neutrophils and endothelial or epithelial cells is minimal;
- essential matrix degradation is localized and highly controlled;
- neutrophil release of granule enzymes and ROI during phagocytosis and digestion of bacteria is minimized;
- neutrophil exudation ceases promptly and extravasated neutrophils (mostly intact) are rapidly removed.

Although the mechanisms controlling many of these events are only poorly understood, it is likely that any loss of their efficiency could tip the balance towards excessive tissue injury and the development of chronic inflammation, cardinal features of inflammatory disease (Fig. 10.18). That endothelial and epithelial injury do occur, even in beneficial, self-limited inflammation implies that this balance is normally precarious and that endothelial and epithelial cells may be at particular risk in poorly controlled inflammation, a concept supported by the histological appearances in many inflammatory and allergic diseases.

The mechanisms whereby neutrophils may cause excessive injury to host cells are coming under more rigorous scruntiny (Fig. 10.19). Firstly, it is likely that close apposition between the neutrophil and 'target cell' is necessary for injury. This may be mediated by surface adhesion molecules. However, in some vascular beds, such as the lung, factors reducing neutrophil deformability would also promote cell contact. The kinetics of the dynamic events of intercellular interactions are also likely to be important factors determining injury, greatly prolonged cell–cell contact obviously increasing the potential for injury.

- close contact between neutrophils and endothelial cells may favour injury by a number of mechanisms;
- the local concentration of histotoxic agents may reach very high levels;
- histotoxic agent inhibitors and scavengers, particularly those of high molecular weight, would be relatively excluded from this microenvironment;
- highly reactive ROIs may be more likely to exert their toxic influences over short distances;
- some of the potentially injurious neutrophil enzymes may be presented on the neutrophil surface which makes contact with the endothelial cell.

The concept that close contact favours injury is supported by *in vitro* experiments where even the presence of anti-proteinases, e.g. α-1-anti-proteinase, fails to prevent tissue degradation (see Fig. 10.19). The secretory state of the adherent neutrophil, the influence of priming and activation agents and state of the surface with which the neutrophil makes con-

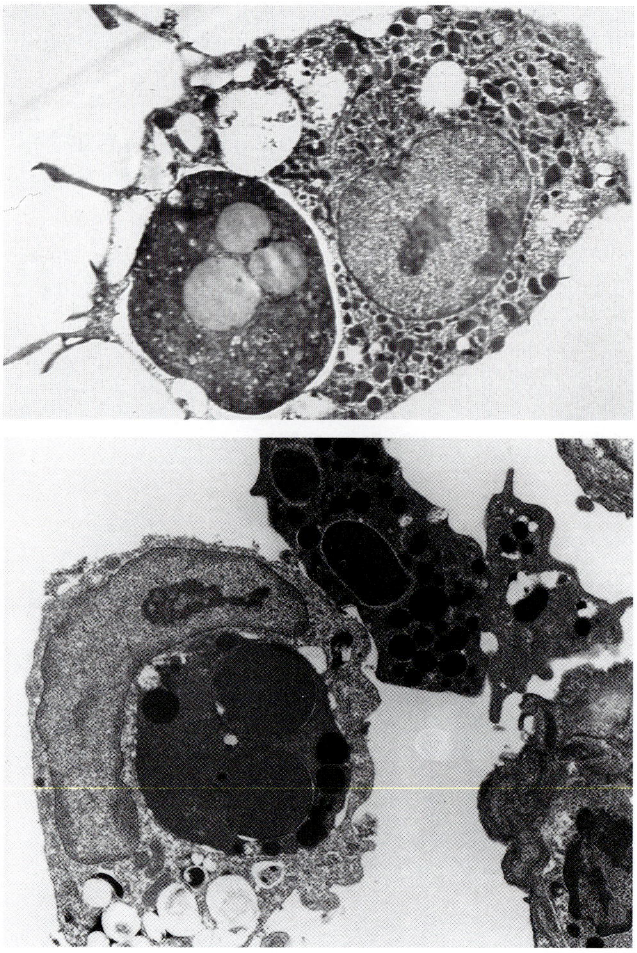

Fig. 10.17 Evidence for neutrophil apoptosis and macrophage removal: [above] a macrophage which has ingested an apoptotic neutrophil *in vitro*; [below] EM of resolving streptococcal pneumonia, showing a macrophage containing an apoptotic neutrophil.

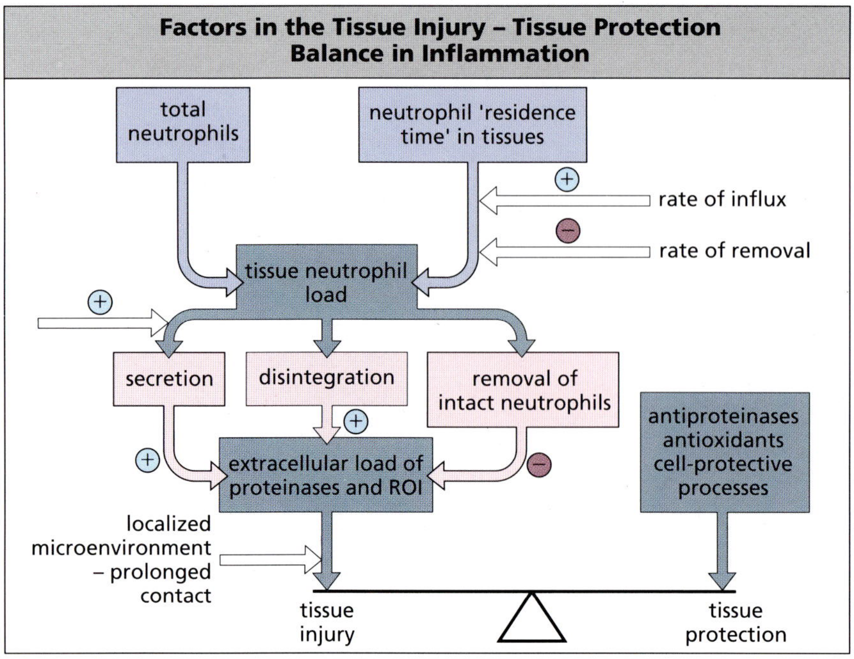

Fig. 10.18 The balance of injurious influences and tissue defences in inflammation.

tact may all influence the degree of neutrophil secretion. For example, immune complexes presented on a non-phagocytosable surface may induce massive secretion of granule enzymes, an event termed 'frustrated phagocytosis'.

One of the most difficult problems at present is to identify which of the plethora of potentially injurious neutrophil products are centrally involved in mediating tissue injury *in vivo*. Many of these, even if secreted in small amounts, may prove highly toxic if presented on the surface of adherent neutrophils. Much attention in the last decade has been focussed on a primary role for ROIs. However, the most toxic ROIs are so ephemeral and reactive that they are likely to be rapidly inactivated, even within the intercellular adhesive microenvironment. Neutrophil elastase is widely believed to play a prominent role in neutrophil-mediated tissue injury. It is capable of digesting a variety of proteins in addition to elastin and is a highly cationic molecule. It is certainly toxic to endothelial cells *in vitro*, but whether its effects are mediated by an enzymatic activity or by other properties, such as its cationicity, is uncertain. Its effects in the intercellular microenvironment may be inhibited by large molecules, such as α-1-antiproteinase. However, anti-proteinases may be rendered locally ineffective by the action of ROIs.

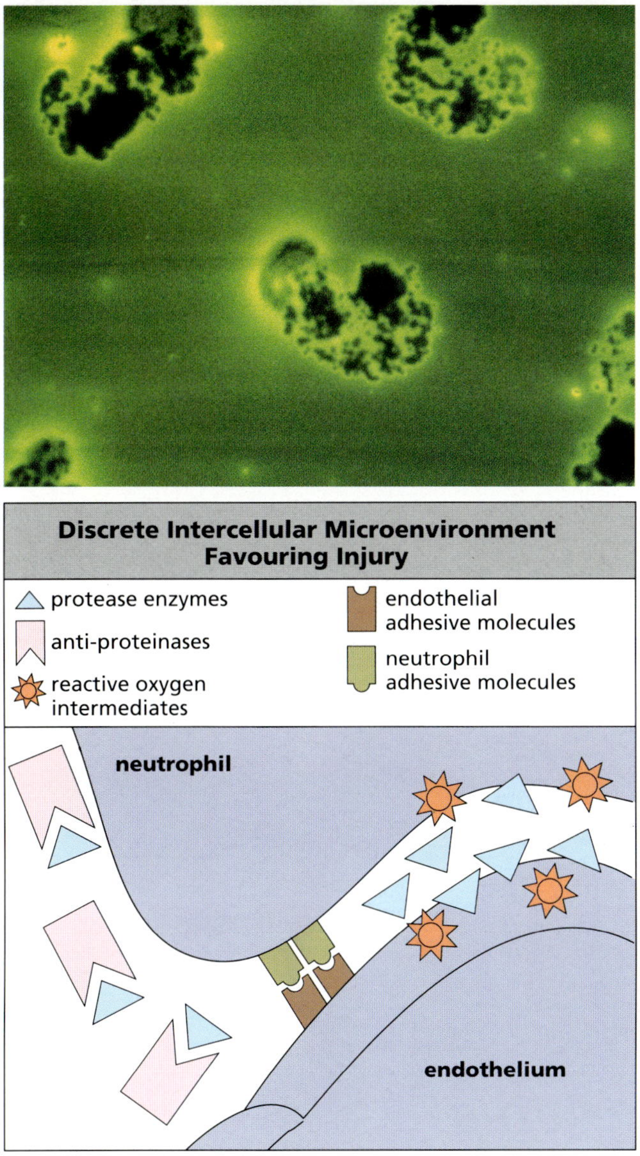

Fig. 10.19 The concept of a discrete pericellular microenvironment which favours tissue degradation and cell injury by neutrophil products. [above] Proteolytic activity of neutrophils, despite the presence of a proteinase inhibitor. Immunofluorescent staining of fibronectin, which had been coated onto the surface of a glass slide, shows green. Human neutrophils were added, in the presence of α-1-antitrypsin, then incubated for 45 minutes. α-1-antitrypsin has generally protected the fibronectin from being degraded by proteinases released by the neutrophils. Each of the dark areas corresponds to the path of a single neutrophil, where fibronectin has been degraded in sharply localized zones, despite the presence of the inhibitor. (Courtesy of Dr E Campbell.) [below] Exclusion of large molecular weight anti-proteinases, apposition to the endothelium of enzymes presented on the neutrophil surface and greater effectiveness of labile ROI (acting either on the endothelium itself or indirectly on anti-proteinases) may increase the likelihood of neutrophil-mediated injury.

New Opportunities for Therapy

The neutrophil is implicated in the pathogenesis of a wide variety of inflammatory and allergic diseases: lung diseases include chronic bronchitis and emphysema, adult respiratory distress syndrome (ARDS), asthma and a variety of chronic interstitial scarring diseases. Inflammatory diseases of the kidney are the commonest cause of renal failure requiring transplantation. Inflammatory skin diseases include psoriasis, acne and urticaria. These diseases, which represent only a small fraction of the total number in which neutrophils have been implicated, are characterized by the persistent accumulation of neutrophils (and other inflammatory cells) and a spectrum of tissue perturbations, ranging from oedema to permanent architectural disruption and scarring. Oedema and scarring in the skin are distressing and unsightly, but in delicate exchange organs, such as lung, kidney and meninges, these processes may cause catastrophic loss of organ function.

The use of non-specific anti-inflammatory agents, such as corticosteroids, has often proven disappointing in many of these diseases. However, the continued expansion in our knowledge of molecular mechanisms of neutrophil behaviour in inflammation should provide novel and specific therapeutic strategies (see Fig. 10.20). These might include the development of:

- agents which specifically inhibit the mediators which initiate inflammation (e.g. C5a, TNF, IL-8, etc.);
- agents directed against specific cell adhesion molecules;
- inhibitors of specific secretion mechanisms;
- agents directed against injurious products such as neutrophil elastase.

However, these exciting possibilities should not obscure the central paradox of inflammation as a host defence mechanism and a pathogenetic process. Firstly, the effectiveness of the inflammatory response lies, at least in part, in the redundancy of many of its mechanisms. Thus, the inhibition of a

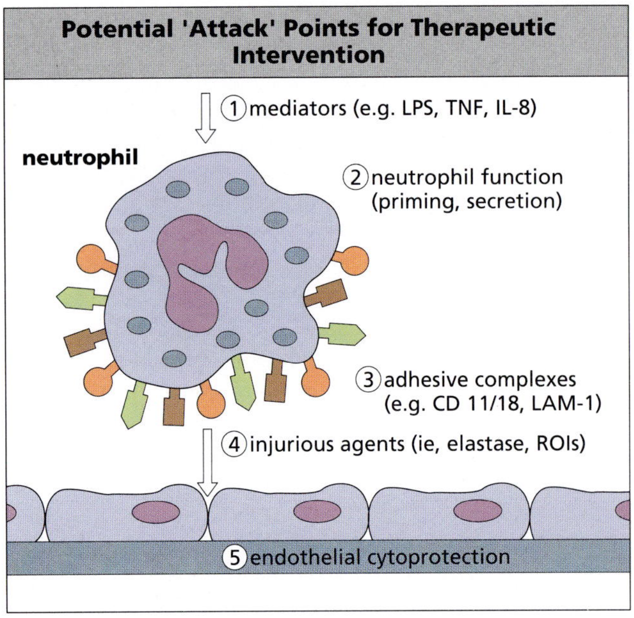

Fig. 10.20 Possible areas of development in anti-inflammatory therapy, using neutrophil-mediated endothelial injury as a model. (1) Mediators – the use of inhibitors and antibodies against important mediators which orchestrate the inflammatory response. (2) Strategies to 'de-activate' or 'de-prime' neutrophils. (3) Sequestration and adhesiveness – approaches designed to block specifically the molecular mechanisms of neutrophil adhesion to and transmigration of endothelial cells. (4) Strategies, e.g. enzyme inhibitors, directed against injurious neutrophil products. (5) Boosting the cytoprotective defences of endothelial cells against enzyme and oxidant attack.

single mediator, or possibly even of a single cell, is not likely to render the whole response ineffective. This redundancy is a great advantage in host defence, but, when this principle is turned against the host in inflammatory disease, the development of rational therapeutic strategies is likely to be a formidable task. Secondly, it appears that the neutrophil employs mechanisms in inflammatory diseases that are similar, or identical, to those required for host defence. Thus, interference with the many apparently histotoxic processes which have probably evolved to aid the neutrophil's rapid passage through tissues (e.g. proteinases) or killing of bacteria (e.g. MPO, ROIs) is likely to compromise host defences against bacterial infection, as exemplified by the major problems ensuing from genetic defects in some of these processes. However, progress is likely to be made by a combination of, firstly, precise elucidation of injurious mechanisms to distinguish between mainly injurious and mainly beneficial mechanisms and, secondly, clearer definition of the temporal stages of inflammatory diseases to identify phases during which a particular cell, or process, is more critical to disease pathogenesis than it is to host defence.

Further Reading

Henson PM, Henson JE, Fittschen C, Kimani G, Bratton DL, Riches DHW. Phagocytic cells: degranulation and secretion. Ch. 22

Klebanoff SJ. Phagocytic cells – products of oxygen metabolism. Ch. 23.

Snyderman R, Uhing RJ. Phagocytic cells: stimulus response coupling mechanisms. Ch. 19.

Unkeless JC, Wright SD. Phagocytic cells: FCγ and complement receptors. Ch. 21.

All in: *Inflammation : Basic Principles and Clinical Correlates*. Gallin JI, Goldstein IM, Snyderman R, eds. New York: Raven Press Ltd, 1988.

Haslett C, Savill JS, Meagher L . The neutrophil. *Curr Opin Immunol* 1989; **2**: 10–18.

Hugli TE. Chemotaxis. *Curr Opin Immunol* 1989; **2**: 19–27.

Springer TA. Adhesion receptors of the immune system. *Nature* 1990; **346**: 425–434.

Weiss SJ. Tissue destruction by neutrophils. *N Eng J Med* 1989; **320**: 365–376.

Chapter 11

Diagnostic Tests for Allergy

Introduction

Allergy, in a strict sense, is an IgE-mediated inflammation often included in the condition described as 'atopy'. However, not all 'allergic' complaints from patients can be ascribed to an IgE-mediated inflammation ('non-allergic condition'). We also have to deal with 'hyperreactivity' as a state of general hyperresponsiveness defined as strong reaction to everyday stimuli and irritants, such as dusts, tobacco smoke, smog, cold air, milk, eggs, perfume, preservatives, and pets, which give rise to abnormal reactions characterized by the patient as allergy. Each year, more than 10 per cent of the population will complain of a condition considered to be of an allergic nature; 25 per cent of people will consult their doctor about an allergic condition at some time in their life. Both the allergic and non-allergic hyperreactivity diseases are increasing in industrialized societies. The hyperreactivity disease state may be considered an imbalance between the individual and the environment.

The doctor may explain to a patient that he or she is 'sensitive', but that it is necessary to test the degree of sensitivity and to evaluate whether the sensitivity is due to allergy (IgE-mediated inflammation, or atopy) or to non-allergy (non-IgE-mediated condition). The grouping of patients into IgE-allergic and non-IgE-allergic is represented in Fig. 11.1.

One adult in four will have a positive skin test to one or more of the commonly inhaled allergens, but not all of these will have an IgE-allergic disease. These IgE-sensitive patients have a subclinical sensitization ('latent allergy') and represent a risk group in whom an IgE inflammation may later appear as a consequence of special exposure and conditions. Hyperreactive diseases and their triggers are listed in Fig. 11.2.

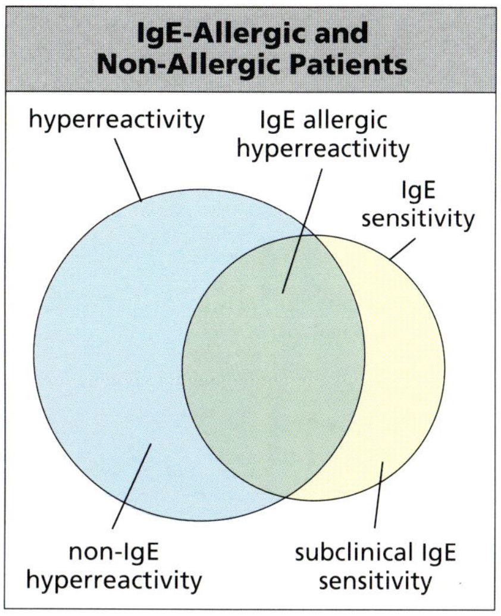

Fig. 11.1 Patients with hyperreactivity disease may be subdivided into IgE-allergic and non-IgE-allergic patients. A smaller risk group has IgE sensitization of the skin without symptoms so far.

Reasons for Testing

A diagnostic test should not be performed unless the doctor is willing to take action based on the result. The distinction between IgE and non-IgE hyperreactivity is important because there are different treatment modalities for the two types of conditions. In the case of IgE-mediated allergy, allergen avoidance and allergen-specific immunotherapy are major supplements to the pharmacological and symptomatic treatment given for the non-IgE-mediated hyperreactive states. The doctor should be able to determine whether a patient's hyperreactivity is IgE-mediated and, if so, to identify the relevant allergen.

The Distribution of Allergy and Hyperreactivity

IgE inflammation makes its first appearance early in life (Figs. 11.3 and 11.4). Most IgE allergies last at least 10–20 years, and the IgE-allergic condition is therefore present for many years in children and adults. On the other hand, the many allergy-like conditions which are not IgE-mediated appear later in life. Tests for IgE sensitivity are therefore valuable in children and young adults, but later in life they may often be negative, and the frequency of negative test results increases with age.

Triggers of Hyperreactive Diseases

Specific IgE triggers	Symptoms (prevalence % population)	Non-specific triggers
insect venom	anaphylaxis (0.001%)	exercise
pollen	asthma (5%)	acetylsalicylic acid
mould spores	rhinitis and conjunctivitis (10%)	tobacco
animal dander	urticaria (10%)	pollution
food allergens	gastrointestinal (1–2%)	sulphur dioxide
		cold air
		temperature
		pressure
		water
		food items

Fig. 11.2 Examples of exposures which may elicit symptoms in hyperreactive patients.

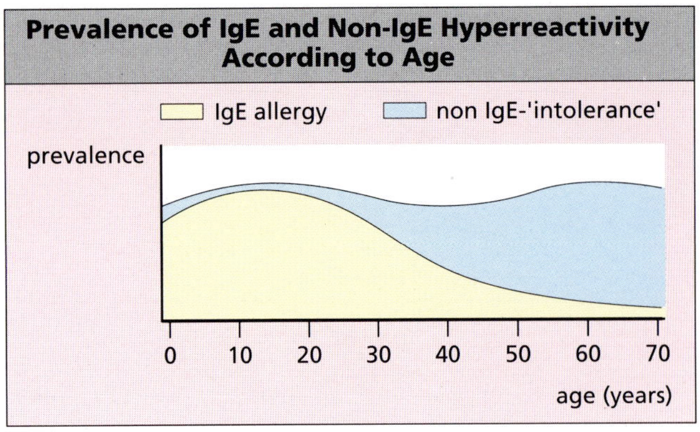

Fig. 11.3 The first appearance of IgE and non-IgE mediated hyperreactivity disease.

The hyperreactive diseases present differently according to age (Fig. 11.4):

- in the neonate, dermatological symptoms and IgE-mediated conditions caused by foods are the most common ones;
- later in childhood, airways symptoms appear as a result of sensitivity to airborne allergens;
- in young adults, symptoms from the airways prevail, with an increasing frequency up to 10–15 years, and the yearly prevalence increases after the age of 15;
- in adults, hyperreactivity from the airways still constitutes the majority of allergic problems, but after the age of 30 an increasing number of patients experience skin reactions, non-IgE mediated reactions from the airways, and non-specific symptoms from the connective tissue of the gastrointestinal tract, brain, etc. Surprisingly, venom allergy and allergic problems due to venom most often appear in adults.

This information is essential for the understanding of the mechanisms and the allergy testing that should be performed in the different age groups.

The Medical History

The medical history will supply much information suggesting IgE sensitivity (Appendix 11.1, p. 11.8). A panorama of the diagnostic tests available, and important features of the medical history are given in Fig. 11.5.

Assessment of Tests

Every test needs to be assessed before being taken into daily practice (Fig 11.6). This applies to all kinds of tests, be it a standardized questionnaire providing help for the medical history, or a laboratory test measuring a new inflammatory parameter. Assessment implies two steps:

- a technical one, in which the test is evaluated with regard to its own properties: precision, reproducibility, sensitivity, and specificity.
- a clinical one, in which the test is compared to an established clinical diagnosis. Making this comparison, one should bear in mind the prevalence of the disease. In other words, an adequate number of subjects with and without the disease should be tested and the clinical sensitivity and specificity calculated on this basis.

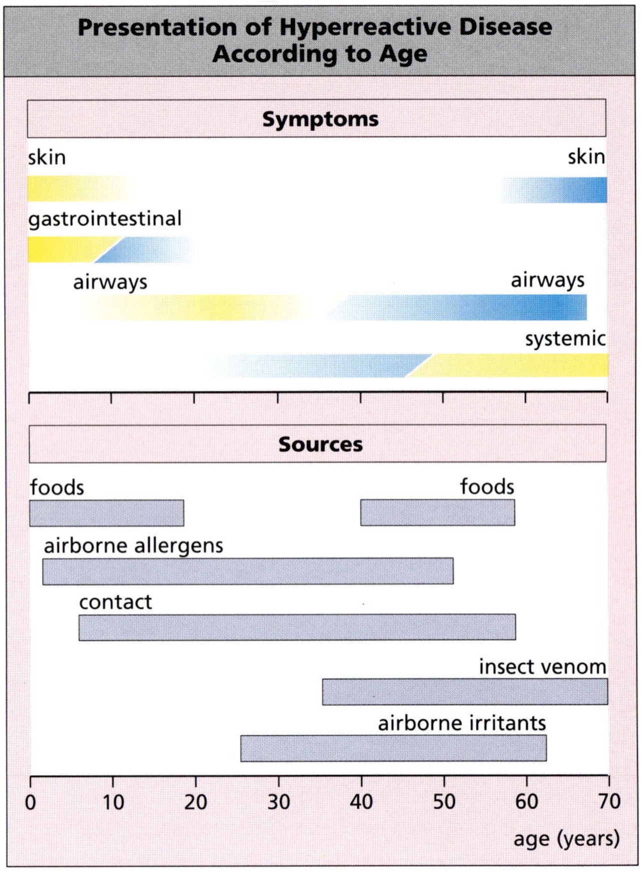

Fig. 11.4 The hyperreactive diseases look different throughout life.

When considering which tests to choose, it is important to remember that a test cannot have both a high clinical sensitivity and specificity. By changing the cut-off level, i.e. the test result defined to discriminate between a negative and a positive test, it is possible to change the two parameters of the test.

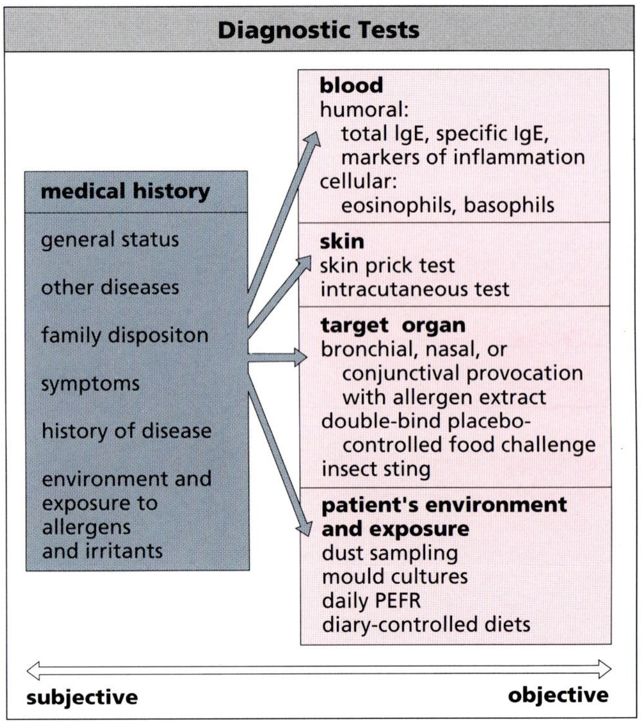

Fig. 11.5 Overview of diagnostic tests.

Assessment of Diagnostic Tests

technical validation

relevant and standardized allergens or irritants
analytical sensitivity,
e.g. ability to determine small amounts of specific IgE
analytical specificity,
e.g. lack of interference from non-specific IgE or specific Ig of other isotypes (blocking antibodies)
accuracy
reproducibility

clinical interpretation

should we aim at sensitivity or specificity?
different cut-off levels for varying age groups?
different cut-off levels for varying clinical situations?

comparison to other diagnostic procedures

cost-benefit analysis

Fig. 11.6 Assessment of diagnostic tests.

Criteria for Diagnosis of IgE-Allergic Disease

symptoms from target organ

positive provocation in the target organ with the allergen

occurrence/aggravation of symptoms due to natural exposure to the allergen source in the patient's everyday life

Fig. 11.7 The requirement for the true diagnosis of an IgE-mediated allergy

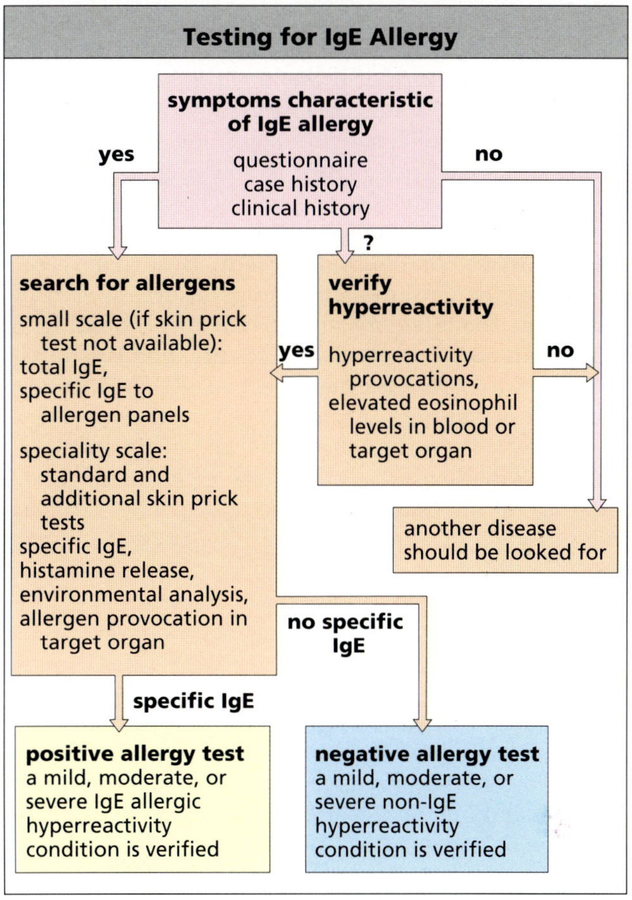

Fig. 11.8 The strategy for IgE testing.

Testing for Allergy

Strategy for Allergy Testing

The true diagnosis of an IgE-allergic disease should be based on the three conditions described in Fig. 11.7. In real life, it is not always possible to extend symptom registration over a long period, or to perform bronchial provocation tests with a large number of suspected allergens. Thus we have to rely on more practical and convenient procedures.

As shown in Fig. 11.8, the flow chart for the allergy testing is based on the demonstration of a hyperreactive disease (see Fig. 11.12), evaluation of an IgE sensitivity and allergen exposure.

The Blood

Total IgE measurement

The concentration of serum IgE is approximately 10,000 times less than that of serum IgG and therefore requires sensitive tests for its determination. The basic principle of tests for total IgE is shown in Appendix 11.2. A number of different solid-phases and labelling of the detection antibody are available. IgE concentration is approximately 1 $ng.ml^{-1}$ in cord blood and increases throughout life to concentrations around 200 $ng.ml^{-1}$ in non-allergic adults. It is still questionable whether an increased IgE concentration in cord blood is of any prognostic value. Approximately half of the IgE allergic patients will have a total IgE within the normal range, and therefore the predictive value of the test is rather limited, but an elevated total IgE should stimulate further investigations for IgE sensitivity. Increased total IgE occurs in a number of conditions (Fig. 11.9). Higher serum IgE are seen in hyperreactivity diseases in which larger parts of skin and/or mucosa are involved.

Allergen-specific IgE (see Appendix 11.2)

Determination of allergen-specific IgE in serum is often made by immunoradiometric assays, ELISAs or

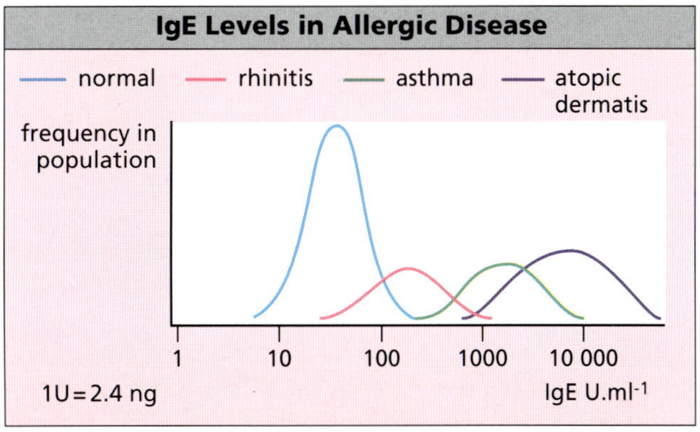

Fig. 11.9 Determination of total IgE in serum and cord blood is of some value in allergy testing, but there is great overlap between normal and IgE-allergic patients. In general, the more severe the IgE inflammation and the greater the surface of IgE mucosa, the higher the serum IgE.

chemiluminometric methods, of which the radioallergosorbent test (RAST) is best known. The allergen extract is a mixture of protein antigens – there are often between 20 and 50 antigens in the extracts. The antigens are chemically bound or adsorbed to a sorbent, the patient's serum is added, and the allergen-specific IgE binds to the allergens in the extract. Only the antigens capable of binding the patient's IgE are allergens for that patient. By using serum from over 20 patients, the major allergens can be defined as the allergens giving rise to IgE binding in more than 50 per cent of the patients, and the minor allergens as those giving rise to IgE binding in a minority of patients. From the point of view of IgE sensitivity, the other antigens are of no interest. Finally, labelled anti-IgE – very often monoclonal antibody to the human IgE – is added. The antibody is labelled by means of radioactivity, enzymes, use of the colour staining reaction in the medium or the output of photons in chemiluminescence.

Using crossed radioimmunoelectrophoresis (CRIE), to be described later, it is possible to identify and quantify the different allergen extracts, and radiolabelled anti-IgE can be used to visualize the precipitation lines. This technique is essential for the standardization of the allergen extract and the use of the radioimmuno assay (RIA) technique for determination of allergen-specific IgE.

The sensitivity of the techniques for detection of specific IgE varies with the different extract systems. A high-quality allergen extract and an optimal detection system are necessary to obtain a high sensitivity and specificity. Today, an increasing number of allergen systems have been optimized by isolation of one or more of the allergens and the application of these in isolated systems.

For inhalant allergies, the sensitivity of the RAST system is 60–80 per cent and the specificity is higher than that of the skin prick tests, often as high as 90 per cent. The technique is not, therefore, the best means of selecting the total number of IgE-sensitive patients, but if the RAST is positive, most patients will be IgE-sensitive, indicating high specificity.

Histamine release from basophils
Analysis of the histamine released from blood basophils after addition of allergen extract is used in the histamine release technique (see Appendix 11.2). This test uses fluorescence or an RIA to determine the amount of released histamine. It requires only a 20 μl blood sample for each allergen, and the analysis takes only a few hours. Like the specific IgE assays, it can be used for allergy screening.

The result can be semiquantified on the basis of the concentration of the allergen extract which gives rise to a certain amount of histamine released. Results are often quantified as negative tests to strongly positive tests class 3. About 5 per cent of the population will be non-responders to anti-IgE testing, so this technique cannot be applied to them (positive control).

The sensitivity and specificity of the test are similar to those of the RAST technique.

The Skin

The skin prick test
The skin prick test is currently the commonest way of demonstrating a skin sensitivity to an allergen. This test is usually performed on the volar aspect of the forearm and up to 25 skin tests may be performed on each arm (Appendix 11.3). The back may also be used for skin prick testing.

An aqueous extract of the allergen extract is applied, often in 50 per cent glycerol, using a special prick lancet with a 1 mm stylus. A small needle may also be used to penetrate the skin at an angle of 30°. The weal-and-flare reactions depend on the degree of sensitivity, the number of mast cells, and the potency of the allergen extract. A weal diameter exceeding 3 mm is often expressed as positive. In the Nordic countries a positive control, often histamine dihydrochloride 10 $mg.ml^{-1}$ producing a weal of average 6mm diameter, is used. A negative reaction to this control will appear if the patient has been treated with an antihistamine or corticosteroids. A buffer without allergen extract is applied as negative control. A positive reaction to the negative control shows a labile skin as occurs in urticaria factitia. Late reactions sometimes occur six to 12 hours after skin prick testing, manifesting as indurated skin reactions.

Skin prick testing is of great help in the evaluation of IgE allergy. It may be performed at any time of life, but the skin reaction is less pronounced in smaller children and the elderly. Late reactions sometimes occur six to 12 hours after skin prick testing, manifesting as indurated skin reactions.

The sensitivity and specificity of the skin prick test relies heavily on the allergen extract and the lancet. In the majority of cases, a very sensitive skin prick test is the best tool for detecting an IgE sensitivity (sometimes it has up to 100 per cent sensitivity as a diagnostic tool). On the other hand, the specificity of this test can be less, (70–80 per cent), indicating that too many patients will be detected by a positive test ('latent allergy'). After the medical history, skin testing is therefore a good diagnostic test for detecting positive patients. Subsequently, a supplementary test with higher specificity, but excluding the patients with a positive skin test who are not clinically allergic, is needed. Such tests include specific IgE or histamine release provocation.

Determination of the sensitivity of the skin by means of skin prick testing can be performed by titration. Different allergen solutions are used, and the concentration which gives rise to a particular positive reaction can be used as the skin sensitivity. This can then be correlated to a positive histamine control or to an end-point titration with the lowest concentration giving a positive reaction exceeding 3 mm. Determination of skin sensitivity can be used as a follow-up on treatment of the patient with allergen-specific therapy (allergen elimination or immunotherapy).

The intracutaneous skin test
Intracutaneous tests are still used in some parts of the world. They are especially indicated if the allergen

extract is not strong enough to give a positive skin prick test reaction (see Appendix 11.3). The method is around 10,000 times more sensitive than the skin prick test.

Intracutaneous tests often give false positive reactions as compared to skin prick tests, and they carry more risk owing to possible systemic reactions. The technique can be used if the deposition of greater amounts of allergen extract is required.

Target Organs

In approximately 10 per cent of all the patients examined in the allergy clinic it is not possible to reach a conclusion based on the different allergy tests without performing an allergen provocation in the organs involved. In certain situations it may be necessary to exclude a particular allergen – for example, conjunctival provocation with cat allergen to indicate whether the patient's cat is the source of eye symptoms.

By increasing the concentration of the allergen extract used for provocation, the allergen concentration necessary to produce a positive reaction can be demonstrated. The sensitivity of the organ to a specific allergen is utilized in this titration technique. A high sensitivity in the provocation will correspond to many symptoms due to minor exposure in everyday life, and is characteristic of the hyperreactive allergic mucosa. The technique can be used as a control during treatment with allergen elimination and immunotherapy (Appendix 11.4).

The reaction due to allergen exposure is frequently read as the reaction occurring minutes (early) to hours after the exposure. A wash-out period of one to two weeks is needed between two provocation tests in the bronchi, nose, or eyes.

In many challenge tests, a late-phase reaction occurring six to 12 hours after the allergen exposure can be measured. In clinical practice, demonstration of late-phase reactions is considered to be of special significance in the pathogenesis of allergic tissue responses and for assessing the influence of different types of therapy, e.g. steroids, immunotherapy, and anti-allergic drugs. The selection of patients with easily demonstrated late-phase reactions may also be of importance to those likely to benefit from immunotherapy.

As will be shown later, examination of the mediators in inflammation will give additional information about immediate and late-phase reactions. In most situations, the local mucosal production of mediators can be measured, as opposed to taking blood for determination of these mediators.

The Patient and the Environment

A number of naturally occurring protein antigens in the patient's environment may give rise to sensitization and stimulation of IgE production. Many of these allergens are well known or visible; others are hidden and have to be determined by a thorough medical history and analysis of the environment.

Different biological and immunochemical methods are presently available for the demonstration of allergens in the air, in foods, and in contacts. Determining the relationship between symptoms and allergens, and the decrease in symptoms during allergen reduction makes up a part of the testing for allergy.

Dust sampling

A simple technique for sampling dust is to use a vacuum cleaner with a special filter which retains small particles found in the dust. The dust is extracted 1:3 (w/v) in saline for an hour and the allergen content is identified and quantified by immunochemical techniques. This is illustrated in Appendix 11.5. For some purified allergens, monoclonal antibodies have been produced, thereby enabling a quantification (ng of major allergen per gram of dust). Other devices for collecting airborne allergens are available, e.g. stationary high volume air samplers and portable air samplers.

Mould cultures

Mould spores can be identified and quantified in the home, the working place of the patient or the outdoor air (see Appendix 11.5).

Conclusion

What combination of allergy tests should be used?

The combination of allergy tests to be recommended varies with the allergen system, the sensitivity of the patient to the allergen in question, and the availability of allergy tests of the examiner.

Fig. 11.10 shows a simplified system for assessing a patient with a suspected allergic disorder. Each of the allergy tests is scored from 0 to 2; 0 being a negative test, 1 positive, and 2 strongly positive. By combining two or more allergy tests, the necessary sum of points must be collected to reach a final conclusion. If four or more points are obtained, the diagnosis is assured; if zero or one points are obtained in two or more tests, the diagnosis is negative. If two or three points are obtained in a number of tests, a provocation test is required. Provocation will also be necessary if, despite negative test results in a number of tests, the patient still has doubts about the diagnosis (e.g. he has a dog at home, but negative test results). Only in a few cases does the medical history *per se* allow a firm, conclusive diagnosis. An example of this is allergy to birch pollen, where the symptoms appear in the birch pollen season in northern Europe, against a background of perennial intolerance to nuts and fresh fruit.

Scoring System for Allergy Testing

							total
case history	0	1	2				
skin prick test	0	1	2				
specific IgE in serum/ histamine test	0	1	2				
total	0	1	2	3	4	5	6
diagnosis	negative		?		strongly positive		
provocation in target organ indicated							

Fig. 11.10 A simplified scoring system for allergy testing.

Why is allergy testing so important?
It is necessary to select IgE-allergic patients and to determine sensitivity to one or more allergens so that correct treatment can be started at an early stage and the risk of chronic inflammation and tissue destruction reduced (Fig. 11.11). This is particularly important for the prognosis of the hyperreactive state.

Testing for Hyperreactivity

As shown in Fig. 11.12, examination of hyperreactivity is the first step in allergy testing. Much information about hyperreactivity can be obtained from medical histories, clinical and paraclinical examinations.

A number of subjective symptoms and objective measurements are characteristic of hyperreactivity. Complaints are most frequently due to strong reactions to several non-specific irritants in the air (tobacco smoke, smog, dust, perfume, strong odours, etc.), to foods containing histamine, or to pressure, cold, or heat affecting the skin. Eosinophilia in the blood and local eosinophilia in the disease organ is a common characteristic of hyperreactivity; therefore it is important to look for this (see Fig. 11.14).

Hyperreactivity provocation with mediators or physical/chemical stimuli can be demonstrated, and hyperreactivity confirmed (Appendix 11.6). A positive provocation means a hyperreactive condition. If negative test results for eosinophilia and provocation are obtained, this test may have to be re-evaluated. Otherwise another disease should be looked for.

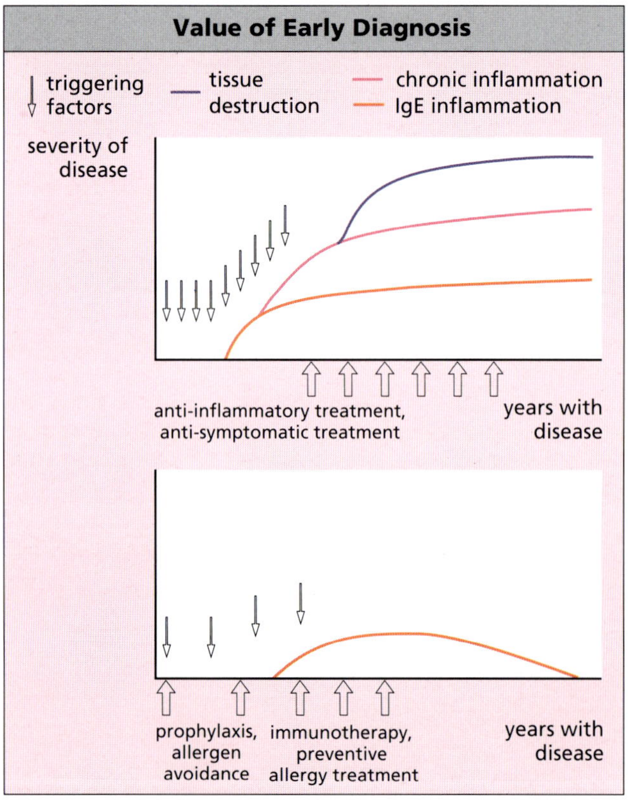

Fig. 11.11 The specific diagnosis of IgE allergy is very important in the early phase of the disease. By prophylaxis and early treatment, it is possible to alter the natural history of the disease. However, if the disease is already well established, anti-inflammatory and anti-symptomatic treatments will become dominating.

Testing for Inflammation

Cells and Mediators in Hyperreactivity

A number of cells and released mediators are involved in the hyperreactive state of a mucosa and can be looked for both locally and in the blood (Fig. 11.13).

Various cytokines are thought to play a role in the development and recruitment of the cells involved in the allergic inflammation. The cells and the mediators have been described in the preceding chapters and are at present not available for routine diagnosis. In this chapter only the eosinophil count will be described.

Eosinophils

Blood eosinophilia is present in both IgE-allergic and non IgE-allergic hyperreactivity (Fig. 11.14). The degree of eosinophilia is correlated closely to the severity of the hyperreactivity disease. Detemination of the eosinophil count should be carried out specifically, and should not be calculated from differential counts and leukocyte concentration (Appendix 11.7).

Eosinophilia in the blood is an expression of mobilization of the eosinophils which are transported via the blood from the bone marrow to the disease organ. Blood eosinphilia will be particularly pronounced if the extension of the disease is very great and the inflammation severe. For example, only about 10 per cent of patients with a combination of rhinitis and conjuntivitis have blood eosinophilia, and then only for a few days after exposure to the allergen; nearly

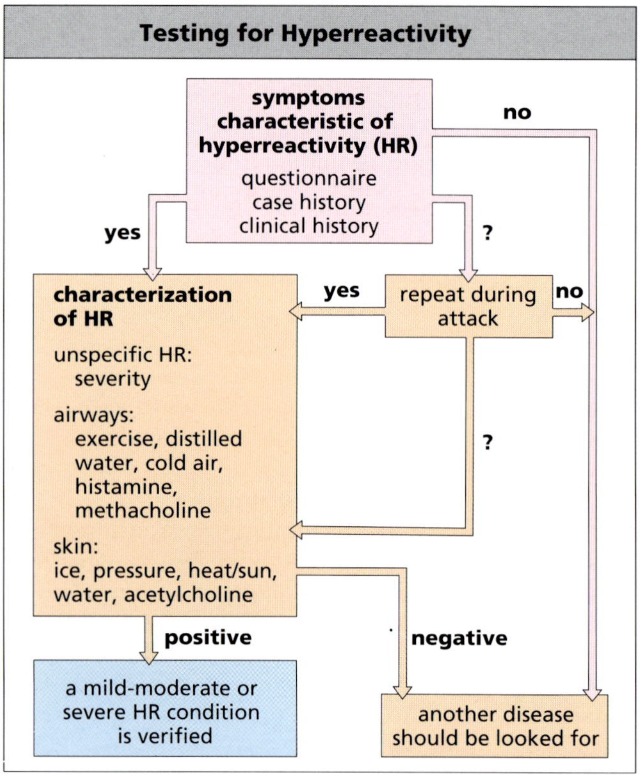

Fig. 11.12 The strategy for hyperreactivity testing.

all patients with a combination of rhinitis and asthma have blood eosinophilia, though again only for a few days after exposure to the allergen; and nearly all patients with rhinitis, asthma, and atopic dermatitis will have blood eosinophilia. So blood eosinophila is an expression of the presence and degree of hyperreactivity.

The number of eosinophils in the blood is also influenced by the time of the day, and use of systemic of local steroids.

Although blood eosinophilia is variable and is not always present in hyperreactive disease, topical eosinophilia will almost certainly be present in the inflamed mucosa of the affected organ. Demonstration of local eosinophilia in the nose is of great importance in the local treatment of rhinitis with steroids; demonstration of local eosinophilia in the eyes or bronchi is however of no great diagnostic importance.

Recently a number of eosinophilic proteins have been described, and assays are available. Their diagnostic value is currently being investigated.

Sophisticated Tests

All the diagnostic tests which are based on allergens are influenced by the quality of the allergen extract. There are several research methods for standardization of allergens by means of a serum of known specificity. These same techniques can be applied for detailed determination of the antibody response to the individual allergens in the extract based on known allergen extracts.

These techniques include CRIE, SDS-PAGE followed by immunoblot, and RAST-inhibition (Appendix 11.8).

Determination of IgG-subclasses by means of RIA and CRIE is listed in Appendix 11.9. These techniques have been used for monitoring allergen-specific immunotherapy, but their value in determining the clinical outcome has been limited.

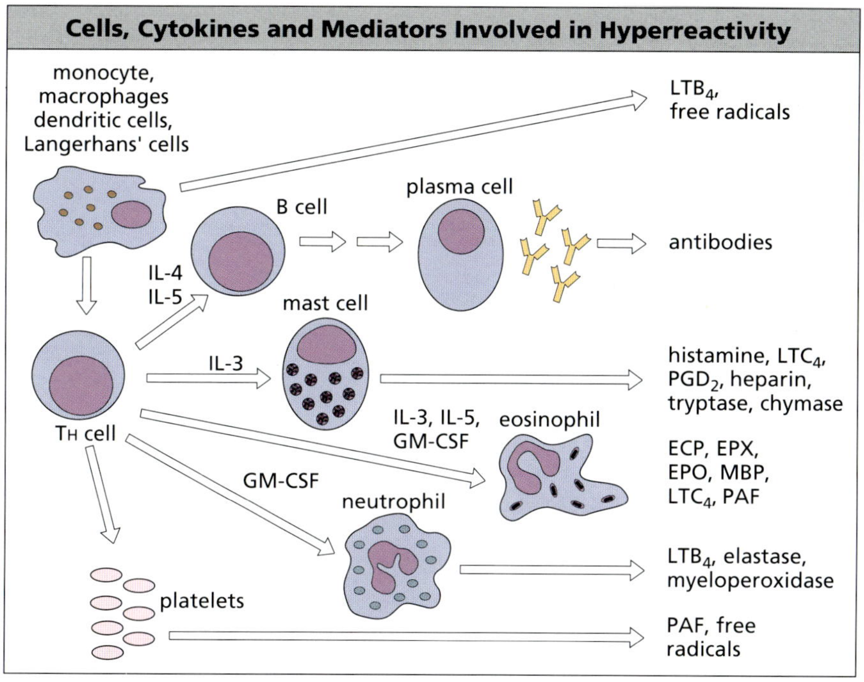

Fig. 11.13 Cells, cytokines and mediators involved in hyperreactivity.

Eosinophils

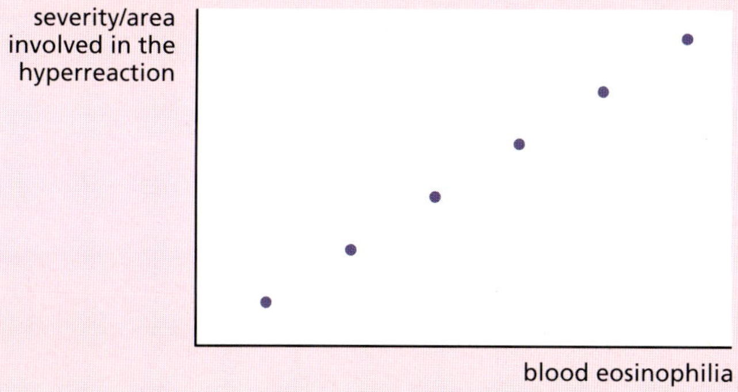

effected organs	blood eosinophilia (% of all cases)
nose	10
lung	50
nose and lung	80
nose and lung and skin and GI	100

Fig. 11.14 The number of eosinophils in the blood depends upon the severity of the infection and the surface area of the mucosa involved. Increased eosinophils in the blood are independent of IgE allergy and non-IgE allergy.

In nearly all hyperreactive conditions, a local increase in eosinophils can be demonstrated. The diurnal variation in blood eosinophils has to be taken into consideration.

Name of Test	Principle	Quantification	Capacity (patients per day)	Economy	Time before result
Medical history	structured interview or questionnaire covering: general status; symptoms; history of disease; other diseases; family disposition; environment and exposure to allergens and irritants; any known coincidence between exposure and symptoms	at best semiquantitative. Based on the answers, it is possible to assign a statistical estimation of probability of disease	10–15	*	20–30 minutes

Appendix 11.1 Medical history in diagnosis.

Total IgE in serum	1. solid-phase or sorbent antibody against human IgE 2. serum sample incubating IgE (hours – day) 3. labelled detection antibody to human IgE	IgE units per ml (WHO) = 2.4 ng IgE per ml	> 100	***	> 1 day
Allergen-specific IgE	1. solid-phase or sorbent antigens 2. serum sample incubating IgE (hours – day) 3. labelled detection antibody to human IgE	expressed relative to a reference allergen system and a standard; often semiquantified: 0–4 (or 5, 6)	> 100	** for each allergen	> 1 day
Histamine release from basophil	1. reaction of allergen and basophils with IgE 2. released histamine bound to paper on tubes 3. histamine liberated and coupled with OPT to a fluorescent substance	semiquantitative classes based on the quantity of allergens necessary to produce a significant histamine release	50	** for each allergen	> 4 hours

Appendix 11.2 Diagnostic tests which target the blood.

Skin prick test (SPT)	1. allergen molecules are pricked into the skin 2. allergen–IgE bridging activates cells and mediators are released 3. 10–20 minutes later the mediators activate vessels, nerves, and skin	area of wheal (or flare in USA) is calculated; semiquantitative compared to a wheal produced by a histamine reference, e.g. 10 $mg.ml^{-1}$	20–30	*	20 minutes
Intracutaneous test	1. allergen molecules are injected intracutaneously into the skin using a syringe 2. allergen–IgE bridging activates mast cells and mediators are released 3. 10–20 minutes later the mediators activate vessels, nerves, and skin	area of wheal (or flare in USA) is calculated; semiquantitative compared to a wheal produced by a histamine reference, e.g. 1 $mg.ml^{-1}$	10–15	*	20 minutes

Appendix 11.3 Diagnostic tests which target the skin.

Bronchial provocation test with allergen extract	1. allergen molecules are inhaled into the bronchi 2. allergen–IgE bridging activates mast cells; mediators are released 3. a few minutes later the mediators activate vessels, nerves, and muscles, resulting in bronchoconstriction	the allergen concentration causing 20% increase in airways resistance	6–8	***	1 hour
Nasal provocation test with allergen extract	1. allergen molecules are sprayed into the nose using a spraying device 2. allergen–IgE bridging activate mast cells; mediators are released 3. a few minutes later the mediators activate vessels, nerves, and the mucosa, with itching, watery secretion, and obstruction	the allergen concentration producing 2 of 3 positive: > 5 sneezes > 0.5 ml secretion > 50% fall in PEFR	10	**	1 hour

Appendix 11.4 Diagnostic tests which target specific affected organs (continues over).

Key * – least expensive *** – most expensive

Sensitivity and Specificity	airways	skin	anaphylaxis	GI	Skill	Equipment	Advantages	Drawbacks
sensitivity	++++ (depends on allergen)	++	++++	+	specialized training in allergy	pollen and spore counts for the region may be used. Questionnaire may be used as a supplement	direct contact to patient. Non-invasive. An informative history will reduce further costs of diagnosis. Computerized and standardized questionnaires are available	subjective and depends on patient compliance
specificity	+++ (depends on allergen)	+	++	+++				
sensitivity	+	++	+	+	clinical chemistry	laboratory facilities	serum samples can be stored	not allergen specific; other diseases (e.g. parasitic infections) may give high IgE concentrations
specificity	–	–	–	–				
sensitivity	+++	++	++++	+	clinical chemistry	laboratory facilities required	serum samples can be stored; mixtures of several allergens can be tested in one assay for screening purposes	after successful immunotherapy the test may still be positive; very dependent on a standardized allergen extract; many unassessed tests on the market today
specificity	+++	++	++++	+				
sensitivity	+++	++	++++	++	clinical chemistry	laboratory facilities required	possible to use extracts made from samples from patient's environment; *in vitro* provocation of a biological system	fresh blood (< 24h) required; few non-responders to anti-IgE for which reason the test is inconclusive
specificity	+++	++	++++	++				
sensitivity	++++	++++	++++	++	educated staff, medical profession	special reagents and needles, emergency kit	50% glycerol extracts can be used (easy storage); patient compliance high; informative to the patients; can be done in office	antihistamine and steroid systemically or topically may suppress the wheal-and-flare reaction
specificity	+++	++	++	++				
sensitivity	++++	++++	++++	++	educated staff, medical profession; requires more exerience than SPT	special reagents and syringes; emergency kit particularly important	better for late-phase reactions	risk of anaphylactic side effects; traumatic and inconvenient for the patients; contagious potential; anti-histamines, and systemic and dermatological steroids may suppress the reaction
specificity	+	+	+	+				
sensitivity	++++	NA	NA	NA	educated staff, medical profession	emergency facilities, nebulizer, lung function measurement	basis for the 'true' diagnosis; can be used for longitudinal studies, control of allergen avoidance, or therapy including immunotherapy	inconvenient; potential danger of severe asthma attacks; risk of late-phase asthmatic reactions
specificity	+++	NA	NA	NA				
sensitivity	++++	NA	NA	NA	educated staff, medical profession	emergency facilities, nebulizer, rhinomanometer or nasal peak flow meter (inspiratory or expiratory)	basis for the 'true' diagnosis; technically easy to perform; more convenient to the patient than bronchial provocation test	dependent on the drug treatment; low potential for systemic side effects
specificity	+++	NA	NA	NA				

Name of Test	Principle	Quantification	Capacity (patients per day)	Economy	Time before result
Conjunctival provocation tests with allergen extract	1. allergen molecules are installed on the conjunctiva by a droplet 2. allergen–IgE bridging activates mast cells; mediators are released 3. a few minutes later the mediators activate vessels, nerves and the mucosa with itching, swelling, redness, and tears	the allergen concentration producing 2 of 3 symptoms: redness, itching, running eyes	20	**	30 minutes
Sting by living insect	1. venom allergens are deposited in the skin by a stinging insect 2. allergen–IgE bridging activates mast cells; mediators are released 3. a few minutes later the mediators activate vessels, nerves, and the mucosa with itching, swelling, redness, and occasionally systemic reactions	clinical evaluation of symptoms due to sting from a living bee, wasp, or other insect (the insects may be 'stored' for days in the refrigerator)	5	***	30 minutes
Food challenge	1. food allergens are placed in the GI tract via the oral route. 2. allergen–IgE bridging activates mast cells, and mediators are released 3. a few minutes later the mediators activate vessels, nerves, and muscles, giving rise to colics, vomiting, diarrhoea, and meteorism	clinical evaluation of symptoms due to increasing doses of food; the amount giving rise to positive reactions (grams of food)	10	***	2 hours

Appendix 11.4 Diagnostic tests which target specific affected organs (continued).

Dust stampling followed by allergen detection	1. dust is collected using a vacuum cleaner 2. elution of allergens from the dust by a few hours extraction in saline (1:3 w/v) 3. determination of the allergens by means of counter current immunoelectrophersis (CCIE) or RIA/ELISA	semiquantification based on a standard extraction procedure and quantification of allergens in twofold dilutions 1:2, 1:4, 1:8, 1:16 etc; the dilution still producing a precipitation line in CCIE is the end result; a few major allergens can be expressed as nanograms per gram of dust	20	**	> 1 day
Culturing and identification of mould spores	1. a petri dish with a special medium is exposed to the air (indoors or outdoors) 2. culture of the mould spores for 1–2 weeks at 25°C 3. identification and counting of mould colonies by microscopy	identification based on the morphology, colour, and smell of the colonies; semiquantification based on the number of colonies during the culturing procedure, e.g. 15 colonies of *Cladosporium herbarum*	20	***	> 1week
Symptom and medication recording used in conjunction with pollen and spore counts	1. the daily pollen or mould spore counts, in particles per m^3 2. the daily use of rescue medicine expressed arbitrarily in scores 3. the daily symptom scores given by the patient for one or more target organs and symptom categories	a significant correlation between symptoms, use of rescue medication, and the exposure to allergens (e.g. pollen and spores per m^3) is useful in the diagnosis of allergy	20	*	days–weeks

Appendix 11.5 Diagnostic tests which assess the patient's environment.

Bronchial provocation test with mediators, irritants, or exercise	1. the 'triggering' compound is inhaled in increasing doses 2. histamine, mediators, exercise trigger the bronchoconstriction within a few minutes 3. the dose or the exercise giving rise to a certain fall in lung function is the sensitivity	the histamine concentration that produces 20% increase in airway resistance	10	**	1 hour

Appendix 11.6 Diagnostic tests involving provocation with mediators or physical or chemical stimuli (continues over).

Sensitivity and Specificity	airways	skin	anaphy-laxis	GI	Skill	Equipment	Advantages	Drawbacks
sensitivity	++++	NA	NA	NA	educated staff, medical profession	sterile allergen extract in physiological, isotonic solution	basis for the 'true' diagnosis; very simple and reproducible; minimal inconvenience to the patient; in-office test	influenced by antihistamines
specificity	+++	NA	NA	NA				
sensitivity	NA	NA	+++	NA	emergency training highly important; medical profession	emergency facilities; living insects	basis for 'true' diagnosis; psychologically convincing for the patient; control of efficacy of immunotherapy with insect venom	intravenous route necessary; patient fear of systemic reactions
specificity	NA	NA	+++	NA				
sensitivity	NA	NA	NA	++++	educated staff, medical expertise; emergency kit	reagents for oral challenge, capsules, tubes, target organ measurement	basis for the 'true' diagnosis; the controlled challenge excludes many unnecessary suspicions	time-consuming; often three positive and three placebo challenges with wash-out periods of days
specificity	NA	NA	NA	+++				
sensitivity	++	+	NA	NA	technical staff	clinical chemistry	allergen exposure; the daily load; the effect of chemical cleaning procedures; demonstration of unknown exposure	dust analysis, not airborne allergens (mostly the same)
specificity	+	–	NA	NA				
sensitivity	++	NA	NA	NA	technicians with special experience in micro-biological techniques	micro-biological facilities and culture media	mould exposure of known and unknown origin; the effect of cleaning procedures	time-comsuming, expensive; specially trained personnel needed
specificity	+	NA	NA	NA				
sensitivity	++	+	NA	NA	specialist staff	diary; pollen and spore counts	inexpensive; natural exposure	high patient compliance needed; subjective symptom scores
specificity	++	+	NA	NA				
sensitivity	+++	NA	NA	NA	educated staff, medical profession	emergency facilities; nebulizer, lung function measurement, exercise equipment	a fast result compared to the daily PEFR registration for weeks	inconvenient for the patient; influenced by anti-asthmatic drugs
specificity	+++	NA	NA	NA				

Name of Test	Principle	Quantification	Capacity (patients per day)	Economy	Time before result
Nasal provoction test with mediators or irritants	1. the mediators or irritants are installed in the nose by a spray 2. the mediators or irritants trigger the nerves, glands, and the vessels and give rise to rhinitis symptoms. 3. a few minutes later symptoms like sneezing, watery secretion, itching, and stuffy nose appear (fall in PEFR > 50%)	the mediator concentration producing 2 or 3 positive: > 5 sneezes > 0.5 ml secretion > 50% fall in PEFR	20	**	1–2 hours

Appendix 11.6 Diagnostic tests involving provocation with mediators or physical or chemical stimuli (continued).

Blood eosinophilia	1. blood is taken by micropuncture or venepuncture 2. transferred to a counting chamber and stained with eosin for identification of the eosinophils 3. the number of eosinophils per mm^3 is counted manually or automatically	the number of cells per μl (normal < 400)	> 100	*	2 hours

Appendix 11.7 Blood eosinophilia.

Crossed radio immuno-electrophoresis (CRIE)	1. the allergen extract is examined in CIE and the individual allergens are presented as precipitation lines 2. serum IgE to the individual allergens is bound, and radiolabelled anti-IgE is finally used 3. the dried gel with 125-I activity is placed on an X-ray film for days or weeks. Radiostaining identifies the allergen	the X-ray exposure time giving rise to visible radiostaining is a semi-quantitative method for expressing the amount of IgE bound to the allergens; an internal standard is used with a reference antigen–IgE system	20	***	> 1 week
Immuno-blotting	1. dialysis membrane filter paper; SDS/PAGE gel NC membrane filter paper 2. serum IgE to the individual allergens is bound, and radiolabelled anti-IgE is finally used 3. the dried gel with 125-I activity is placed on an X-ray film for days or weeks. Radiostaining identifies the allergen	the X-ray exposure time giving rise to visible radiostaining is a semi-quantitative method for expressing the amount of IgE bound to the allergens; an internal standard is used with a reference antigen–IgE system	20	***	> 1 week
RAST-Inhibition	1. serum with increasing amounts of allergen extract 2. non-bound IgE is examined in a RAST system and the inhibition of the result is expressed in inhibition units 3. an unkown extract can be examined for total allergenic activity using a reference RAST-inhibition	comparing a reference extract and an unknown extract, the 50% inhibition is oftern used; the concentration of the extract giving 50% inhibition is the difference in allergenicity	20	***	> 1 day

Appendix 11.8 Sophisticated diagnostic tests for allergy.

Allergen-specific IgG subclasses	1. allergens are immobilized in CIE or on polysyrene tubes 2. serum incubation and binding of human allergen-specific IgG, monoclonal anti-IgG or other solid phase and detection by anti-monoclonal antibodies 3. identification and semiquantification of IgG subclasses in CRIE and RIA/ELISA	IgG subclass CRIE gives information about the individual allergen responses while IgE subclass RAST gives the total antibody response	5 (CRIE) 50 (IgE subclass RAST)	***(CRIE) **(IgE subclass RAST)	1 week (CRIE) 2 days (IgE subclass RAST)

Appendix 11.9 Determination of IgG-subclasses by means of RIA and CRIE.

Sensitivity and Specificity	airways	skin	anaphy-laxis	GI	Skill	Equipment	Advantages	Drawbacks
sensitivity specificity	++++ ++ +	NA NA	NA NA	NA NA	educated staff, medical profession	emergency facilites; nebulizer, rhinomano-meter (inspiratory or expiratory)	easy to perform and reasonably reproducible	influenced by drugs like antihistamines
sensitivity specificity	++ +	++ +	– –	+ +	haemato-logical expertise	clinical chemistry	one of the only markers of inflammation; can be used for monitoring therapy with local and systemic steroids	small target organs do not often cause blood eosinophilia; fresh blood needed; blood eosinophil count increased in other diseases as well
sensitivity specificity			like allergen-specific IgE		clinical chemistry	laboratory facilities; rabbit antibodies against the allergens; facilites for handling 125-I and X ray film	serum samples can be stored, unknown allergen systems can be examined using a known serum reference and vice versa	time-consuming; rabbit antibodies against the allergen extract are required
sensitivity specificity			like allergen-specific IgE		clinical chemistry	laboratory facilities; special SDS/PAGE techniques; facilities for handling 125-I and X-ray film	serum samples can be stored; unknown allergen systems can be examined using a known serum reference and vice-versa; a known marker with molecular weight is included; no rabbit antibodies	time-consuming; the allergen pattern is still arbitrary and variable; the semiquantification is more difficult than CRIE
sensitivity specificity			like allergen-specific IgE		clinical chemistry	laboratory facilities; special RAST techniques; facilites for handling 125-I	serum samples can be stored; unknown allergen systems can be examined using a known serum reference and vice versa	time-consuming; the inhibition curve needs at least 4 double inhibition points in order to describe the curve and 50% inhibition
sensitivity specificity			depends on immunization status of patient group		clinical chemistry	laboratory facilities; special CRIE/RIA techniques; facilities for handling 125-I or enzyme labelling	serum samples can be stored; IgG subclasses and other immunoglobin classes and subclasses can be detected (e.g. during immunotherapy)	IgE -subclass CRIE (and immunoblot) have the same drawbacks as the corresponding IgE techniques (of Appendices 2 and 8)

Further Reading

Axelsen NH, ed. Handbook of immunoprecipitation-in-gel techniques. *Scandinavian Journal of Immunology*, Suppl 10 1983.

Bousquet J. In vivo *methods for study of allergy: skin tests, techniques and interpretation*. Ch. 19. In: Middleton E, Reed R, Ellis EF, eds. Allergy: Principles and Practice. CV Mosby, 1988.

Drebourg S, ed. Skin test used in type I allergy testing. Position paper of the European Academy of Allergy and Clinical Immunology. *Allergy* 1989; 44 Suppl. 10.

Homburger HA, Katzman JA. Methods in laboratory immunology; prinicples and interpretation of laboratory text for allergy. Ch. 18. In: Middleton E, Reed R, Ellis EF, eds. *Allergy: Principles and Practice*. CV Mosby, 1988.

Mosbech H, Dirksen A, Madsen F, Stahl Skov P, Weeke B. House dust mite asthma. Correlation between allergen sensitivity in various organs. *Allergy* 1987; **42**: 456.

Mygind N. *Essential Allergy*. Part 3. Oxford: Blackwell Scientific Publications, 1986, pp. 91–133.

Naclerio RM, Norman PS, Fish JE. In vivo methods for study of allergy: mucosal tests, techniques and interpretation. Ch. 20. In: Middleeton E, Reed R, Ellis EF, eds. *Allergy: Principles and Practice*. CV Mosby Co, 1988.

SEPCR Working Group 'Bronchial Hyperreactivity'. Eiser NM, Kerrebijn KF, Quanjer PH, eds. Guidelines for standardization of bronchial challenges with (nonspecific) bronchoconstricting agents. *Bull Europ Physiopath Resp* 1983; **19**: 495–514.

Chapter 12

The Classification and Epidemiology of Asthma

Definition and Classification

There is no clear and unequivocal rule for deciding whether an individual has asthma or not. There are, however, many descriptions of asthma and a few approximate rules of thumb for diagnosis. Most of these include as one criterion the minimum amount of variability in airflow (usually 15 per cent) to be demonstrated before a diagnosis of asthma is confirmed.

The lack of a definition is related to the lack of any single agreed hypothesis about the nature of the disease and how it relates to other obstructive lung diseases. According to the 'Dutch hypothesis' there is relatively little to distinguish these different conditions and chronic obstructive lung disease in later life is a natural progression from asthma in earlier life. In the same way 'wheezy bronchitis' of childhood is seen as prodromal asthma.

This identification of wheezy bronchitis with asthma was given support by the difficulties in distinguishing between the two conditions in childhood, and the generally good response of wheezy conditions in childhood to standard treatment for asthma. In addition a number of studies reported persistent increases in bronchial reactivity following viral infections of the lower respiratory tract. However there are reasons for distinguishing between the common wheezy conditions of childhood. Firstly, there appears to be a difference in prognosis between different groups of wheezy children, atopic children in particular appearing to have a worse prognosis and being much less likely to remit in later childhood. Secondly, the clinical correlates of disease seem to change with age. Childhood wheeze is much more likely to be associated with viral respiratory tract infections than is adult wheeze.

Adult chronic bronchitis also has similarities to adult asthma. Both asthmatic and bronchitic patients suffer from wheeze and increased sputum production. Both groups also show increased variation in peak flow measurements and increased bronchial hyperresponsiveness. Finally, both groups have increased serum IgE. It is not surprising to find, as in childhood, that there appears to be quite arbitrary use of the two diagnoses that cannot be justified in terms of history, smoking habits, or the results of tests. However, there do seem to be important distinctions to be made. The bronchial hyperresponsiveness associated with smoking is strongly associated with the baseline lung function, obstructed patients being markedly more responsive to histamine. This is not so noticeable among the hyperresponsive patients whose condition appears to be associated with atopy. This increasing responsiveness in smokers appears to be strongly associated with the continued loss of lung function – those who continue to smoke experience a greater loss of lung function and greater increases in hyperresponsiveness, and those who stop smoking experience a deceleration in the progress of both conditions, though there is no improvement.

Problems of clinical definition, and their apparent arbitrariness, have led to the search for more precise and more easily standardized definitions. Standardization is particularly important in epidemiological studies because they rely so heavily on accurate comparisons and often aim to pick up relatively small differences between large populations. The interest of epidemiologists in relatively small differences arises from two considerations. Firstly, epidemiologists study only natural variation in a measurement and do not artificially increase this variation as in experimental studies. Secondly, it is frequently the case that in public health terms a relatively small risk, because of the large number of people exposed to it, may be responsible for a high proportion of disease when compared to exposures that may be more obvious in small groups of exposed individuals but to which only a small part of the population is exposed.

A principal attempt to find a more reliable and objective definition of asthma has been the development of measurements of bronchial hyperresponsiveness. There is now a large selection of these which includes bronchial challenge with a wide range of pharmacological agents, bronchial challenge with physical agents such as cold air or anisotonic saline solutions, exercise challenge, and measurement of the natural variation in the peak flow rate. Most people who would be characterized as unequivocally asthmatic show enhanced bronchial responsiveness, and the degree of responsiveness has been linked to the requirement for specific anti-asthma medication. However, these measurements are not specific tests for asthma. Apart from the other groups already mentioned who show increased bronchial responsiveness, a number of other groups who do not show any of the symptoms or signs generally associated with a diagnosis of asthma may be hyperresponsive on testing. A further problem is that the different measures of hyperresponsiveness do not correlate very closely, and measure slightly different aspects of the same process (Fig. 12.1). Which of these aspects is most important is unclear, as is the relative suitability of each measure of reactivity. In so far as they may relate to different aetiological factors and may have different implications for prognosis, these differences may be of great importance and require further research. Nevertheless, providing that they are not interpreted as defining asthma, they may be worth studying in their own right in the same way that blood pressure or other physiological variables subject to complex mechanisms of control are studied.

It is not always possible to use tests of bronchial reactivity, particularly when surveying very widely distributed populations or populations with little incentive to cooperate with time-consuming tests. For this reason there is still a need for criteria for asthma based on questionnaires. The principle difficulty with this approach is the lack of a definition of asthma against which these tests can be developed. Questions about a history of asthma are biased by medical care and are therefore not appropriate; though they are specific for asthma, they probably fail to detect a large and variable proportion of asthmatics who have not been given the diagnosis. Questions on wheeze also seem to be relatively non-specific, picking up large numbers of people with trivial problems. Other questions relating to bronchial hyperresponsiveness include waking at night with shortness of breath, and shortness of breath when coming into contact with animals, dust, or feathers. Wide self-reported variations in symptoms also relate to wide variations in peak flow rate. As with measures of bronchial hyperresponsiveness, these symptoms may well be detecting different components of disease. Which will prove the most meaningful remains to be evaluated.

Distribution

The confusion over definition leaves much of the literature on the distribution of asthma difficult to interpret with any confidence. The lack of standardization between studies makes any comparison between studies difficult. Comparisons of data from within studies is much more reliable. Wheeze is very common in early life, declines in prevalence during childhood and increases again through adult life. In childhood the pattern is significantly different if only 'serious' or persistent wheeze is considered. In this case the prevalence during childhood remains much more constant with increasing age. Wheeze is more common in early life in boys, but this excess in boys evens itself out and then reverses in adolescence. An exception to this pattern was reported from one study in East Africa which showed that schoolgirls were reported to have a higher prevalence of wheeze and exercise intolerance than schoolboys. In adult life reactivity and symptoms are more common in men than women, but this is accounted for by the increased prevalence of smoking among men. When non-smokers alone are considered hyperresponsiveness is more common among women.

Large variations in the prevalence of symptoms and hyperreactivity have been noted. These are particularly marked in developing countries where it is a frequent observation that asthma-like conditions are rare in the most deprived areas and become common only in the urban areas. There are fewer comparative studies in the Western world, but there is some evidence of regional variations here too, though they are less dramatic. Many of these studies rely on self-reported asthma which may for reasons already given be unreliable.

Variations in time are often even more difficult to document. Seasonal variations in hyperresponsiveness have been documented, with increases noted between spring and summer, and further increases in the autumn. There also appear to have been large changes over time. Local increases in symptoms and diagnosed asthma have been noted in Birmingham

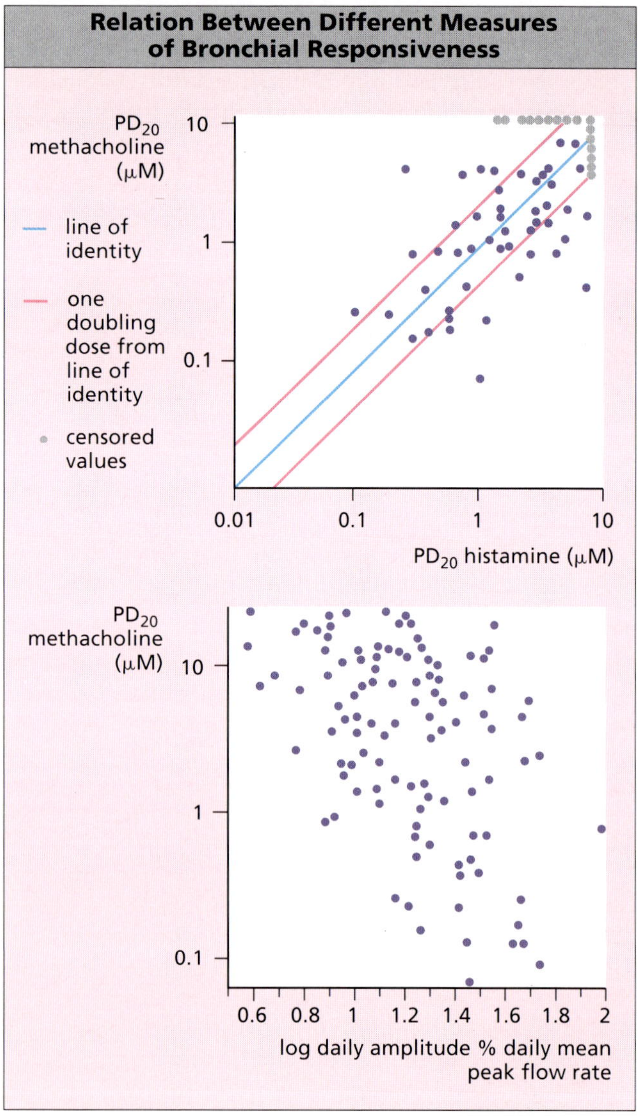

Fig. 12.1 While there is fair agreement between the bronchial responses to histamine and methacholine, the agreement is not so good with the spontaneous variation in peak flow. (Data reproduced from [top] Higgins B *et al.* *Thorax* 1988; **43**:605–10 and [below] Higgins B, unpublished.)

(UK), Lower Hutt (New Zealand), Geneva, Paris, Taipei, Finland, and Sweden. There were large increases not only in symptoms and reported diagnosis of asthma, hay fever, and eczema, but also in the response to exercise among 12-year-old children in Caerphilly between 1973 and 1988. This suggests that the reported changes are not due simply to alterations in reporting of symptoms or to changes in diagnostic categories. More recently information from a national sample of primary school children aged 5–11 in England has shown similar increases in persistent wheeze 'on most days and nights'. National increases in diagnosed asthma are also clear from general practice records and from the National Health and Nutrition Surveys of the USA, though here the only marked increase was among the black population.

Causes

The Genetics of Asthma

It has long been realized that atopic disease runs in families, but until recently it has been impossible to show a convincing Mendelian pattern that could be attributed to a single 'atopic' gene. Much of this work has concentrated on predicting the 'high' and 'low' IgE responders. More recently the study of large lineages with high proportions of atopic members have revealed a dominant pattern of inheritance taking a more complex definition of atopy as either a high IgE, or positive skin tests, or clinical disease. Linkage analysis has localized this dominant gene to the long arm of the eleventh chromosome. There is also evidence that the response to highly purified allergens, particularly in low IgE responders, is linked to the HLA phenotypes.

There is a question of whether there is a further gene that is important in asthma and that predicts hyperresponsiveness. This suggestion was first raised in some small family studies which suggested that wheeze was inherited independently to atopy. Further studies which have assessed bronchial response to histamine have seemed to confirm this, with hyperresponsiveness being bimodally distributed in atopic genealogies. Although no Mendelian mode of inheritance has yet been suggested it would seem that this distribution is not explained by either smoking or atopy, two major determinants of reactivity. Breeding experiments in mice suggest that one or more such genes are indeed likely. The distribution of atopic disease, and particularly the very rapid increases that have been noted in the prevalence of eczema, asthma, and probably allergic rhinitis, suggest that there is also an important environmental component to the aetiology of these diseases.

The Environmental Causes of Atopy

The presentation of antigen

Without the presence of allergen in the environment people would not become sensitized and there would be no atopic disease. As there is always likely to be some allergenic substance around however, the more important question is whether the quantity and presentation of antigen are important in determining whether sensitization will take place. Current evidence suggests that it is. In the case of house dust mites, for instance, it has been suggested that children exposed to greater than 10 000 ng of allergen per gram of dust are much more likely to develop an atopic response to the allergen. In addition, there is preliminary evidence that the early presentation of antigen may be particularly important. Children born into homes with high levels of antigen are at particular risk of persistent sensitization to the antigen. Mothers at risk of having atopic children may be able to reduce the risk by a strict avoidance of allergenic food during pregnancy.

Breast feeding

There has been considerable discussion as to whether breast feeding protects against sensitization to allergen, and in particular whether it protects against the subsequent development of asthma. Most of the large studies have failed to show any association with asthma, but these have not always been adjusted for important potential confounding factors, nor have they always measured sensitization directly, but have relied on a mother knowing of a diagnosis. More recently, experimental evidence has suggested that breast feeding may be protective against sensitization, and one of the few studies to make very full adjustment for other confounding factors has shown a protective effect of breast feeding, however briefly this continued.

Smoking

Smoking has a number of observable effects on immune responses, including a small increase in the serum IgE. For the most part, however, smokers do not have increased skin sensitivity to the common inhaled allergens. On the other hand there is an increased liability for smokers to become sensitized to occupational agents, and there has also been a reported increase in the atopic sensitivity of children born to women who smoked during pregnancy (Fig. 12.2). One possible interpretation for these findings is that smokers are more liable to become sensitized to allergens that they have not previously encountered, and to which they have not developed tolerance.

Air pollution

Some animal experiments, as well as human experiments, have shown an increased probability of sensitization against airborne allergens when these are presented in the presence of ozone or diesel exhaust fumes, and this has led to speculation that air pollution may increase the liability to sensitization. There are a number of studies that have shown associations between living in air-polluted areas and the prevalence of atopy. Many of these are based on small numbers of areas and are therefore unreliable, but there are some intriguing results. In Japan the likelihood of sensitization to Japanese cedar pollen has

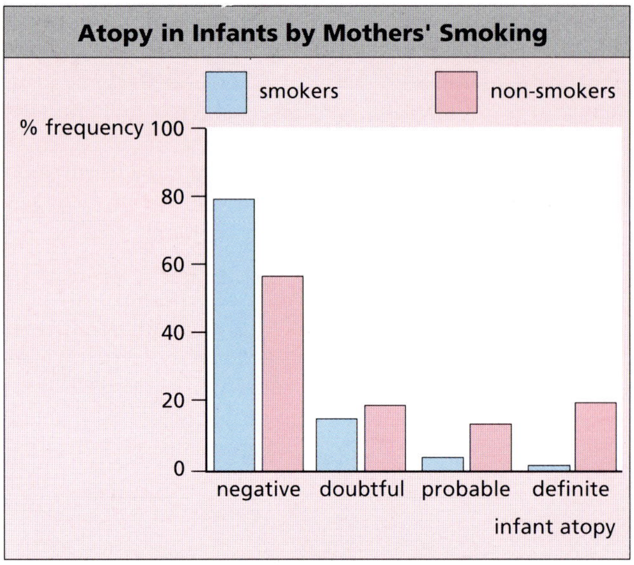

Fig. 12.2 The incidence of atopic disease appears to be higher among the children of women who smoked during pregnancy. Other researchers have failed to reproduce these results. (Data reproduced from Magnusson CG. *J Allergy Clin Immunol* 1986; **78**:898–904.)

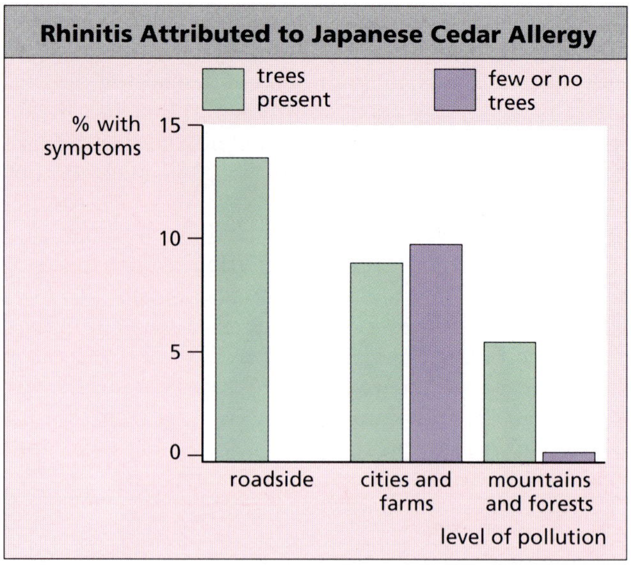

Fig. 12.3 The prevalence of rhinitis attributed to Japanese cedar allergy appears to be dependent on the level of pollution as well as on the presence of cedar trees. (Data reproduced from: Ishizaki T *et al. Ann Allergy* 1987; **58**:265–70.)

Persistent IgE Against RSV 5 Weeks After Onset of Disease

		Present	Absent	Total	Incidence
Personal or family history of wheezing	+	9	6	15	60%
	–	3	12	15	20%

Fig. 12.4 The persistence of cell-bound IgE in subjects with respiratory syncytial virus infections is more likely in those with a personal or family history of wheezing episodes. (Data reproduced from: Welliver R, Kaul T, Ogra P. *N Engl J Med* 1980; **303**:1198–1202.)

been shown to be associated with living in an area with a high density of traffic almost as strongly as it depends on living in an area with large amounts of cedar pollen (Fig. 12.3). In the Erie County studies, the admission rates with eczema were related to the 'air pollution' levels in the 136 residential areas studied after adjusting for social class differences between the areas. The second result is particularly difficult to assess as the air pollution at the time of this study was predominantly $S0_2$ and particulates. This form of air pollution has declined very rapidly over the last three or four decades and yet there is mounting evidence of an increase in the prevalence of atopic disease. Such seemingly contradictory trends are not however entirely incompatible in a disease with a complex aetiology.

Infection

There is evidence both from animals and man that viral infections can affect the production of IgE and that specific anti-viral IgE can be produced. Both these observations might support the hypothesis that viral infections are important in determining the atopic status of an individual. Direct evidence on this question is hard to come by, and the evidence that does exist suggests that this is not a particularly important determinanat of atopic sensitization. Welliver, Kaul, and Ogra showed evidence that cell-bound IgE might well be an important part of the pathogenetic mechanism in viral respiratory tract disease in children, but they also showed that the proportion of subjects with persistent IgE after RSV infection was strongly determined by a personal or family history of wheezing (Fig. 12.4). Cogswell and colleagues followed a cohort of children at high risk of developing atopic disease for the first year of life and found no association between recorded respiratory tract infections and the development of atopy.

The Induction of Bronchial Hyperresponsiveness

Atopy and allergen

Those with positive skin tests to common airborne allergens, particularly young adults, are much more likely to show bronchial response to agents such as histamine and methacholine. The association between 'asthma' and serum IgE is even greater and persists throughout life. In subjects with clearly defined sensitization to seasonal allergens, such as ragweed, bronchial hyperresponsiveness increases during the period of exposure, and uncontrolled studies suggest that removal from exposure to allergen will lead to reduction of hyperresponsiveness.

Infections

Studies have shown that both normal and rhinitic patients will respond to viral infections with an increase in bronchial hyperresponsiveness lasting a few weeks. These changes have also been shown to

Identification of Viral Infection				
	Yes	No	Total	Prevalence
Wheezing exacerbation	8	76	84	9.5%
Routine visits	8	235	243	3.3%

Fig. 12.5 In adults, unlike in children, viruses are not very commonly isolated during exacerbations of asthma. This study could suggest that about 6 per cent of wheezing exacerbations are due to viral infections. (Data reproduced from: Hudgel D, Langston L, Selner J, McIntosh K. *Am Rev Respir Dis* 1979; **120**:393–7.)

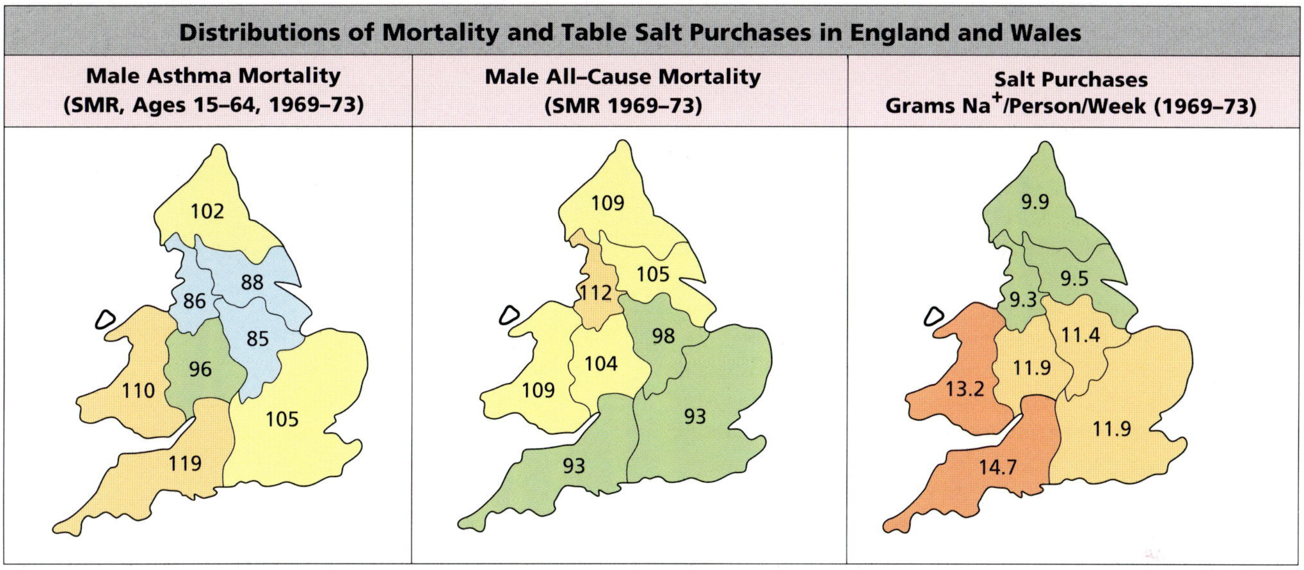

Fig. 12.6 Asthma mortality in adult males [left] is distributed very differently from all-cause mortality [middle], but is similar to purchases of table salt [right]. The same pattern is seen with children, but not with adult women. SMR = standard mortality ratio. (Data reproduced from: Burney P. *Chest* 1987; **91**:143s–148s.)

follow immunization with live but not with killed vaccines. The importance of this in determining the prevalence of disease at any one time is more difficult to evaluate. In children respiratory tract infections are probably an important cause of wheezing illness and a high proportion of these illnesses are probably attributable to infections. This seems to be less true in adults (Fig. 12.5).

Cross-sectional data relying on histories of respiratory tract infections do not show very much influence on current levels of reactivity, and longitudinal studies also tend to show only a small proportion of wheezing events to be associated with infections in adults.

Smoking

Smoking has a small transitory effect in increasing the reactivity of the bronchi. Much more important than this is the long-term effect of smoking on bronchial hyperreactivity. Over the age of about 40, smokers show increasing bronchial hyperresponsiveness. This appears to be related largely to the loss of lung function in these people, which probably explains why it is not seen to the same extent in younger smokers. The increase in reactivity continues as long as the smoking continues but is arrested if smoking ceases. This is probably the most important cause of bronchial hyperresponsiveness in older subjects.

Diet

A high dietary sodium increases bronchial hyperresponsiveness. It is also likely that this is an important source of variation both between people and between different populations in the prevalence of bronchial hyperresponsiveness. There is even some indirect evidence that dietary salt may be an important source of variation in asthma mortality (Fig. 12.6). So far the evidence seems to indicate that children of both sexes and adult men are sensitive to salt consumption but that adult women are not. Low serum magnesium levels have been associated with severe asthma but this seems to be a rare condition, often associated with chronic alcohol abuse. Other dietary factors associated with asthma include low selenium levels.

The Incitement of Bronchial Constriction

Stimuli other than allergens can induce bronchoconstriction. The list is very long and may include many of the agents already mentioned. High levels of air pollution can increase symptoms and lead to a fall in lung function in asthmatics as demonstrated in laboratory experiments and some epidemiological studies. Stress can also cause bronchoconstriction, though the mechanism for this is still disputed.

Prognosis

Wheezy illness is commonest in early childhood, decreases with age and increases again thereafter. Wheezy illness in early childhood therefore has a relatively good prognosis. Memories of a past history of asthma or wheezing in childhood are selective. Data

Prevalence of Asthma or Wheeze recalled by Parents			
		Illness ever	
Age	Illness in last 12 months	Recalled at current interview	Recalled at current or previous interview
7	8.3	18.3	18.3
11	4.7	12.1	21.9
16	3.5	11.6	24.7

Fig. 12.7 The prevalence of asthma or wheezing declines rapidly with age. Asking about cumulative prevalence provides very misleading data. (Data reproduced from: Anderson HR, Bland JM, Patel S, Peckham C. *J Epidemiol Community Health* 1986; **40**:121–9.)

from the National Child Development Study in which parents were interviewed when their children were 7, 11, and 16 years old, they found that 18.3 per cent of parents remembered their child ever having asthma or wheeze at age 7. At 11, only 12.1 per cent of the parents remembered their child ever having asthma or wheeze, where the linked records from the two interviews showed that 21.9 per cent had reported such a history on at least one of the two occasions, and at 16 years 11.6 per cent of parents remembered their child having had such a history, whereas the linked data showed that 24.7 per cent had reported asthma or wheeze on at least one of the three occasions (Fig. 12.7). Studies of the prognosis of childhood asthma should, for this reason, be based on prospective studies of cohorts of children with reliable data and should not rely on memories of illness.

Most prospective studies of asthma and wheeze in childhood begin in middle childhood around the age of 5–7. Two markers have been relatively consistent in their association with persistence of disease into adolescence and adult life, the severity of the disease as defined by early onset, frequent attacks, and hospitalization, and the presence of atopy as defined by the presence of another atopic diagnosis. The extent to which these two markers are independent of each other must be in doubt as wheezy illness in the presence of atopy is generally more severe.

Among adults, as among children, studies are confounded by the wide variation in definition and diagnosis of disease. Decline in lung function with age, however, does not seem to be related to the presence of atopy as measured by skin sensitivity of serum IgE though a couple of studies have suggested a relation between a higher blood eosinophil count and a more rapid loss of lung function. There is an association between bronchial response to histamine and decline in lung function, but it seems that the direction of this association lies in the declining lung function bringing about an increase in reactivity rather than the other way about.

Several studies have estimated the survival of adults with a diagnosis of asthma. In a British study, 2457 patients aged 25–64 consulting selected general practices with asthma during the National Morbidity Survey between 1970 and 1976 were followed up to 1 October 1985, together with 2457 controls who did not have asthma, and all deaths recorded (Fig. 12.8). The risk of death in the asthmatics was 1.69 times greater than in the controls, most of the excess deaths being due to respiratory disease and more of these being ascribed to chronic obstructive airway

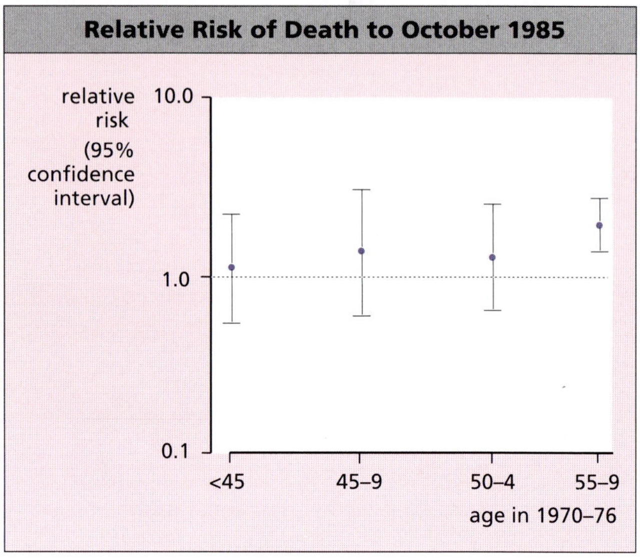

Fig. 12.8 Patients diagnosed as having asthma have an increased risk of dying, but this is only noticeable over the age of 55 years. (Data reproduced from: Markowe H, Bulpitt C, Shipley H, Rose G, Crombie D, Fleming D. *Br Med J* 1987; **295**:949–52.)

disease than to asthma. Almost all of the excess mortality was in those aged over 54, and there was virtually no excess below the age of 45. An American study followed 14 404 adults aged 25–74 examined in the NHANES I survey in 1971–5 and followed up in 1982–4, the mean follow-up period being 9.1 years. Overall, those with self-reported asthma had an increased risk of death that was only marginally increased to 1.2 times that of the rest of the population after adusting for age, sex and race. Interpretation of both of these surveys is complicated by the diagnostic assumptions in the definition of the cohorts in the first instance.

Mortality

Death Certification

International attempts to standardize the way that deaths are certified date from the latter part of the 19th century and the introduction of the first international classification of disease (ICD). In 1948, the World Health Assembly adopted the sixth revision of the ICD as mandatory for all member countries, and introduced a standard death certificate, together with coding rules defining the cause of death, for administrative purposes, as the 'underlying' rather than the 'immediate' cause of death. Despite these advances in

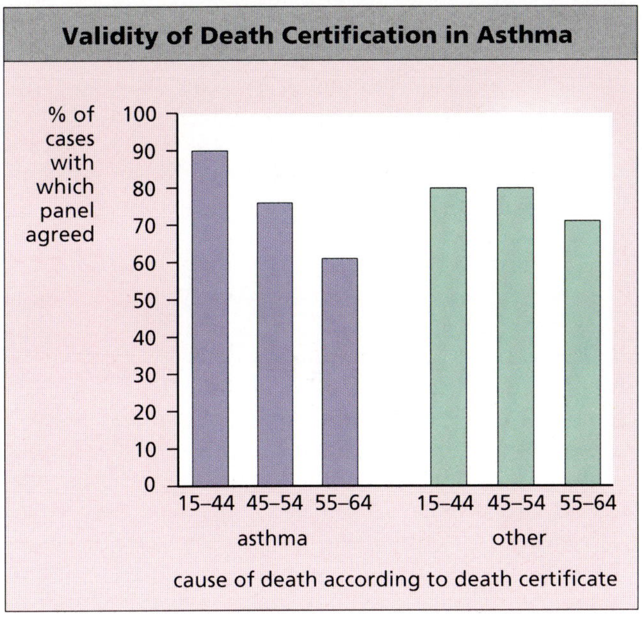

Fig. 12.9 Coding of deaths from asthma has been judged by panels of experts to be accurate in the younger age groups but increasingly inaccurate as age increases. (Data reproduced from: British Thoracic Association. *Thorax* 1984; **39**:505–9.)

standardization there remain considerable differences between countries in the rules relating to who can sign a death certificate and under what circumstances; in some cases local coding rules may introduce further variation.

Several major studies have been undertaken to validate the causes of death on death certificates and these include large post-mortem studies that have compared autopsy results with death certificates. These studies have contained few if any deaths ascribed to asthma and have therefore shed little light on the accuracy of death certificates in asthma. Most of our knowlege of this comes from comparisons of death certificates with the opinion of panels of experts provided with as much information as is available about the illness prior to death. The British Thoracic Association identified 147 people aged 15–64 years who had died and had 'asthma' written at some point on their death certificate (Fig. 12.9). Of these, 101 (69 per cent) had been coded as being due to asthma. On review the panel agreed with the coding on 36 (24 per cent) of the certificates and concluded that 89 (61 per cent) had died of asthma. Thus, although the panel agreed with the conclusion from the death certificate in only 24 per cent of cases, their estimate of the proportion of subjects dying of asthma was only 9 per cent different from that derived directly from the death certificates. This arises because misclassifications occur in both directions and tend to cancel out.

The second important result from this survey was that the accuracy of the certificates depends on age. While the overall disagreement was 24 per cent, disagreement in the 15–44 age group was 10 per cent, that in the 45–54 age group was 24 per cent, and that in the 55–64 age group was 39 per cent. This result has justified the general tendency to analyse mortality only in the younger age groups. A similar study in

European Commission Study

Case History 8

A smoker who is also a retired cement worker. Regular cough and sputum for many years. His breathing then gets rapidly worse and he wakes during the night with wheezing. During a trial of prednisolone he improves to some degree with maximal peak flow rate 140 l/min. He is maintained on oral prednisolone but dies after worsening of his breathlessness over several days with night time waking.

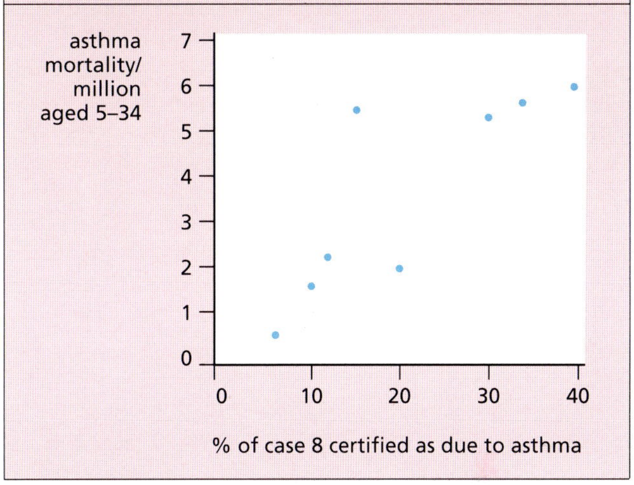

Fig. 12.10 When doctors who had signed death certificates recently in eight European countries were asked to certify the cause of the death of this patient [top], the proportion in each country assigning the death to asthma agreed well with the death rate from asthma reported for each of the countries [below, left]. (Data reproduced from: Burney P. *Rev Epidem Sante Publ* 1989; **37**:385–9.)

Auckland, New Zealand, confirmed the general accuracy of death certification in the younger age group. This study examined the deaths of almost all deaths in the age group 5– 34, omitting only those that could not have been due to asthma. Of 94 certificates, 18 (19 per cent) attributed certificates of asthma and the panel agreed that all these were correct. In a further two cases not attributed to asthma on the certificates the panel could not exclude the possibility that the deaths were due to asthma.

Despite these encouraging results, there are significant variations between countries in the way that cause of death is attributed on death certificates. Representative samples of physicians who had recently signed death certificates in eight European countries were sent case histories and asked to fill in death certificates (Fig. 12.10). The recorded mortality rates for asthma in each of the eight countries were compared to the proportion of doctors in each country certifying two of the standard histories as due to asthma. Coding of the case history that was intended to represent a clear case of asthma showed little clear relationship to local recorded asthma mortality, but there was a strong relationship between coding of the more ambiguous case and locally recorded asthma mortality. More disturbing than this is that the association is seen even in the 5–34 year age group. It appears that at least some of these differences are due to systematic differences in the way that asthma is defined in the different countries.

Geographical Variation

There are clear variations between countries in the recorded asthma mortality (Fig. 12.11). For reasons already given it is difficult to interpret these. However it is also true that within countries there are also well-documented variations in asthma mortality and it is less likely that these are due to differences in the way that death certificates are completed. Significant variation has been documented for England and Wales, France, Germany, and Belgium. The differences within Belgium may be due to variation between the two traditions of medicine practised in that country; the others are more likely to be due to true variations in asthma mortality.

So far there have been few studies of these geographical variations, and this is probably for three reasons. There have been few specific and testable hypotheses to explain the differences; the numbers of deaths due to asthma are small, so requiring the study of relatively large populations; and there are difficulties in interpreting ecological studies. In the UK, sales of table salt have been associated with regional asthma mortality rates for children of both sexes and adult men, but not for women, associations compatible with what is known of the effect of dietary sodium on bronchial hyperresponsiveness.

Time Trends in Mortality

Time trends may also be confounded by changing definitions. Changes may be due to a gradual change in the practice of those signing death certificates or to changes introduced by revision of the ICD. The former changes are very difficult to study, the latter changes can be studied either by double coding by the old and new revisions of the classification in the year that the new classification is introduced – the so-called bridge code exercises – or by looking for sudden discontinuity in trends at the time the new classification is introduced. Both these methods suggest that there was little effect of changing from the eighth to the ninth revision of the ICD in the way that younger subjects were classified as having died from asthma, but that

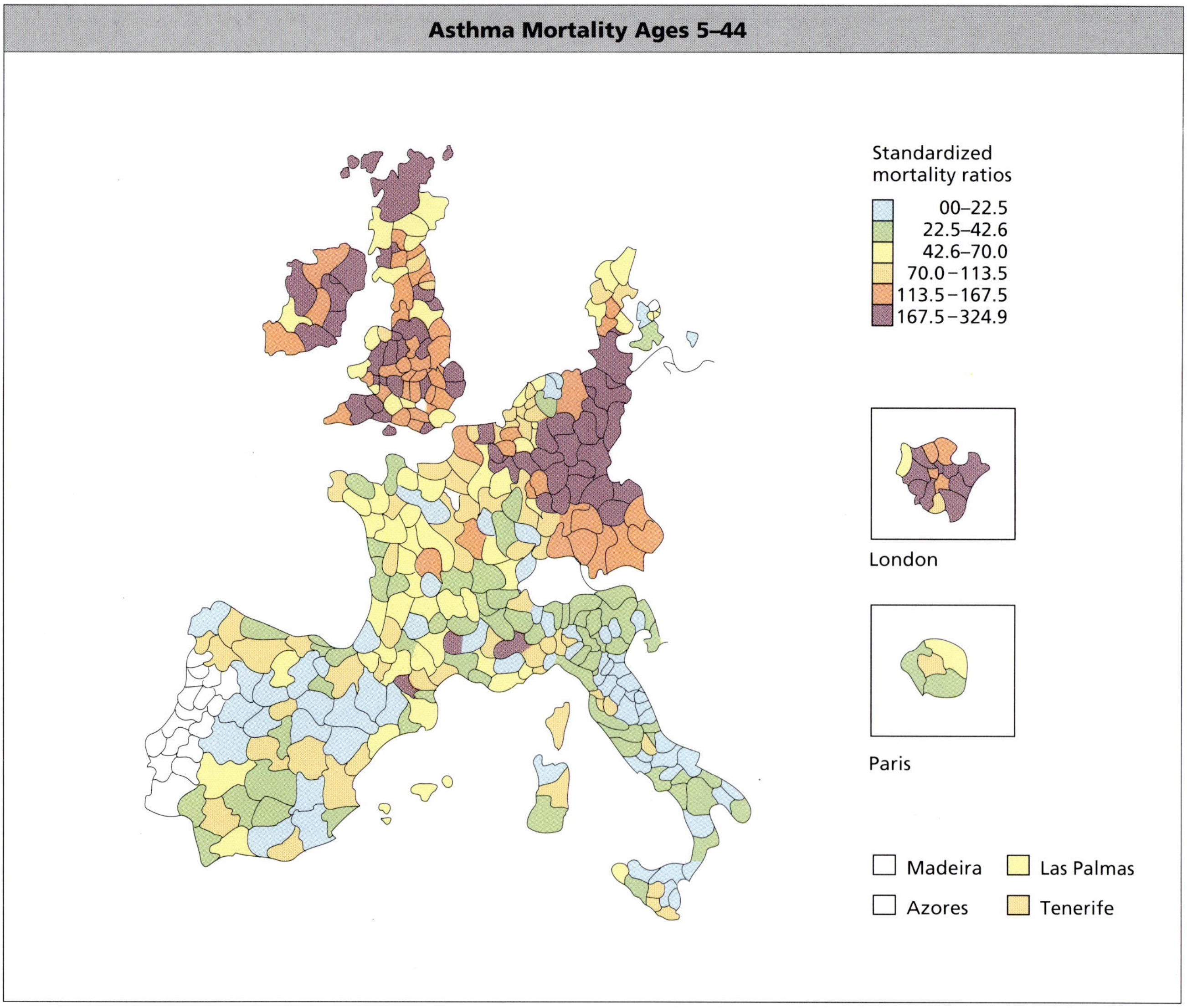

Fig. 12.11 Mortality rates from asthma in the European Community vary not only between countries but also within countries. These variations are less likely to be due to differences in death certification. (Data reproduced from: Holland WW, ed. *European Community Atlas of Avoidable Death.* Oxford: OUP, 1988.)

there were considerable changes in the way that older subjects were classified, changes that led to an important increase in the proportion certified as dying of asthma.

In England and Wales mortality from asthma has been relatively stable over the century with the exception of a large increase in mortality in the 1960s. However since the mid-1970s there has been a tendency for mortality to increase in many countries (Fig. 12.12). Several explanations have been put forward for these increases: artefacts due to changes in coding; increases in prevalence or severity; and increased case-fatality due to use or abuse of medications. Analysis of trends in asthma mortality in England and Wales have suggested that there are two components to the increases: an increase that is related to mortality changing from generation to generation – a so-called cohort effect; and changes that are related to the period of death and which affect all generations living at that period. Because the cohort effects characterize a generation from the age of 5 to the age of 34, they are likely to originate close to the time of birth and may well represent a long-term increase in the prevalence or severity of disease. Evidence that such increases may have taken place (see above) suggest that changes in prevalence may explain this component of the increase in mortality.

The sudden increase in the 1960s was attributed at the time to the widespread use of isoprenaline aerosols, particularly the high-dose sprays. The principal evidence for this was that the start of the 'epidemic' coincided with the introduction of the drug onto the market, and the end of the epidemic began when a warning went out that the drug might be responsible for the increase in deaths. Furthermore, increases in mortality were most marked in those countries that introduced the high-dose aerosols. Counter arguments have been raised. It has been pointed out that the decline in mortality was more rapid than would have been expected if the use of the high-dose isoprenaline inhalers were responsible for the excess deaths, and it has been shown that in Australia the same decline in mortality occurred without the corresponding decline in sales of isoprenaline. It has also been argued that high-dose isoprenaline was introduced into countries that had a high mortality in the first instance and that the increase in mortality in these countries would be expected to be in proportion to the baseline mortality and so higher in absolute terms than in other countries. Notwithstanding these arguments, no more coherent explanation has so far been put forward for the 'epidemic' of the 1960s.

Studies of Asthma Deaths

There have been a number of studies of individual asthma deaths as distinct from analyses of the patterns of mortality from asthma. The earliest of these began to appear around the 1930s, as case reports apparently contradicting the textbook teaching that asthmatics did not die of asthma. Some reports began to note associations with particular modes of treatment, especially with the use of sedative drugs.

Case reports and case series were superceded by more systematic audits of asthma deaths. These were attempts to collect specific information on all those who died of asthma during a particular period and in a particular region or area. The more sophisticated studies employed panels of experts to make judgments about the care received by the dead patients and to attribute death to identifiable failures in the health care system. Though these studies, which included the British Thoracic Association's audit of deaths in two Regions of England and the New Zealand Medical Research Council's national enquiry, collected a great deal of useful clinical information on the circumstances surrounding the death of patients with asthma, interpretation of that information is inconclusive. Without a control group, it is not possible to say whether the inadequacies

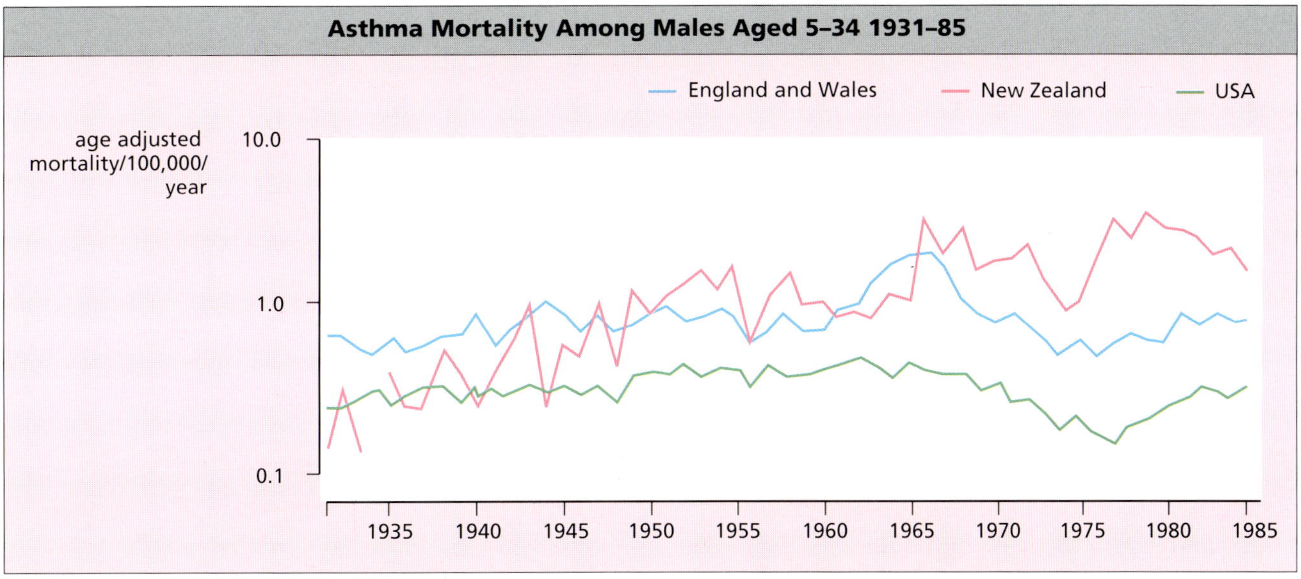

Fig. 12.12 Trends in mortality from asthma in England and Wales, the USA, and New Zealand. Analysis of these trends suggests that some of the increase is due to 'cohort' effects associated with year of birth, as well as changes in risk of death in different time periods.

identified in the treatment of the dead patients really did contribute to their deaths. In fact, having defined 'adequate treatment', the researchers were bound to find 'inadequacies', but it did not follow that these were the cause of the deaths.

An advance on these studies was provided by the case control studies of asthma deaths. An early study from the 1940s comparing dead and surviving patients with asthma showed an association between mortality and the use of adrenaline spray (Fig. 1.13). Subsequent case-control studies include those of Cochrane and Clark, Strunk et al, Rea et al, Markowe and Eason, and, more recently, a series of studies from New Zealand which assess the possible association between asthma mortality and the use of fenoterol. These have suggested associations between asthma mortality and severity of disease, poor compliance, psychosocial problems in the patients, poor management, including lack of assessment and poor patient education, underuse of beta-agonists in hospital, and use of fenoterol. Though these studies do contain comparison groups, the principal discussion has been over whether there has been adequate control for potential confounding. In particular with studies that suggest an association between increased use of drugs and increased mortality, there is the problem of knowing whether the association is due to the effect of the drugs, or whether use of the drugs is simply a marker of more severe disease.

Assocation Between Death and Use of Adrenaline Spray

		Died	Survived	Total	Fatality rate
Use of Adrenaline Spray	yes	48	600	648	7.4%
	no	22	1566	1588	1.4%

Fig. 12.13 An early association between inhaled medication and death from asthma. Potential differences between those taking the medication and the other patients makes for difficulties in interpreting such associations. (Data reproduced from: Benson R, Perlman F. *J Allergy* 1948;**19**:129-40.)

Further Reading

Clark TJH, Godfrey S, ed. *Asthma*. London: Chapman Hall Medical, 2nd Ed, 1983.

Holgate ST, eds. *The Role of Inflammatory Processes in Airway Hyperresponsiveness*. Oxford: Blackwell Scientific Publications, 1989.

Brewis RAL, Gibson GJ, Geddes DM, eds. *Respiratory Medicine*. London: Baillière Tindall, 1990.

Marsh D, Blumenthal M, eds. *Genetic and Environmental Factors in Cinical Allergy*. Minneapolis: University of Minnesota Press, 1990.

Chapter 13

Asthma – Pathophysiology

Introduction

In clinical terms, asthma is described operationally as reversible airflow obstruction. While limited knowledge of the pathogenesis of the disordered airway function in asthma precludes a precise definition of the disease, it is clear that asthma in its various forms comprises a syndrome of bronchial inflammation, hyperresponsiveness and airflow obstruction.

Clinical Classification

With an increasing awareness of factors that can induce an asthmatic state, including acute attacks of airways obstruction, clinicians have found it useful to classify asthma according to different aetiological factors (Fig. 13.1). Most asthma in children and young adults is found in association with atopy. Occupational sensitizing agents are also an important cause of asthma. However, for those patients in whom an underlying cause cannot be shown, the unsatisfactory term 'intrinsic' or 'cryptogenic' asthma is used.

Bronchial Hyperresponsiveness

Irrespective of the type of asthma, the majority of patients with this form of airway dysfunction experience attacks of bronchoconstriction, provoked by a

Classification of Asthma

	Characteristics	Examples
Extrinsic		
atopic	onset in childhood, associated with other allergic diseases	perennial and seasonal allergic asthma
non-atopic		
IgE-dependent	late onset, often occupational	acid anhydrides, animal handlers
non-IgE-dependent	late onset often, occupational	dilsocyanates, red cedar
Intrinsic		
early onset	often severe, with highly reactive airways	–
late onset	often presents with cough and sputum, sinusitis and nasal polyps	–
complicating chronic obstructive airways disease	a reversible component develops on top of smoking-induced lung disease or bronchiectasis	–
Precipitating factors		
exercise-induced	more frequent in children and young adults	–
aspirin-induced (and related NSAIDs)	more frequent in adults, associated flushing and nasal obstruction form a triad	–
Complicated asthma		
bronchopulmonary allergic aspergillosis	restrictive immunological reaction leads to bronchiectasis	–
Churg-Strauss syndrome	associated with a very high eosinophilia	–
polyarteritis nodosa	manifestation of an arteritis	–

Fig. 13.1 Breakdown of asthma according to aetiology.

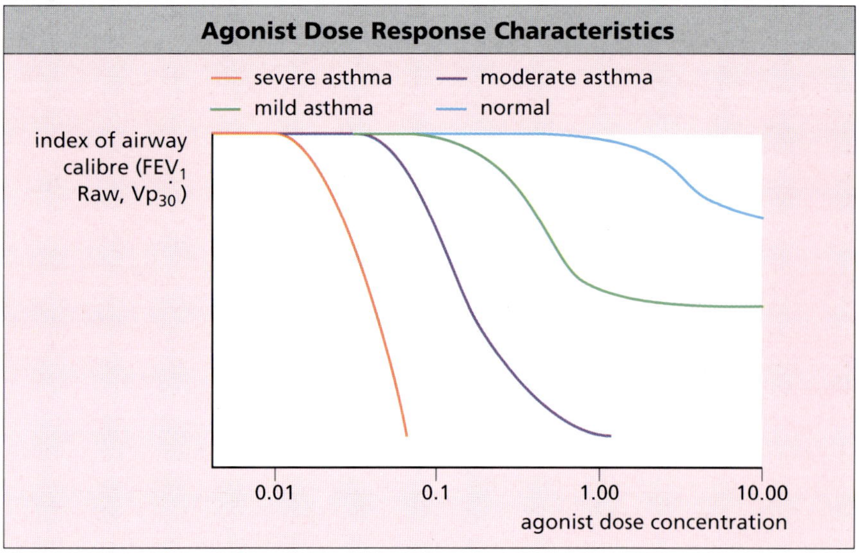

Fig. 13.2 Change in the shape of the agonist/airway calibre/dose response characteristics for normal to severely asthmatic subjects. Note the change in the maximum fall with increased stimulation.

wide variety of chemical and physical stimuli. Clinically this denotes a state of bronchial irritability. In the laboratory a wide range of different stimuli have been used in a dose-response manner to quantify bronchial hyperresponsiveness (Fig. 13.2). Broadly these stimuli provoke the airways either directly, through stimulation of specific receptors linked to excitation-contraction coupling of airways smooth muscle, such as histamine (H_1), methacholine (muscarinic M_3), or indirectly, by stimulating afferent neurones with recruitment of cholinergic and peptidergic reflexes (e.g. bradykinin, SO_2, metabisulphite) or by triggering mediator-secreting cells, particularly mast cells (e.g. exercise, isocapnic hyperventilation, non-isotonic aerosols, adenosine) (Fig. 13.3).

The airways of asthmatic subjects not only respond to lower levels of a provoking stimulus than those of normal subjects, but also show excessive narrowing. These factors can be described by constructing complete dose-response curves to an inhaled stimulus. The position of this curve denotes the airway sensitivity, while the presence of a plateau, and its configuration, denotes the extent of maximal airway narrowing (see Fig. 13.2). The dimension most frequently used to describe responsiveness of the airways to a provocative stimulus is the inhaled concentration (or dose) that is able to reduce FEV_1 by 20 per cent of baseline, while for the patient what is probably more important is the magnitude of maximal bronchoconstriction that can be achieved with the stimulus. The possible mechanism, or mechanisms, that can account for the plateau and relative position of the dose-response curve are depicted in Fig. 13.4. Both in experimental animals and in lungs obtained from patients who have died from asthma, airway swelling caused by oedema and inflammatory cell infiltration is likely to have a major influence in increasing the effect of smooth muscle shortening on airway calibre without there necessarily being any abnormality of the smooth muscle itself. Indeed, there are many published studies to indicate that contractile response of smooth muscle from patients with hyperactive airways *in vivo* behaves normally *in vitro*, although in many of these one might question whether clear examples of asthma were analysed. Recently Dutch investigations have reported that in 'pathologically defined' asthma, airway smooth muscle responses *ex vivo* do exhibit increased responsiveness to agonists while others have shown reduced relaxant responses to ß-agonist stimulation.

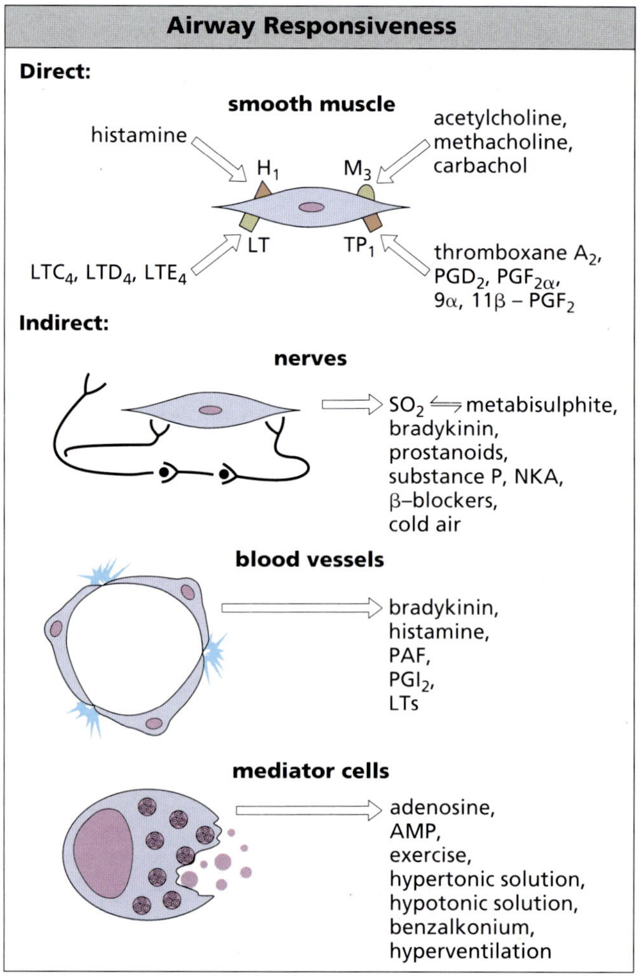

Fig. 13.3 Possible routes for producing pathways for direct and indirect bronchial hyperresponsiveness.

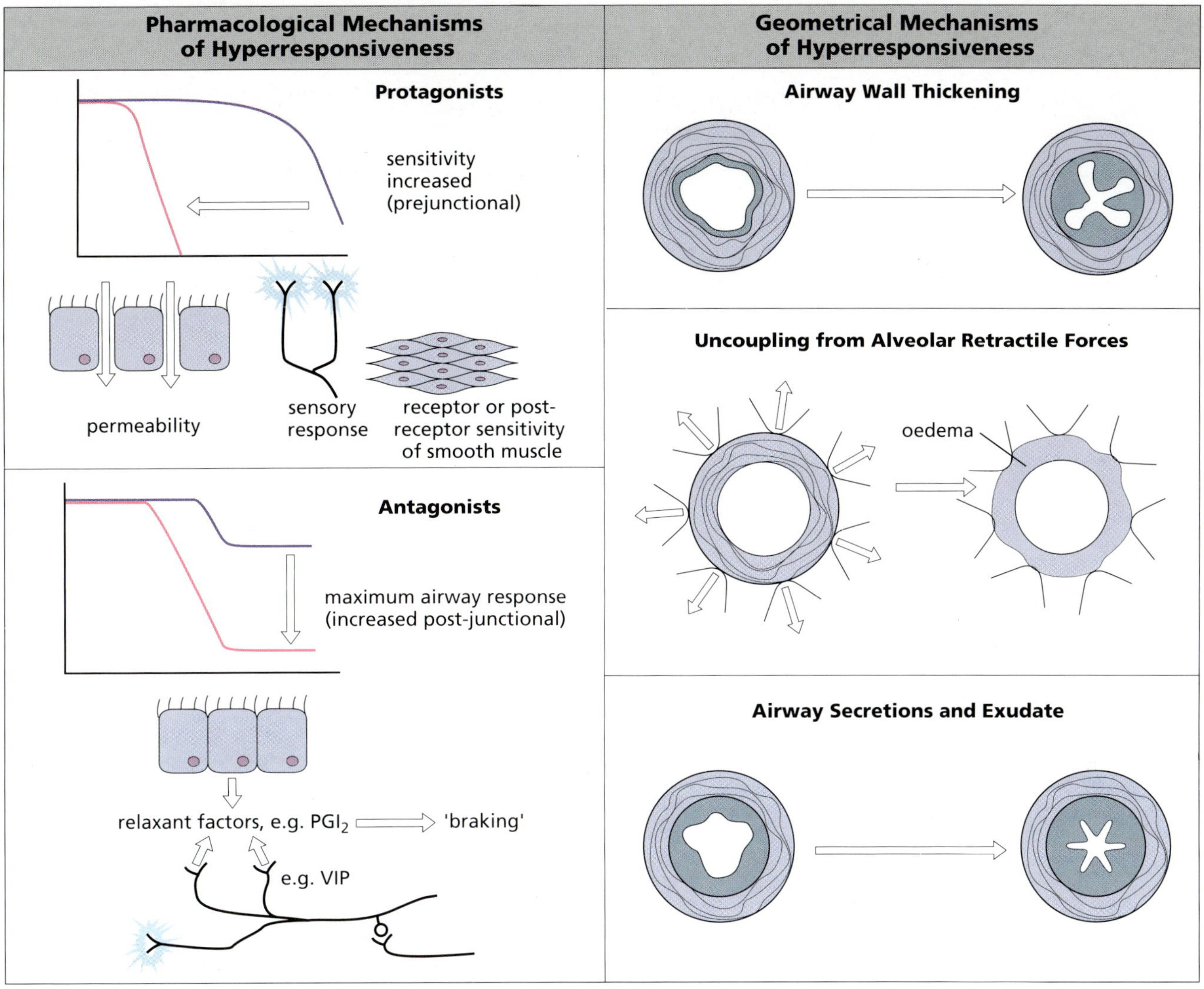

Fig. 13.4 Proposed mechanisms to explain hyperresponsiveness in asthma.

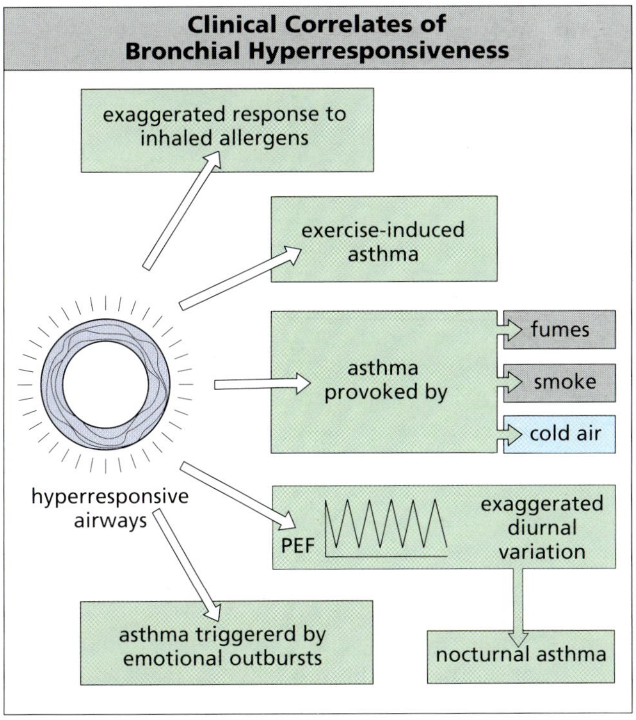

Fig. 13.5 Clinical consequences of bronchial hyperresponsiveness.

Pathology of Asthma

It would be a mistake to believe that the symptomatology of asthma can be accounted for solely on the basis of hyperresponsiveness. However, there are several clinical features that relate closely to it (Fig. 13.5). While instability of the airways is a characteristic of asthma there also occur more prolonged periods of airway obstruction which are relatively refractory to inhaled bronchodilators and probably result from airway swelling and hypersecretion of mucus. During severe exacerbations, occlusion of both small and large airways with a mixture of inspissated mucus, cell debris and plasma protein produces extended periods of airway obstruction that may require systemic corticosteroids to achieve resolution. Most patients who die during a severe episode have post-mortem evidence of widespread and extensive blockage of their airways with tenacious plugs (Fig. 13.6). This secretory process probably accounts for the observed refractoriness of severe asthma to inhaled bronchodilators. The characteristic pathological features found in an asthma death are shown in Fig. 13.7, which serves to emphasize the importance of inflammation as a major contributory event in this disease. While considerable information may be

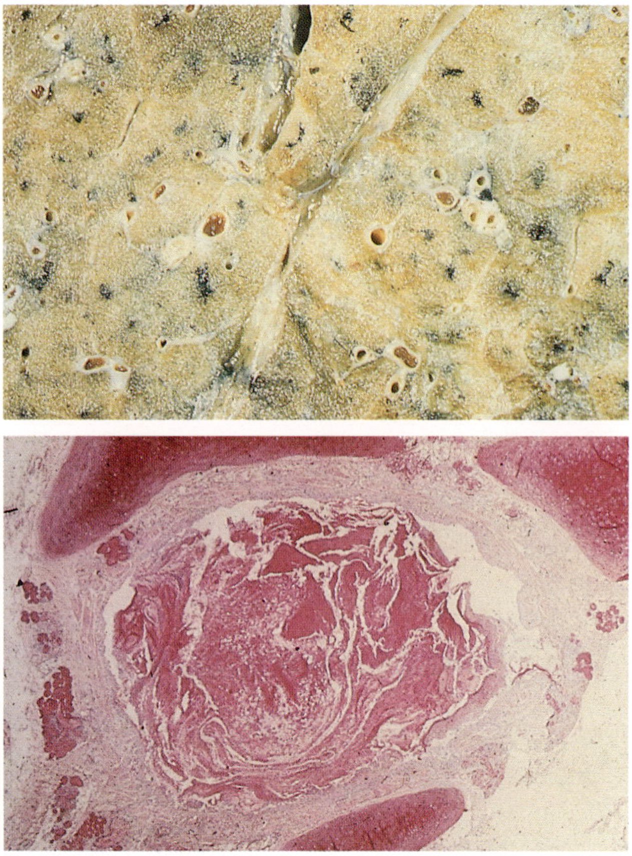

Fig. 13.6 [above] Cut section of lung from subject who has died from asthma, showing white mucous plugs projecting from the airways. [below] Complete occlusion of a cartilagenous airway by a large mucous plug.

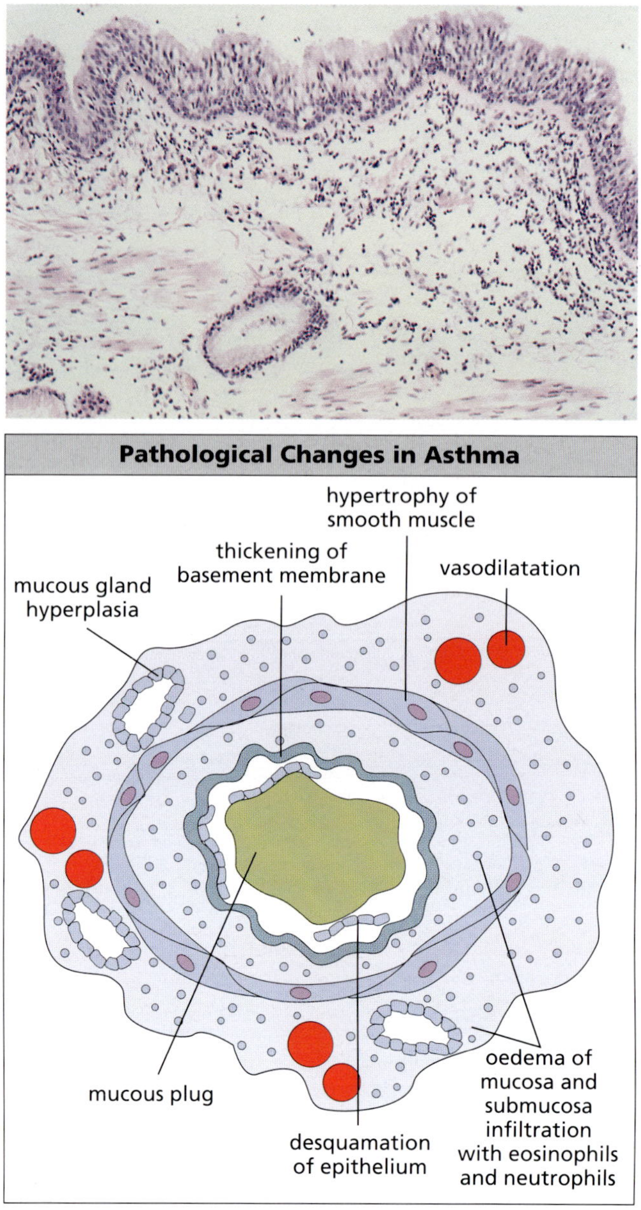

Fig. 13.7 [above] Histological appearance of the bronchial mucosa in an asthma death showing extensive inflammatory changes and a thickened basement membrane. [below] Cross-section of an airway in severe asthma to illustrate the characteristic pathological changes.

gained from post mortem studies, the application of fibreoptic bronchoscopy with lavage and endobronchial biopsy has provided additional insights into the role of inflammation in clinical asthma.

Bronchoalveolar lavage

The introduction of prewarmed physiological solutions into the airways of asthmatic patients enables retrieval of surface cells and mediators. Most studies have been conducted in atopic mildly asthmatic subjects, using comparisons with normal controls. The characteristic cellular features of bronchoalveolar lavage (BAL) in asthma are shown in Fig. 13.8. Data drawn from a large number of studies show the presence of increased numbers of ciliated epithelial cells often in clumps, mast cells and eosinophils. In mild asthma, T lymphocytes ($CD3^+$) and their subclasses ($CD4^+$ helper, $CD8^+$ suppressor/cytotoxic) are not increased, although using activation markers such as CD25 (α-chain of IL-2 receptor) and HLA-DR (MHC Class II molecule), there is accumulating evidence of T-cell activation. When assessed by a variety of techniques, macrophage and neutrophil function is also enhanced. Even in mild disease the degree to which macrophages respond to allergen by generating cytokines such as IL-1ß and IL-8 may reflect an important change to their phenotype (Fig. 13.9). Both mast cells and eosinophils are also present in the airway lumen in a secretory mode. Further evidence for the active participation of mediator secreting cells in asthma has been gained by measuring inflammatory products in the fluid phase of BAL. A wide variety of different mediators from many cell types have been described but paramount among them are histamine; prostaglandin (PG) D_2 (and other prostanoids); 15-hydroxyeicosatetraenoic; leukotrienes (LT) B_4, C_4, D_4, E_4; lysosomal enzymes; and a number of basic proteins from the eosinophil (Fig. 13.10). Many of these mediators originate from activated mast cells and eosinophils, but platelets, macrophages and monocytes also contribute to the autocoid pool.

Target effects of mediators

Many of these products have well-defined pharmacological actions. Histamine, PGD_2, 9_α,11ß–PGF_2, thromboxane (Tx) A_2, LTC_4, LTD_4, LTE_4 and potent contractile agonists of airways smooth muscle. Prostaglandins I_2 and E_2 are vasodilators while

Composition of Bronchoalveolar Lavage in Asthma							
	Total cells	**Macrophages**	**Mast cells**	**Eosinophils**	**Neutrophils**	**Lymphocytes**	**Epithelial cells**
Cell number	→	→	↑	↑↑↑	↑→	→	↑
Cellular activation		↑	↑ releasability	↑	↑	↑(TH_2)	?
Mediators		β-glucuronidase	histamine	MBP	O_2^-	IL-3	endothelin 1,
		LTD_4/E_4	tryptase	ECP		IL-4	neutral
		IL-1β	PGD_2	LTD_4/E_4		IL-5	endopeptidase
		TNF_α	LTD_4/E_4	O_2^-		GM-CSF	IL-1β
		IL-8	IL-4				IL-8
		GM-CSF	IL-5				GM-CSF

Fig. 13.8 Cellular and mediator composition of BAL in asthma compared with normal subjects.

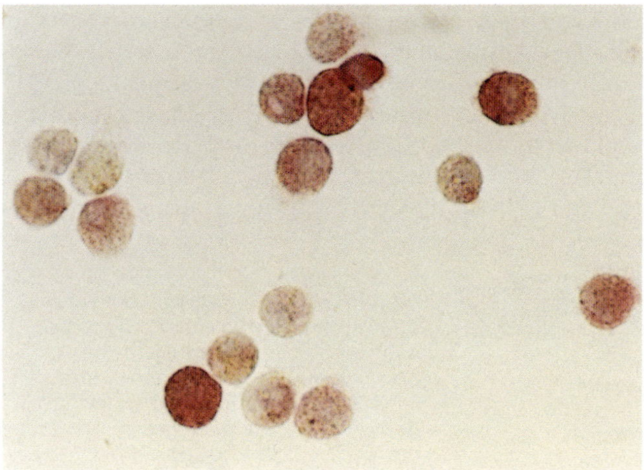

Fig. 13.9 Effect of 24 hours' exposure to specific allergen (grass pollen extract) on the intracellular production of IL-1ß by bronchoalveolar macrophages from a patient with atopic asthma. Immunohistochemistry is used to demonstrate upregulation of IL-1ß production (red).

platelet-activating factor (PAF), the sulphidopeptide leukotrienes (LTC_4, LTD_4 and LTE_4), bradykinin, histamine and TxA_2 increase microvascular leakage from post-capillary venules. Platelet-activating factor is a potent chemoattractant for eosinophils and LTB_4 a chemotactic factor for neutrophils. The relative potency of these mediators differs widely. For example, bradykinin, PGD_2 and LTD_4 are 10, 30 and 100–1,000 times more potent at causing bronchoconstriction in asthma than is histamine.

Many of these pharmacologically active mediators produce their effects by interaction with specific receptors on airways smooth muscle and the vasculature. A common receptor has been identified for many of the contractile prostanoids (TP_1- or PGH_2-receptor) and another for the three sulphidopeptide leukotrienes. Careful studies both *in vitro* and *in vivo* have shown that different mediators interact to reduce airways calibre, e.g. LTC_4 and histamine, while others enhance airways responsiveness, e.g. $PGF_{2\alpha}$, PGD_2, PAF and LTE_4. Released lysosomal enzymes such as tryptase, kallikrein and ß-glucuronidase probably serve to loosen the connective tissue matrix. In addition, through their capacity to attack epithelial attachment proteins and the basement membrane, proteolytic enzymes will lead to the

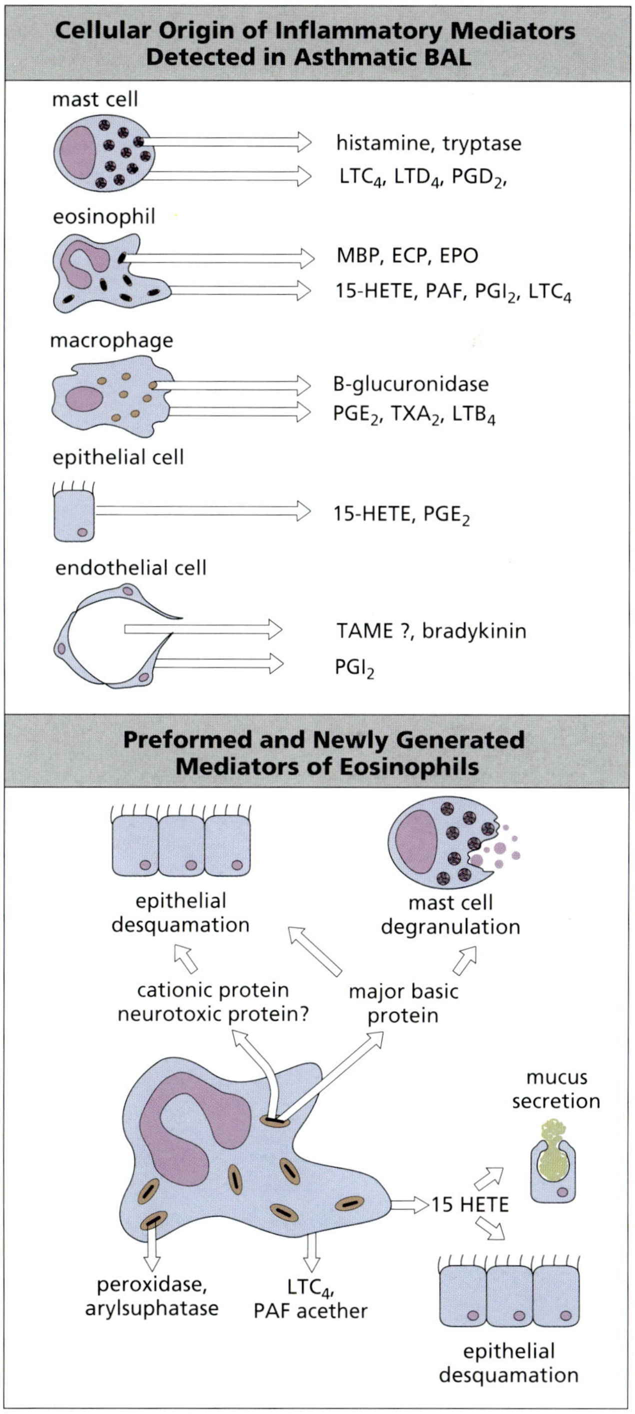

Fig. 13.10 Cellular origins of mediators.

observed increase in epithelial permeability to high molecular weight molecules and loss of the ability to control the electrolyte and protein composition of the airways lining fluid (Fig. 13.11). Other mediators are reported to be cytotoxic toward bronchial epithelial cells. In this regard the arginine-rich proteins of the eosinophil granule – major basic protein (MBP), eosinophil cationic protein (ECP), eosinophil-derived neurotoxin (EDN) and eosinophil peroxidase (EPO) are considered important. Immunofluorescent staining of the airway wall of post mortem lung from subjects who have died from asthma demonstrates extensive deposition of MBP and ECP in relation to regions of epithelial loss. MBP and related proteins have been shown to damage epithelial cells, increase smooth muscle responsiveness and enhance epithelial cell expression of leucocyte adhesion molecules. The mechanism(s) of basic protein-induced injury to the epithelium is not known, although a cognate interaction between eosinophils and epithelial cells is needed for optimal destruction of the permeability barrier. One possible mechanism is the capacity of eosinophils to communicate with epithelial cells, resulting in the release of metaloproteases with their capacity to loosen junctional cell adhesion molecules and components of the basement membrane.

A targeted attack on the bronchial epithelium has led to the view that removal of this protective barrier enhances the underlying response of the airways through loss of muscle relaxant factors secreted by these cells (see Fig. 13.4) and by augmentation of neural reflexes. The walls of the airway are rich in sensory nerves that extend their receptors between and beneath the epithelium (Fig. 13.12). These sensory nerves contain a wide array of neuropeptides with potent mediator functions (Fig. 13.13). It is suggested that in asthma an imbalance occurs between some of the peptides in favour of those that increase vascular permeability and contract airways smooth muscle. Such an imbalance might arise from the selective action of nerve growth factors, the enzymatic degradation of the relaxant peptides, e.g. VIP by tryptase and other lysosomal proteases, and the removal of epithelial cells along with their content of metalo-endoproteinases capable of degrading substance P, NKA and CGRP. However, while being the-

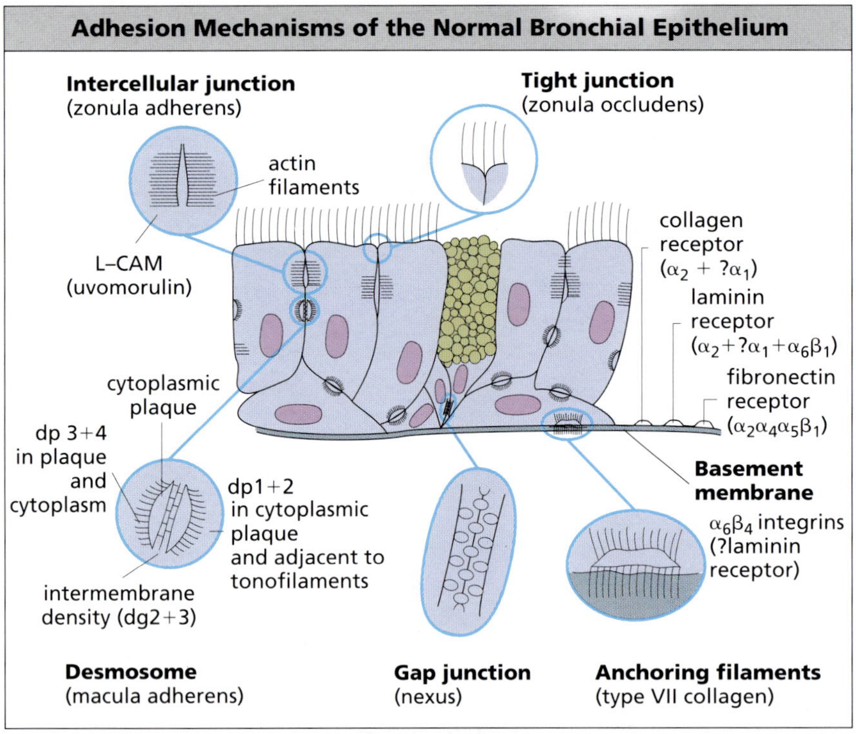

Fig. 13.11 [left] Intercellular adhesion molecules responsible for maintaining the integrity of the bronchial epithelium. [below, left] Fluorescent immunohistochemistry to demonstrate the presence of desmosomes on the suprabasal epithelial cells, and on the apex of the basal cells. [below, right] Epithelial disruption in asthma, showing separation of suprabasal epithelial cells from the basal cells attached to the basement membrane.

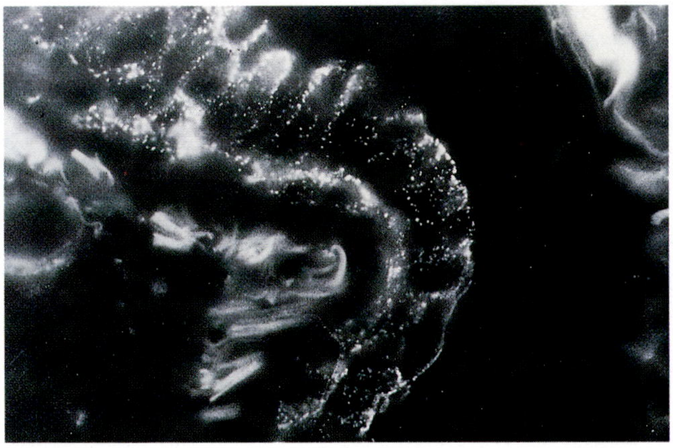

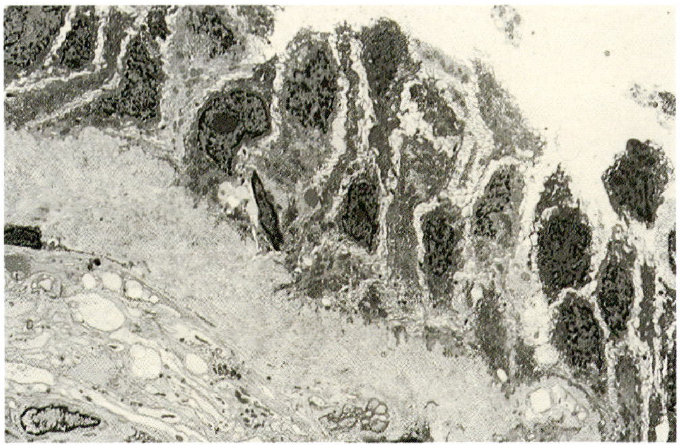

oretically attractive, it is not known how important this amplification pathway is for propagating an airway inflammatory response in asthma. The known pharmacological actions of many neuropeptides and the observation that some are co-released with more classical mediators, e.g. VIP with acetylcholine, might suggest that they serve a modulatory role over the neural regulation of smooth muscle, blood vessels and mucus secretion in a manner analogous to the role of the axon reflex in the skin.

Inflammation of the Airway Wall in Asthma

While the demonstration of desquamated epithelial cells (Creola bodies), eosinophils and their cell products (Charcot-Leyden crystals – eosinophil lysolecithinase) and the presence of metachromatic staining cell (mast cell/basophils) in the sputum of patients with asthma, provides evidence for ongoing mucosal inflammation during exacerbations, it has proved difficult to obtain an accurate picture of the inflammatory response in clinical asthma. The presence of inflammatory cells in the BAL of asthmatics (see Fig. 13.8) indicates that inflammatory mechanisms are operative even in mild disease, but this technique only provides information about the cells lining the airways and not about events within the airway wall.

The recent application of bronchoscopy to obtain mucosal biopsies has provided a new insight into the potential role of inflammation as an underlying pathogenetic mechanism of asthma. When comparing biopsies obtained from atopic asthmatics and normal subjects major differences are apparent (Fig. 13.14). These include epithelial fragility, sub-basement membrane thickening and infiltration of the epithelium and submucosa with inflammatory leucocytes. In atopic asthma, mast cells in the epithelium and submucosa may increase, but more noticeable is the presence of large numbers of eosinophils both in extravascular and intravascular spaces (Figs 13.14

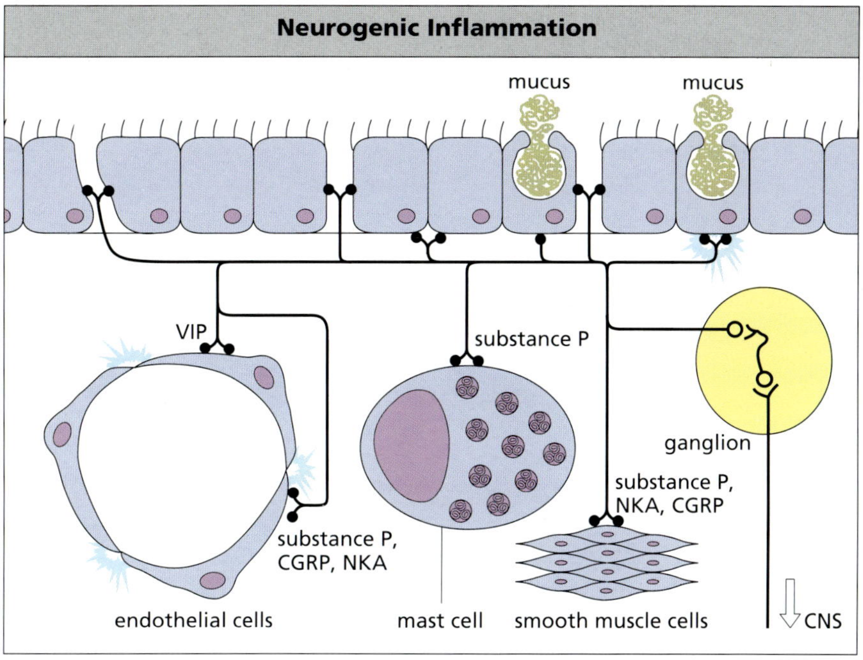

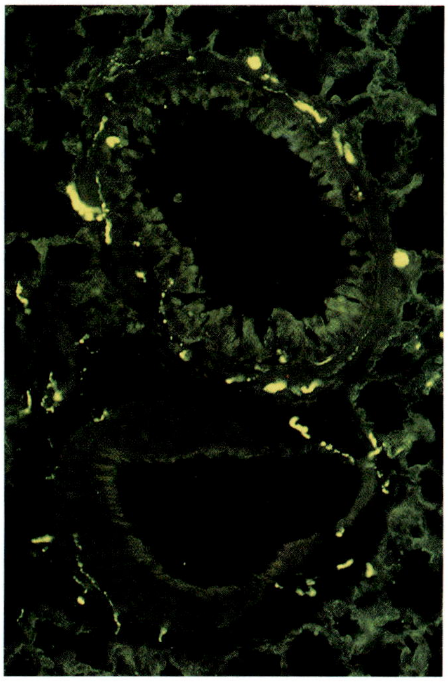

Fig.13.12 [left] Neurogenic inflammation. [right] Immunofluorescent localization of VIP to the nerves of an airway and adjacent blood vessel

Peptide Neurotransmitters Implicated in Neurogenic Inflammation

Neuropeptide	Receptor	Function
substance P	NK_2	smooth muscle contraction
	NK_1	microvascular leakage, goblet cell secretion, submucous gland secretion
calcitonin gene-related peptide (CGRP)	CGRP receptor	prolonged vasodilatation, smooth muscle contraction
vasoactive intestinal polypeptide (VIP)	VIP receptor	smooth muscle relaxation, vasodilation
endothelin 1	ET_1 receptor	smooth muscle contraction, vasodilation

Fig. 13.13 Peptide neurotransmitters implicated in neurogenic inflammation.

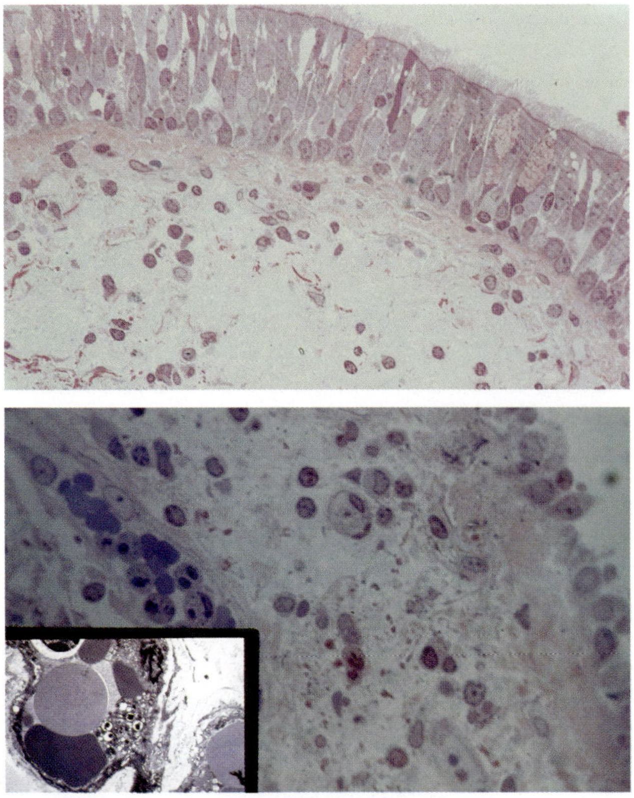

Fig. 13.14 Characteristic appearance of the bronchial mucosa obtained by fibreoptic bronchoscopy from [above] normal and [below] asthmatic subjects. Note the extensive inflammatory infiltrate of the asthmatic biopsy and the presence of eosinophil-endothelial interaction (inset).

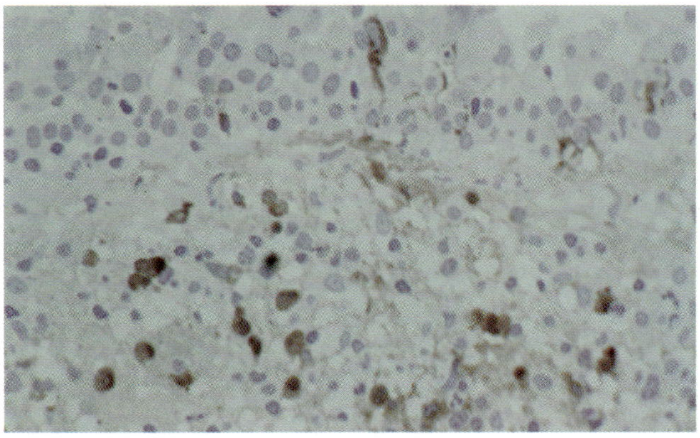

Fig. 13.15 Immunohistochemical demonstration of eosinophil staining for ECP in asthma showing migrating eosinophils (brown).

and 13.15). When eosinophils are seen within post-capillary venules they are found in close association with post-capillary venule endothelial cells, with which they interact through the mutual expression of specific adhesion proteins. A large number of these have now been identified, but of particular importance is intercellular adhesion molecule-1 (ICAM-1), expressed both on endothelial and epithelial cells, and its ligand LFA-1 on T-cells and VCAM with its ligand VLA-4 on eosinophils (Fig. 13.16).

In symptomatic asthma, the secretory granules of both mast cells and eosinophils appear heterogeneous in size and electron density, suggesting that these cells are activated to secrete their mediators (Fig. 13.17). Eosinophils are seen migrating out of venules

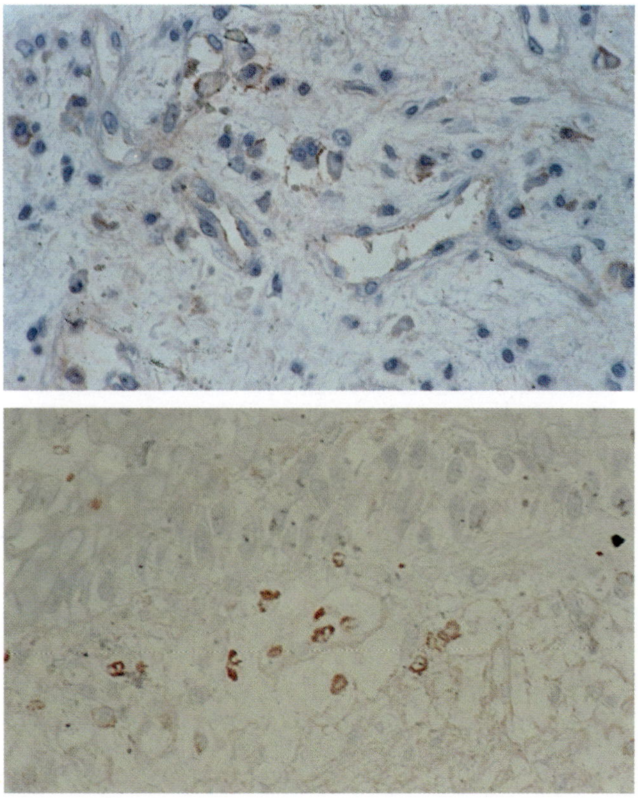

Fig. 13.16 [above] Basal expression of ICAM-1 on endothelium of subepithelial blood vessels in a patient with symptomatic asthma. [below] The expression of the complementary receptor for ICAM-1, LFA-1 on T-cells and eosinophils in an asthmatic bronchial biopsy.

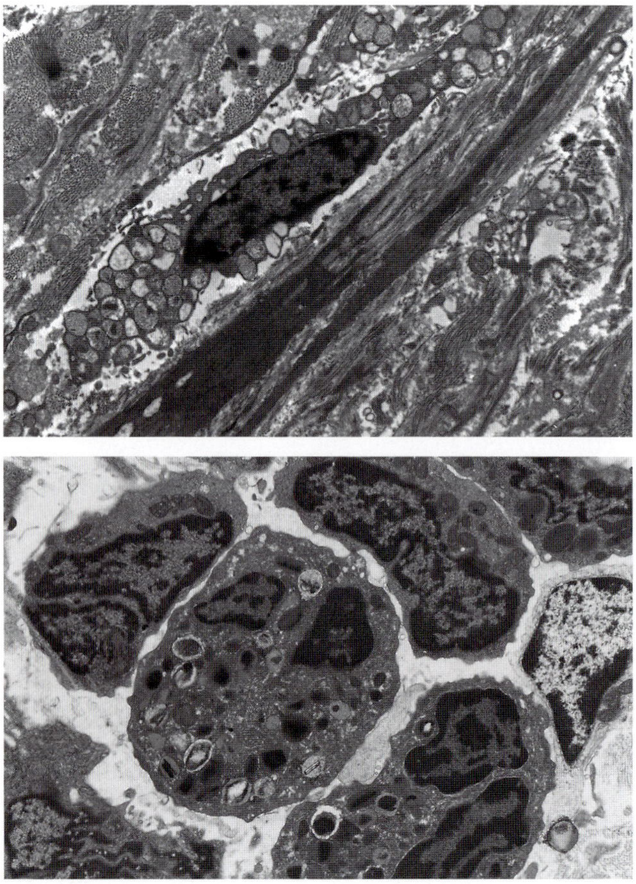

Fig. 13.17 Transmission electron micrographs of [above] an activated mast cell and [below] eosinophil from an allergic asthmatic subject.

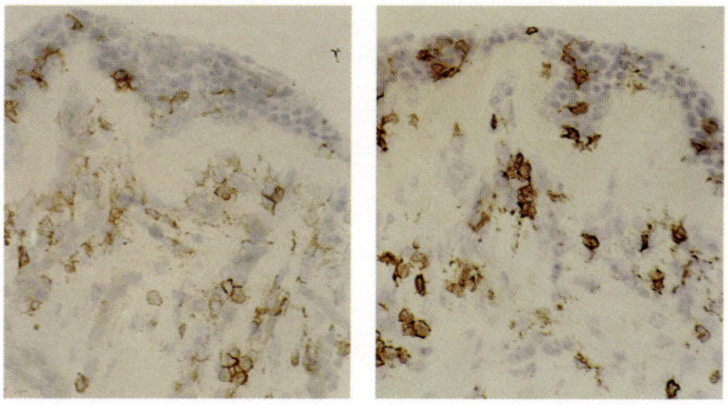

Fig. 13.18 Epithelial and subepithelial T-cell subsets ([left] $CD4^+$, [right] $CD8^+$) in a bronchial biopsy from a subject with mild asthma. While T-cells may be activated in mild-moderate disease, their total numbers are not changed.

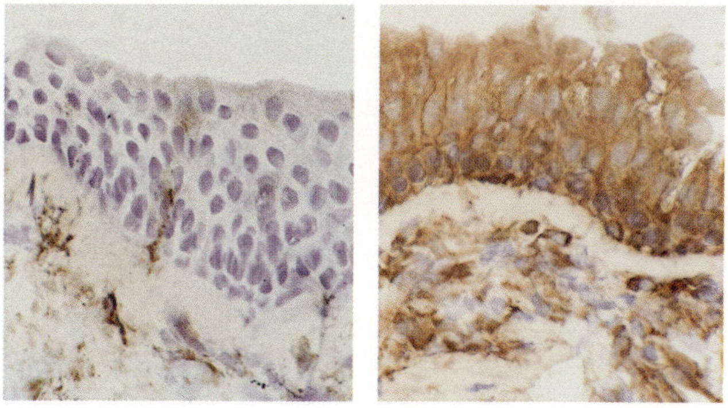

Fig. 13.20 Immunoperoxidase demonstration of HLA-DR on the bronchial epithelim of [left] normal and [right] asthmatic subjects, showing upregulation of this heterodimer in asthma.

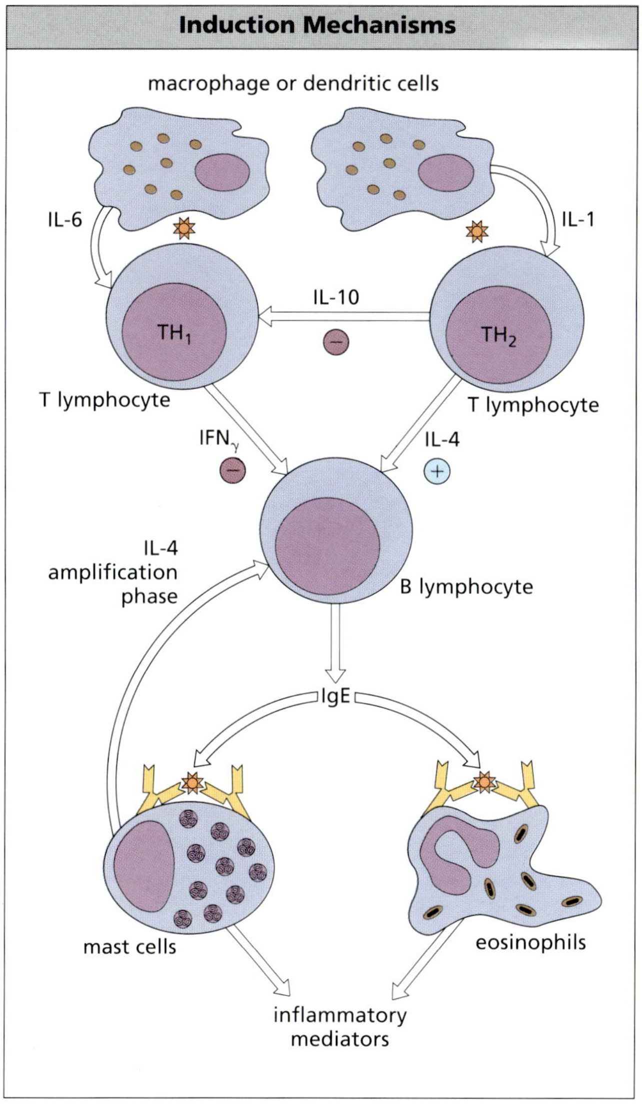

Fig. 13.19 Interrelationship between inducer and effector mechanisms of allergic inflammation in asthma.

and through the submucosal tissues and epithelium towards the luminal face, suggestive of directed migration.

The predominant lymphocyte in both normal and asthmatic airways is the T-cell. However, in asthma of mild-moderate severity, neither T-cell numbers nor their subtype ($CD4^+$ and $CD8^+$) are increased in either the epithelium or submucosa (Fig. 13.18). In intrinsic asthma, T-cell numbers are increased, representing largely $CD4^+$ cells. In bronchial biopsies and BAL of both atopic and non-atopic asthmatics there is increased expression of the T-cell activation markers, IL-2 receptor and HLA-DR. This supports the view that T-cells are involved in the control of mast cell and eosinophil recruitment into the airways and their function as mediator-secreting cells. In mice, there is convincing evidence for the existence of at least two populations of $CD4^+$ T-cells with differing cytokine repertoires. The TH_1 cell elaborates interferon-α, lymphotoxin and IL-2 while the TH_2 cell produces IL-3, IL-4, IL-5, GM-CSF and IL-10. From a functional standpoint, TH_1 cells are utilized in the classical delayed hypersensitivity response (Type IV), while TH_2 cells are upregulated in allergic and parasitic responses. Recent evidence suggests that similar T-cell phenotypes may exist in humans, with TH_2-like cells being utilized to promote the allergic inflammatory response as occurs in asthma. TH_1 and TH_2 cells are under negative feedback control, one subtype producing factors which suppress the other (Fig. 13.19). Most recently human mast cells have been shown to contain IL-4, IL-5, IL-6 and TNF_{α}, probably in a preformed state, which upon IgE-dependent stimulation are released. Since IL-4 is able to induce VCAM expression on endothelial cells and IL-5 is a potent chemoattractant and activator of eosinophils, it is possible that the release of these cytokines from mast cells is responsible for the allergen-induced late-phase response and the associated acquired increase in bronchial responsiveness with T-cell recruitment to maintain and prolong the inflammatory response, as occurs with continued allergen exposure.

Normal bronchial epithelium contains dendritic cells with a high expression of HLA-DR identifying their capacity to recognize and present allergens to T-cells. In a high proportion of asthmatic – but less so in normal – biopsies, HLA-DR is also expressed on the surface of the ciliated and non-ciliated epithelial cells (Fig. 13.20), but the function of this is not known.

Another prominent feature of mucosal biopsies in

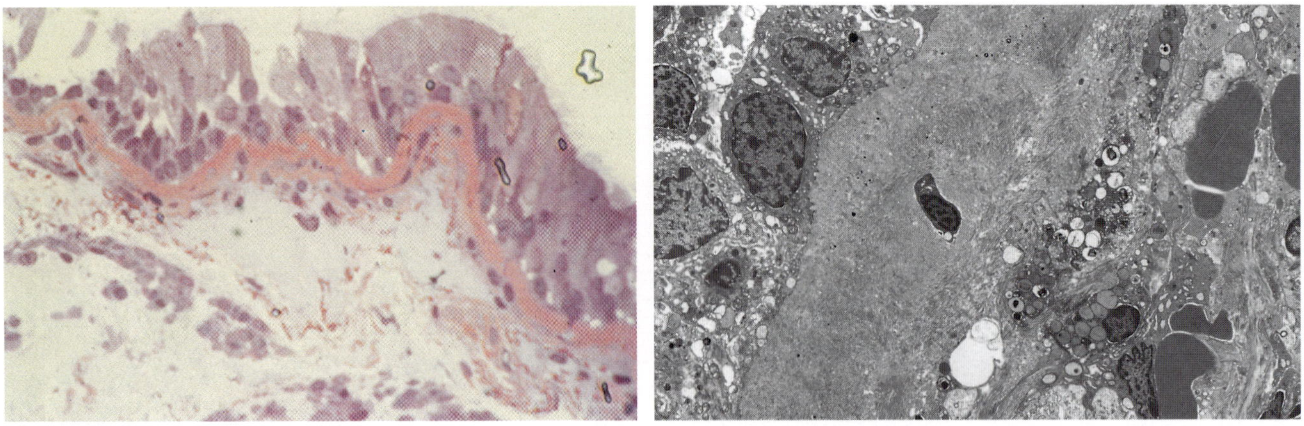

Fig. 13.21 [left] Light and [right] electron microscopical appearance of sub-basement membrane collagen deposition in asthma.

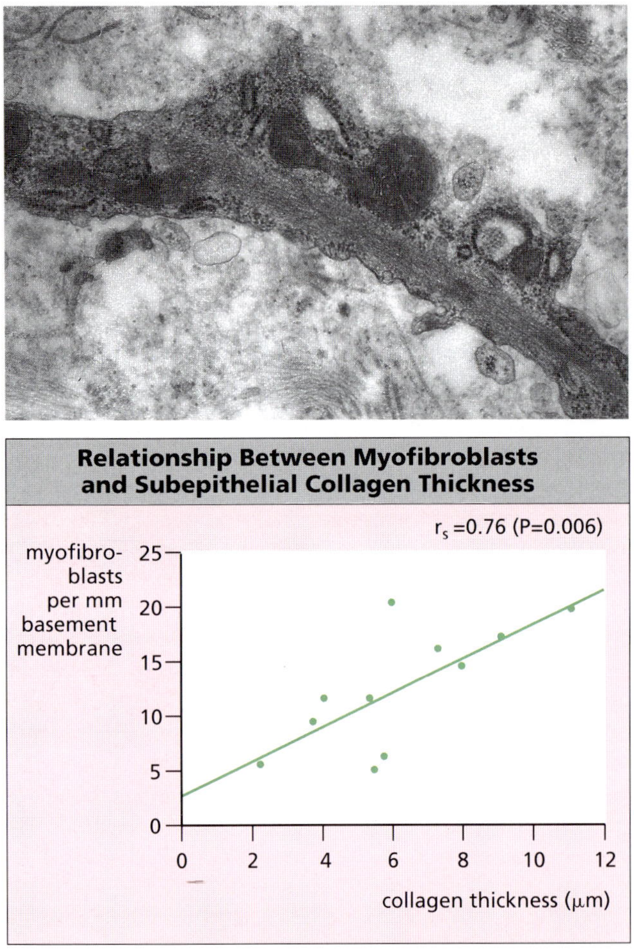

Fig. 13.22 Transmission electron micrograph of epithelial myofibroblast in asthma, showing [above] contractile actin filaments and [below] relationship between the number of these cells determined by the monoclonal antibody PR2D3 and subepithelial collagen thickness in asthma.

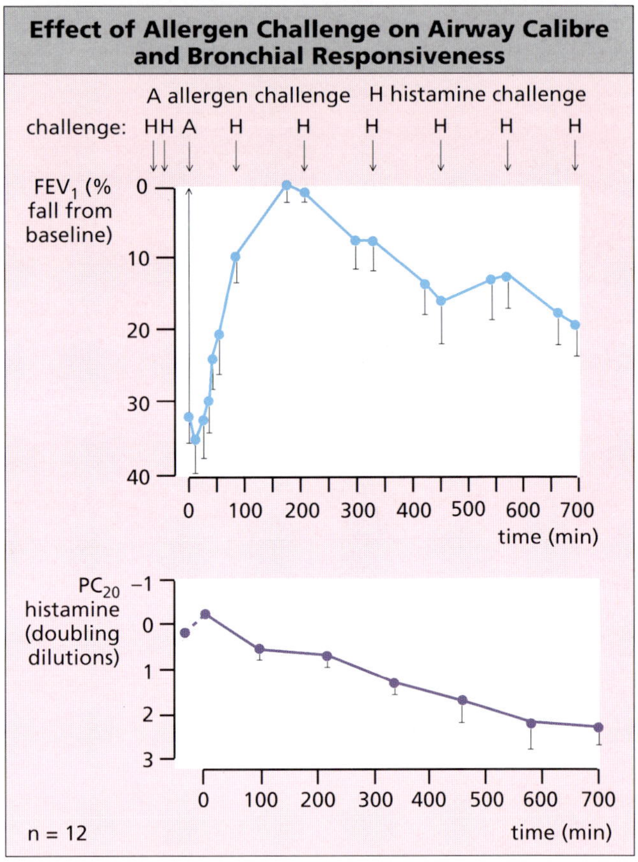

Fig. 13.23 The influence of allergen provocation on the early- and late-phase airway responses to inhaled allergen in allergic asthma.

asthma is thickening of the subepithelial basement membrane (Fig. 13.21). Transmission electron microscopy has shown that this is due to the deposition of dense cross-linked collagen. Immunohistochemical stains, using monoclonal antibodies directed against different collagen subtypes, confirm the presence of Type IV collagen in the basement membrane of the epithelium, blood vessels and smooth muscle, but not in the thickened sub-basement membrane region. At this site and spreading through the submucosa there is excessive deposition of Types I, III and V interstitial collagens, derived from a special form of fibroblast that proliferates in asthma, the myofibroblast. Identification of these cells using the monoclonal antibody PR2D3 has shown that their numbers are increased in proportion to the extent of sub-basement membrane thickening (Fig. 13.22). In chronic severe asthma, it is possible that this fibrotic response extends further into the airway wall, leading to an irreversible component of airways obstruction. These cells may also be important in maintaining the inflammatory response through the secretion of cytokines.

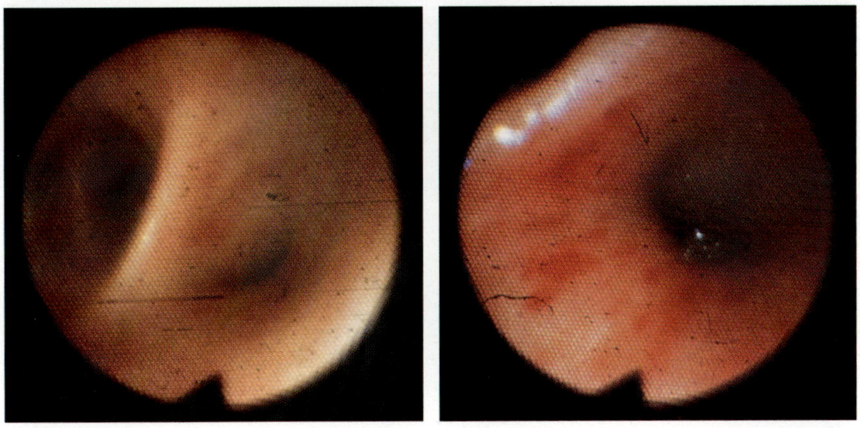

Fig. 13.24 Bronchoscopic appearance of [left] early and [right] late asthmatic reactions. The EAR is characterized by a mast cell-dependent smooth muscle contraction, while the LAR also encompasses airway oedema.

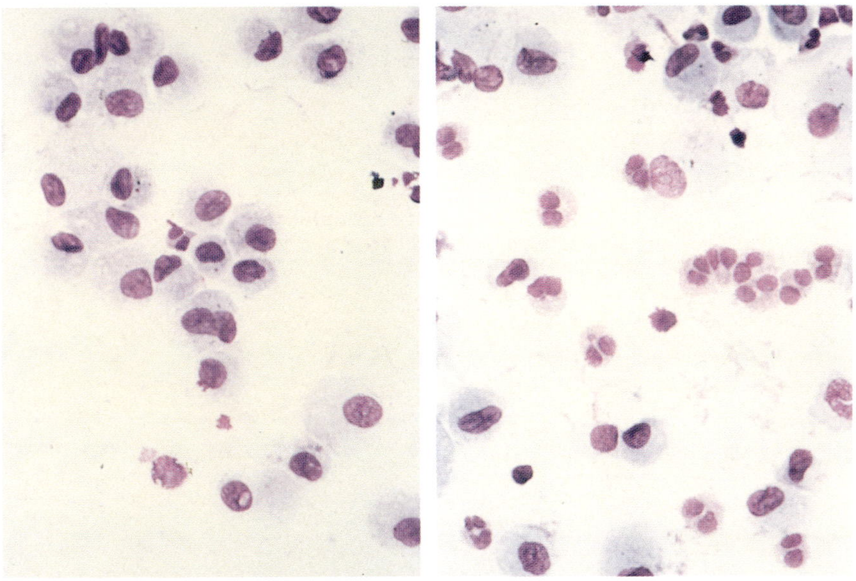

Fig. 13.25 Cellular profile of BAL [left] before and [right] four hours after allergen challenge of an atopic asthmatic subject. The dominant cells are macrophages, although after allergen there is a selective recruitment of eosinophils.

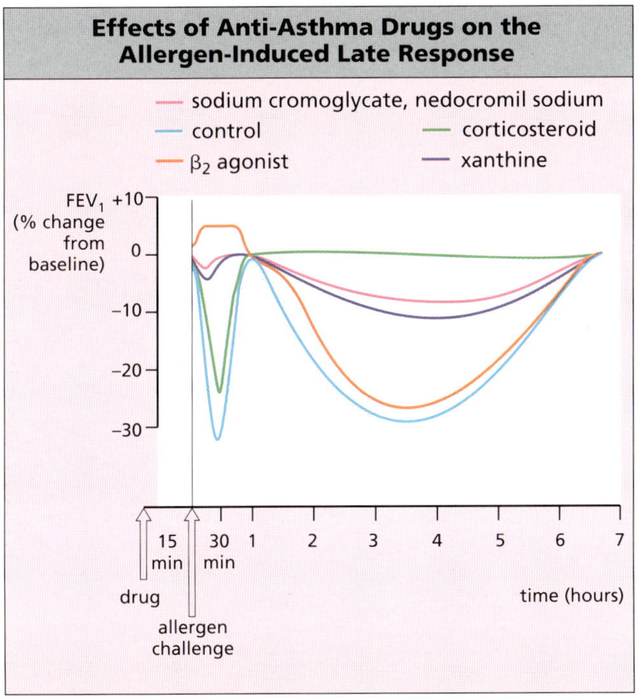

Fig. 13.26 The effect of a β_2-agonist (salbutamol) on anti-allergic drug (sodium cromoglycate or nedocromil sodium), an inhaled corticosteroid (beclomethasone diproprionate) and a xanthine (theophylline). On the early - and-late phase response to allergen challenge. The drugs were given 15 minutes prior to challenge.

Clinical Implications of Considering Asthma as an Inflammatory Disease

In atopic asthma, and probably in other forms of the disease, much of the symptomatology can be related directly to the presence of airway inflammation. It is clear that mast cell and eosinophil mediators have the capacity of producing bronchoconstriction through their effects on the bronchial smooth muscle and microvasculature. Some aspects of this response can be modelled in the form of the early and late asthmatic reactions (EAR, LAR). Provocation of the airways with a sensitizing allergen produces a rapid bronchoconstriction, which lasts for about 1 hour (EAR), followed by a more prolonged phase of airway narrowing (LAR) accompanied by a progressive increase in bronchial responsiveness (Fig. 13.23). The EAR results mostly from airway smooth muscle contraction following the release of mast cell autocoids (histamine, PGD_2 and LTC_4), while the LAR has an important oedema component (Fig. 13.24) produced by mediators released from recruited eosinophils (Fig. 13.25). These challenge responses have proved of some value in dissecting the mechanisms of action of anti-asthma drugs, although it cannot be said that they truly represent the pattern of clinical disease (Fig. 13.26). It is becoming increasingly apparent that a second level of inflammation is important in asthma which leads to proliferative and repair responses (Fig. 13.27). Included in this is the targeted destruction of the bronchial epithelium, the expansion and activation of fibroblasts, hypertrophy and hyperplasia of smooth muscle and the proliferation of neuropeptide-containing nerves. All of these events are likely to be under the control of specific cytokines, some being responsible for the more acute responses (IL-3, IL-4, IL-5 and GM-CSF) and some for the chronic phase (TNF_{α}, IL-1, platelet-derived growth factor (PGDF), transforming growth factor-ß (TGF_{β}) and nerve growth factors).

If asthma is viewed primarily as an inflammatory disorder then the use of β_2-agonists and other bronchodilators to treat symptoms alone should be discouraged in favour of introducing drugs which reduce airway inflammation such as corticosteroids and sodium cromoglycate (see Fig. 13.26). In adopting such a strategy β_2-agonists should then be reserved for breakthrough symptoms. This philosophy has been adopted in guidelines for the management of asthma drawn up by a number of countries and for the first time provides a rational basis for management based on the known disease mechanisms.

Mast Cell, Eosinophil and Fibroblast Interactions

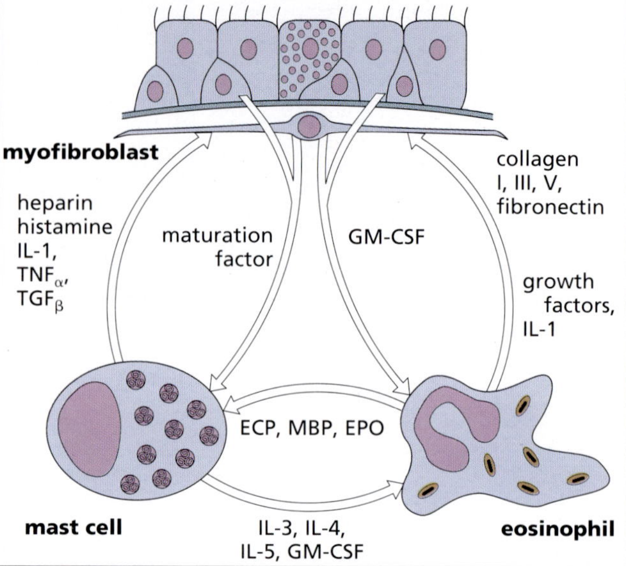

Fig. 13.27 Mast cell, eosinophil and fibroblast interactions.

Further Reading

Barnes PJ. Nerves, neurotransmitters and asthma. In: Seymour CA, Summerfield JA, eds. *Horizons in Medicine*, No. 3. Cambridge: Cambridge University Press, 1991, pp. 14–29.

Bierman WC, Lee TH, eds. Allergic inflammatory mediators and bronchial hyperresponsiveness II. In: *Immunology and Allergy Clinics of North America*, Vol. 10, No. 3. Philadelphia: WB Saunders, 1990.

Bray MA, Anderson WH, eds. Mediators of pulmonary inflammation. In: Lenfant C (executive ed.), *Lung Biology in Health and Disease*, Vol. 54. New York: Marcel Dekker, 1991.

Djukanovic R, Roche WR, Wilson JW, Beasley CRW, Twentyman OP, Howarth PH, Holgate ST. Mucosal inflammation in asthma. *Am Rev Respir Dis* 1990; **142**: 434–57.

Holgate ST, ed. *The Role of Inflammatory Processes in Airway Hyperresponsiveness*. Oxford: Blackwells, 1989.

Kobayashi S, Bellanti JA, eds. Advances in Asthmology 1990. Amsterdam: Excerpta Medica, 1991.

Mygind N, Pipkorn U, Dahl R, eds. *Rhinitis and Asthma*. Copenhagen: Munksgaard, 1990.

Piper PJ, Krell RD, eds. Advances in the understanding and treatment of asthma. *Annals of New York Academy of Sciences*, Vol. 629, 1991.

Chapter 14

Asthma – Diagnosis, Management and Outcomes

Introduction

Asthma is a disease of the airways which makes them narrow excessively to a wide range of inhaled stimuli. The episodic nature of the airway narrowing, referred to as an attack if it lasts for minutes, or as an exacerbation if it lasts for hours or even days, is characteristic of the disease.

As described in the previous chapters, it is clear that the airways of patients with persistent chronic asthma have inflammatory changes characterized by the presence of eosinophils, mast cells, and lymphocytes. The histopathological changes in patients with intermittent asthma are less well defined.

Tests of spirometric function, including forced vital capacity (FVC), the one-second forced expiratory volume (FEV_1), the ratio of these two measurements, and peak expiratory flow rate (PEFR) are useful for monitoring an attack, but isolated values are of no help in deciding the overall severity of the disease. For this, a knowledge of the variability of PEFR readings (PEFRvar) during the day, including the response to a bronchodilator, is essential.

Fig. 14.1 outlines some clinical criteria that can be used to classify a patient with asthma. These criteria apply to patients who are not already enrolled in a management plan and who are not experiencing an exacerbation. As it is not realistic to do bronchial biopsies for diagnostic purposes, it is necessary to rely on indirect information including the frequency and severity of symptoms and the PEFRvar to determine the nature and severity of the inflammation present. The shape and position of dose response curves to non-specific stimuli, often loosely referred to as bronchial responsiveness, can also help in assessing asthma severity, but this information is not necessary for classification.

The classification of asthma shown in Fig. 14.1 has little to do with the allergic state of the patient, although most patients in the first three groups are allergic to inhaled substances. The presence or absence of atopy or sensitivity to inhaled substances does not affect the classification or the overall treatment plan to any great extent.

Life-threatening attacks can occur in patients in groups 2 to 4. Within group 4 there is a small group of patients with apparently severe asthma who have largely fixed airways obstruction with little reversibility, a prominent cough and poor response to steroids. No satisfactory name has been given to this abnormality because its causes and pathological basis are not known.

Classification of Asthma

Grade	Nature	Severity	Clinical Description
1	intermittent	mild	occasional attacks, often after exposure to known allergen or sensitizer; PEFRvar normal between attacks; includes subjects with seasonal and early occupational asthma.
2	persistent	mild to moderate	attacks of varying frequency and severity, easily reversed; PEFRvar >10 per cent <30 per cent between attacks; symptoms usually controlled without steroids.
3	persistent – normal lung function	severe	frequent attacks, which may take hours to days to reverse; often nocturnal symptoms; PEFRvar >30 per cent. Steroids needed for control; normal FEV_1 possible.
4	persistent – abnormal lung function	severe	as for Grade 3 but FEV_1 never reaches predicted value.

Fig. 14.1 Classification of asthma. These grades are based on clinical criteria. This classification is useful in planning the longterm management and for thinking about outcomes. One aim of management is to prevent a Grade 1 patient deteriorating to Grade 4. A guide to assessing the severity of asthma itself in individual patients is shown in Fig. 14.9. PEFRvar = variability of daily Peak Expiratory Flow readings.

Diagnosis of Asthma

Symptoms

Typical symptoms observed with increasing severity of asthma are shown in Fig. 14.2. Wide variations exist in practice and these are only guidelines.

The diagnosis of asthma rests largely on the history. Wheeze and chest tightness are the most common symptoms. Classically symptoms are episodic and frequently occur in response to a recognized 'trigger'. Sometimes, however, no trigger can be identified. The symptoms are due to episodes of airway irritation or narrowing, and may last minutes, hours, days, or weeks. Patients with poor lung function may have dyspnoea on exertion unrelated to attacks of asthma.

Airway narrowing which occurs acutely (e.g. during a provocation test) causes chest tightness and sometimes wheeze. The symptoms are interpreted in different ways by different patients, and the perception of narrowing, for a given fall in lung function, is extremely variable between patients. This makes it difficult to assess the severity of asthma from the symptoms alone, and measurement of PEFR variability or bronchial responsiveness are also required.

Signs

The physical signs of asthma are rarely useful in making a diagnosis, in assessing the severity of the disease, or in assessing a particular attack–except when the attack is very severe. The sign of widespread airway narrowing is audible ronchi, and, if the narrowing is severe, there may be overinflation, tachypnoea and tachycardia. In elderly patients presenting for the first time, the presence of left ventricular failure should be excluded.

Confirming the Diagnosis

Spirometric Function (FEV1)

Fig. 14.3 (left) shows typical forced expiratory curves from a 30-year old female before and after an inhaling a bronchodilator. The increase in the FEV_1, which is more than 15 per cent of the predicted values, is diagnostic of asthma. The decreased FVC as well as the decreased FEV_1 indicates that many airways are closing prematurely during the expiration. It is stressed that the severity of the disease cannot be derived from these tracings. Furthermore, failure to respond acutely to a bronchodilator does not exclude the diagnosis.

Fig. 14.3 (middle and right) shows spirometric function from the same patient on a different occasion. Initially she had poor spirometric function and no response to bronchodilator. After a week of treatment with oral steroids, the obstruction became almost fully reversible.

Variability of PEFR

Fig. 14.4 shows typical PEFR values from a patient presenting with a history suggesting asthma. Values before and after bronchodilator in the morning (red) and evening (blue) have been recorded. The most useful way to analyse these results is to calculate the variability–the range for the day divided by the highest value, expressed as a percent and averaged for 10 to 14 days. It is important to use values before and after bronchodilator in the calculation. This value has been shown to correlate with the severity of bronchial hyperresponsiveness to methacholine and histamine. Studies in normal children and adults show that values for PEFR vary by less than 6 per cent in a 24 hour period.

Symptoms of Asthma, According to Grade of Severity

Grade	Chest Tightness/Wheeze	Cough	Exertional Dyspnoea *
1	frequency = <1 month duration = <2 hour response to bronchodilator = rapid & complete triggers = known	dry; day and/or night; may be only symptom	–
2	frequency = weekly duration = <1 hour response to bronchodilator = rapid & complete triggers = known	dry; day and/or night; may be only symptom	–
3	frequency = daily ** duration = hours to days response to bronchodilator = slow but complete triggers = known and unknown	dry or productive; often at night; not sole symptom	during exacerbations
4	frequency = daily ** duration = hours to days response to bronchodilator = incomplete triggers = often unknown	often productive; never sole symptom	often present between exacerbations

* not due to exercise triggered attacks with wheeze
** unless on daily medication

Fig. 14.2 Symptoms of asthma. Based on the four grades, typical symptoms are listed. Great individual variability in the perception of symptoms means that the assessment of severity requires objective measurements as well as symptoms.

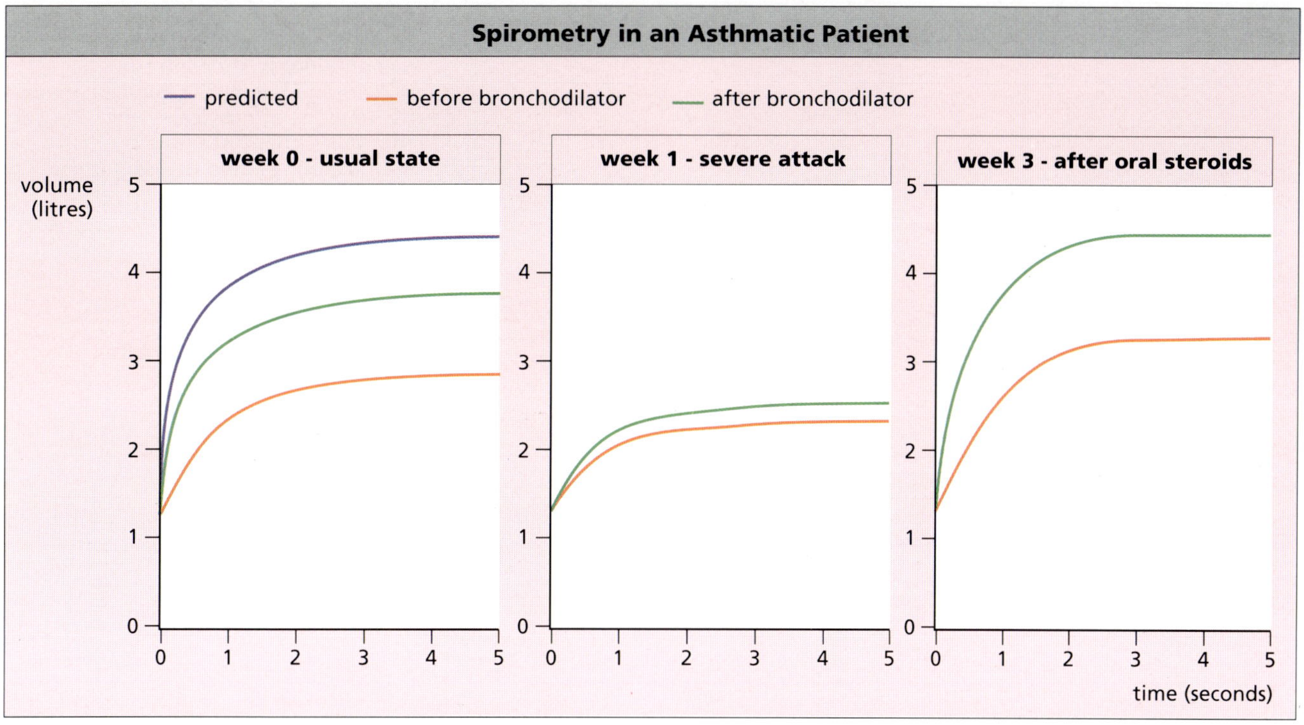

Fig. 14.3 Spirometric function in a patient with asthma. [Left]. The response of the FEV_1 and the FVC to inhaled bronchodilator are shown, together with the predicted value. [Middle and Right]. The response to bronchodilator before and after a week of treatment with oral steroids. The subject is a 30-year old female, height 165 cm.

In Fig. 14.4, the mean value for the initial 10 days was 32 per cent. With the introduction of inhaled corticosteroids, this value began to decrease and the overall level of the PEFR improved. It must be stressed that PEFRvar is diagnositic of asthma only in patients with fully reversible lung function. Patients with abnormal PEFR values for any reason, e.g. chronic airflow limitation, are likely to have increased PEFR variability, probably due to thickened airway walls.

Non-specific bronchial responsiveness

There is some confusion about the place of challenge tests in the diagnosis of asthma; see Fig. 14.5 which shows typical dose response curves in a normal subject, a patient with grade 2 asthma, and a patient with grade 4 asthma. The dose or concentration of the provicant that causes a 20 per cent fall in the FEV_1 is called the PD20 or PC20 respectively. For histamine and methacholine, the most commonly used provicants, these values are usually less than 1 μmol or 2.0 mg/ml in people who have current symptoms of asthma. Such curves can be obtained with many agonists that act on receptors on the airway smooth muscle.

The interpretion of the dose response curves requires knowledge of the current understanding of their characteristics:

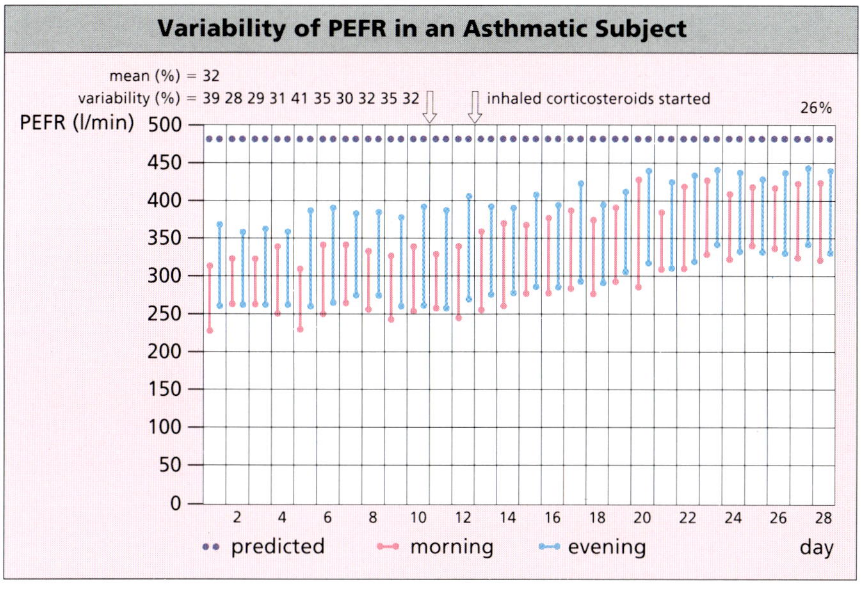

Fig. 14.4 Daily peak flow records. These records, before and after bronchodilator in the morning and evenings for a month, show the effect of inhaled steroids which were introduced after 10 days. The lower bullet in each pair of readings represents the value before bronchodilator, the upper bullet represents the value after bronchodilator. These records are from the same patient as in Fig. 14.3

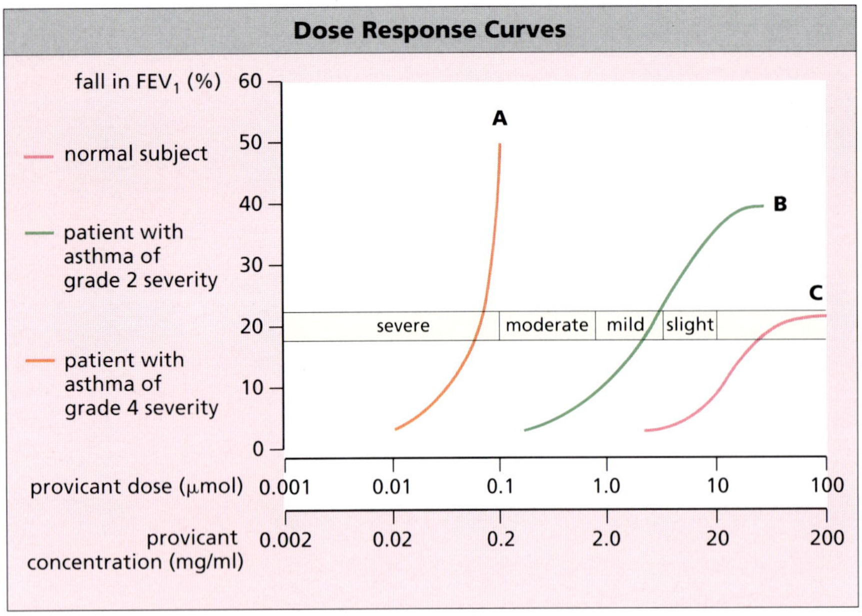

Fig. 14.5 Typical dose response curves from tests of bronchial responsiveness, showing the percentage fall in FEV_1 plotted against the amount of provicant which causes that fall. Either histamine or methacholine could be used as the provicant.

(1) Normal people, i.e. those without airways disease, have dose response curves which are well to the right and always have a plateau (subject C in Fig. 14.5).

(2) Patients with established, persistent asthma have dose response curves which are shifted to the left and do not have a plateau. Their position correlates, to some extent, with the amount of therapy needed to control symptoms (eg subject A in Fig. 14.5).

(3) In patients with chronic airflow limitation, the position of the curve is related to the degree of underlying airway obstruction as measured by the FEV_1. The curves to methacholine usually have a plateau.

(4) Some patients with classical symptoms of asthma have normal dose response curves.

(5) Some people with normal FEV_1 values and no symptoms of asthma have dose response curves shifted to the left. Curve B in Fig. 14.5 could be from a mild asthmatic or from someone without symptoms.

In patients with symptoms of asthma, obtaining a dose response curve, particularly with methacholine, gives useful information because it seems likely that thickening of the airway walls causes the shift and also the loss of the plateau. Thus a normal curve implies no wall thickening and suggests complete resolution of airway inflammation between attacks. People with normal curves between attacks usually do not respond to non-specific challenges such as exercise, hyperventilation, osmotic changes and sulphur dioxide. A large shift to the left with a steep curve suggests that, in addition to wall thickening, the bronchial smooth muscle has altered contractility. The nature of this alteration is unknown.

Increased sensitivity of the airways to histamine or methacholine in the absence of symptoms is commonly found in epidemiological studies of children. There are several likely explanations for this common observation. Firstly, in everyday life the airways may not be narrowing sufficiently (i.e. the dose response curve has a plateau) to cause symptoms. Secondly there may be narrowing but this is poorly perceived by the subject. Thirdly, the mediator-releasing cells are normal and do not suddenly release large amounts of constrictor mediators. Fourthly, the narrowing is occurring in the small

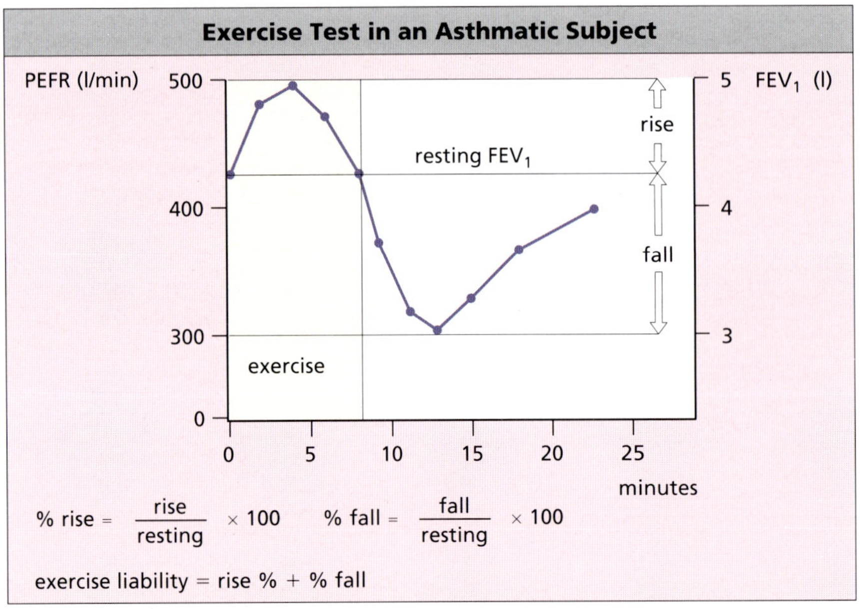

Fig. 14.6 A typical asthmatic response to an exercise test, showing an initial rise in FEV_1, caused by bronchodilatation, followed by a fall in FEV_1, caused by bronchoconstriction.

rather than in the large airways. It is clear that a shift of the dose response curve to the left cannot be used to make a diagnosis of asthma.

The main reasons for testing for increased bronchial responsiveness are:

(1) To help determine the severity of the disease, especially if PEFR variability and symptoms are discrepant.
(2) To define the position and shape of the curve. These factors are useful for determining those likely to be at risk from a life-threatening attack.
(3) To exclude a serious abnormality in someone with symptoms and normal lung function.
(4) To chart progress of treatment and to educate and encourage the patient.

Other useful tests

(1) Response to exercise. This requires a standard procedure as shown in Fig. 14.6 and may be more readily available than challenge tests with histamine or methacholine. A fall of 15 per cent or more in the FEV_1 is diagnositic of asthma but a negative result does not exclude the diagnosis. The typical response shown in Fig. 14.6 is one of bronchodilatation followed by bronchoconstriction. It is essential that the exercise has been sufficient to increase the ventilation to 80 per cent of maximum. A good guide to this is running or cycling until the heart rate is more than 80 per cent of the predicted maximum. Breathing of warm moist air during the exercise will diminish or abolish the response.
(2) The response to inhaled suphur dioxide, more easily documented than the response to inhaled metabisulphite, is emerging as a useful test to distinguish patients with asthma from those with chronic airflow limitation, and from normal subjects. All asthmatics appear to respond to this stimulus, although the response is not cumulative as with histamine and methacholine and may not involve release of mediators.
(3) Lung Function. Measurement of the diffusing capacity is helpful when the lung function remains abnormal after treatment. A normal or high value makes asthma a more likely cause of the problem than smoking-related lung disease. Measurement of the lung volumes is useful to determine the severity of hyperinflation but abnormal values are not diagnostic of asthma.

Important alternative diagnoses

Fig. 14.7 shows how different diagnostic labels may overlap with asthma, and gives an example of a patient from each of these groups to illustrate specific diagnostic problems. In all of these examples, the diagnosis will become clear with time and sometimes two conditions will be present and each will require treatment.

It is extremely uncommon for patients with allergic angiitis, the Churg–Strauss syndrome or eosinophilic pneumonia to present as asthma, even though these conditions are commonly mentioned in textbooks as diagnostic problems.

Differential Diagnosis of Asthma

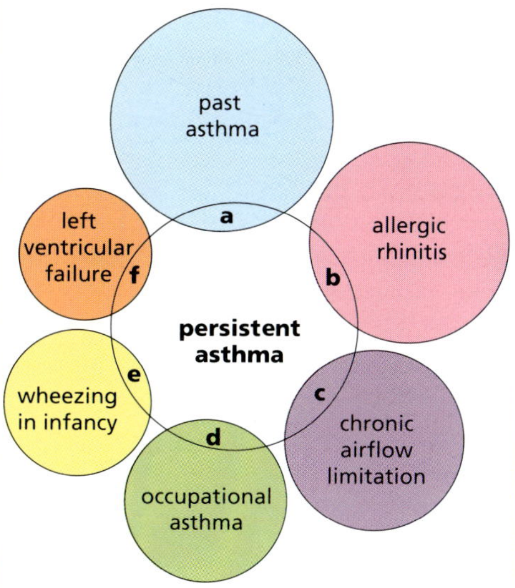

a	Presentation	An adult presenting with an isolated attack of wheezing and the history strongly suggests asthma in the past.
	Question	Is this patient in the process of developing persistent asthma of adult life?
b	Presentation	Patient with allergic rhinitis during the pollen season complains of chest tightness and wheeze but the lung function and variability of PEFR are normal.
	Question	Are the symptoms caused by airway narrowing?
c	Presentation	A heavy smoker with abnormal lung function develops symptoms of wheezing in adult life.
	Question	Is this chronic airflow limitation alone or has the patient now developed asthma?
d	Presentation	A patient presents with asthma symptoms at night or after exposure to known sensitizing agents; he refuses to leave that environment and symptoms become more frequent and induced by known triggers such as exercise.
	Question	Does he have occupational or classical persistent asthma?
e	Presentation	A one-year old has had two attacks of wheezing associated with respiratory infections in the last three months.
	Question	Is this wheezy bronchitis of infancy that will disappear by the age of five or are these the first attacks of asthma?
f	Presentation	A 70-year old lady with a history of rheumatic heart disease presents with an attack of breathlessness in the middle of the night during a flu epidemic.
	Question	Is this left ventricular failure or the onset of asthma in old age?

Fig. 14.7 [Left]. Diagram illustrating common problems in diagnosing asthma. The size of the circles indicates the relative frequency with which these diagnostic problems arise. [right]. An example of a patient from each of the groups a–f, to illustrate specific diagnostic problems.

Management of Asthma

Aims
To establish a management plan that reduces the severity, and thus the associated risks, of asthma in each individual. Where possible, the disease should be reversed.

The risks are discussed below. In planning management, it is important to know the risks to the individual asthmatic patient.

Risks
(1) Death from an acute attack. This is difficult to predict. Theoretically any patient in Groups 2–4 in Fig. 14.1 is at risk from death but the risk is significantly higher in Group 4. Also, a steep dose response curve, (A in Fig. 14.5) implies that the airways are able to narrow easily and to an excessive degree.
(2) Disability due to abnormal lung function or constant attacks. This is most frequent in group 4 but also occurs in group 3. The group of patients most at risk for developing abnormal lung function has not been well documented.
(3) Complications of drug therapy, especially of corticosteroids.
(4) Altered lifestlye. This may appear to be the least important of the long-term risks but it is the problem than most concerns that patient.

Asthma Management Plan
Step 1. Find the 'best' or 'target' lung function
Step 2. Assess severity of the asthma (not during an attack)
Step 3. Maintain best lung function with prescribed drugs
Step 4. Introduce regular home monitoring of PEFR
Step 5. Reduce trigger and aggravating factors
Step 6. Write an action plan for exacerbations.
Step 7. Educate the patient and family
Step 8. Review regularly

Fig. 14.8 Outline of an asthma management plan.

Management Plan
The steps are outlined in Fig. 14.8.

Step 1. Achieve 'best' or 'target' lung function

If the lung function is abnormal at the time of the first assessment or if there is large response to bronchodilator, the patient should be treated for 10 days with high doses of oral corticosteroids as well as an inhaled bronchodilator. The 'best' value is then recorded and becomes the 'target'. If maintaining the 'best' value involves using excessively large amounts of systemic corticosteroids, then the 'target' may be set at a slightly lower value than the 'best'. The 'target' is the value to be reached each day if possible.

Step 2. Assess the severity

Fig. 14.9 shows a scoring system that can be used to assess the severity of the disease in individual patients. The information can be obtained in about one to two weeks and can also be used for diagnosis. Severity cannot be assessed at the first visit as the variability of the PEFR is required. This should not be assessed during an exacerbation of disease.

In patients with abnormal lung function, oral corticosteroids can be prescribed along with regular doses of inhaled bronchodilator while the PEFR values are recorded for a 10 day period.

Step 3. Prescribe therapy to keep the PEFR value close the 'target'.

Fig. 14.10 suggests the most appropriate drugs for patients with asthma of differing severity.
Inhaled corticosteroids are essential if the symptoms and PEFR variability cannot be controlled with sodium cromoglycate, and are probably needed for all patients with severe disease, but the doses suggested are largely empirical. Long-term trials, to determine the most appropriate doses based on severity, have yet to be undertaken.
Sodium cromoglycate prevents the worsening of bronchial hyperresponsiveness during the pollen season and prevents both early and late asthmatic reactions. It has a dose related protective effect

Asthma Severity Score*

Symptoms	Score	Bronchodilator use	Score	PEFR variability**	Score
waking at night with wheeze/cough/choking	4	>4 × day	4	>50%	4
daily symptoms	3	3–4 × day	3	30–50%	3
symptoms more than 3 days/weeks	2	1–2 × day	2	15–30%	2
symptoms rare or only on exercise	1	not every day	1	10–15%	1
no symptoms	0	never	0	<10%	0

* over the previous three months
** see text

Fig. 14.9 Guildelines for the assessment of asthma severity.

Treatment of Asthma According to Severity Score							
P	Score	Inhaled corticosteroids (μg/day)	Sodium cromglycate	Bronchodilator (β agonist)	Oral corticosteroids	Iprotropium bromide	Theophylline
1	1–3	not necessary	during pollen season	a) if symptoms b) before known triggers	not necessary	not necessary	not necessary
2	4–5	a) if PEFRvar >20% b) if Sodium Cromoglycate ineffective	a) children b) before known triggers including exercise	a) if PEFR <80% b) symptoms	rarely for severe attacks	not necessary	not necessary
3	6–8	yes a) ⩾800 until PEFR stable b) 400-800 as maintenance	a) worth a trial if atopic b) needs frequent and high doses	twice daily and as required if symptomatic	only for acute attacks (PEFR <70% best)	not necessary	occasionally helps
4	9–12	yes a) >1500 until PEFR stable b) 800-1500 as maintenance	helpful in some patients	twice daily and if symptomatic	may need low dose continuously	a) if smoker b) chronic bronchitis c) β-agonist side effects	may benefit especially if on oral corticosteroids

Fig. 14.10 Guildelines for treatment of asthma according to severity score, as calculated from Fig. 14.9.

against exercise induced asthma. It controls asthma in many children and is a useful adjunct to inhaled steroids for controlling symptoms in many adults. It needs to be given in adequate dosage and frequency (four times a day) to be fully effective.

Bronchodilator aerosols available at present probably have no anti-inflammatory action. They are needed to control symptoms and to both prevent or reverse episodes of airway narrowing. When the PEFR is less than 80 per cent of the 'target', it seems logical to inhale a bronchodilator before inhaling steroids or sodium cromoglycate to improve distribution in the lungs.

Fig. 14.11 shows the relative anti-asthma and anti-trigger effects of the commonly used asthma medications. It is clear that to treat asthma and to prevent attacks a combination of drugs is necessary.

Step 4. Home monitoring and tight control

It is not sufficient to assess the severity and prescribe the appropriate drugs. It is necessary to keep the patient well, with PEFR values close to the 'target'. This can only be done by home monitoring – there is no alternative if the aims outlined above are to be achieved.

Step 5. Treatment of exacerbations

Each patient within the management plan must have a written plan of how to deal with exacerbations. (See Fig. 14.12 which shows such an example.) If the PEFR does not reach 80 per cent of the 'target' over a period of 24 or sometimes 12 hours, more treatment is needed. Usually instructions are given to introduce

Properties of Some of the Drugs Commonly Used to Treat Asthma							
Drug	Reduces severity	Broncho-dilates	Protects against				Frequency of doses (daily)
			Exercise	Early asthmatic response	Late asthmatic response	Sulphur dioxide	
inhaled corticosteroids	++++	–	+	–	+++	?	twice
oral corticosteroids	++	–	–	–	+++	?	once
sodium cromoglycate	+	–	+++	+++	+++	+++	four
bronchodilator	–	++++	++++	++++	–	+++	varies
ipratopium bromide	–	+++	++ or –	–	–	±	varies
theophylline	–	+++	±	–	+	?	twice

Fig. 14.11 Properties of drugs commonly used for asthma treatment, indicating their relative efficiency either at reducing the severity of asthma , or preventing attacks induced by common triggers. Ipratropium bromide protects in some people to some extent whereas the inhaled β-agonist bronchodilators protect in virtually all patients.

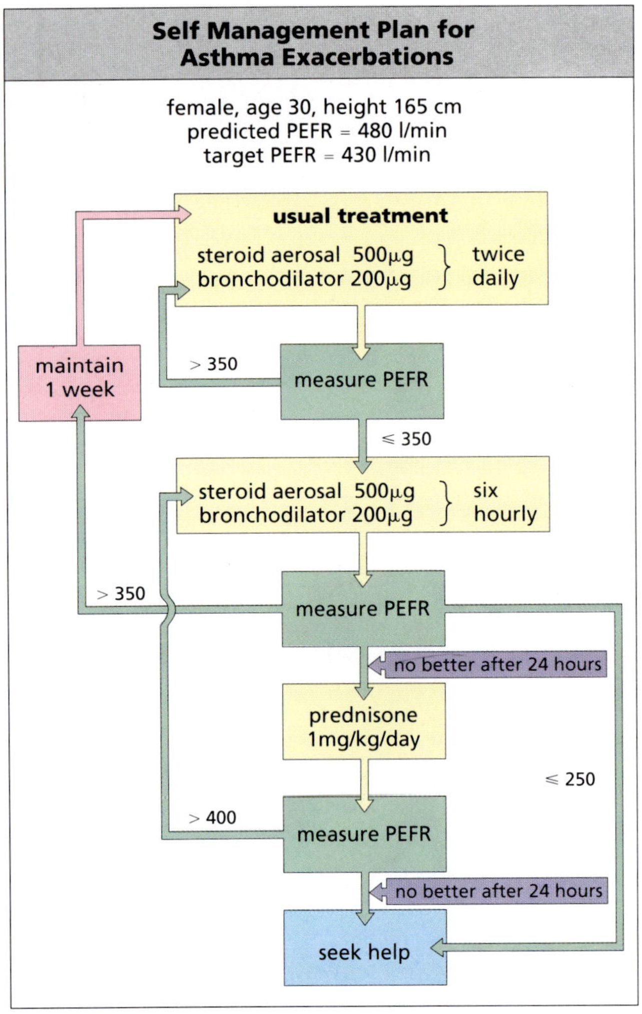

Fig. 14.12 Self management plan for exacerbations. This is an example taken from the patient whose data are shown in Figs. 14.3 and 14.4. The value for PEFR at which drugs are changed and the length of time the higher doses are needed will vary between patients, and is arrived at by trial and error.

or increase the dose of inhaled steroids. If the PEFR is less than 70 per cent of the 'target' then oral steroids are usually needed. Experience shows that a few high doses (0.8mg/kg/day) are more effective than low doses over many days. Some patients need a low maintenance dose of oral steroids. These patients should also be given a trial of theophylline.

If the patient is outside the management plan, or if the plan described above fails then emergency treatment at a clinic or hospital is necessary.

The action which should be taken here is described in Fig. 14.13

Step 6. Triggers and aggravating factors

Fig. 14.14 lists the important trigger and aggravating factors. It is obviously not sensible to administer high doses of inhaled corticosteroids when an allergic or sensitized subject continues to be exposed to an inhalant that can be removed. This applies to occupational agents, house dust mites, cockroaches and animals. Evidence for these allergens playing a role in the severity of the asthma in an individual comes from the history, from skin tests, from specific IgE measurements, and sometimes from specific challenge tests. Practical methods to measure and to reduce aero-allergens in the home are not yet well developed. It is likely that techniques for monitoring allergens in the home will become part of the management of asthma, especially of young children. Nevertheless, once the allergens are identified, they should be removed as far as possible from the home environment.

The aggravating factors for which there is evidence of an effect on asthma severity are bronchopulmonary aspergillosis, gastric reflux, rhinitis, and severe snoring. All of these conditions can be treated with specific measures. Treatment of these conditions often has a considerable effect of the overall severity of asthma as well as improving the well-being of the patient.

Emergency Treatment of Asthma
Immediate
a. Given oxygen until severity of the attack can be assessed. b. Measure FEV_1 or PEFR and the blood gas tensions. c. Give β-agonists (with or without ipratropium bromide) via nebuliser at frequent intervals. d. Give systemic corticosteroids in appropriate dose. e. Continue to monitor until improved.
Longer term
a. Monitor every few hours with PEFR and/or arterial blood gas tensions. b. Introduce high dose aerosol steroids. c. Reduce the systemic steroids - rapidly if the onset of the exacerbation was rapid. d. Maintain intensive therapy until 'best' PEFR achieved. e. Introduce a long-term management plan.

Fig. 14.13 Outline of the immediate and the longer term emergency treatment of asthma.

Triggers of Asthma Attacks	
Triggers that make asthma worse	
allergens	pollen, house dust, animal proteins, moulds
viral Infections	Rhinovirus, respiratory syncitial virus
occupational sensitizers	isocyanates, plicatic acid, platinum salts
Triggers that cause attacks but no worsening of the disease	
osmotic Stimuli	exercise, hyperventilation
acid Irritants	metabisulphite, sulphur dioxide
psychomotor	emotional upsets, psychosuggestion
non-specific irritants	tobacco smoke, bad smells

Fig. 14.14 Some of the important triggers of asthma attacks.

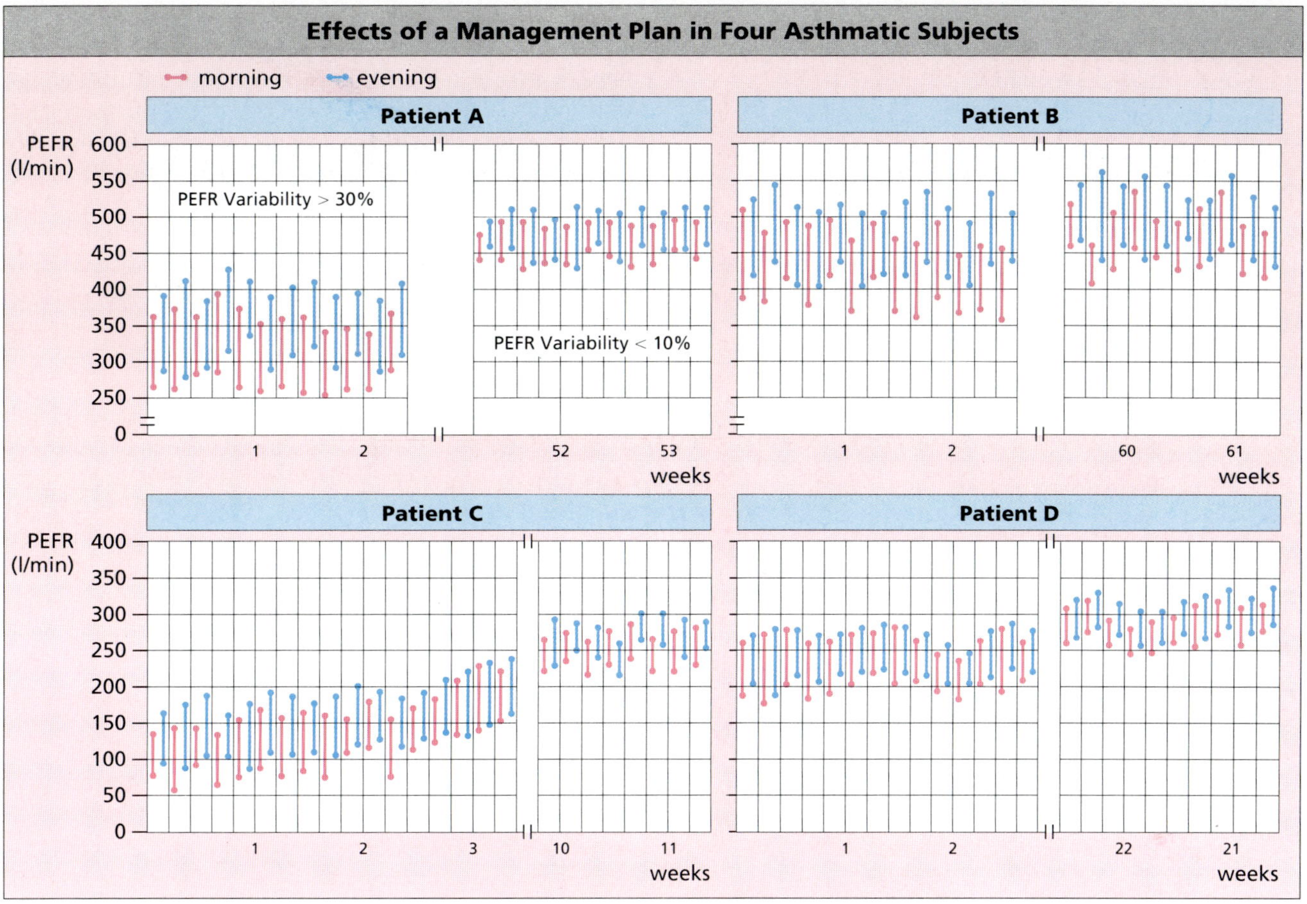

Fig. 14.15 Peak flow charts, before and after use of an asthma management plan in 4 patients. The details are explained in the text.

Step 7. Educate

This treatment plan will only work if the patient and the family understands the nature of the disease, the trigger factors, how each of the drugs that are prescribed work and their side effects.

Step 8. Review regularly

Management and education must be continued indefinitely. An essential part of the plan involves explaining that those with persistent asthma have a disease that is not just going to 'go away'. The chronic nature of this disease is not appreciated by patients or doctors in most countries.

Problems

- Patient acceptance of the disease and the management plan. This usually takes time and, in many patients, great persistence is needed to achieve a full understanding of the disease and the plan. However, most patients do comply once they understand that the disease is not just going to 'disappear'. There are, however, a large group who fail to acknowledge the problem and drift from attack to attack and from doctor to doctor.
- Refractory disease. Some patients who have severe disease respond only to unacceptably high doses of corticosteroids. This is a continuing problem for all physicians. However, if the management plan is used carefully, and with proper doses of inhaled corticosteroids and intermittent doses of oral steroids, these patients constitute a small group. The usefulness of methotrexate and other steroid-sparing drugs such as cyclosporin A is still being evaluated.
- Side effects of drugs. This applies especially to corticosteroids. Some patients get excessive shakiness from the β-adrenoceptor agonists. The side effects of theophylline can be avoided by simply not using it, or taking great care to use the appropriate dose in those who do require it as a steroid-sparing drug.
- Long-term compliance. It is common for patients to abandon the plan of management once symptoms are controlled. Usually the symptoms recur and the plan must be restarted.

Likely Outcomes of Management Plans

Fig. 14.15 illustrates the outcome of the management plan outlined above in four patients of different ages and severities, based on PEFR readings. Patients A and B are from Group 3 as defined in Fig. 14.1. Patient A is the patient whose data are shown in Figs 14.3 and 14.4 and in whom good control was achieved after one year of therapy. Patient B had severe asthma which was not completely controlled after more than a year or treatment. Patient C is a child presenting with under-treated asthma and abnormal lung function. As with most children, improvement occurred within a few weeks. Patient D is a Grade 4 patient whose disease showed little or no response to high-dose inhaled steroids.

Outcomes of Asthma

Long-term Outcomes in Children

Longitudinal studies of children in Western societies show that asthma commonly begins before the age of two and increases in prevalence up to the age of nine or 10 when it begins to decrease. In most populations of children it is more common and more severe in boys, but this sex difference is not present in teenage and adult life. Factors associated with an increased risk of childhood asthma are atopy, a history of early respiratory illness, and parental smoking. Furthermore, the occurrence of frequent wheezing episodes in early childhood is often associated with persisting lung function abnormalities later in childhood.

Figure 14.16 is derived from the data of Kelly *et al.*, showing the long term outcome of asthma of varying

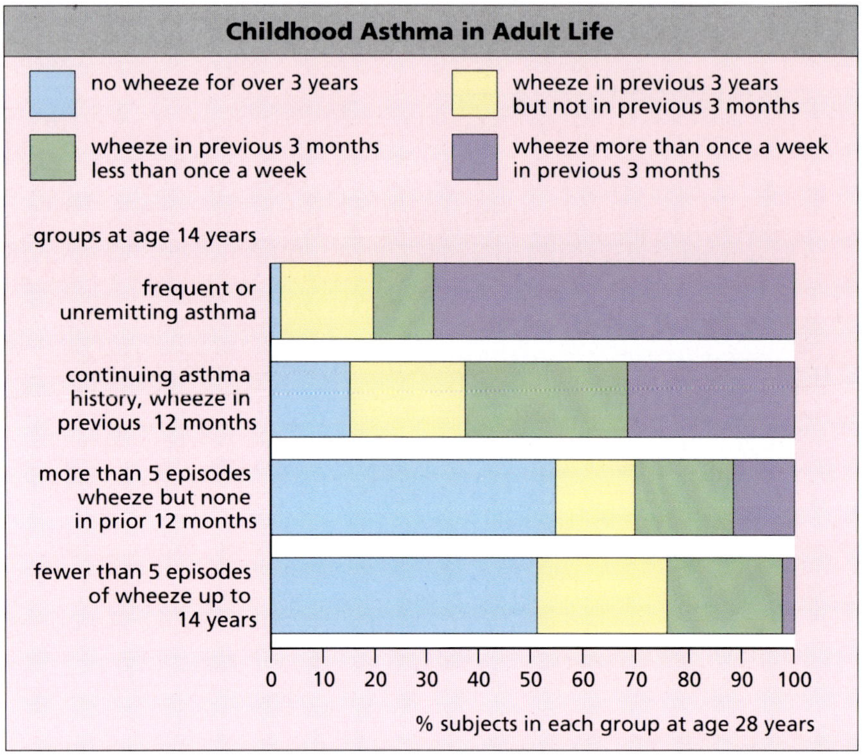

Fig. 14.16 The proportion of subjects with symptoms at the age of 28 in relation to their symptoms at the age of 14 years. Diagram redrawn from the data of Kelly, WJ, Hudson I, Phelan PD, Main MCF, Olindi A, *Br Med J* 1987; **294**; 1059–1062 .

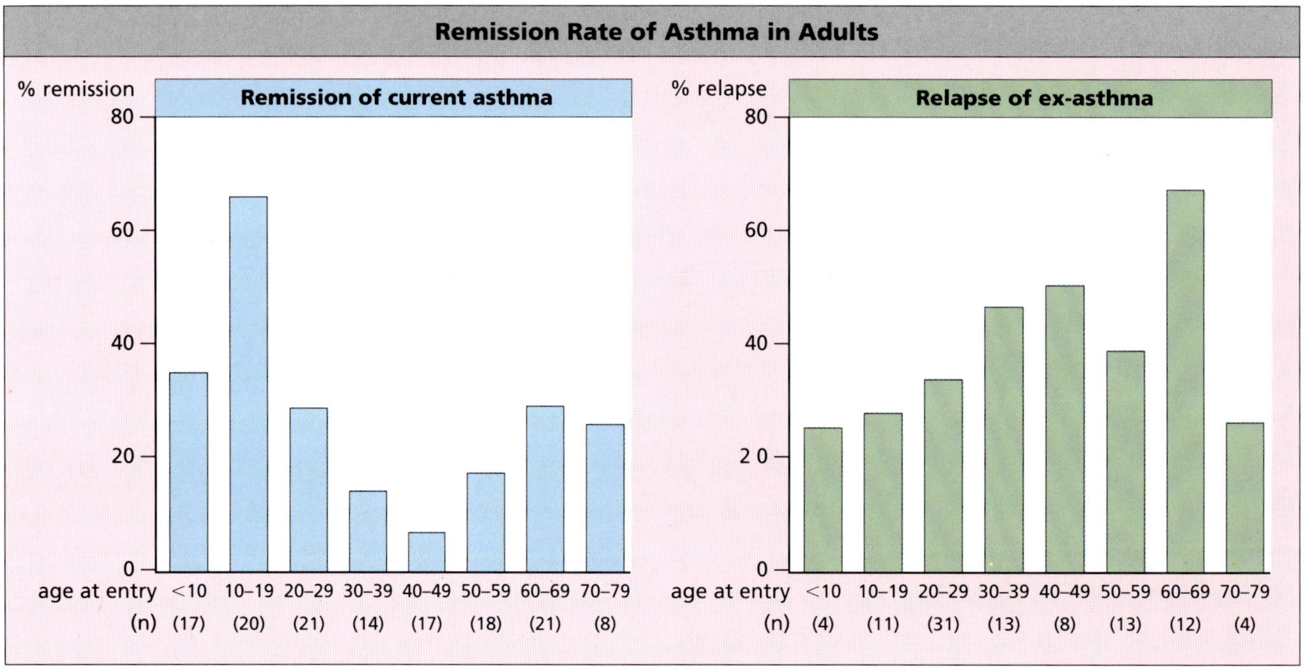

Fig. 14.17 These data show that relapses are common and remittance uncommon in adult Americans living in Tuscon. Diagram based on data of Bronniman and Burrows.

severity in children assessed from age seven years up to the age of 28 years. By the age of 14 years, over half of those who had not wheezed in the previous year were asymptomatic and had normal lung function. At 28 years, of those with a continuing asthma history at 14, only 10 per cent were asymptomatic. As might be expected, these subjects showed the greatest deterioration in lung function since childhood, and had the most severe bronchial hyperresponsiveness. Thus, moderate and severe childhood asthma is likely to continue into adult life.

Long-term Outcomes in Adults

Although there is a high rate of remission of asthma during adolescence, up to 60 per cent of those who become asymptomatic and 'grown out' of asthma have evidence of persisting bronchial hyperresponsiveness if provocation tests are performed. Not only is there a high rate of relapse of asthma in adults with histories of childhood wheezing, but in adults remission is uncommon. Fig. 14.17 illustrates data obtained by Bronniman and Burrows and shows the low remission rate of asthma in adult life. As in children, the probability of remission in adulthood is closely related to the severity of the disease. Remission is less likely in patients with frequent symptoms, lung function abnormalities, and coexisting smoking-related lung disease. The effect of smoking is graphically illustrated in Fig. 14.18 which shows the gradual decline of lung function, as measured by FEV_1, in a population survey in a small rural town in Australia. It should also be noted that patients with persistent asthma also have a more rapid decay in their lung function than normal subjects, and that the decrease is similar in magnitude to that found in smokers.

From the data shown in these last three figures, it is concluded that asthma is a serious disease associated with a number of long-term risks. These risks make it essential to have a scheme for each patient that includes objective assessment of asthma severity and the introduction of a management plan designed to reduce the severity and the accompanying risks.

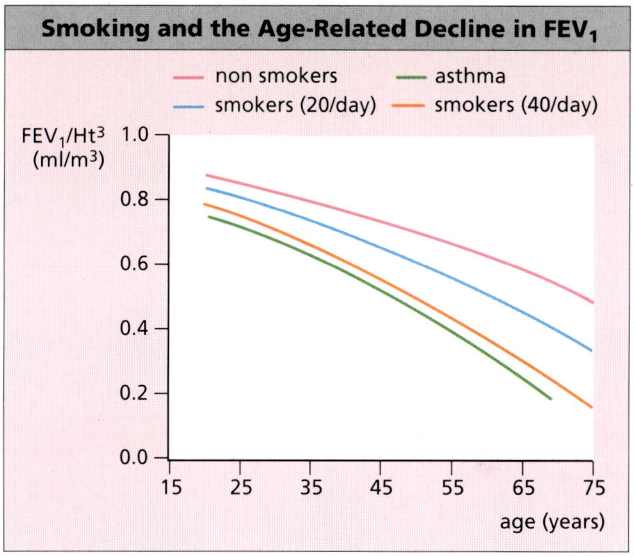

Fig. 14.18 Decline in the FEV_1 in asthmatic and smoking subjects living in Busselton, a rural town in Australia. The data were collected over a period of 20 years.

Further Reading

Anderson SD, Tessier P, Smith CM, Malo, JL. Exercise and hyperventilation provocation challenges. In: *Methods in Asthmology* Ed: Braga PC. New York: Review Press (in press).

Beaseley R, Cushley M, Holgate ST. A self management plan in the treatment of adult asthma. *Thorax* 1989; **44**:200–204.

Bronniman S, Burrows B. A prospective study of the natural history of asthma: remission and relapse rates. *J Allergy Clin Immunol* 1986; **90**:480–484

Burrows B. The natural history of asthma. *J Allergy Clin Immun* 1987; **80**:373–377.

Chan-Yeung M. Occupational asthma update. *Chest* 1988; 93:407–411

Cockcroft DW, Killian DM, Mellon JJA, Hargreave FE. Bronchial reactivity to inhaled histamine: a method and clinical survey. *Clin Allergy* 1977; **7**: 235–243

FitzGerald JM, Hargreave FE. The assessment and management of acute life-threatening asthma *Chest* 1989; **95**:888–894.

Kelly WJW, Hudson I, Raven J, Phelan PD, Pain MCF, Olinsky A. Childhood asthma and adult lung function. *Am Rev Respir Dis* 1988; **138**:26–30.

Kelly WJW, Hudson I, Phelan PD, Pain MCF, Olinsky A. Childhood asthma in adult life: a further study at 28 years of age. *Br Med J* 1987; **294**: 1059–1062.

McFadden ER (Clinical physiological correlates in asthma. *J Allergy Clin Immunol* 1986; **77**:1–5.

Sears MR, Beaglehole R. Asthma morbidity and mortality: New Zealand. *J Allergy Clin Immunol* 1987; **80**:383–388.

Toogood JH. High-dose inhaled steroid therapy for asthma. *J Allergy Clin Immunol* 1989; **83**:528–536

Weiss ST, Tager IB, Munoz A, Speizer FE The relationship of respiratory infection in childhood to the occurrence of increased levels of bronchial responsiveness and atopy. *Am Rev Respir Dis* 1985; **131**:573–578.

Woolcock AJ, Yan K, Salome CM The effect of therapy on bronchial hyperresponsiveness in the long term management of asthma. *Clin Allergy* 1989; **18**:165–176.

Woolcock AJ, Rubinfeld AR, Seale JP, Landau LL, Antic R, Mitchell C, Rea HH, Zimmerman P. Thoracic Society of Australia and New Zealand: asthma management plan, 1989. *Med J Aust* 1989; **151**:650–653.

Chapter 15

Drugs in Asthma Treatment

Introduction

Asthma is a complex disease in which episodic exacerbations or attacks are superimposed on a chronic inflammatory condition in the lung. The armamentarium of drugs used to treat the disease is therefore diverse, since it is aimed at various components of the disease. Furthermore, the development of drugs from a historical standpoint has been somewhat empirical as it is only recently that a true understanding of the mechanisms of the disease is beginning to emerge. In this chapter, an attempt has been made to classify anti-asthma drugs into those which are aimed primarily at the relief of symptoms and those which are primarily anti-inflammatory. Several drugs do not fall satisfactorily into either of these categories as they share aspects of both. This has necessitated the use of a further category of drugs which provide relief from immediate symptoms and yet appear also to influence the underlying inflammation.

Symptom-Relieving Drugs

β-Adrenoceptor Stimulants

The use of adrenaline in the relief of asthma symptoms or as a life-saving drug in systemic anaphylaxis has been established for almost 90 years. In the latter use, the ability of adrenaline to stimulate both α- and β-receptors, as illustrated in Fig. 15.1, contributes to its beneficial effects. Of particular note are its bronchodilator properties, its capacity to inhibit mast cell mediator secretion and its restoration of a satisfactory circulation by its action on the heart, blood vessels and renin-angiotensin system. However, in the treatment of bronchial asthma, many of these effects are not desired, with the cardiovascular effects – particularly stimulation of cardiac arrhythmias – being of particular concern. Many of those problems have now been overcome by chemical modifications of the adrenaline molecule and by developing preparations with a satisfactory pharmacokinetic profile when administered to the lung by inhalation.

The first clue that chemical modification of adrenaline may modify its receptor selectivity came in 1941 when the terminal methyl group on the side chain was replaced by an isopropyl group (Fig. 15.2).

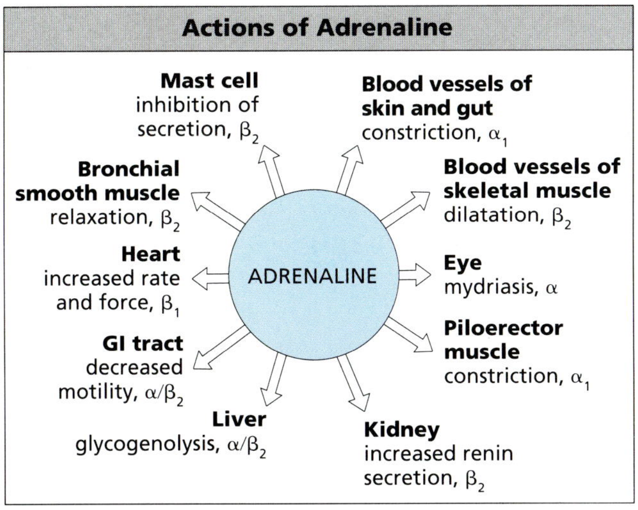

Fig. 15.1 Actions of adrenaline.

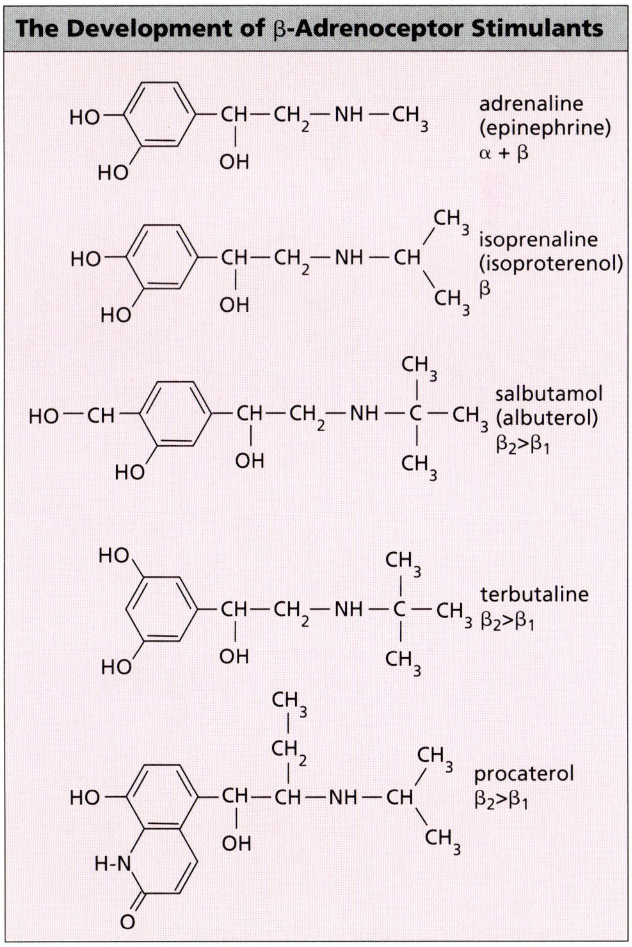

Fig. 15.2 Chemical development of β-adrenoceptor agonists.

This manipulation, which increased the bulk of the side chain, produced isoprenaline, a drug which acts almost exclusively at β-receptors. Further increases in the bulk of this substituent have produced drugs which, although having decreased absolute potency, have a degree of selectivity for β_2-receptors over β_1-receptors. Examples of such drugs are shown in Fig. 15.2. It should be emphasized, however, that such chemical manoeuvres do not confer an absolute specificity for β_2-receptors but only a selectivity, thus with high systemic concentrations β_1-receptor mediated effects on the heart may become apparent.

A second objective of chemical manipulation has been to increase the duration of action of sympathomimetic bronchodilators. Adrenaline is rapidly inactivated by two enzymatic process, monoamine oxidase (MAO) in neuronal tissue and catechol-O-methyl transferase (COMT) in extraneuronal tissues. Besides conferring β-receptor selectivity, increasing the bulk of the side chain also precludes neuronal uptake of the drugs, thus preventing its access to MAO. To prevent metabolism by COMT, drugs have been synthesized in which the native catechol group has been substituted or removed (see Fig. 15.2). Metabolism of these drugs occurs in the liver.

Chemical modifications, such as those described above, have extended the duration of action of β-stimulants to 4–5 hours when given by inhalation and 4–8 hours when given orally. More recently further chemical modification has extended the duration of action of inhaled bronchodilators to 8–12 hours with formoterol and to more than 12 hours with salmeterol.

Action

More is known about the biochemical mechanism of action of β-adrenoceptor stimulants than probably any other of the drugs used in the treatment of allergic diseases. These are summarized in Fig. 15.3. Briefly, binding of a β-stimulant to the receptor unit initiates the binding of guanosine triphosphate (GTP) to the α_s sub-unit of the regulatory G-protein leading to its dissociation from the G-protein complex. This sub-unit then complexes with adenylate cyclase (AC), the catalytic unit of the complex, activating it to generate cyclic AMP from ATP. Cyclic AMP then acts as a second or intracellular messenger to activate a series of cyclic AMP-dependent protein kinases (cAMP dPK) which phosphorylate a number of proteins crucial to many intracellular biochemical events.

By these mechanisms, β-stimulants are potent relaxers of bronchial smooth muscle, from which the term bronchodilator is derived. As this is a direct action, β-agonists are able to relax bronchial smooth muscle regardless of the contractile stimulus, thus giving rise to the term functional antagonists. Similarly, β-adrenoceptor stimulants prevent the activation of mast cells, but not basophils, to release histamine, tryptase and eicosanoids. In this respect, β-stimulants are considerably more effective than the archetypal mast cell stabilizer, sodium cromoglycate. As the highest concentration of β-receptors in the lung is found on the luminal aspect of bronchial epithelial cells, it is postulated that β-agonists stimulate these cells to release their bronchorelaxant factors.

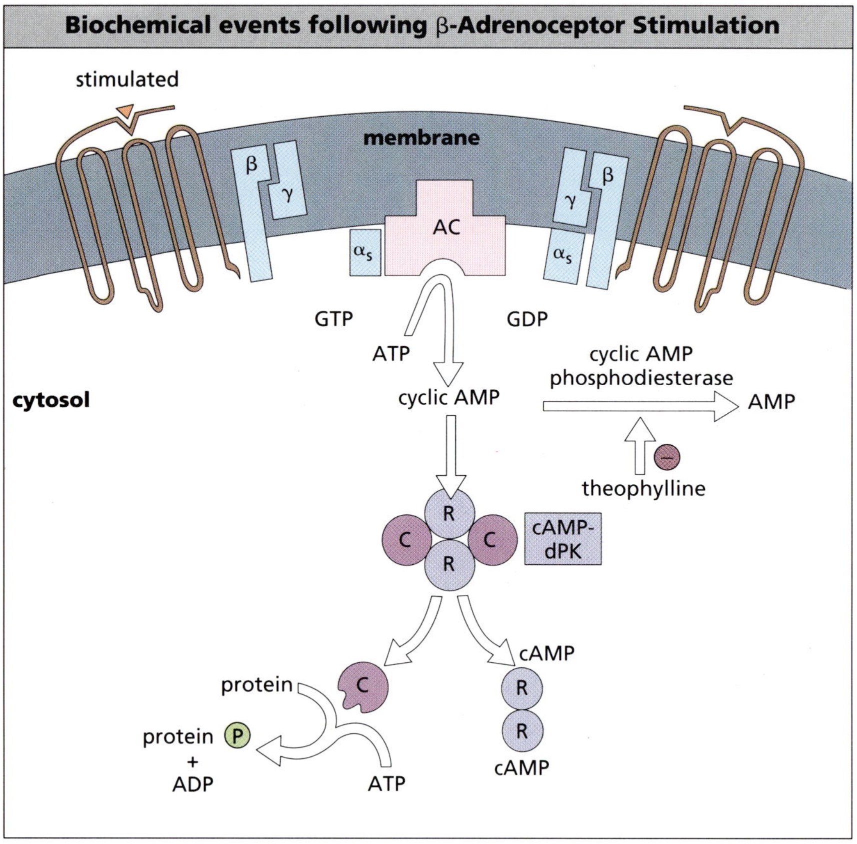

Fig. 15.3 Activation of adenylate cyclase and protein kinases. The diagram shows two β-adrenoceptor molecules, each of which is composed of three transmembrane loops. Stimulation of the receptor (left) causes its activation in which the α_s unit of the heterotrimeric G_s protein binds GTP and dissociates from the complex to the adenylate cyclase catalytic unit (AC). Activated AC catalyses the formation of cyclic AMP (cAMP) which binds to the regulatory units (R) of cAMP-dependent protein kinases (cAMP dPK), thus freeing the catalytic units (C) to phosphorylate specific proteins. The activated state exists only transiently, ATP hydrolysis to ADP leading to reassociation of the $\alpha_s\beta\gamma$-complex of G_s, inactivation of AC, receptor regeneration and the breakdown of AMP by phosphodiesterases.

All of these events contribute to the effectiveness of β-stimulants as inhibitors of the early asthmatic response, indicative of their ability to provide symptomatic relief in asthma. As such they are the first-line treatment used on an 'as required' basis for the reversal of acute asthmatic attacks. Recently much debate has raged about the suitability of β-stimulants to suppress the long-term bronchial inflammation associated with asthma. The consensus of opinion at present is that they are not suitable. Indeed two recent studies in which β-stimulants were given on a regular basis, have shown a small deterioration rather than an improvement in objective parameters of airways function over a prolonged period. For this reason, it is advisable to treat the inflammatory aspects of the disease with an anti-inflammatory agent, such as an inhaled corticosteroid, while providing β-stimulants for their bronchodilator actions on an 'as required' basis during periods of enhanced bronchoconstriction.

Administration

The choice of the most appropriate route of administration is of paramount importance with β-stimulants as it is with all anti-asthma drugs. In all but the severest asthma, inhalation of an aerosol provides an effective topical treatment by delivering the drug directly to the luminal surface of the bronchus where it can act on superficial mast cells and gain ready access to the bronchial smooth muscle. Onset is rapid, within 5–15 minutes, a vital factor when trying to reverse a developing or established bronchoconstriction. With the older bronchodilators, the duration of action of 4–6 hours proved to be a drawback in that it was not long enough to allow the nocturnal asthmatic a full night's sleep. This problem has now been overcome with the newer long acting drugs which can be given on a twice daily basis. The major drawbacks to inhalation therapy are problems of poor administration techniques by the patients, particularly young children and geriatric patients, and poor penetration into the airways of patients with severe obstruction. Systemic side effects of β-adrenoceptor therapy are usually minimal with inhaled drugs, but may become a problem with overusage, a point which must be stressed to the patient. These include:

- skeletal muscle tremor to which tolerance develops;
- hyperglycaemia in diabetes;
- cardiovascular effects, cardiac arrhythmias acutely and a possibility of myocardial ischaemia in the long term.

β-Adrenoceptor stimulants may also be given orally, although the use of this route is declining with the introduction of long-acting inhaled agents. Oral administration may be advantageous when patients cannot use an inhaler effectively or when prolonged duration of action is required. The obvious disadvantages are the unwanted systemic effects. Parenteral administration is usually reserved for acute severe asthma (status asthmaticus) where it may have life-saving potential when used in conjunction with other appropriate supportive therapy.

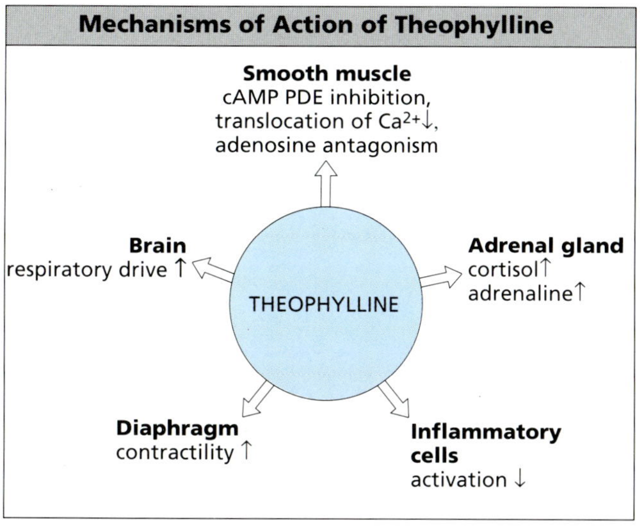

Fig. 15.4 Proposed mechanisms of action of theophylline.

Methylxanthines

Methylxanthines, in the form of coffee and extracts from the tea plant, have been used for the treatment of bronchial asthma for almost 700 years. Today the predominant methylxanthine in clinical use is theophylline, given either as the native drug, as its water-soluble ethylene diamine salt, aminophylline, or as a long-acting conjugate such as choline theophyllinate. The use of these drugs is somewhat enigmatic: they are the drug of choice in North America and some parts of continental Europe, while rarely used in the UK and Australasia.

Action

The precise mechanism by which theophylline acts as an anti-asthma drug is still somewhat obscure. Clearly it has the potential to inhibit cyclic AMP phosphodiesterase (PDE), thus allowing it to elevate intracellular levels of cyclic AMP by preventing its breakdown (see Fig. 15.3). The theory for this mechanism of action in asthma has been based on biochemical and *in vitro* studies that use concentrations of theophylline which would be toxic *in vivo*. Consequently a variety of alternative mechanisms have been proposed which are summarized in Fig. 15.4. However, the PDE inhibition theory has recently gained more credence from two lines of evidence. First is the observation that at therapeutic doses there is evidence in leucocytes *in vivo* of increased levels of cyclic AMP suggesting that even a small and subtle action on PDE at these concentrations may be sufficient to confer clinical activity. Second is the identification of PDE enzymes and the synthesis of specific inhibitors for them (Fig. 15.5). Of particular note is that bronchial smooth muscle and inflammatory cells, including mast cells, have type IV PDE. Initial studies with inhibitors of this isoenzyme indicate that they carry the beneficial actions of theophylline while being devoid of many of the side effects. Clearly this is a potential area of future drug development.

Cyclic Nucleotide Phosphodiesterase Enzymes		
Isoenzyme family	**Nucleotides hydrolysed (characteristics)**	**Selective inhibitors**
I	cAMP and cGMP (Ca^{2+} and calmodulin dependant)	vinpocetine
II	cAMP and cGMP (cAMP hydrolysis stimulated by cGMP)	no selective inhibitors
III	cAMP and cGMP (cAMP hydrolysis stimulated by cGMP)	milrinone pimobendan piroximone
IV	cAMP (no known regulator)	rolipram denbufylline
V	cGMP (multiple forms)	zaprinast dipyridamole

Fig. 15.5 Phosphodiesterase enzymes and their functions.

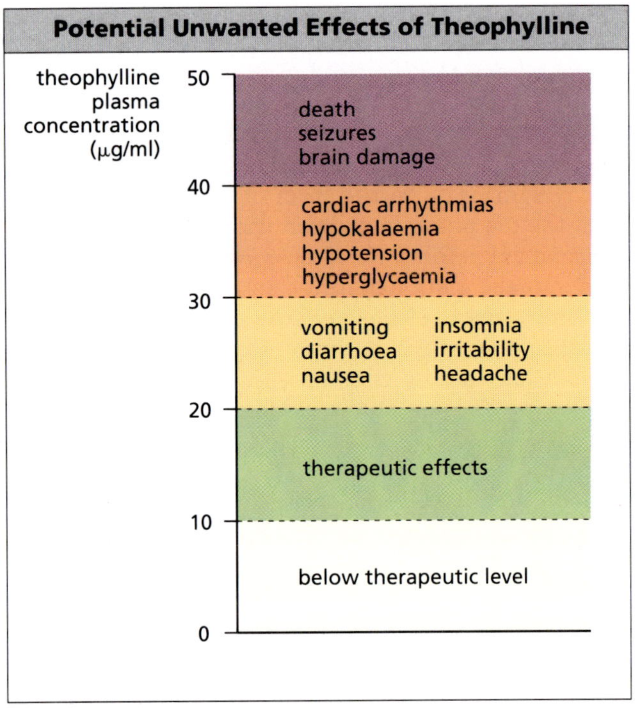

Fig. 15.6 Dose-related therapeutic and toxic effects of theophylline.

The major disadvantage with theophylline is its narrow therapeutic window (Fig. 15.6). The beneficial effects of the drug are observed only with plasma levels in the range of 10–20 μg/ml. Below 10μg/ml, the drug is comparatively ineffective and above 20 μg/ml toxic effects are observed which increase in number and in severity with increasing plasma concentrations. Because of this relationship, the prudent physician will regularly monitor serum theophylline levels and adjust the dose so that possible life-threatening toxicity is avoided.

Administration

Theophylline is only weakly active and of transient duration when given by inhalation and is, therefore, given routinely by oral administration. Rectal preparations of aminophylline are available and may well be suited for young children. Theophylline and aminophylline are rapidly and completely absorbed from the intestinal tract. Theophylline is metabolized in the liver with a half-life of approximately 6 hours in normal individuals. Because of this relatively short duration of action, many slow-release preparations have been formulated to extend its duration to 8–12 hours. However, care must be taken with such preparations, as large fluctuations in plasma concen-

Receptor-Mediated Effects of Histamine		
Target tissue	**Effect**	**Receptor**
Airways		
bronchial smooth muscle	contraction	H_1
bronchial epithelium	increased permeability	H_1
secretory glands	increased glycoprotein secretion	H_1, H_2
	secretion	H_1
	stimulation	
	cough receptors	
Blood vessels		
post-capillary venules	dilatation	H_1
	increased permeability	
Nerves		
sensory nerves	stimulation	H_1
central nervous system	neuroregulation	H_3
Nose	rhinorrhoea	H_1
	oedema	H_1
Leucocytes	increased proliferation	
	chemotaxis and activation	H_2

Fig. 15.7 Receptor-mediated effects of histamine.

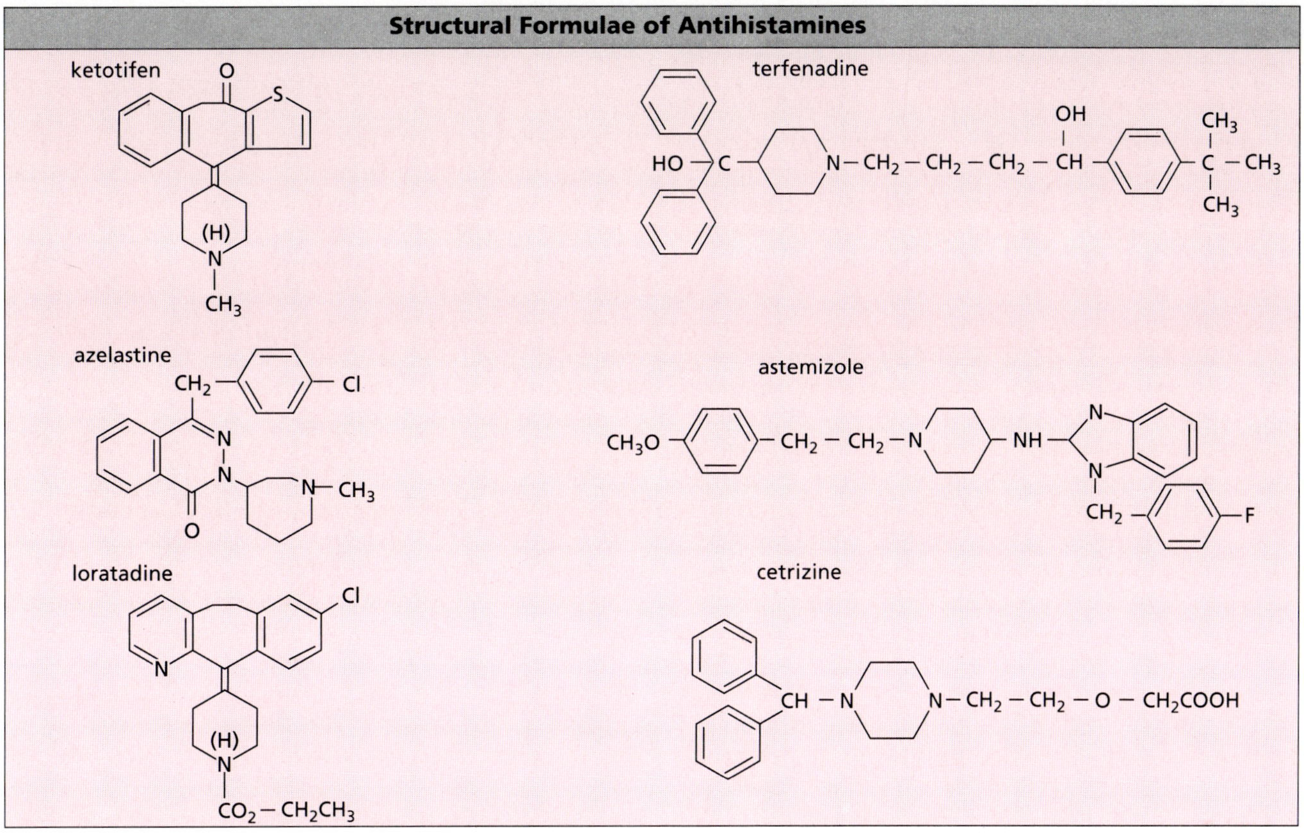

Fig. 15.8 Structural formulae of some antihistamines.

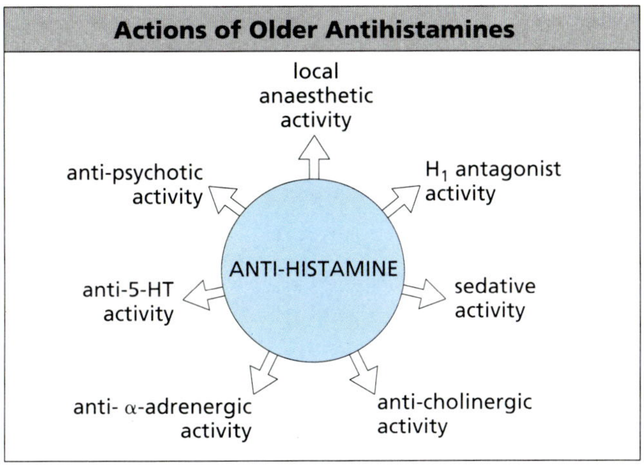

Fig. 15.9 Some unwanted effects of antihistamines.

trations may occur, bringing with them either lack of efficacy or potential toxicity. These problems may arise in two ways. Firstly, the presence of food in the gastrointestinal tract may lead to erratic absorption with changes in gastric emptying, so causing 'dumping' of enteric-coated preparations into the intestine. Secondly, other disease processes or the use of drugs may markedly alter the rate of metabolism of theophylline, the half-life being around 20 hours in hepatitis and 4 hours in heavy cigarette smokers. As a consequence, a conservative approach to therapy should be adopted, and the dose titrated to suit individual patients. In acute severe asthma, intravenous theophylline may be used by infusion, rather than by bolus injection, with a view to obtaining plasma levels within but not above the therapeutic range.

Histamine Receptor Antagonists

As histamine is one of the major mediators released from the mast cell in allergic reactions, prevention of its ability to stimulate target organs has presented an obvious goal in drug development. Over the last two decades it has become obvious that not all the actions of histamine are mediated by the same receptor but rather two, or even three, distinct receptors. Examples of organs stimulated by histamine and the subtype of histamine receptors mediating these effects are shown in Fig. 15.7.

Action

Two classes of histamine H_1-antagonists, the structures of some of which are shown in Fig. 15.8, are available on the market today. The older agents, including mepyramine, diphenhydramine, chlorpheniramine and ketotifen all penetrate well into the central nervous system (CNS) where they induce sedation. It is claimed, however, that tolerance rapidly develops to the sedative effects of ketotifen. Although this sedative effect may have some clinical benefit in the treatment of night-time asthma, especially in children, it severely compromises their use in ambulatory patients in whom doses capable of causing only a 3–5 fold shift of the histamine dose-response curve may be given. Then potential to enhance the central effects of alcohol and other CNS sedatives further limits their use. In addition to sedative properties, many of these drugs also have other unwanted actions, including an atropine-like effect blockade of α-adrenergic and 5-hydroxytryptamine receptors (Fig. 15.9).

Newer H_1-antagonists, including astemizole, terfenadine, cetirizine, mequitazine, loratadine and acrivastine are essentially free of CNS sedation at doses recommended for the treatment of rhinitis or urticaria. Furthermore, these drugs have little or no atropine-like activity or effects at other receptors. There is no evidence that H_2- or the newly developed H_3-receptor antagonists have therapeutic benefit in asthma.

Administration

All H_1-antagonists are well absorbed from the gastrointestinal tract after oral dosage. With most, symptomatic relief is observed within 15–30 minutes and peaks within 1 hour. Their extensive metabolism by the cytochrome P450 system of the liver also limits the duration of action to 3–6 hours. There are, however, some notable exceptions to this rule; mequitazine, loratadine and acrivastine have biological activity for 12–36 hours following a single dose. With astemizole, the maximum effect is not achieved until 16–18 hours after a single oral dose and activity can still be perceived for up to 21 days afterwards. The prolonged duration is due in part to the slow clearance of astemizole and in part to the exceptionally strong binding of the drug to the H_1-receptor.

Although ketotifen is widely used as an anti-asthmatic drug in Japan, the use of H_1-antagonists as first-line drugs for the treatment of asthma is questionable. Clearly these drugs may have a small (10–20 per cent) bronchodilator affect, especially when inhaled, and may reduce the bronchoconstrictor symptoms following acute provocation with allergen. However, to have a demonstrable benefit in clinical asthma, they have to be used at high doses when unwanted effects, including sedation, are again observed. As not all H_1-antagonists are equally effective in asthma, additional properties have been claimed for some drugs (Fig. 15.10). At present the clinical relevance of these additional properties, or even their presence in normal therapeutic doses, is unclear and further studies are necessary to optimize their effects.

Non-Steroid Anti-Inflammatory Drugs

The use of cyclooxygenase inhibitors, such as indomethacin or flurbiprofen, to inhibit the production of the mast cell-derived bronchoconstrictor, PGD_2, is a theoretical form of therapy. While they have some beneficial effects in acute antigen provocation, they appear to have little benefit in clinical asthma. Furthermore, these drugs may precipitate the so-called 'aspirin-induced' asthma in a small percentage of patients, a property which precludes their indiscriminate use in asthma.

Anti-Cholinergic Agents

Anti-muscarinic agents, particularly the smoking of leaves of stramonium, belladonna and hyoscyamus, have been used for the treatment of asthma for centuries. Certainly the inhibition of the muscarinic M_3-receptor actions of acetylcholine, which are linked directly with cyclic GMP-mediated contractile events in bronchial smooth muscle, represents an attractive target for drug intervention.

There is a large literature covering the use of atropine in asthma. In summary, this agent is a bronchodilator but its inhibitory effects on the parasympathetic nervous system, particularly the heart, make its use unjustified today. More recently ipratropium bromide and oxitropium bromide, potent topical anti-cholinergics with poor systemic absorption and hence few systemic side effects, have been introduced while affording some bronchodilator action. These agents have found little place in asthma treatment in competition with β_2-adrenoceptor stimulant bronchodilators.

Drugs with Symptom-Relieving and Anti-Inflammatory Properties

Sodium Cromoglycate and Nedocromil Sodium

Drugs of this class are often termed 'anti-allergic drugs' which is defined here as drugs capable of inhibiting both the early phase response and chronic allergic-inflammatory reactions. Sodium cromoglycate was originally introduced as a 'mast cell stabilizer'. Clearly, this aspect of its effects is responsible at least in part for its prophylactic activity against immediate hypersensitivity responses. Its effects in chronic asthma, however, are probably mediated by effects on the influx and activation of inflammatory cells, including eosinophils. Nedocromil sodium has been introduced more specifically to treat pulmonary inflammation associated with asthma.

Both sodium cromoglycate and nedocromil sodium (Fig. 15.11) are acidic drugs with pKa values of 1.0–2.5 and, consequently, exist almost exclusively in

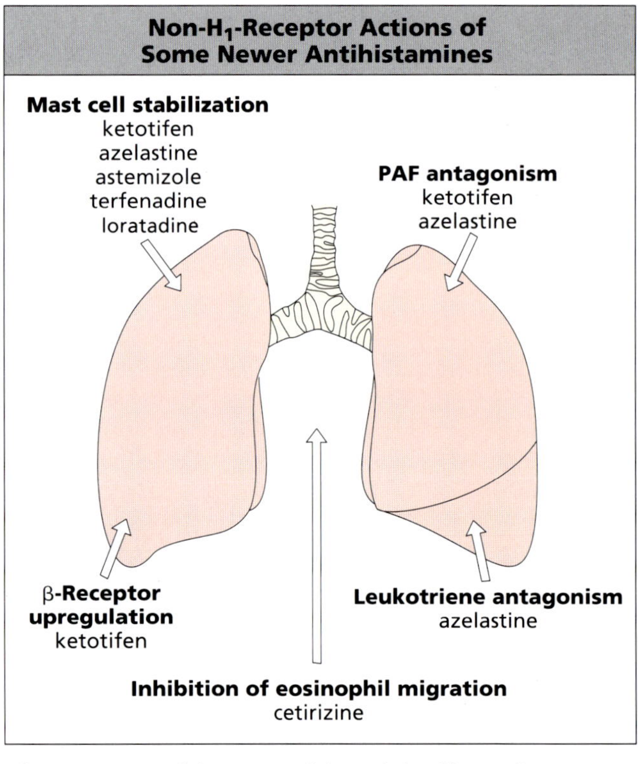

Fig. 15.10 Possible non-antihistaminic effects of antihistamines.

the ionized form of physiological pH (~7.4). These physicochemical characteristics carry both advantages and disadvantages.

Advantages:

- retained on site of action at the bronchial mucosa;
- swallowed drug poorly absorbed from intestine but voided in faeces;
- remains in extracellular compartment giving it a low toxicity.

Disadvantages:

- cannot be given as an oral preparation for asthma.

Action

The possible sites of action of anti-allergic drugs are shown in Fig. 15.12. Sodium cromoglycate was originally marketed as a 'mast cell stabilizer'. The mechanism by which the drug reduces the release of histamine, PGD_2 and LTC_4 from mast cells is still unclear, despite more than 20 years' research. Phosphorylation of a 78 kDa protein, a substrate for protein kinase C, is the currently purported drug target. While an action on mast cells may explain the action of sodium cromoglycate on bronchoconstriction induced by allergen, exercise and cold air, its effect on that induced by irritant agents, such as sulphur dioxide, cannot. An effect on neuronal reflexes, possibly involving C-fibre sensory neurones, has been postulated. The ability of nedocromil sodium to inhibit bronchoconstriction induced by bradykinin and capsaicin would support this theory. Thus, there are probably two complementary mechanisms by which sodium cromoglycate and nedocromil sodium may exert their beneficial effects against the early phase of acute asthma attacks.

Besides inhibiting the early response, sodium cromoglycate and nedocromil sodium also protect against allergen-induced late phase responses and the acquisition of bronchial hyperresponsiveness. As these events are associated with the accumulation and activation of inflammatory cells, particularly eosinophils, an inhibition effect on these aspects of asthma must be considered. *In vitro* studies have shown that sodium cromoglycate inhibits the accumulation of eosinophils in the lung both following allergen challenge and in clinical asthma. *In vivo*, activation of eosinophils, neutrophils and macrophages is reduced by sodium cromoglycate and nedocromil sodium, the latter again being approximately ten times more potent. Furthermore, nedocromil sodium, rather than sodium cromoglycate, inhibits platelet activation in aspirin-sensitive patients.

Administration

Both sodium cromoglycate and nedocromil sodium have achieved a well-established place in the control of mild to moderately severe asthma but are less effective in severe asthma. The major advantage is their relative freedom from systemic toxicity – transient cough and mild wheezing following inhalation of the drug powder preparations are the most common side effects. Their ability to treat both immediate and late-phase bronchoconstrictor events and to prevent the acquisition of bronchial hyperresponsiveness provides a unique wide spectrum of activity. However, the major drawback of sodium cromoglycate is its relatively weak action since it is ineffective in approximately 30 per cent of patients. The usefulness of nedocromil sodium is likely to be greater.

When used for the prevention of an early-phase allergic response, a single prophylactic inhaled dose has been shown repeatedly to be effective. However, to have an effect against bronchial hyperresponsiveness, courses of at least 1–2 months are necessary

Structural Formulae of Sodium Cromoglycate and Nedocromil Sodium

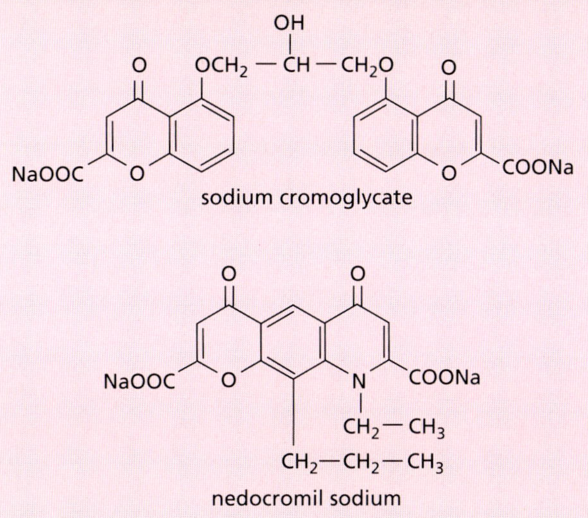

Fig. 15.11 Structures of sodium cromoglycate and nedocromil sodium.

Actions of Sodium Cromoglycate and Nedocromil Sodium

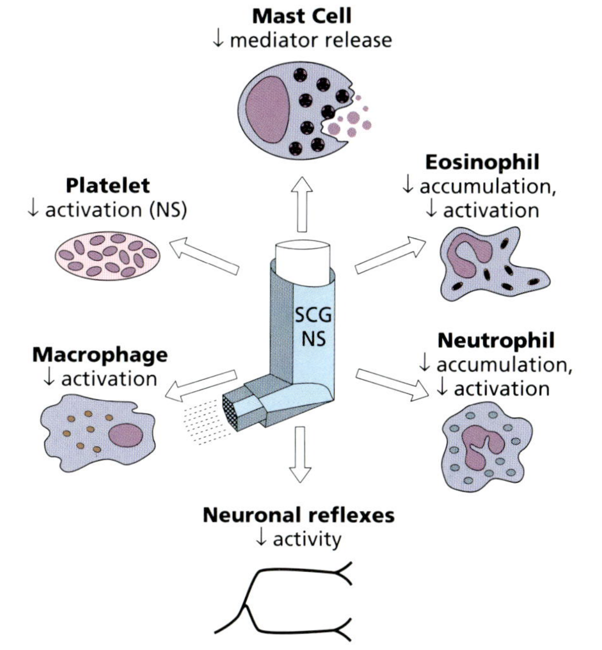

Fig. 15.12 Target tissues for sodium cromoglycate and nedocromil sodium.

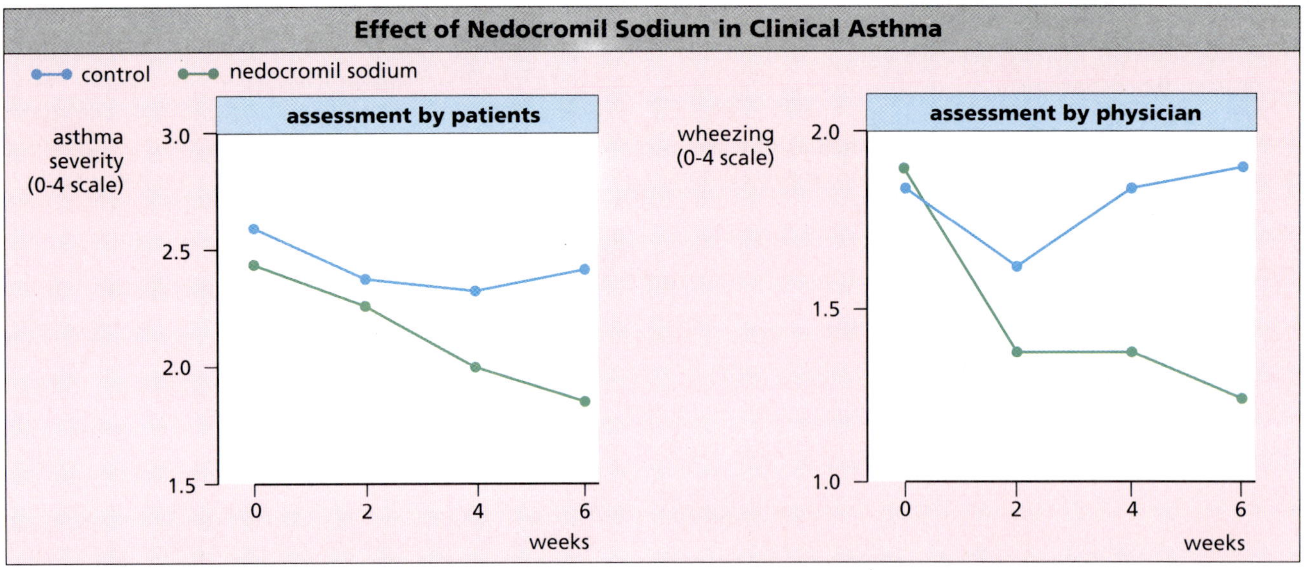

Fig. 15.13 Nedocromil sodium in clinical asthma.The subjective asthma score made by the patients and the wheezing severity score made by the physician of 45 asthmatic patients receiving nedocromil sodium, 4 mg twice daily, and 45 controls. (Adapted from Van As A, et al. *Eur J Respir Dis* 1986; **69** suppl. 147:143–148.)

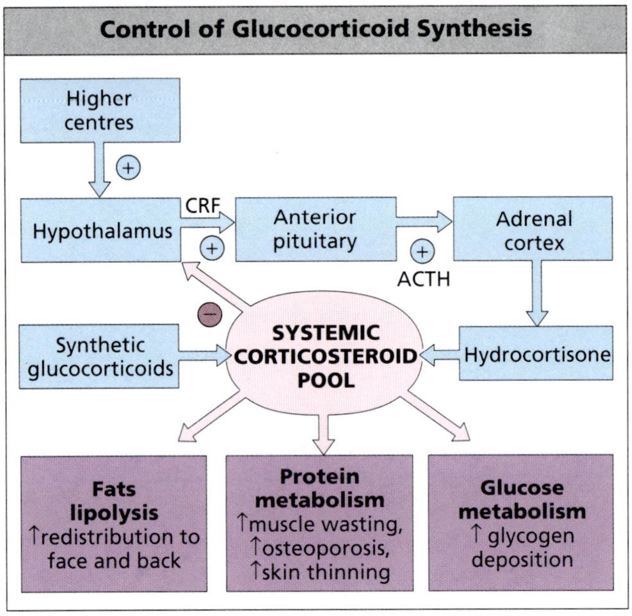

Fig. 15.14 Control of secretion and metabolic effects of glucocorticosteroids. In normal individuals, the positive signals of corticotrophin releasing factor (CRF) and adrenocorticotrophic hormone (ACTH) from the hypothalamus and pituitary gland respectively induce the secretion of hydrocortisone from the adrenal cortex. Both hydrocortisone and exogenous glucocorticoids exert a negative effect on the hypothalamus to reduce natural hydrocortisone secretion.

(Fig. 15.13). The unwillingness of patients and physicians to wait for this length of time before experiencing the beneficial effects of the drugs is one of the major reasons why anti-allergic drugs are often considered to be ineffective. However, skilled management of patients with sodium cromoglycate or nedocromil sodium may provide a single asthma therapy which is free from the potential hazards associated with β-stimulants, corticosteroids or theophylline. Sodium cromoglycate and nedocromil sodium may, therefore, be particularly useful drugs in young children or others where the unwanted effects of other drug classes may be a problem.

Anti-Inflammatory Agents

Corticosteroids

Corticosteroids have been the drug of choice for the treatment of chronic severe asthma since their introduction in 1950. More recently it has been recognized that the treatment of milder asthma with corticosteroids may also help to reduce bronchial inflammation and control the progression of the disease. However, it must be stressed that corticosteroids have potentially debilitating unwanted effects when used incorrectly or inappropriately.

The natural glucocorticoid released from the zona fascicularis of the human adrenal cortex is hydrocortisone. When considering its use as a drug to treat asthma, this molecule is a potent anti-inflammatory but carries with it considerable effects on glucose metabolism (Fig. 15.14) and mineral absorption by the kidney. Chemical manipulation of the steroid molecule has essentially removed the mineralocorticoid action but, to date, has been unable to separate anti-inflammatory and glucocorticoid effects. Further chemical manipulation has led to an optimization of their pharmacokinetic profile. For systemic activity, chemical manipulations have been made to increase potency and extend duration of action. For local administration to the lung as an aerosol, a different pharmacokinetic profile is required, namely, slow absorption from a mucosal surface and rapid metabolism on entering the systemic circulation. The first of these criteria were met with the introduction of the dipropionate ester of beclomethasone (Fig. 15.15) which has been used in aerosol form for several years without overt systemic effects. The second

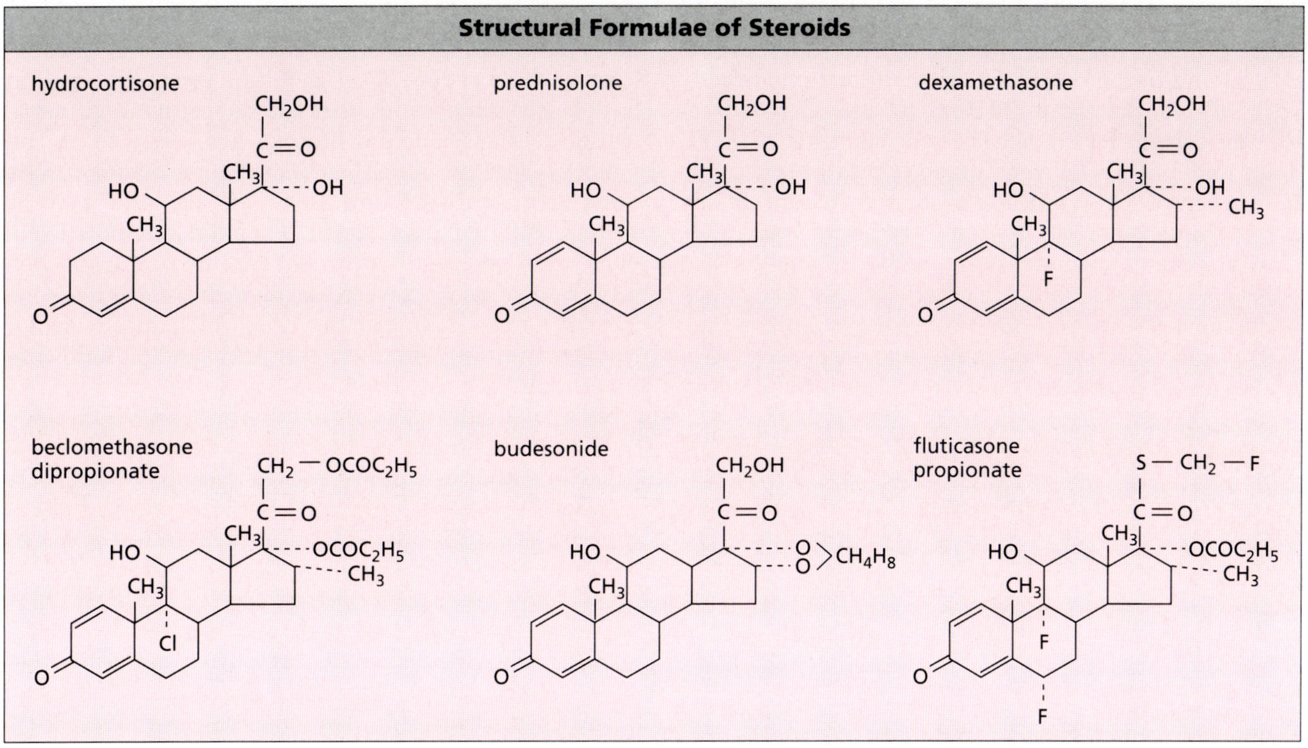

Fig. 15.15 Structural formulae of common corticosteroids.

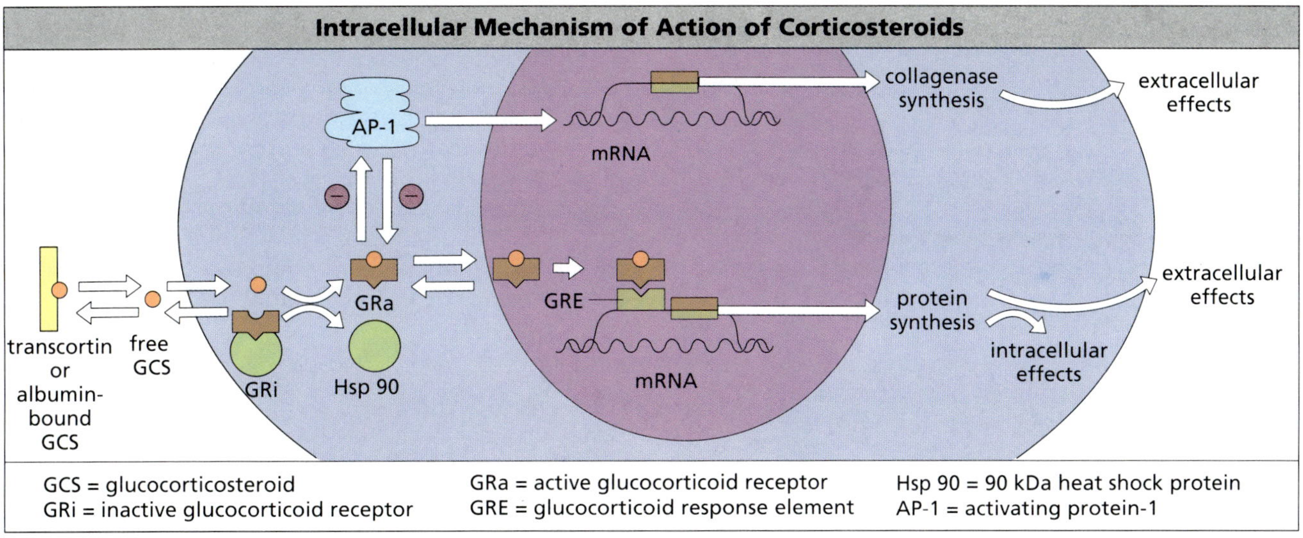

Fig. 15.16 Intracellular mechanisms of action of corticosteroids (see text).

of these criteria is now being achieved with the introduction of budesonide and fluticasone propriate (see Fig. 15.15), both of which undergo rapid systemic metabolism.

Action

Both natural and synthetic corticosteroids are highly lipophilic and largely bound to either of two plasma proteins; transcortin, a specific corticosteroid binding globulin which binds hydrocortisone and prednisolone with high attempts, and albumin which binds all steroids with low affinity. Free steroid molecules diffuse across the cell membrane where they interact with glucocorticoid receptors (GR) in the cytoplasm (Fig. 15.16). Inactive GR (GRi) are maintained in their resting state by being bound to a 90 kDa heat shock protein; when they interact with a glucocorticosteroid molecule, this protein is shed to expose the active site. The resultant activated receptor (GRa) then diffuses into the nucleus where it interacts with a specific glucocorticoid response element (GRE) on the chromatin of the DNA to influence transcription and consequently *de novo* synthesis of steroid-susceptible proteins. An example of a protein whose synthesis is upregulated is lipomodulin which exerts an anti-inflammatory activity by inhibiting the activity of phopholipase A2. Glucocorticoids may downregulate transcription by one of two mechanisms. First, the GRa may combine with a GRE which downregulates transcription directly. Second, the GRa may inactivate proteins which themselves stimulate transcription. An example of the latter is the inhibition of collagenase synthesis which is stimulated by activating protein-1 (AP-1). Both in the cytosol and in the nucleus, GRa may combine directly with AP-1 to inactivate it. However, this is a selfregulating system for the consistuent elements of AP-1, *c-jun* and *c-fos*, both combine with CRa to inactivate it. The complexities of these processes account for the considerable time delay, often 6–12 hours, even after intravenous administration, before the beneficial effects of corticosteroids are observed.

At the cellular level, glucocorticoids suppress both acute and chronic inflammation, irrespective of cause, by inhibiting many steps in the inflammatory process. Some cellular actions pertinent to asthma are shown in Fig. 15.17. Of these, the ability of corticosteroids to reduce T-cell cytokine production and to reduce eosinophil and mast cell deposition and maturation of the bronchial mucosa are likely to be the mechanisms by which corticosteroids achieve their long-term anti-inflammatory effects and benefit chronic asthma (Fig. 15.18). Their life-saving effects, which are apparent within 8–12 hours of intravenous injection in acute severe asthma, are more likely to be due to the ability of the drugs to reduce oedema, reduce the local generation of eicosanoids following lipomodulin generation, reduce inflammatory cell activation and reverse adrenoceptor downregulation.

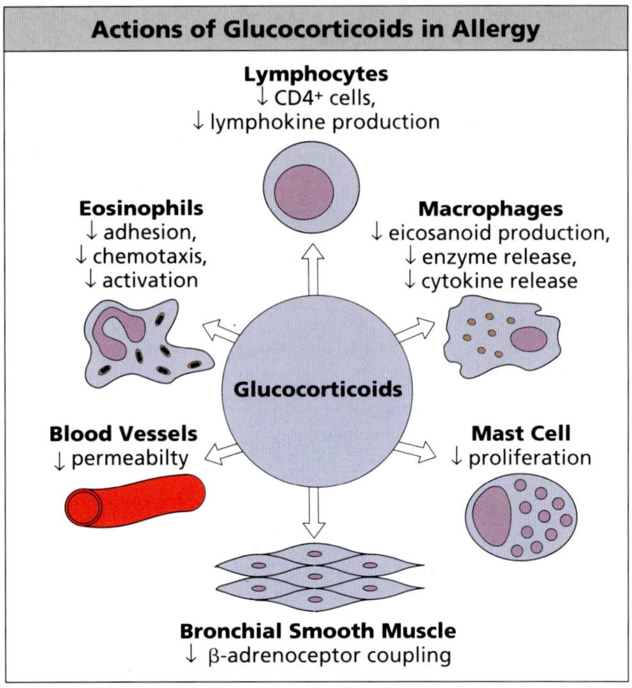

Fig. 15.17 Possible mechanisms by which corticosteroids reduce allergic diseases.

The intracellular events which are responsible for the anti-inflammatory effects of glucocorticosteroids cannot be separated from their effects on glucose, protein and lipid metabolism and their suppressive effects on the hypothalamo-pituitary-adrenal (HPA) axis. These effects are summarized in Fig. 15.14. It should be noted that all synthetic or natural corticosteroids used in the treatment of asthma will exert these effects when present in the systemic circulation. Furthermore, the magnitude of the side effects is dependant on:

- the dose of the drug absorbed systemically;
- the duration of its systemic effect;
- the duration of treatment.

With systemic treatment this means that treatment should be instigated, bearing in mind the balance between beneficial and harmful effects of corticosteroids and that suppression of the HPA axis is likely to lead to adrenocortical atrophy, particularly with prolonged treatment. While adrenocortical atrophy is reversible, this occurs only slowly, thus making it potentially dangerous to withdraw corticosteroids from a chronically treated patient.

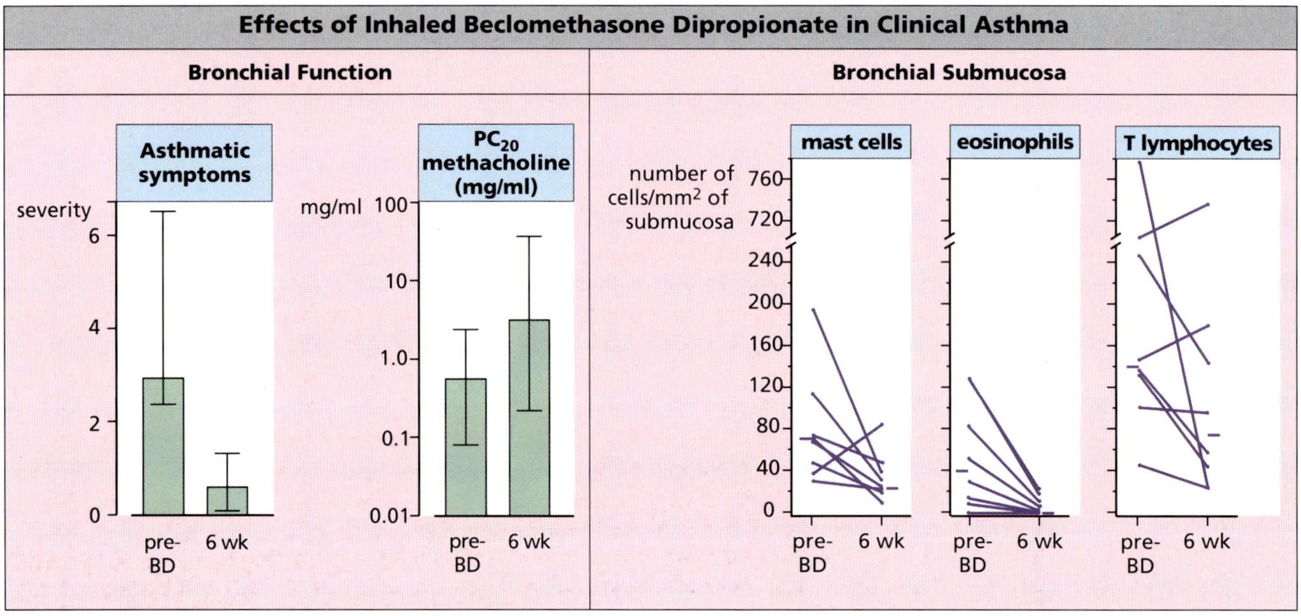

Fig. 15.18 The effect of beclomethasone dipropionate in asthma. Patients were examined before and after treatment with beclomethasone dipropionate (BD), 1 000 μg/day by inhalation. Improvements were observed in subjective symptoms and bronchial hyperresponsiveness to methacholine. These were parallelled by significant falls in submucosal mast cell and eosinophils as assessed in bronchial biopsies.

Administration

The choice of individual corticosteroid for treatment will depend on its route of administration. For oral use in chronic severe asthma or for intravenous use in acute severe asthma, the drug should be rapidly absorbed and distributed, have a high affinity for the receptor, be slowly metabolized and be devoid of mineralocorticoid action. These criteria are best met by beclomethasone and dexamethasone and, to a lesser extent, by prednisolone and prednisone. To minimize unwanted effects and maximize effectiveness, large initial doses should be used followed by systematic reduction to the lowest possible maintenance dose. Alternatively, intermittent high dose therapy may be used, thus allowing the body periods of recovery between administrations.

In less severe chronic asthma, corticosteroids should be administered locally to the lung surface by inhalation whenever possible. The ideal pharmacokinetic properties of such a drug, of slow absorption from the site of deposition and rapid metabolism once absorbed systemically, are met most closely by beclomethasone dipropionate, budesonide and fluticosone. With experience of inhaled steroids now established since the early 1970s, it is evident that original fears about long-term adverse effects appear not to have been borne out with only occasional reports of candidiasis and reversible dysphonia and rare reports of systemic effects. Only with inhaled doses of around 1000–2000 μg/day have mild systemic effects and some degree of HPA suppression been reported. Thus, the increasing tendency to use inhaled corticosteroids as anti-inflammatory agents in mild asthma appears to be a logical and safe development of therapy. However, it should still be a maxim of the practising physician to use as low a dose as possible, particularly in children.

Drugs in Development

Even with our present drug range the prevalence of asthma and the incidence of asthma deaths is still rising. Our current therapy is not reaching its objectives to reverse the progression of the disease in addition to treating the symptoms. Thus, the quest for newer and more effective drugs must continue. For the details of drugs in development, the reader is referred to more specialized texts. They are described in general terms here.

There are a number of approaches towards achieving bronchodilation and symptomatic relief. *Calcium antagonists* aim to reduce the stimulus-induced entry of calcium into bronchial smooth muscle and thus decrease its contractility. The major problem with such drugs so far is their lack of specificity, effects on the cardiovascular system being of major concern. A more attractive proposition appears to be *potassium channel opening drugs* which lead to a hyperpolarization and, consequently, a reduction in contractile sensitivity of bronchial smooth muscle. One of these agents, cromakalim, has been shown to reduce morning dipping in human nocturnal asthma by an action more likely to involve reduction in cholinergic affector mechanisms than a direct effect on bronchial smooth muscle. The possibility of delivering such drugs to the airways by aerosol inhalation presents a viable drug entity. As mentioned earlier, *type IV phosphodiesterase inhibitors,* aimed at increasing cyclic AMP levels in bronchial smooth muscle and inflammatory cells, are under active investigation as anti-asthma agents. The recent observations that the contractile effects of PGD_2, its metabolite 9α, 11β, PGF_2 and TXA_2 all stem from an interaction with the TP_1-receptor make *thromboxane receptor antagonists* an attractive proposition. Preliminary tests with such drugs are, however, disappointing.

The lipoxygenase products of arachidonic acid, namely the leukotrienes, HETEs and lipoxins, are involved in many aspects of the asthmatic response by virtue of their various bronchoconstrictor and pro-inflammatory properties. Consequently *leukotriene antagonists* and *lipoxygenase inhibitors* provide an attractive option for drug development. Although the first generation of compounds, yielded little encouragement, more recent compounds which are more potent and have an improved bioavailability, have given rise to optimism. Examples of leukotriene antagonists are ICI-204,219 and MK-571 which cause a 30–100-fold displacement of the LTD_4 dose-response curve in reducing FEV. MK-571 in particular produces a bronchodilation which is additive with that of β-stimulants and reduces the severity of exercise-induced asthma. Both compounds prevent early and late phase asthmatic responses and bronchial hyperresponsiveness following allergen provocation. A 5-lipoxygenase inhibitor, A-64077, has a similar profile while being somewhat less effective. Its 5-lipoxygenase inhibitory activity has been demonstrated in the clinical environment by its ability to reduce the generation of LTB_4 in the nose following allergen provocation and in the colon in inflammatory bowel disease.

Another lipid-derived product which emanates from many inflammatory cells, platelet activating factor (PAF), has been shown to be associated with increased bronchial reactivity, particularly in animal models. Many *PAF antagonists,* including derivatives of the naturally occurring ginkgolides and synthetic hetrazepines, such as WEB-2086, have been shown to be potent inhibitors of PAF and allergen-induced bronchoconstriction and acquired bronchial hyperresponsiveness in the guinea-pig. In man, PAF antagonists, used in doses which suppress responses to intradermally injected or inhaled PAF, have shown little effect on experimental asthma induced by allergen inhalation. Whether or not this may be interpreted as a minor role for PAF in human asthma will become clear when the results of phase 2 trials are available.

Further Reading

Anderson KE, Persson CGA, eds. *Anti-Asthma Xanthimes and Adenosine*. Amsterdam: Excerpta Medica, 1985.

Church MK, Polosa R, Rimmer SJ. Cromolyn sodium and nedocromil sodium: mast cell stabilizers, neuromodulators or anti-inflammatory drugs. In: *Asthma: Its Pathology and Treatment*. Kaliner MA, Barnes PJ, Persson CGA, eds. New York: Marcel Dekker, 1991, pp. 561–593.

Corticosteroids: their biological mechanisms and applications to the treatment of asthma. *Am Rev Respir Dis* 1990;**141** (supplement):S1–S96.

Kerrebijn KF. Beta agonists. In: *Asthma: Its Pathology and Treatment*. Kaliner MA, Barnes PJ, Persson CGA, eds. New York: Marcel Dekker, 1991, pp. 523–559.

Murphy S, Kelly HW. Cromolyn sodium: a review of mechanisms and clinical use. *Drug Intell Clin Pharm* 1987; **21**: 22–35.

Pearce FJ, Foreman JC. Cromolyn. In: *Allergy : Principles and Practice*. Middleton E, Reed CE, Ellis EF, Adkinson NF, Yuninger JW, eds. St Louis: Mosby, 1988, pp. 766–781.

Rimmer SJ, Church MK. The pharmacology and mechanisms of action of histamine H_1-antagonists. *Clin Exp Allergy* 1990; **20** (suppl. 2): 3–17.

Chapter 16

Extrinsic Allergic Alveolitis

Introduction

Extrinsic allergic alveolitis (AA), or hypersensitivity pneumonitis, describes a broad spectrum of pulmonary interstitial and alveolar diseases caused by repeated, intense exposure to a wide variety of inhaled organic dusts or related occupational antigens. The primary sources of antigen in the classic forms of this disease, among which are Farmer's lung and bagassosis, are actinomycetes-laden composts, especially mouldy hay and bagasse (the residue of sugar cane fibre).

It is likely that any organic dust of appropriate particle size can induce pulmonary lesions characteristic of AA under conditions of sufficiently intense or prolonged exposure. This fact is of great importance to medicine, agriculture, and industry, since knowledge of the aetiological agents and removal of the individual from the source of exposure can either prevent the disease or result in a cure.

Thermophilic actinomycetes are the main sources of antigen in several classic forms of the disease. They have been shown to possess certain common properties, such as potent immunological adjuvant activity. This finding might be expected since actinomycetes are members of the same botanical order as *Mycobacterium tuberculosis*, namely the *Actinomycetales*.

Epidemiology

Many forms of AA have a world-wide distribution. The diseases are seen in many occupational and environmental settings, but occur particularly in areas given over to farming, growth of sugar cane, and cultivation of mushrooms.

Farmer's lung has been well studied from the epidemiological viewpoint and it has been determined that the highest incidence occurs in early spring, the time of year when farmers handle mouldy hay. There is a male to female incidence of the disease of approximately 10:1, which probably reflects the greater number of males involved in farming. Curiously, cigarette smoking is associated with a lower incidence of this disease.

Patients, and to some extent exposed asymptomatic individuals, develop serum precipitating antibodies (precipitins) against epitopes expressed on inhaled organic dust. Surveys of farmers have shown that approximately 10 per cent have this serum precipitating antibody and 50 per cent are symptomatic, have abnormal pulmonary function tests, or X-rays suggestive of pulmonary disease. The incidence of precipitins against offending thermophilic actinomycetes organisms has been determined to be more than 100 per 100,000 in farmers, as opposed to approximately 10 per 100,000 in the population at large.

Clinical History and Physical Findings

The disease may present in acute, subacute, or chronic forms. Major symptoms are an unexplained productive cough, dyspnoea and weight loss. In the acute (or episodic) forms of the disease there is often haemoptysis and the patient is usually febrile. Chronic disease often causes general malaise, though the patient is usually afebrile.

All patients with symptoms suggestive of recurrent bacterial pneumonia and patients with chronic unexplained cough, dyspnoea, and sputum production should be suspected of having the disease. Without careful investigation of the patient's occupational or environmental background, the diagnosis may be missed or mistaken as viral pneumonia, primary atypical pneumonia, or bacterial pneumonia. Relief of symptoms away from a particular environment may be an important diagnostic clue, although occasionally pulmonary symptoms persist even after avoidance of exposure for a relatively prolonged period.

Acute recurrent symptoms characteristically occur within several hours of exposure to the offending agents in the classic of form of the disease and recur with progressively increasing severity after repeated exposure. They may, at times, be associated with striking weight loss, malaise and weakness.

In the chronic form of the disease, individuals have often been exposed to small amounts of antigen for prolonged periods, e.g. from contaminated home humidifiers, or sometimes from avian or animal foreign protein. These insidious forms of AA are characterized predominantly by chronic non-productive cough and dyspnoea, and pulmonary fibrosis is often noted.

Host Susceptibility

Only a small proportion of the exposed population develops the disease. This suggests a host susceptibility factor. Yet studies attempting to implicate genetic factors and susceptibility to the disease have not demonstrated an association between specific

HLA antigens and overt disease in patients with Pigeon Breeder's disease or Farmer's lung. Studies of farmers in the United Kingdom have shown an incidence of approximately 7 per cent, and other studies of office workers exposed to contaminated air-conditioning systems revealed a 15 per cent incidence of pulmonary symptoms associated with sensitization to thermophylic actinomycetes. Studies of members of pigeon-breeding clubs have shown that between 6 and 21 per cent of exposed breeders may develop the disease.

These diseases are not mediated by IgE, and atopy is not a predisposing factor. In an experimental animal model of granulomatous pulmonary inflammation following injection of BCG, some high-responder strains of mice developed intense pulmonary granulomatous lesions, whereas low-responder strains showed significantly smaller lung granulomas (Fig. 16.1). The intensity of this granulomatous response is linked to the immunoglobulin heavy chain locus (IgH) and has been shown to be a dominant and polygenic trait. The indication of linkage to the IgH haplotype in these models is not well understood, but these studies do suggest a genetically determined predisposition toward development of granulomatous lung disease in this species. If this experimental pulmonary granulomatous disease can be construed to be similar to AA in humans, then additional studies should be undertaken to uncover similar genetic predispositions in humans.

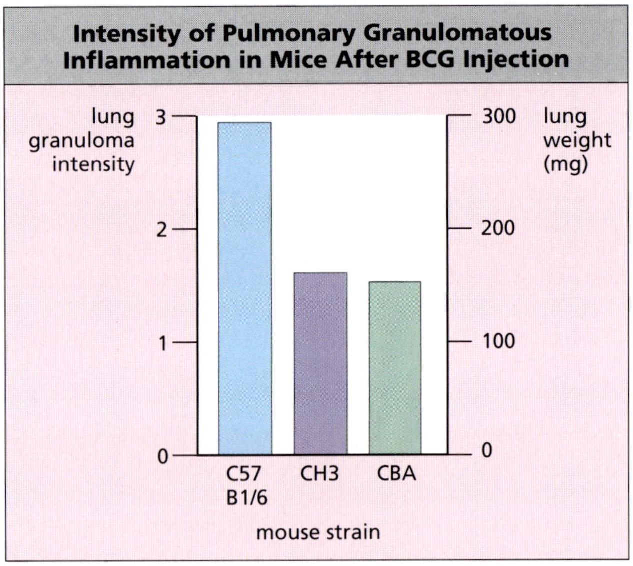

Fig. 16.1 Intensity of pulmonary granulomatous inflammation in mice after inoculation with BCG.

Radiologic Findings

Chest X-ray findings are variable and non-specific. During acute episodes there are often diffuse, fine, micronodular deposits or patchy pneumonitis (Fig. 16.2). Infiltrates are often bilateral, and usually spare the apices. However, they may occasionally be predominantly unilateral (Fig. 16.3).
In more subacute cases, linear interstitial changes are often superimposed upon the fine acinar deposits, resulting in a mixed acinar-interstitial appearance. A variety of patterns may however be noted, including hilar haze patterns and symmetric ground glass densities resembling those seen in pulmonary oedema.

In the chronic forms of the disease, diffuse interstitial fibrosis with classic honeycombing patterns can be seen. Secondary loss of lung volume and cardiac enlargement also occur.

Pulmonary Function Studies

During acute episodes the vital capacity is decreased, and carbon monoxide diffusing capacity D_{CO} and lung compliance are also reduced. Airways resistance usually remains normal. There is usually arterial oxygen desaturation and a mild reduction in the arterial carbon dioxide due to chronic alveolar hyperventilation.

Chronic forms of the disease are characterized by a decrease in lung volumes and diffusing capacity, but there may be an element of airways obstruction manifesting as decreased expiratory flow rates. The characteristic changes in pulmonary function studies and in cell analyses of peripheral blood after acute exposure are illustrated in Fig. 16.4.

Diagnosis

History

The diagnosis of AA should be considered in all patients presenting with acute or chronic symptoms

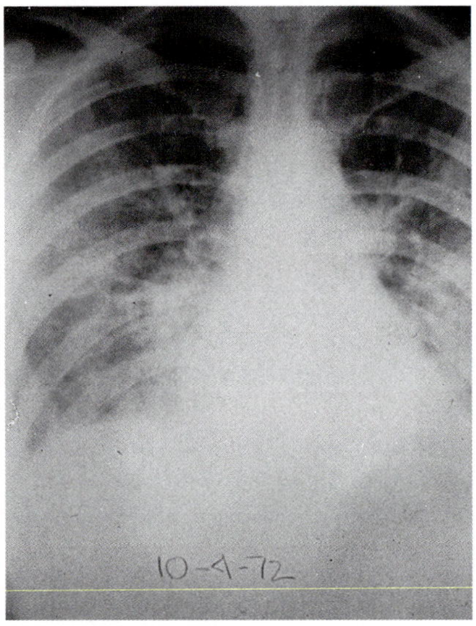

Fig. 16.2 Patchy bilateral infiltrates in patient with humidifier lung. Lesions cleared after removal of duct work, cleaning and replacement of the humidifier and the residual water pan which contained heavy growth of actinomycetes, bacilli, and other micro-organisms.

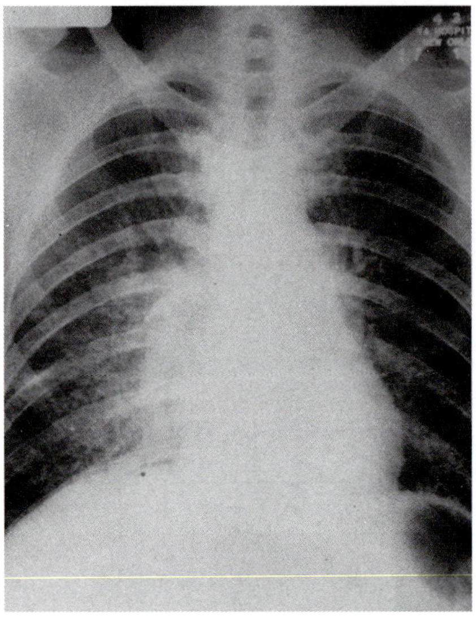

Fig. 16.3 Predominantly unilateral, fine and course micronodular infiltrate in patient with acute AA.

associated with the inhalation of organic dusts or foreign animal proteins in an appropriate environmental, occupational or avocational setting. A careful history may be complemented by demonstration of remission of symptoms after extended removal from the source of antigen.

Precipitating antibody

High levels of precipitating antibody which react with the offending antigen are detectable by simple double gel diffusion, particularly during the acute form of the disease.

However, many exposed people who are presumably well also have detectable serum precipitating antibodies and neither the presence nor the quantity of precipitins seems to correlate with disease severity. Other techniques, more sensitive than double gel diffusion, such as enzyme-linked immunosorbent assay (ELISA), complement fixation, radioimmunoassay, and countercurrent electrophoresis, have proven to be sufficiently sensitive to detect activity against organic dust antigens in virtually all patients. However, because of the increased sensitivity of these tests, they also detect antibody in large numbers of asymptomatic people.

Considering the limitations of the antigens involved, the wide range of potential sources of antigen, the presence of occasional non-specific reactions, and the finding of precipitins in many asymptomatic subjects, it is still reasonable, for screening purposes, to check any suspected organic dust for antigenic activity by simple double gel diffusion in agar. If precipitins are demonstrable, the crude dust extract can be presumed to contain the suspected antigen and further, more refined precipitin or other specific immunoglobulin assays can be employed using well defined-antigens.

Skin tests

The use of skin tests as diagnostic aids can be performed with certain antigens, such as serum proteins or partially characterized fungal extracts though, in most cases, non-irritant allergenic extracts are not commercially available for skin testing in humans. When positive, the skin test often reveals an early

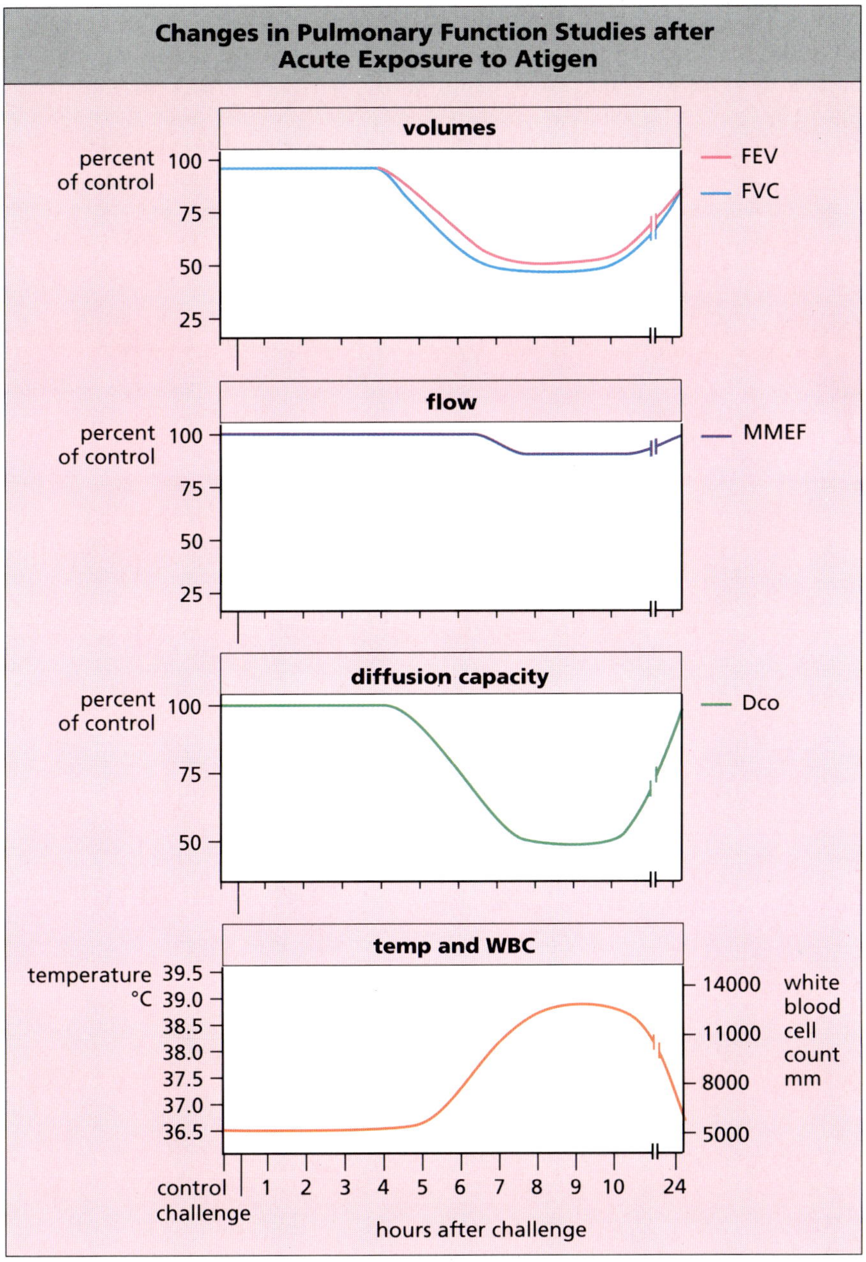

Fig. 16.4 Characteristic changes in pulmonary function studies and peripheral blood cell analysis following acute exposure to antigen in patient with Pigeon Breeder's disease. Note decrease in FEV_I and FVC and MMEF plus D_{CO}, commencing five hours after exposure. Typical rise in temperature and total white cell count were also noted at this time.

immediate wheal and flare reaction followed by a late phase response at four to six hours, and occasionally delayed skin reactivity at 24 to 72 hours. Delayed skin reactivity has been demonstrated in experimental animal models of the disease, but is more difficult to demonstrate in humans, possibly because of the removal of antigen during the associated immediate skin reaction. As in the case of serum precipitins, positive skin reactivity may be demonstrated in exposed but asymptomatic subjects.

Environmental assessment

Identification of aetiological agents occasionally requires direct assessment of the environment with sophisticated microbiologic analysis of suspected sources of antigen, including dust samples collected from work or home environments.

'Natural' or 'biologic' inhalation challenge testing may, at times, be important in obtaining presumptive diagnostic evidence of these diseases. Such 'natural' challenges (in which the patient is simply allowed to return to the suspected environment in an attempt to reproduce symptoms) are helpful in acute cases, particularly when a cause and effect relationship is not apparent, or when the antigens are not identified (Fig. 16.5). In chronic cases, exacerbation of symptoms may not occur after such brief exposure.

Assays for cell-mediated immunity

Other *in vitro* tests to demonstrate cell-mediated immune responses have been employed in the diagnostic evaluation of AA. Among these are assays for lymphocyte transformation (blastogenic factor production), and assays for production of other lymphokines such as macrophage migration inhibition and aggregation factors (MIF and MAF). These tests generally do not have any practical clinical application. As is the case with serum precipitins and skin testing, they have been shown to be positive in some exposed, asymptomatic subjects.

Lung biopsy

Although non-specific, biopsy may be of diagnostic help in chronic cases, when considered together with clinical and laboratory findings. Lesions are characterized histologically by alveolar and interstitial infiltrates of granulomatous mononuclear cells. The lung appears to be the sole site of inflammation; lesions in liver, bone, and other reticuloendothelial tissues, such as are often observed in sarcoidosis, are not present. Activated alveolar macrophages (Fig. 16.6) and infiltrates of lymphocytes (particularly suppressor T cells) are prominent in the loosely formed, non-caseating granulomas.

In acute stages, there is thickening of the alveolar septi with predominant lymphocytic and plasma-cell infiltrates, as well as extensive accumulation within the alveoli of cells having the morphology of immature alveolar macrophages (Fig. 16.7). Langhans' giant cells may be prominent, particularly in subacute or chronic stages of the disease. During more chronic stages of the disease, there may at times be marked narrowing of bronchial walls, characteristic of bronchiolitis obliterans. This is reflected by mild but persistent airways obstruction in some chronic cases.

Most immunofluorescent studies in animal models and in human lung biopsy specimens have not revealed pulmonary vasculitis as seen in classical Arthus (Type III) reactions. In some cases when biopsies have been taken within 10 days of an acute episode, nodules containing acute vasculitic lesions involving both alveolar capillaries and arterioles have been noted. Immunofluorescent studies from patients with AA have also revealed actinomycetes antigen in bronchial walls, along with large numbers of antibody-forming cells and complement-coated mononuclear cells.

Broncho alveolar lavage (BAL)

Analysis of BAL fluids from patients with AA has shown that the percentage of lymphocytes is often in the range of 70 per cent, with large numbers of suppressor cytotoxic $CD8^+$ T lymphocytes rather than helper $CD4^+$ T lymphocytes. $CD8^+$ cells are usually present in concentrations well above 40 per cent, whereas $CD4^+$ cells constitute at most 30 per cent of the lymphocyte population (Fig. 16.8). (By contrast, in sarcoidosis, the percentage of lymphocytes

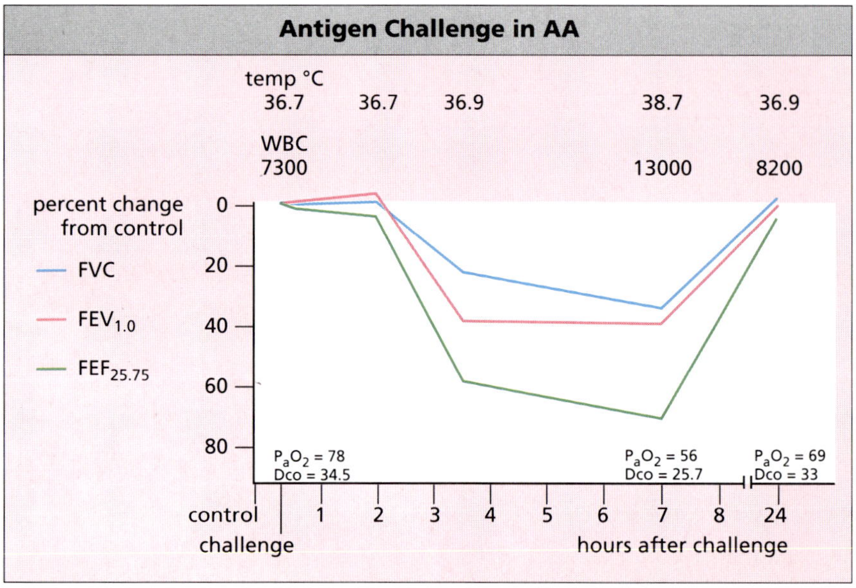

Fig. 16.5 Response to challenge with inhaled antigen in patient with AA caused by toluene diisocyanate (TDI). There is an approximate three-hour delay after exposure before impairment in lung function becomes demonstrable. Onset of fever is also delayed. Improvement in the patient's condition begins after approximately 24 hours or more.

obtained from BAL is often in the range of 40 to 50 per cent, and $CD4^+$:$CD8^+$ ratios are 5:1 or greater.) Of interest is the fact that elevated numbers and percentages of $CD8^+$ cells are present in BAL fluids of asymptomatic subjects exposed to the antigen as well as in BAL fluids of those who develop clinical disease.

The presence of T cells bearing class II histocompatibility antigen (HLA-DR), and of activated T-cell markers (MLRI-3) in the BAL effluent of patients with AA, indicates that these cells are activated. Since activation markers are not necessarily related to the regulatory or effector function of lymphocytes, and can be detected on activated lymphocytes of both helper and suppressor T-cell subclasses, the presence of these cells probably reflects an ongoing, local, T-cell-dependent immune process and not necessarily disease. However, these cells are present in lesser numbers in subjects who are exposed but remain asymptomatic.

Increased gallium uptake has been noted in most patients, even those receiving corticosteroid treatment, and is likely to indicate infiltration of the alveoli with activated macrophages.

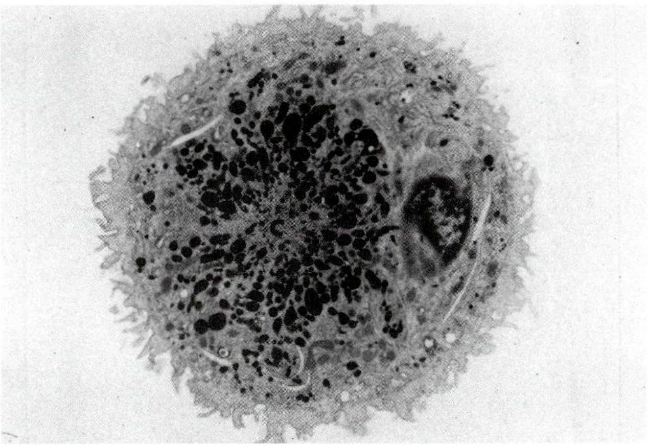

Fig. 16.6 Electromicrograph of a typical macrophage, obtained by bronchoalveolar lavage from rabbits which had been immunized with *Micropolyspora faeni* 14 days earlier by the respiratory tract route. Note the rosetting of lysosomal bodies in the perinuclear area which has been described as an indication of cellular activation. Typically, such free alveolar cells also demonstrate less variation in size than those obtained only a few days after immunization, with increased numbers of phagocytic inclusions. This suggests a maturing population of phagocytes. (Uranyl acetate and lead citrate stain, original magnification × 1390).

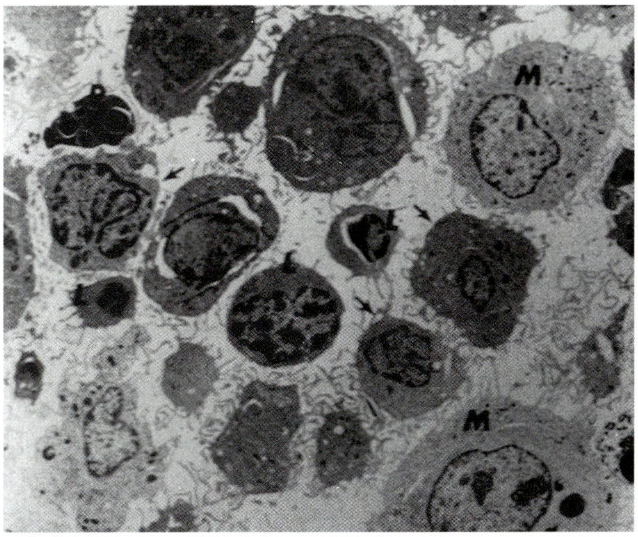

Fig. 16.7 Free alveolar cells obtained from bronchoalveolar lavage in rabbits, eight days after immunization with *Micropolyspora faeni*. There is considerable variation in the size of macrophages (M) and there are more lymphocytes (L) and polymorphonucleated neutrophils (P). It is difficult to tell whether many of the smaller mononuclear cells are lymphocytes or monocytes. A smaller number are phagolysosomes, and many of these cells appear to be immature phagocytes that have been recruited in response to immunization. (Uranyl acetate and lead citrate stain, original magnification × 1390).

Pathogenesis

Organic dusts that cause AA are known to possess a variety of biological effects, and in particular they can serve as potent immunological adjuvants: they stimulate alveolar macrophages and they directly activate the alternative pathway of complement by providing the necessary mediator stimuli for increasing vascular permeability and promoting chemotactic migration of neutrophils and other cells into the lung. They also contain toxic substances, many of which have enzymatic activities, while other agents induce non-specific precipitins, mediator release, and lymphocyte blastogenesis. The inflammatory consequences of these direct injurious effects, and of those modulated by complement and macrophages, could be important factors in the pathogenesis of AA (see Fig. 16.9).

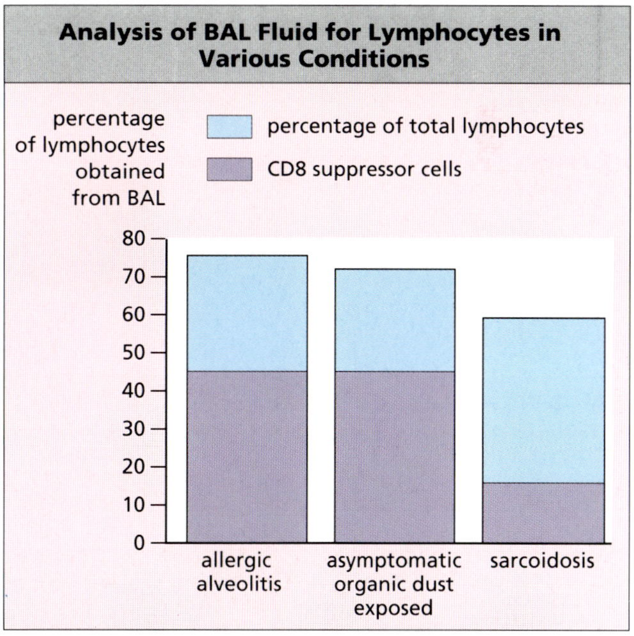

Fig.16.8 Comparison of bronchoalveolar fluids from patients with AA, asymptomatic subjects exposed to organic dust, and patients with sarcoidosis. It can be seen that patients with AA and asymptomatic patients exposed to organic dusts have a preponderance of $CD8^+$ suppressor cells. Conversely, patients with sarcoidosis exhibit a significantly smaller number of suppressor cells with large numbers of $CD4^+$ helper lymphocytes.

Many animal models have been developed in an attempt to help understand the pathogenesis of the various forms of granulomatous pneumonitis which characterise AA. In some of these models, aerosol challenge with particulate organic dust or related antigens after systemic immunization has resulted in early neutrophilic infiltrates, followed by granulomatous lesions compatible with cell-mediated (Type IV) tissue injury (Fig. 16.10). In the rabbit and guinea pig, intraperitoneal transfer of specifically sensitized lymph node and spleen cells, followed by aerosol antigen challenge , has resulted in production of lesions closely resembling those observed in humans (Fig. 16.11). Local lymphokine production (specifically MIF, MAF, and blastogenic factors) together with the presence of activated alveolar macrophages in lesions, have repeatedly been demonstrated in BAL fluids and in serum from these experimental animal models. In animal models of Pigeon Breeder's disease, long-term aerosol exposure to the appropriate antigens has resulted only in antibody formation without detectable pulmonary inflammation. However, when the lung had been primed with BCG and then exposed to the appropriate antigens by aerosol, granulomatous lesions resembling those of AA have occurred in association with demonstrable T-cell-dependent hypersensitivity to the inhaled antigens. This model might have relevance for humans, since many people are apparently exposed to aetiological agents of the disease for long periods of time with consequent development of precipitating antibodies, but display no detectable inflammatory changes in the lung.

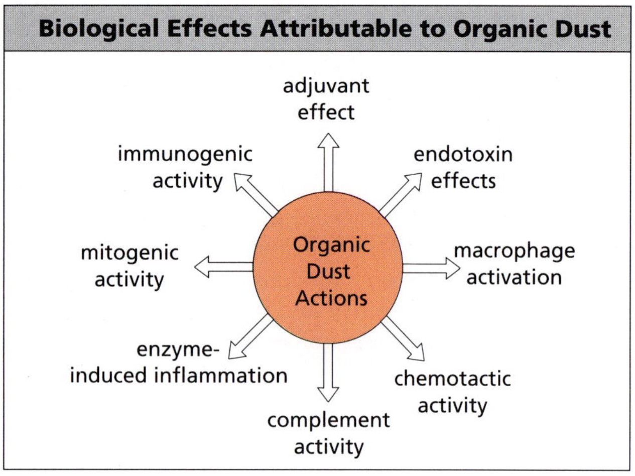

Fig. 16.9 A variety of biologic effects attributable to organic dusts.

Very few longitudinal studies have been performed to assess the immunological and phagocytic competence of the mononuclear cells which infiltrate the lung parenchyma in AA. In one recent study, BAL cell populations and biopsies of lung parenchymal tissue from patients with well-characterised AA were investigated during a prolonged follow-up. Initially, a high number of $CD8^+$ suppressor T cells were seen, with a subsequent persistent reversal of the $CD4^+$:$CD8^+$ ratio in individuals who continued to be regularly exposed to relevant antigens while at work.

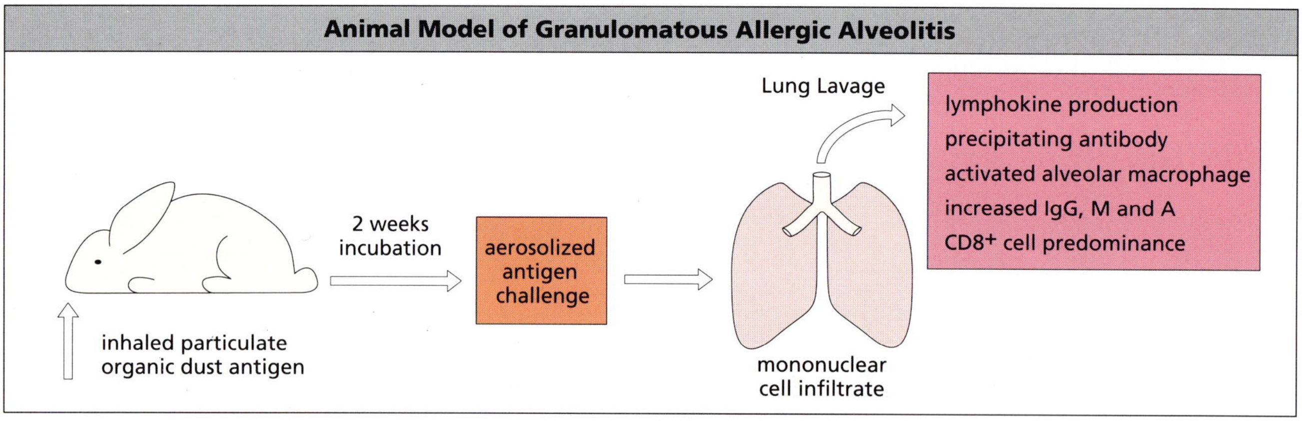

Fig. 16.10 Animal model of granulomatous AA. Aerosol challenge with particulate organic dust or related antigens after systemic immunization results in early neutrophilic infiltrate followed by granulomatous lesions compatible with those in cell-mediated allergic tissue injury. Presence of lung lesions is also associated with lymphokine production, precipitating antibody formation, and the presence of activated alveolar macrophages plus a predominance of $CD8^+$ suppressor cells.

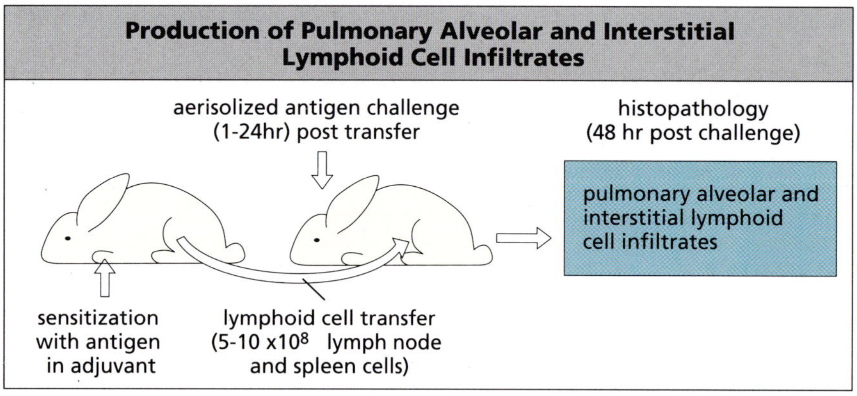

Fig. 16.11 Production of pulmonary alveolar and interstitial lymphoid cell infiltrates by the intraperitoneal transfer of specifically sensitized lymph node and spleen cells, with subsequent aerosol antigen challenge.

An increase in natural killer (NK) lymphocytes was also demonstrated in these patients. Immunohistochemical analyses of lung tissue has also demonstrated a diffuse infiltration of the lung parenchyma with $CD8^+$ T cells in patients with AA. Interestingly, those subjects who discontinued exposure to the specific work-related antigens, but continued to live in normal agricultural environments, demonstrated a decrease in $CD8^+$ T cells and a recovery of the $CD4^+$ T-cell population within a period of six months (Figs 16.12 and 16.13). There is also evidence for participation of mast cells in the development of AA, but the role of this mediator-secreting cell in disease pathogenesis is not known.

These results suggest that lymphocytic alveolitis is a chronic event in patients with AA and that its intensity might be modulated by the extent and degree of exposure to appropriate causative antigens. Other BAL studies in asymptomatic healthy farmers who were non-smokers revealed elevated levels of albumin, fibronectin, and angiotensin converting enzyme, which suggests that healthy farmers exposed to appropriate mould-laden composts may exhibit subclinical alveolitis including an accumulation of inflammatory cells in the airways.

Elevated levels of IgG, IgA and IgM in BAL fluid have been demonstrated repeatedly in experimental animal models of AA. High levels of Interleukin-1 (IL-1) are present in aqueous extracts prepared from pulmonary granulomatous lesions induced in BALB-c mice following the intratracheal injection of antigen-coated agarose beads. The presence of large amounts of IL-1 in these experimental pulmonary granulomatous infiltrates indicates that macrophages and T cells within the lesions are active in cytokine production. IL-1 may be involved in the expression and maintenance of the pulmonary granulomas by acting as a maturation signal which prepares T cells to be responsive to the specific antigens. IL-1 also probably participates in the inflammatory response as an inducer of B-cell differentiation and as a stimulator of IgG secretion. IL-6 has also been shown to be elevated in BAL fluid from patients with AA, but the possible role of other interleukins (IL-3,-4,-5,-7, and-8) in disease pathogenesis has yet to be studied. These experimental data all suggest an important role for T-cell-dependent responses in disease pathogenesis.

Lipoxygenase products derived from macrophages also appear to play a role in the induction of experimental pulmonary granulomatous inflammation. In studies employing a model of pulmonary granulomas induced in mice by *Schistosoma mansoni* eggs, it was noted that the development of hypersensitivity-type lung granulomas was associated with the synthesis of the macrophage-derived lipoxygenase derivatives leukotriene C4 (LTC4), LTD4, and 5-hydroxyeicosatetraenoic acid (5-HETE) (see Fig. 16.14). Marked suppression of these experimental pulmonary granulomas was achieved with the use of 5-lipoxygenase inhibitors, but granulmata were not inhibited by cycloxygenase inhibitors.

5-Lipoxygenase inhibitors also suppressed the *in vitro* kinetics of Ia antigen expression by alveolar macrophages in this mouse model. Thus, certain products of arachidonic acid breakdown may play an important role in the induction of tissue inflammation associated with chronic hypersensitivity granulomas. The ability of macrophages to express Ia antigens is an absolute requirement for the presentation of macrophage-mediated antigen to T cells in the mouse, and probably reflects the stage of macrophage maturation.

Lipoxygenase inhibitors have also been shown to suppress cell-mediated immune mechanisms, mitogen- and antigen-induced lymphocyte blastogenesis, and effector T cell cytotoxicity. The finding that these inhibitors can also suppress the expression of Ia antigen on alveolar macrophages within the granuloma, suggests yet another mechanism whereby macrophages can regulate or modulate the formation of granulomas.

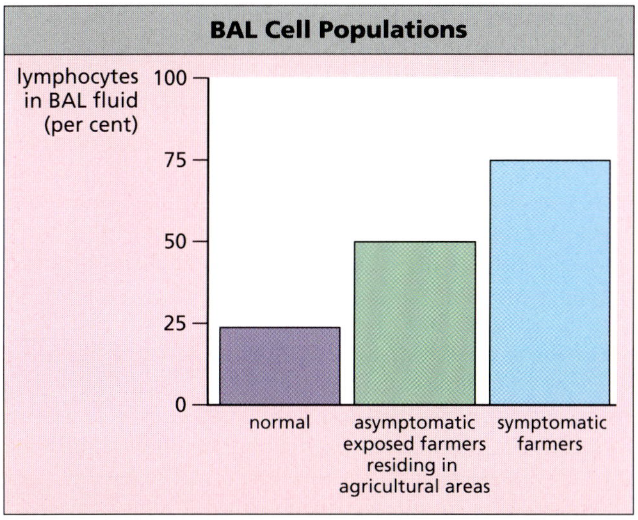

Fig. 16.12 Study of BAL cell populations in symptomatic farmers and asymptomatic exposed farmers.

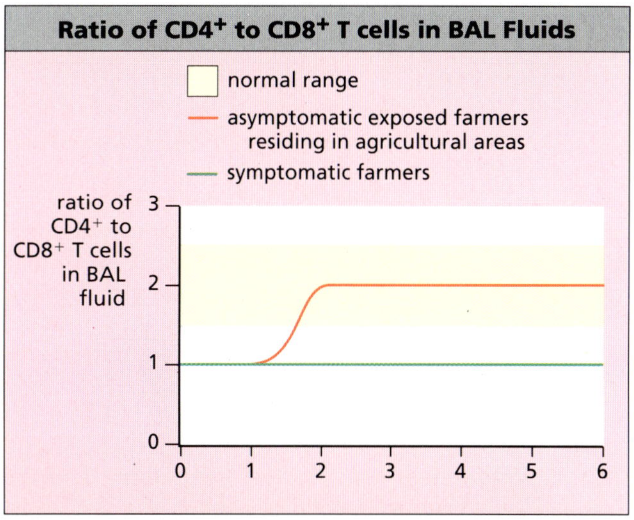

Fig. 16.13 Those study subjects who discontinued exposure to specific antigens in a farm workplace environment but continued to live in normal agricultural environments, demonstrated a decrease in $CD8^+$ suppressor cells and a recovery of the $CD4^+$ helper cell populations within the period of six months.

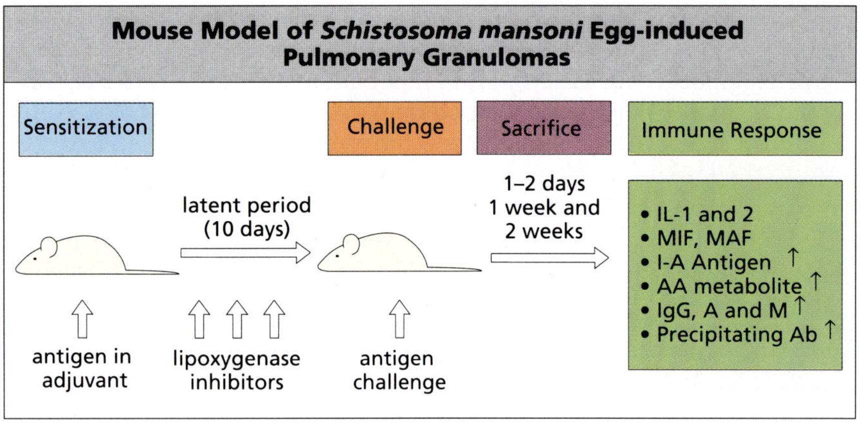

Fig. 16.14 Mice were sensitized with antigen in adjuvant, and left for a 10-day latent period. Subsequent antigen challenge resulted in hypersensitivity-type lung granulomas associated with synthesis of macrophage-derived lipoxygenase derivatives (LTC4, LTD4, 5-HETE, and 12-HETE). Animals also showed increased levels of interleukin and of other lymphokines such as MIF, as well as increased Ia antigen expression by alveolar macrophages. Marked suppression of these experimental pulmonary granulomas is achieved with the use of lipoxygenase anticycloxygenase activity.

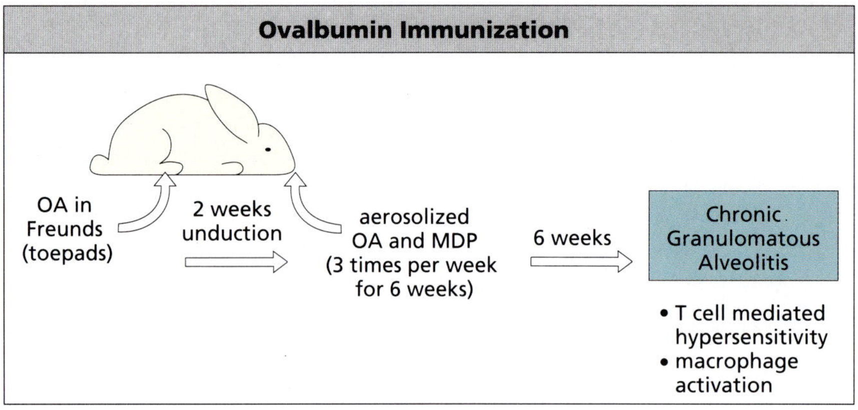

Fig. 16.15 Immunization with ovalbumin in Freund's adjuvant via the toepad, followed by aerosol antigen challenge with muramyl dipeptide on multiple occasions results in the appearance of chronic granulomatous alveolitis with evidence of T-cell-mediated hypersensitivity and macrophage activation.

Immunoregulatory Events in Experimental and Human Allergic Alveolitis

Experimental pulmonary granulomas resembling those seen in human AA have been inhibited by a variety of agents, including corticosteroids, an anti-macrophage serum, neonatal thymectomy, cobra factor venom, and the immunosuppressant cyclosporin. Cyclosporin has also been shown to suppress the anamnestic antibody response in previously sensitized rabbits when it is administered before challenge (Figs 16.15 and 16.16). Experimental pulmonary granulomas have also been associated with the development of anergy (i.e., inhibition of delayed-type hypersensitivity).

Lymphoid cells from anergic granuloma-bearing animals have demonstrated suppressed IL-2 production in response to specific antigens, together with suppressed antigen-induced proliferative responses in studies *ex vivo*. Conversely, delayed-type hypersensitivity responses in several experimental animal models correlate well with enhanced IL-2 production, and IL-2-dependent T helper cells play a prominent role in the production of delayed hypersensitivity responses. Thus, it is significant that suppressor cells which inhibit antigen-induced production of IL-2 by sensitized lymphocytes are prominent in anergic granuloma-bearing mice. A T-cell suppressor/effector factor (TseF) has also been described in certain granulomas induced by schistosome eggs during their chronic modulatory phase. TseF is a soluble protein that induces genetically restricted and antigenically specific suppression of granuloma formation *in vivo*. It has also been reported to inhibit the formation of acute-phase granulomas. In experimental models of AA, other suppressor factors from alveolar macrophages have been shown to inhibit granuloma formation both *in vivo* and *in vitro*. This evidence suggest that granuloma formation and the associated anergy observed in experimental models of AA are the likely result of cell-mediated immunity and associated immunoregulatory events. The data also suggest that the anergy associated with these granulomas may be due to impaired antigen-induced IL-2 production, perhaps caused by suppressor T cells or soluble mediators derived from them.

Experimental animals which demonstrate chronic pulmonary granulomatous inflammation can also be 'desensitized' following a series of antigen challenges given either by aerosol or intravenously (Fig. 16.17). The resulting desensitization is associated with decreased T-cell-dependent hypersensitivity, and is non-transferable with immune serum. It is associated with the diminution of the characteristic pulmonary granulomatous lesions. This type of desensitization appears to be mediated in part by a population of activated antigen-specific suppressor T cells. This negative modulatory effect can also be transferred to normal recipient animals with non-antigen-specific suppressor macrophages or lymphocytes. These desensitization studies provide further evidence that experimental granulomatous pulmonary lesions are modulated by suppressor factors after repeated antigen exposure.

The ability of several agents to inhibit experimental lesions, particularly antilipoxygenase compounds, corticosteroids, and cyclosporine, may also prove to be of practical therapeutic importance in man.

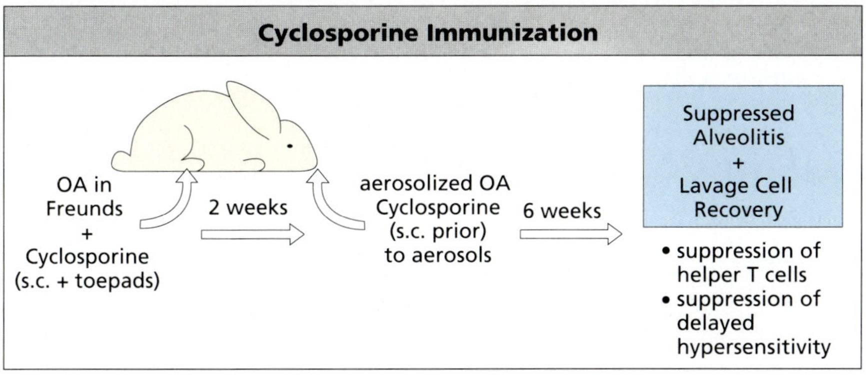

Fig. 16.16 Administration of cyclosporine prior to antigen challenge suppresses the granulomatous pulmonary lesions plus the anamnestic antibody response in previously sensitized rabbits .

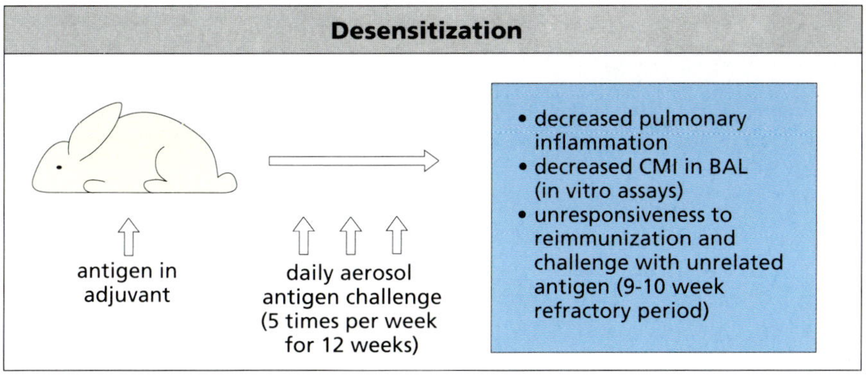

Fig. 16.17 Animals immunized with antigen in Freund's adjuvant followed by daily aerosol antigen challenge over 12 weeks exhibit progressive decrease in pulmonary inflammation, with decreased cell-mediated immunity. They also exhibit unresponsiveness to reimmunization and challenge with an unrelated antigen over a 'refractory period' of nine to ten weeks following this 'desensitization'. Such desensitization is immunospecific and associated with T-cell-dependent hypersensitivity.

Therapy

The correct management of patients with AA necessitates recognition and elimination of the aetiological agents and removal from the offending environment. (Fig. 16.18). Elimination of antigen from the patient's environment will help control the disease (and prevent sensitization in other exposed individuals). For example, simply altering the moisture content or pH of mouldy bagasse has resulted in the diminution and even the disappearance of bagossosis in those areas of the world where it was originally described. Certain other organic dusts can be rendered sterile by exposing the fibres to high temperatures. In the case of humidifier lung, frequent cleaning and changing of the water in the humidifier should prevent growth of micro-organisms. Effective indoor ventilation systems may greatly diminish respiratory dusts. When elimination of the antigen is not feasible, or if the aetiological agent has not been identified, the best approach is to remove the patient from the work environment. An alternative approach (though this is markedly less effective) is the continual wearing of protective face masks by the workers; depending upon the degree of efficiency of the masks, they may diminish the amount of antigen inhaled.

Many mild acute febrile episodes will abate spontaneously when the patient is removed from the offending work environment. Severe attacks require treatment with corticosteroids at doses equivalent to prednisone 40mg or more per day. Other routine supportive measures, including oxygen, bed rest, and bronchodilators, if some element of bronchospasm is present, may be helpful. Prednisolone is often continued for two weeks or longer until significant clinical and radiological improvement is noted and pulmonary function tests return to near normal. The Prednisone dosage is then slowly tapered and eventually discontinued.

Little is known about the natural history and prognosis of AA after chronic long-term exposure. One study of patients with Farmer's lung revealed a five-year morbidity rate of 30 per cent; respiratory disability in these cases was caused mainly by pulmonary fibrosis.

Summary

AA develops as a result of a complex series of events involving initial non-specific inflammation, followed by immunologically specific sensitization, and a genetically-controlled granulomatous inflammatory response. An overview of the complex series of currently known events which are probably operative in the pathogenesis and regulation of AA is shown in schematic form in Fig. 16.19.

The clearly established link between this granulomatous lung disease and evironmental inhaled antigens, as well as the protective reversibility of the

Therapy and Prevention Principles

- Recognition of aetiological agent(s)
- Elimination of aetiological agent(s)
- Alteration of offending microorganism growth
- Removal of patient from offending environment
- Corticosteroids (prednisone 40 mg/day or equivalant)
- Supportive measures (0_2 therapy, bedrest)

Fig. 16.18 Principles of therapy and prevention in allergic alveolitis.

process, emphasises the importance of establishing an early diagnosis, and in particular of taking the necessary steps to identify the offending aetiological agent(s). If left untreated, AA may progress into an irreversible phase characterized by the predominance of pulmonary fibrosis.

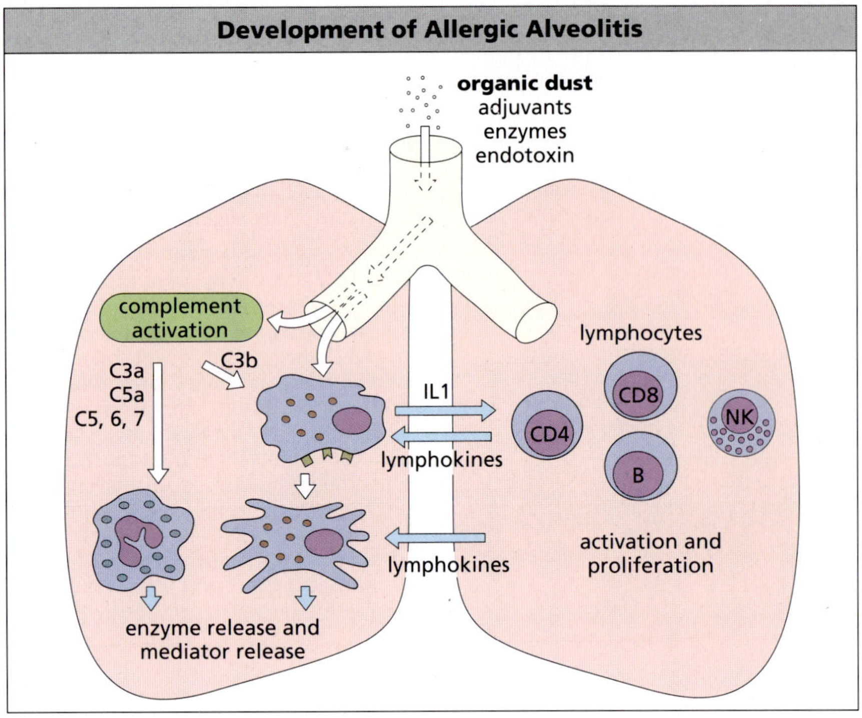

Fig. 16.19 In this simplistic scheme, organic dust antigens, which contain large amounts of enzymes, endotoxin and immunological adjuvant activity are inhaled, resulting in an initial non-specific activation of the complement system in resident alveolar macrophages, leading to early chemoattraction of neutrophils and further recruitment of macrophages into the lesions. Antigen is appropriately presented to resident bronchoalveolar T and B cells by dendritic cells or macrophages and macrophage-derived IL-1; in addition, other cytokines are released. These mediators lead to clonal expansion of T helper/suppressor cells, NK cells, and B cells in the lung. B cells subsequently produce antibody and a wide array of cytokines. Macrophage- and T-cell-derived suppressor factors are also produced, which ultimately modulate or dampen the granulomatous response.

Further Reading

Fink JN, Ventilation pneumonitis. In: *Humidifiers and Air- conditioners Diseases*. Molina C, eds. Paris, Inserm, 1986; 29–36.

Fink JN, Moore VL. Experimental hypersensitivity pulmonary granulomas. In: *Basic and Clinical Aspects of Granulomatous Diseases*. Boros D, Yoshida T, eds. New York, Elsevier North Holland, 1981; 173–178.

Harris JO, Bice D, Salvaggio JE. Cellular and humoral bronchopulmonary immune responses of rabbits immunized with thermophilic actinomycete antigen. *Am Rev Respir Dis* 1976; **114**:29.

Kawai T, Tamara M, Muroa M. Summer-type hypersensitivity pneumonitis: A unique disease in Japan. *Chest* 1984; **85**:311.

Kopp WC, Diercks SE, Butler JE, Upadrashta BS, Richerson HB. Cyclosporine immunomodulation in a rabbit model of chronic hypersensitivity pneumonitis. *Am Rev Respir Dis* 1985; **132**:1027–1033.

Lopez M, Salvaggio JE. Hypersensitivity pneumonitis. In: Murray JF, Nadel HA, eds. *Textbook of Respiratory Medicine*. Philadelphia, W.B. Saunders Company, 1988; 1606–1616.

Pepys J. Hypersensitivity diseases of the lungs due to fungi and organic dusts. In: *Monographs in Allergy*, Vol. 4. Basel: Karger Publishing Company, 1969.

Salvaggio JE. Hypersensitivity pneumonitis. (Robert Cook Memorial Lecture) *J Allergy Clin Immun* 1987; **79(4)**,558–571.

Takizawa H, Ohta K, Hitai K, Misaki Y, Horiuchi T, Kobayashi N, Shiga J, Miyamoto T. Mast cells are important in the development of hypersensitivity pneumonitis. *J Immun* 1989; **143**:1982–1988

Trentin L, Marcer G, Chilosi M, Sci MC, Zambello R, Agostini G, Masciarelli M, Bizzotto R, Gemignani C, Cipriani A, Di Vittorio G, Semenzato G. Longitudinal study of alveolitis in hypersensitivity pneumonitis patients: An imunologic evaluation. *J Allergy Clin lmmun* 1988; **10**:577–585 .

Wilson BD, Mondloch VM, Katzenstein A-L, Moore VL. Hypersensitivity pneumonitis in rabbits. Modulation of pulmonary inflammation by long-term aerosol challenge with antigen. *J Allergy Clin Immun* 1984; **74**:180–184.

Yoshizawa Y, Ohdama S, Tanoue M, Tanaka M, Ohtsuka M, Uetake K, Hasegawa S. Analysis of bronchoalveolar lavage cells and fluids in patients with hypersensitivity pneumonitis: Possible role of chemotactic factors in the pathogenesis of disease. *Int Archs Allergy Appl Immun* 1986; **68(3)**:226–234.

Salvaggio JE. Immune reations in allergic alveolitis. *Eur Respir J* 1991; **4(13).**

Chapter 17

Rhinitis – Pathophysiology and Classification

Introduction

The diagnosis of rhinitis is based on the subjective reporting of nasal complaints in the absence of upper respiratory tract infection, other diseases, or structural abnormalities. Most people will experience nasal symptoms at times as a normal defence mechanism, and the threshold at which such symptoms are perceived as a problem will vary. To date, investigations for rhinitis have low sensitivity and specificity, and thus the diagnosis must be made predominantly on the basis of the clinical history.

Definition of rhinitis

Symptoms of rhinitis lasting for at least one hour a day on most days are considered abnormal, but this may exclude a proportion of cases with mild disease. Diary recording of symptoms and their circumstances over a two-week period may be helpful in borderline cases.

Clinical Features of Rhinitis

Rhinitis is commonest in patients aged 15–25, and is rare in patients over 45. As with other allergic diseases, the prevalence of rhinitis is steadily increasing (Fig. 17.1).

Patients present with nasal irritation, sneezing, rhinorrhoea, and nasal blockage; these may occur in relation to exposure to known allergens, most frequently pollens and household pets. Often an allergic trigger cannot be identified. Many of these patients have perennial symptoms which may be related to allergens like the house dust mite. In some patients there is no evidence of allergy; some of these have vasomotor rhinitis and the major symptom is rhinorrhoea. In the remaining patients, no allergen can be detected but symptoms are similar to allergic rhinitis (Fig.17.2).

It is important to be aware of other diseases which may present with nasal symptoms. Uncharacteristic

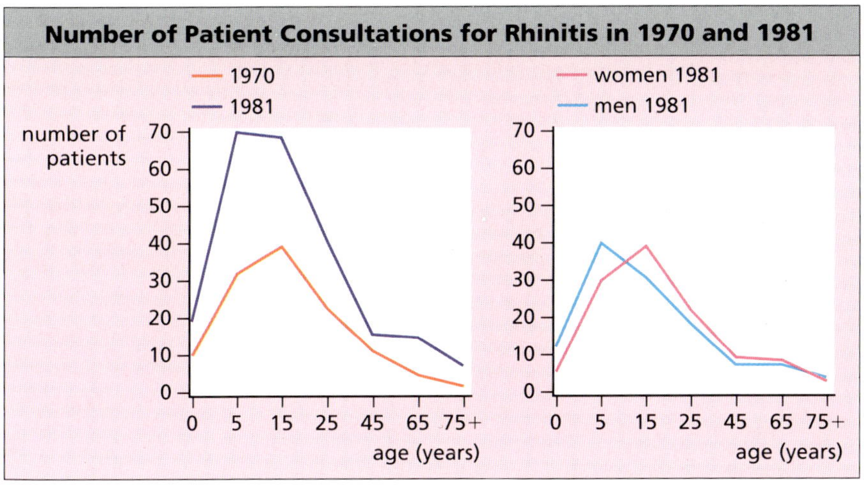

Fig. 17.1 Number of patients consulting their family doctor for treatment for rhinitis in the UK in 1970 and 1981 [left]; number of men and women consulting their family doctor for treatment of rhinitis in the UK 1981 [right]. (From Fleming D M, Crombie DL. *Br Med J* 1987; ***294***: 279–83, with permission.)

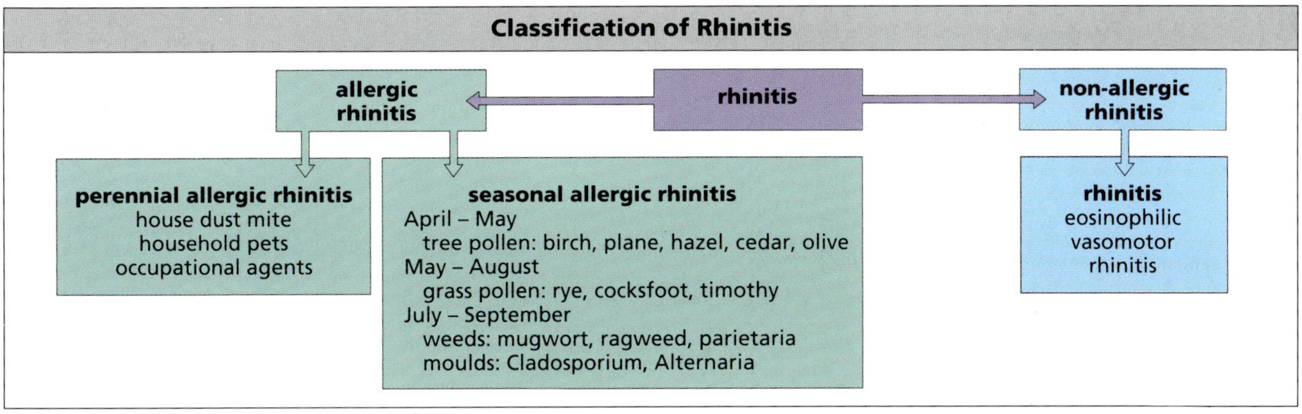

Fig. 17.2 Classification of rhinitis.

features, such as unilateral nasal blockage, bleeding, or pain, may suggest other pathologies – malignant tumours or Wegener's granulomatosis, for example. In infants, unilateral nasal blockage and discharge may also be caused by the presence of a foreign body or, rarely, congenital choanal atresia. Septal deviation, whether congenital or traumatic, may cause nasal blockage, but it is unlikely to be noticed for the first time in adulthood unless there is superadded rhinitis. Chronic infective rhinosinusitis can usually be differentiated by its predominantly greenish secretions and infective exacerbations, although it can occur in association with perennial rhinitis because of impaired drainage from the sinuses.

Allergic Rhinitis

Atopy, defined as the ability to produce high levels of IgE directed against common allergens, is very prevalent in young adults, with approximately 50 per cent of those aged 18–45 having at least one positive skin prick test to common inhalant allergens. The prevalence of allergic rhinitis is around 10 per cent in the 15–25 year age group; approximately half of these seek medical advice (see Fig. 17.1).

Factors Contributing to the Development of Rhinitis

- inheritance of atopy
- predisposition to eosinophil and basophil/mast cell differentiation in atopic individuals
- male gender: raised cord blood IgE at birth
- birth month variation: spring and summer
- viral infection: raises IgE and is associated with onset of allergic disease
- family size and position in the family
- parental smoking: maternal smoking in pregnancy and passive smoking in the home
- damp housing: allergic sensitization to mites and moulds
- urban pollution as an adjuvant to sensitization
- prevalent allergens at different geographical locations
- food additives: metabisulphite
- occupational agents

Fig. 17.3 Factors contributing to the development of rhinitis.

It is likely that allergic sensitization occurs in very early life when the immune system is immature (Fig. 17.3). The inheritance of atopy is likely to be polygenic. Gene linkage studies have suggested an autosomal dominant inheritance for elevated total IgE levels, but there are several levels of genetic control for specific and total IgE, skin test positivity, and disease specificity. There is also a higher prevalence of rhinitis in boys than girls; this may be genetically determined, as IgE levels are higher in boys from birth. Total IgE is also influenced by environmental factors such as cigarette smoking.

Environmental influences in the first year of life are important in the onset of allergic disease. Rhinitis is commoner in those born in spring and summer, which was initially thought to indicate the influence of tree or grass pollen exposure in the first weeks of life; however, non-atopic rhinitis is also commoner in those born in spring and summer, indicating that factors other than environmental pollens are responsible for this seasonality (Fig. 17.4). Infants born in spring or summer might be exposed to winter viral respiratory infection at a vulnerable time when protective maternal immunoglobulins have fallen to a very low level. There is evidence that early respiratory infections have a role in initiating IgE dysregulation, a fundamental feature of allergic disease. The onset of allergic disease in children born to atopic parents is temporally related to early respiratory infections. Detailed studies of infants with respiratory syncytial virus bronchiolitis have shown the presence of virus-specific IgE and raised total circulating IgE, which suggests a direct association of viral infection with IgE production.

Socio-economic factors are also important. A strong inverse relationship of hay fever with family size has been noted, with first-born children being at

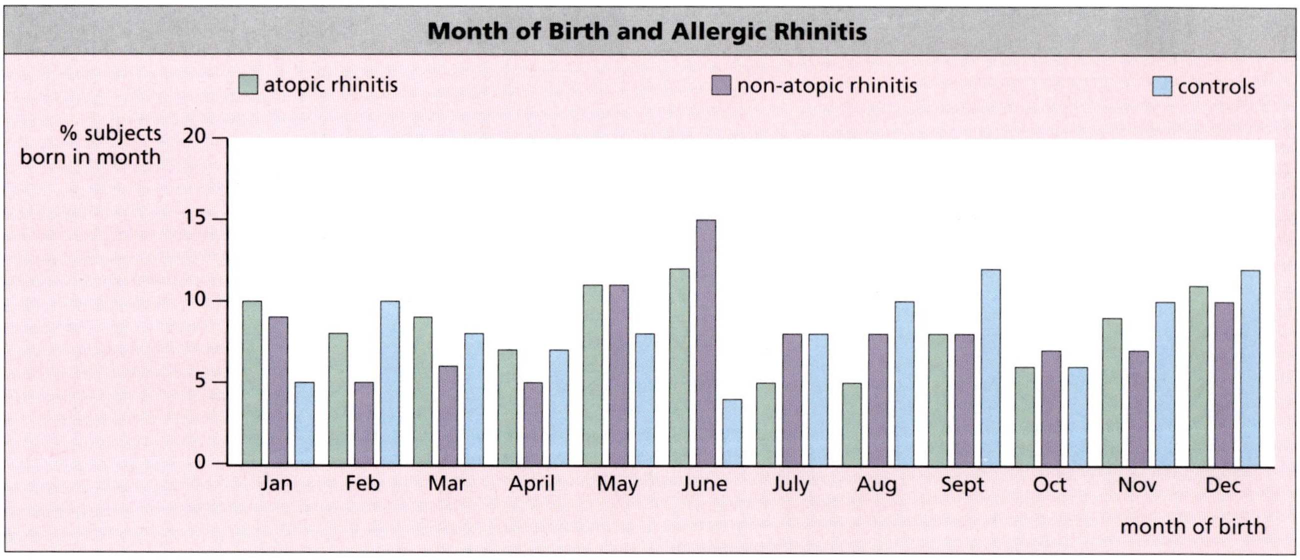

Fig. 17.4 The influence of month of birth on risk of development of rhinitis; showing an increased prevalence of both atopic and non-atopic rhinitis among individuals born in May and June. (From Sibbald B, Rink E. *Clin Allergy* 1990; ***20***: 285–8, with permission.)

greatest risk. Both relationships are independent of the social class of the father. Parental smoking contributes to allergic sensitization. It is associated with wheezing and the risk of rhinitis in infants and young children. The relative risk of rhinitis is doubled for children who live in damp houses and have parents who smoke. Modern energy-efficient 'tight' buildings encourage the growth of house dust mites and moulds because of higher humidity and warmth, and so increase exposure to potential allergens.

Environmental pollution also contributes to allergic sensitization, and epidemiological studies in Japan have shown that the prevalence of Japanese cedar pollen rhinitis is higher in urban than rural environments. Studies in mice have also shown that diesel exhaust particles have an adjuvant effect on sensitization to ovalbumin when both are inoculated intranasally.

The important allergens in allergic rhinitis vary in different parts of the world. Grass pollinosis is commonest in the United Kingdom, whereas in some parts of North America, ragweed predominates, and in Scandinavia, birch pollen is common (Fig. 17.5). Parietaria (a nettle-like weed) and olive tree pollen are common allergens in the Mediterranean. In tropical climates, allergenic pollens may be present all year round; consequently the symptoms of pollen allergy may be perennial. Conversely, classically perennial allergens, such as the house dust mite, provoke seasonal symptoms in temperate climates where there are increased levels of mite allergens during the autumn (Fig. 17.5).

Moulds are uncommon causes of allergic rhinitis. Owing to the small size of the mould spores, they are more likely to be deposited in the lower airway by gravity-dependent sedimentation or inertial impaction than in the upper airway by turbulent airflow. Recently a syndrome of allergic aspergillus sinusitis (AAS) has been recognized, in which patients may have symptoms of rhinitis, sinusitis, and sometimes nasal polyps. The condition is similar to allergic bronchopulmonary aspergillosis (ABPA) and casts are sometimes blown from the nose during exacerbations. Commonly the two conditions co-exist. As with ABPA, AAS responds to corticosteroid administration.

Food allergens are also sometimes a source of symptoms, particularly in children, but rhinitis is very uncommon as an isolated feature of food allergy. Some food additives, such as metabisulphite, can also provoke generalized allergic symptoms, including the symptoms of rhinitis.

Occupational agents also cause allergic rhinitis (Fig. 17.5). In fact, rhinitis is a commoner manifestation of sensitization than asthma, the nasal mucosa being more accessible to deposition of dusts and vapours. Some agents, such as baker's flour, isocyanates, wood dusts, and animal allergens, clearly cause an IgE-mediated response.

Non-Allergic Rhinitis

Non-allergic rhinitis is defined by the absence of positive skin prick tests or radio-allergosorbent test (RAST) to common allergens. In practice, this is dependent on there being no offending allergen apparent from the clinical history. Furthermore, advancing age is associated with a lower IgE and reduced prevalence of skin prick test positivity. This may be a confounding factor when assigning rhinitics into atopic and non-atopic subgroups. Such age-related changes contribute to the fall in the apparent prevalence of allergy among perennial rhinitics from around 80 per cent in childhood to under 20 per cent in elderly people. Epidemiological studies of a population of nearly 3 000 patients in Tucson, Arizona have shown that the prevalence of symptoms of rhinitis is as high as 30 per cent even in those with very low age-adjusted serum IgE scores. This emphasizes that there is a non-allergic subgroup to rhinitis.

The contribution of environmental pollutants and occupational agents to non-allergic rhinitis is uncertain. Well-recognized occupational sensitizers do not necessarily involve an IgE-mediated mechanism. For instance, under 20 per cent of patients sensitized to isocyanates have a raised specific IgE level. It is likely that there are many unrecognized agents which may contribute to development of rhinitis.

Non-allergic rhinitis may be subdivided into eosinophilic and vasomotor subgroups. Some authorities have included all non-allergic rhinitics under the term vasomotor rhinitis. As 'vasomotor' implies a predominantly vascular component to the disease, it seems appropriate to reserve this term for those who cannot be shown to have features of an inflammatory process. The presence of eosinophils in nasal secretions may be demonstrated by light microscopy. Patients with a history of predominantly watery rhinorrhoea who do not have eosinophilic secretions may be included in the vasomotor subgroup. The eosinophilic subgroup is very similar to allergic rhinitis, except for the absence of an identifiable allergen.

Nasal Polyps

Nasal polyps occur most commonly in males aged between 30 and 40. In childhood they are predominantly associated with cystic fibrosis. The polyps of cystic fibrosis differ in that nasal secretions are

Major Allergens Worldwide
Major pollen allergens
Grasses and weeds ragweed (USA) Bermuda grass (USA) timothy grass (UK) cocksfoot (orchard) grass (UK)
Trees silver birch (Sweden) Japanese cedar (sugi tree) (Japan) oak (USA and UK) mesquite tree (South Africa, South America, and Asia)
Domestic and occupational allergens
mite domestic pets flour (bakers) solder (solderers)

Fig. 17.5 Major pollen allergens worldwide.

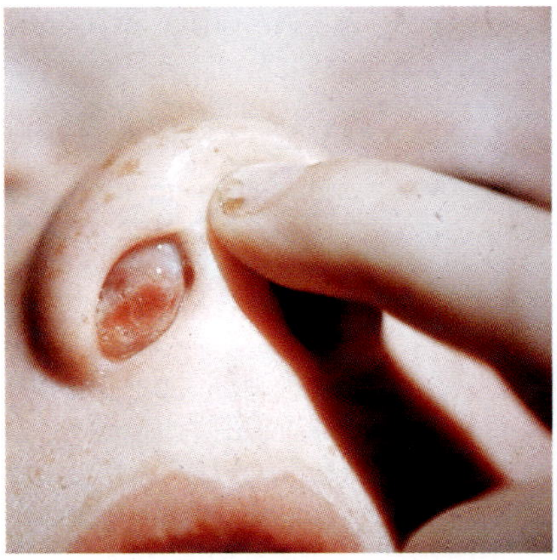

Fig. 17.6. Nasal polyps. (Courtesy of Mr D Gatland, St Bartholomew's Hospital, London.)

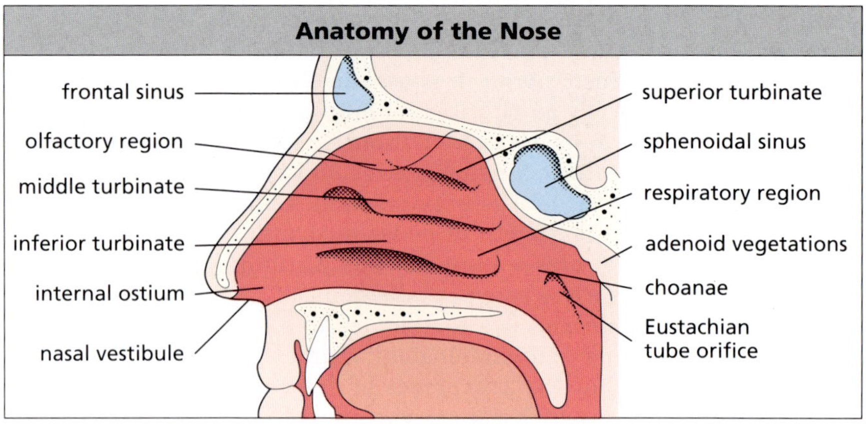

Fig. 17.7 Gross nasal anatomy in a sagittal section.

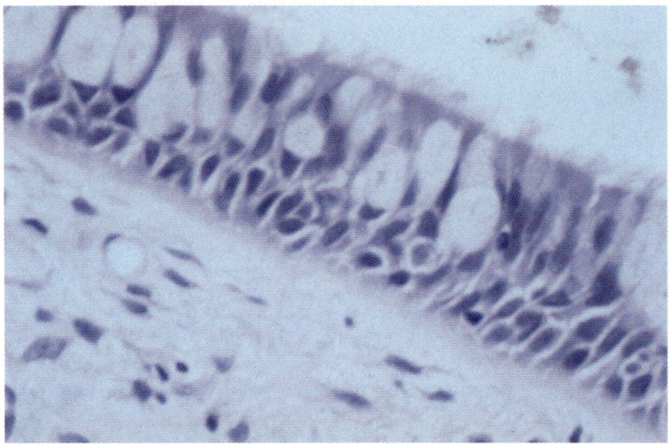

Fig. 17.8 Pseudostratified ciliated columnar epithelium of the nasal mucosa. (Courtesy of Dr M Calderon-Zapata, St Bartholomew's Hospital, London.)

purulent with a high neutrophil content, and they respond poorly to corticosteroids.

The more commonly found nasal polyps may occur in association with both asthma (7 per cent of cases) and rhinitis (2 per cent), but they do not have a clearly allergic aetiology, despite predominant nasal secretion eosinophilia. In fact, polyps are commoner in non-atopic asthmatics than atopic asthmatics. There is an association of nasal polyposis with asthma and aspirin sensitivity, but the mechanism is unknown. The predominant symptoms are nasal blockage and anosmia, sometimes with watery discharge. Symptoms are rarely unilateral, although this may occur with choanal polyps in teenagers, which arise from the maxillary sinuses. More usually, nasal polyps arise from the ethmoid sinuses as well as from the mucosa overlying the turbinates. They can be seen at rhinoscopy as pale grey-yellow rounded masses (Fig. 17.6). They can cause purulent sinusitis due to obstruction of the ostia of the paranasal sinuses.

Normal Nasal Anatomy and Physiology

The nasal cavity commences at the internal ostium, a narrow slit-like orifice about 1.5 cm from the nostrils. The internal ostium is the narrowest part of the respiratory tract with a cross-sectional area of approximately 0.3 cm^2. The inferior, middle, and superior turbinates form the lateral wall, and the nasal septum forms the medial wall of the nasal cavity. The turbinates contribute to the irregular outline of the nasal cavity, which is important to its air-conditioning and air-filtering functions. The nasolacrimal duct opens into the inferior meatus, the portion of the nasal cavity lateral to the inferior turbinate. The orifices of the frontal, maxillary, and anterior ethmoidal sinuses open into the middle meatus, lateral to the middle turbinate (Fig. 17.7).

The epithelium changes from stratified squamous in the nasal vestibule to a squamous and transitional epithelium lining the anterior one-third of the cavity. The remaining portion is lined by ciliated pseudo stratified columnar epithelium typical of the respiratory tract (Fig. 17.8), except in the upper part of the cavity where olfactory epithelium is present. The number of goblet cells is highest in the posterior nasal cavity, similar to that in the trachea and main bronchi.

The epithelium rests on the basement membrane (lamina lucida, lamina densa, and lamina reticularis), a layer of connective tissue composed of collagens type III, IV, and V, laminin, and fibronectin (Fig. 17.9). The underlying lamina propria is characterized by high vascularity. The arterioles have no internal elastic lamina and a porous basement membrane, which increases permeability and allows greater access for pharmacological agents. There is an extensive capillary network, and the capillaries are fenestrated, allowing rapid transit of fluid across the capillary wall. Large cavernous vascular sinusoids are present in the lamina propria on the turbinates. These contribute to heating and humidification of inspired air. Beneath the lamina propria is periosteum and bone.

Innervation

Sensory innervation

The trigeminal nerve supplies afferent (sensory) fibres to the nasal mucous membrane. Activation of these fibres produces the sensations of irritation or pain, which often result in sneezing (Fig. 17.10).

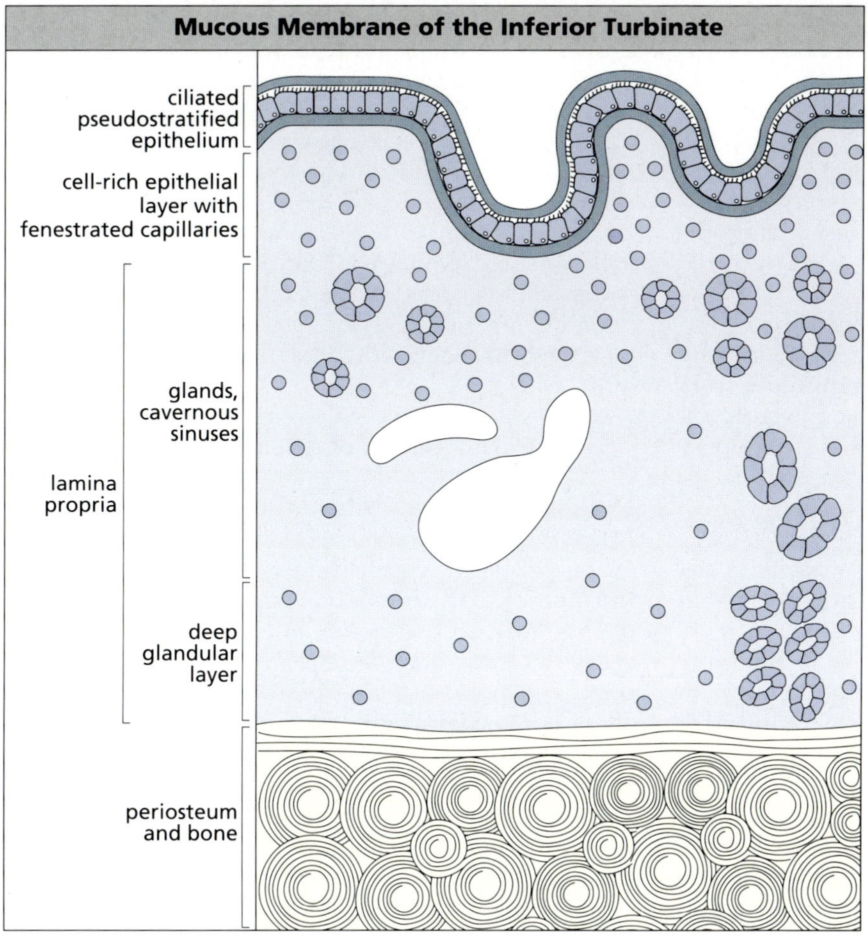

Fig. 17.9 Diagram of the mucous membrane of the inferior turbinate.

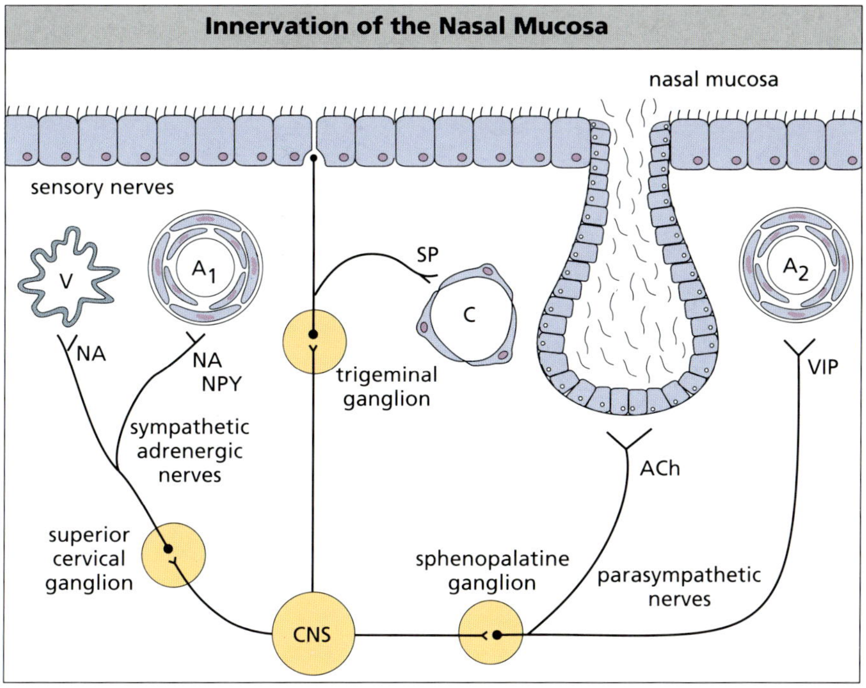

Fig. 17.10 The innervation of the nasal mucosa. SP: substance P; NA: noradrenaline; NPY: neuropeptide Y; ACh: acetylcholine; VIP: vasoactive intestinal polypeptide; C: capillaries; A_1: resistance arteries; A_2: arteries supplying glands; V: venous sinusoids.

Vascular innervation

Sympathetic fibres predominate. Release of co-transmitters noradrenaline and neuropeptide Y causes vasoconstriction. The sympathetic fibres follow the blood vessels and sympathetic tone maintains contraction of the sinusoids. Sympathetic tone fluctuates throughout the day with an increase in patency in alternate nostrils every two to four hours (the nasal cycle).

Parasympathetic fibres, arising in the sphenopalatine ganglion to form the vidian nerve, control vasodilatation and glandular secretion. The parasympathetic co-transmitters are acetylcholine and vasoactive intestinal peptide. Axon reflexes can be powerful in the nasal mucosa, resulting in vasodilatation and transudation with thickening of the mucosa. Axon reflexes may be initiated by the effect of irritants and inflammatory mediators at sensory nerve endings and the transmitters include sensory neuropeptides, substance P, neurokinin A, and calcitonin gene-related peptide. Additionally, sensory nerve activation can cause vasodilatation via neural connections from the trigeminal to the sphenopalatine ganglia and via central nervous reflexes. There are also nasobronchial reflexes which may be activated in asthmatics to promote reflex vasodilatation.

Control of mucus secretion
Mucus is secreted by goblet and serous cells in the epithelium, by submucosal serous glands, and by deep nasal glands. It is diluted by transudate from the blood vessels. Secretion is controlled by parasympathetic cholinergic nerves, but sympathetic stimulation and axon reflexes will also enhance secretion.

Functions of the Nose
Aside from the sense of smell, the nose provides 'air-conditioning' of inspired air and filtration of potentially harmful particulate matter (Fig. 17.11).

The nose has a remarkable capacity to humidify inspired air, raising the temperature of room air to 32°C, and humidifying it to 98 per cent relative humidity before it reaches the lungs. This is effected by fluid shift across the highly vascular mucosa and increasing blood flow through the sinusoids.

The narrow, irregular shape of the nasal cavity promotes turbulent airflow which contributes to impaction of inhaled particles in the upper airway, a protective function against the inhalation of potentially harmful particles into the bronchial tree. Pollen grains which are around 10 μm in size are largely deposited in the nose, whereas turbulent airflow is insufficient to deposit particles less than 2 μm in size in the nose; such particles, e.g. mould spores, will usually reach the distal airways. Particles trapped in the nose are moved into the pharynx by mucociliary transport within 10 to 30 minutes of impaction, and subsequently swallowed. Additionally, 99 per cent of water-soluble gases, such as sulphur dioxide, are prevented from reaching the lower airways because of passage over the nasal mucosa.

Pathogenesis of Allergic Rhinitis

Pathophysiology
Nasal responsiveness
Increased nasal responsiveness can be demonstrated in rhinitics to the inhalation of non-specific challenge agents such as histamine and methacholine. Nasal responsiveness may be measured in terms of symptoms and nasal airway resistance (NAR). Although there is considerable overlap, measurements of NAR show significantly greater histamine responsiveness in rhinitics than in both atopic and non-atopic non-rhinitics (Fig. 17.12). Methacholine does not increase NAR and causes a significant increase in nasal secretion only in rhinitics.

This contrasts with bronchial hyperresponsiveness, in which there is a much closer association with

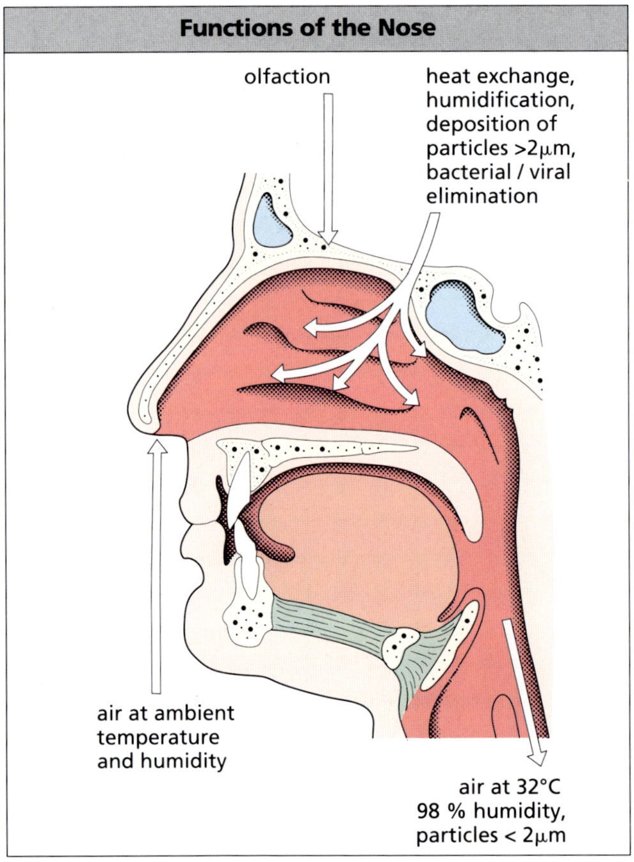

Fig. 17.11 Functions of the nose in warming, humidifying, and filtering inspired air.

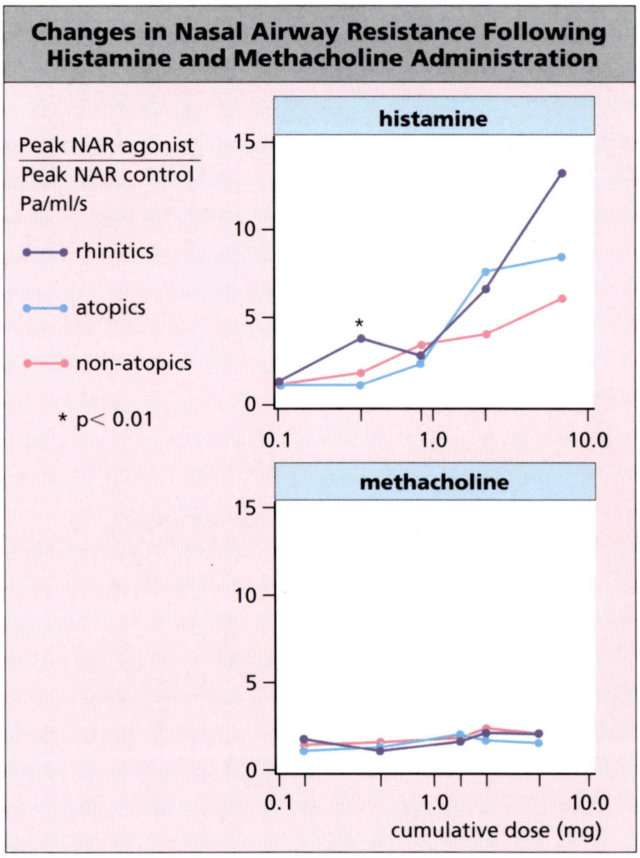

Fig. 17.12 Changes in NAR following the administration of histamine and methacholine (weighted geometric mean change).

symptomatic asthma and a strong correlation between the response to histamine and methacholine (Fig. 17.13). It is likely that the pathogenetic mechanisms of rhinitis and asthma are very similar, with hyperresponsiveness being a cardinal feature in both conditions. The difference in responsiveness of the upper and lower respiratory tract may be explained by the absence of a smooth muscle response in the nose. The action of histamine on the vascular network thus remains effective in reducing airway patency by causing hyperaemia and oedema of the mucosa, whereas methacholine acts predominantly on glandular secretion, with a much less potent effect on vasodilation because of the dominance of sympathetic vasoconstrictor nerves. The importance of vascular congestion as the mechanism of nasal obstruction is demonstrated by the rapid response to vasoconstrictor sprays, which is not a feature of bronchoconstriction in asthma.

Allergen provocation

Early- and late-phase responses may be demonstrated in the nose after inhalation of allergen by sensitized individuals. Late-phase responses occur in approximately 50 per cent of patients between two and eight hours after allergen provocation with an associated increase in symptoms and rise in NAR. The physiological changes of the late phase can be very subtle compared to the intense blockage and symptoms of the early phase (Fig. 17.14). Small increases in NAR during the late phase may be obscured by the nasal cycle. In comparison, the marked late responses which may be demonstrated in the lower airway are probably augmented by a component of smooth muscle constriction.

Priming

During the pollen season, sensitized individuals are exposed for a prolonged time to low levels of pollen. This differs markedly from the artificial conditions of allergen challenge in the laboratory where large doses of allergen are usually required to evoke a response over a short period of time. Thus, during the pollen season, a sensitized person becomes increasingly responsive to allergen, a process known as priming. This may be demonstrated in the laboratory by repeated allergen challenge. The dose of allergen required to elicit a response may be reduced by up to 100 times when challenges are repeated within 24 hours.

Inflammatory Cells and Mediators (see Fig. 17.15)

Mast cells

Studies of the nasal mucosa have shown that the total numbers of mast cells are increased in atopic rhinitics when compared with non-rhinitics. Moreover, the numbers of both mast cells and eosinophils increase in the mucosa during the pollen season. The number of circulating mast cell/basophil progenitors is also increased in such patients and falls during the pollen season, suggesting that these cells are being recruited to the site of allergic inflammation. Atopic individuals are predisposed to the production of cytokines necessary to basophil/mast cell and eosinophil differentiation. In the murine model, mast cells triggered by FcRI cross-linkage secrete interleukins which amplify the inflammatory response through basophil activation (IL-3), IgE synthesis (IL-4), and eosinophil activation (IL-5).

Following allergen inhalation, mast cell degranulation can be shown in nasal mucosal biopsies

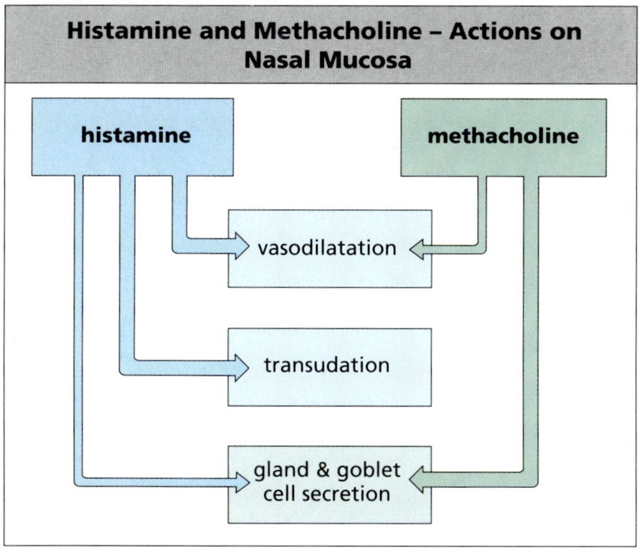

Fig. 17.13 Effects of histamine and methacholine on the nasal mucosa.

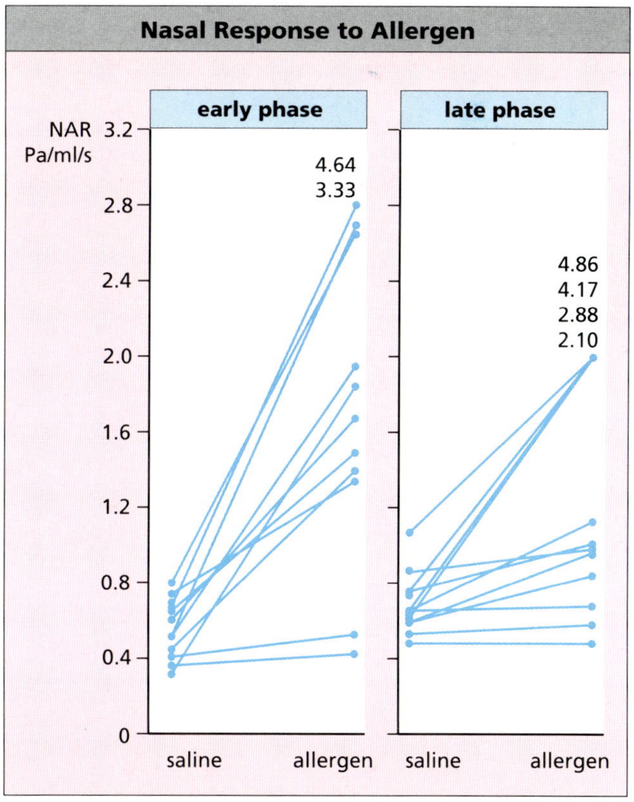

Fig. 17.14 Nasal response to allergen. NAR measurements following saline or grass pollen administration to the nasal mucosa 30 minutes following challenge (early response) and between 2 and 7 hours (late response).

The Effects of Mediators in the Nose		
Mediator	**Action**	**Source**
histamine	vasodilatation, plasma leakage, glandular secretion	mast cells: early phase; basophils: late phase
PGD_2	vasodilatation	mast cells; also platelets, fibroblasts
tryptase	?	mast cells
TAME-esterase	vasodilatation	plasma/glandular kallikrein; mast cell tryptase
LTB_4	eosinophil chemotaxis, neutrophil activation	mast cells; ?neutrophils in late phase
LTC_4 and LTD_4	vasodilatation, increased blood flow	mast cells; eosinophils; neutrophils
kinins	vasodilatation, increased capillary flow	plasma
PAF	vasoconstriction/vasodilatation, eosinophil and neutrophil chemotaxis	macrophages; neutrophils; eosinophils; endothelial cells
ECP, EPO, MBP	epithelial damage	eosinophils

Fig. 17. 15 Mediators which act on the nose, their action, and their source.

(Fig. 17.16) and the presence of mast cell products such as histamine, PGD_2, and tryptase in nasal lavage fluid. Mast cell mediators are responsible for many of the immediate symptoms of nasal allergy. A large number of different mediators have been identified following allergen challenge. Such mediators are derived from mast cell degranulation (histamine, PGD_2) and cell membrane (sulphidopeptide leukotrienes), but also from eosinophils (eosinophil cationic protein, major basic protein), neutrophils (neutrophil peroxidase), platelets (PAF, serotonin), plasma (kinins, complement factors), and nerve endings (VIP, Substance P). The time course of release of some of these mediators is shown in Fig. 17.17, correlating with early- and late-phase responses.

Histamine is the mediator which is most consistently found following allergen challenge. Administration of histamine, albeit at high doses, reproduces the symptoms of nasal allergy, and specific H_1 antagonists reduce such symptoms. The response to other mediators varies; for instance, PAF causes an increase in nasal patency. None of the putative mediators have been shown to cause the ongoing inflammation of a late response. During the late phase, it is thought that basophils are the source of histamine, since it is found in the absence of PGD_2, which excludes the possibility of release from the mast cells. Basophil influx has been demonstrated in nasal lavage fluid during the late-phase response.

TAME-esterase is a non-specific marker of inflammation which represents a mixture of plasma and glandular kallikrein activity and, to a lesser extent, mast cell tryptase activity. Levels of TAME-esterase parallel nasal symptomatology and pollen counts during the pollen season. TAME-esterase is found in nasal secretions following allergen challenge, indicating that plasma leakage is a major component of the allergic response in the nose (Fig. 17.17). It is likely that kinins, complement, and coagulation factors derived from the plasma augment the inflammatory response in the nose. The levels of TAME-esterase and histamine show the features of priming, with an increase following repeated allergen challenge within 24 hours of the initial challenge. The fact that levels of PGD_2 do not increase after repeated allergen challenge is further evidence for the involvement of basophils during the late phase.

Mast cell heterogeneity has been observed in nasal polyp tissue with the tryptase-positive (MC_T) cells predominating in epithelium and the chymase- and tryptase-positive (MT_{TC}) cells being dominant in the lamina propria. The MC_T cells found in the nasal epithelium in rhinitis differ from MC_{TC} cells – they do not stain with saffranin O, which indicates a difference in their granular proteoglycan component, and they do not degranulate in response to the polyamine, compound 48/80. Unlike skin mast cells, those in the nose are sensitive to sodium cromoglycate, which explains the effectiveness of this drug in rhinitis. Mast cells migrate from the lamina propria to the epithelium in response to allergen exposure and differentiate *in situ* under the influence of factors

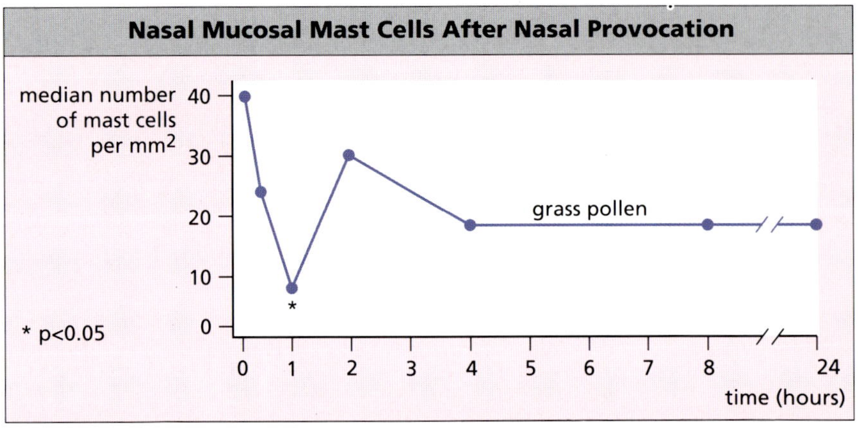

Fig. 17.16 Changes in numbers of mast cells in nasal mucosal biopsies taken at intervals after nasal provocation with grass pollen. The fall in stainable mast cell numbers indicates early degranulation.

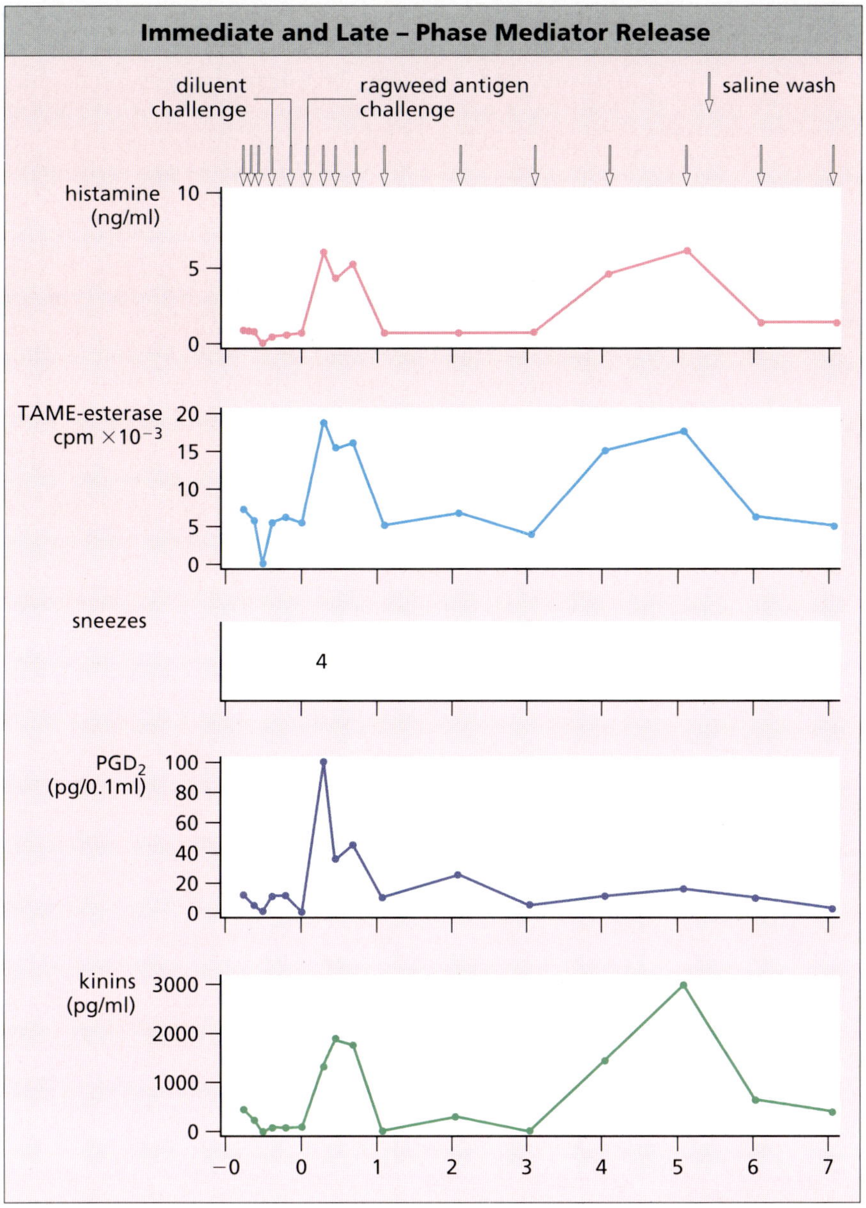

Fig. 17.17 Immediate and late –phasemediator release following nasal provocation with allergen. (From Togias A et al. *Am J Med* 1985; ***79*** (suppl 6a): 26–33, with permission.)

such as cytokines derived from CD4+ T-helper cells, fibroblasts, epithelial cells, and endothelial cells. Their presence at the mucosal surface enhances the rapidity of degranulation following allergen exposure (Fig. 17.18).

Eosinophils

Eosinophil numbers are increased in rhinitics, and rise during the pollen season in pollen-sensitive individuals (Fig 17.19). Eosinophils increase transiently in nasal mucosal biopsies from pollen-sensitive rhinitics 30 minutes after allergen challenge, but the numbers in nasal secretions are persistently raised, and peak at seven to 10 hours. This suggests rapid migration from the mucosa into the secretions. The chemoattractants involved in this process remain to be identified, although they may include leukotriene B4, PAF, and intercellular adhesion molecules (ICAM-1). The eosinophils are activated, with hypodense granules, and can damage nasal epithelial cells cultured *in vitro*, slowing and disorganizing the ciliary beat. The influx of activated eosinophils results in release of toxic granule products, particularly

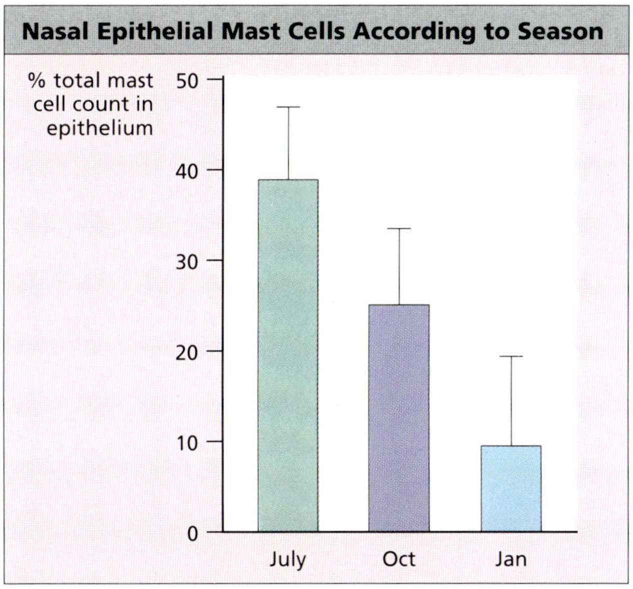

Fig. 17.18 Percentage of total mast cell numbers present in the nasal epithelium in July (in the grass pollen season), compared to October and January, in rhinitics sensitive to grass pollen.

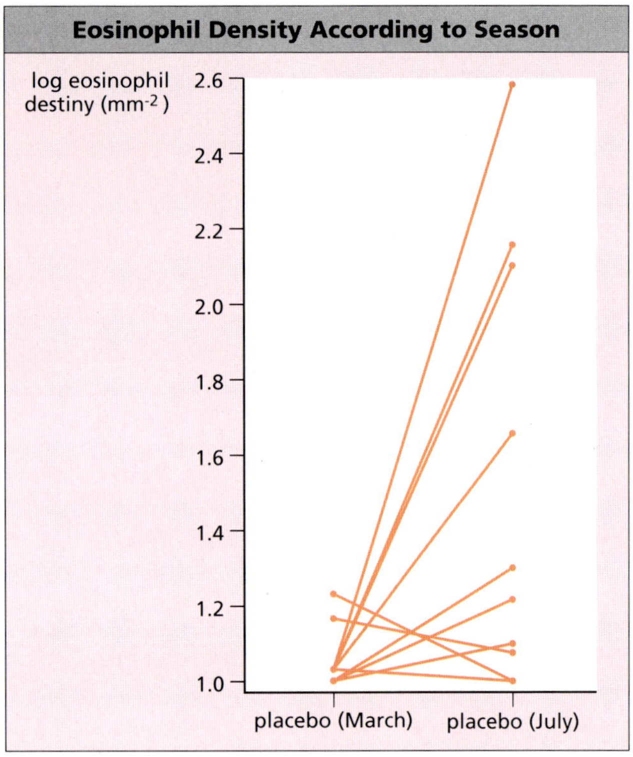

Fig. 17.19 Eosinophil density in rhinitics sensitive to grass pollen before (March) and during (July) the grass pollen season.

eosinophil peroxidase (EPO) and major basic protein (MBP). EPO and MBP are directly toxic to cultured human nasal epithelial cells, causing lysis. Even at low concentrations, MBP can reduce ciliary beat frequency. Such damage may contribute to the inflammatory features of the late-phase response and subsequent nasal hyperresponsiveness.

T cells

There is an imbalance in the cytokine production of T cells from atopics; there is a tendency to produce more IL-4 and IL-5, and less IFN-γ. The number of dendritic or Langerhans' cells at the surface of the nasal epithelium is increased in rhinitics, and these bind allergenic peptides. Interaction of these dendritic cells with T cells promotes differentiation towards the Th 2 type of T cells which produce IL-4 and IL-5, leading to IgE production by plasma cells and eosinophil activation respectively. Indeed, *in situ* hybridization studies show that T cells from atopic asthmatics express messenger RNA for IL-4 and IL-5. In perennial rhinitics, the total number of activated T cells expressing the IL-2 receptor is increased in the nasal mucosa.

Epithelial Cells

Given the similarities between the pathogenesis of asthma and rhinitis, it might be expected that rhinitics would demonstrate evidence of epithelial damage. However, there is no difference between mean epithelial height in pollen-sensitive rhinitics when mucosal biopsies are examined either during or outside the pollen season. The lamina reticularis is not thickened as it is in asthmatics. There is no significant increase in numbers of epithelial cells in nasal lavage specimens following allergen challenge even during the late response. It is likely that epithelial damage only occurs in the context of prolonged inflammation, as with nasal polyps.

Pathogenesis of nasal polyps

The histological features of nasal polyps are more similar to those of asthma than those of allergic rhinitis. There is frequently epithelial damage, epithelial cell shedding, and thickening of the lamina reticularis. There may be squamous metaplasia, and eosinophils and mast cells are present in increased numbers in the epithelium. The stroma of the polyp is grossly oedematous with marked eosinophil infiltration and increased numbers of plasma cells, mast cells, and lymphocytes. Some patients with perennial rhinitis also demonstrate such features to a lesser degree, with evidence of squamous metaplasia, oedema, and increased numbers of inflammatory cells.

Nasal polyp tissue has been used to study local haematopoietic mechanisms. Nasal polyp epithelial cells and fibroblasts are capable of stimulating eosinophil/basophil differentiation in blood from atopic individuals. Additionally, mononuclear cell colonies from nasal polyps yield mainly eosinophil/basophil precursors, indicating an advanced stage of differentiation. High levels of GM-CSF (granulocyte monocyte colony stimulating factor) and also G-CSF (granulocyte-CSF) are present which contribute to this differentiation. Fibroblasts from nasal polyps also demonstrate increased growth *in vitro*.

In contrast to rhinitis, patients with nasal polyps predominantly demonstrate peripheral blood eosinophilia and the counts are increased if asthma is also present. However, such eosinophilia occurs regardless of the presence of allergy. It is possible that secretion of GM-CSF from nasal tissue contributes to differentiation of eosinophil-basophil colonies and to increased eosinophil survival locally or in the systemic circulation.

Further Reading

Davies RJ. Seasonal rhinitis. In: *Rhinitis, mechanisms and management*. Mackay I, ed. Royal Society of Medicine Services Ltd 1989, 97–116.

Mygind N. *Nasal allergy*. Oxford: Blackwell Scientific Publications, 1979.

Mygind N, Weeke B, eds. *Allergic and vasomotor rhinitis: clinical aspects*. Munksgaard: Copenhagen, 1985.

Chapter 18

Allergic Rhinitis – Diagnosis and Treatment

Introduction

The work-up of a patient complaining of upper airway problems consists of the traditional history and physical examination supplemented by critical tests. Sometimes more tedious laboratory, radiological, and morphological examinations are included.

History

A detailed history augmented with specific questions presented either orally on in the form of a written questionnaire is essential to distinguish rhinitis from upper respiratory infections or other nasal complaints. Such a questionnaire should contain the following:

- Is there a family history of atopy?
- What is the symptom profile – is there a dominant nasal symptom such as blockage, sneezes, or nasal secretions?
- Are the nasal problems isolated or are there more extensive symptoms?
- Are there concomitant signs from other parts of the upper airways, such as sinuses or ears?
- Is there a history of lower airway, ocular, or dermatological disease?
- A detailed chronology and description of the symptoms should be obtained.
- Questions about the house environment should include bedding materials, the presence of pets, and the quality of housing.
- Any specific precipitating factors, e.g. flowers.
- Occupation and leisure activities, particularly those which may aggravate symptoms.
- Any relationship to food or drink .

Symptom Presentation

The traditional symptoms are the following: nasal blockage, itching, sneezing bouts, and increased nasal surface fluid, but the dominant symptom may differ from one patient to another. There is also a wide individual variation in terms of the tolerability of nasal symptoms. Some people may find a few bouts of sneezing troublesome, while others do not seek medical advice even when their nasal passage is completely blocked. A detailed symptom score registration may well prove helpful when it comes to assessing the severity of symptoms.

The variability of symptoms may be a result of the difference in the pathogenesis of the major nasal symptoms (see Chapter 17). Nasal blockage is the result of a decrease in the tone of the capacitance vessels and, to a minor degree, tissue oedema. The increase in nasal surface liquid is the result of glandular activity, the leakage of plasma, and the increase in fluids from other sources such as the conjunctiva. Conjunctival symptoms of itching and increase in tear fluid are also very common in association with allergic rhinitis: the term rhinoconjunctivitis is often more relevant.

Physical Examination

Several facial features are associated with the various symptoms of the nasal and ocular disease. These include:

- 'allergic shiners' – infraorbital dark circles, related to venous plexus engorgement;
- 'allergic gape' or continuous open-mouth breathing – a result of nasal blockage;
- 'transversal nasal crease'– a result of the frequent upward rubbing of the nose.

Dental malocclusion and overbite can also result from longstanding upper airway problems.

Rhinoscopic Techniques

A rhinoscopy is essential in the clinical work-up of nasal problems, especially since there are several possible explanations of nasal problems. Simple inspection will reveal any external nasal deformities, but there may also be inner septal deformities. The rhinoscopic examination can be made using the traditional light-mirror, and a nasal speculum to widen the nasal opening. The posterior rhinoscopy is performed with an mirror placed below the soft palate to permit the inspection of the epipharyngeal region. When possible this examination should be supplemented with an endoscopic examination of the nasal cavities and epipharyngeal region. This examination is performed using either a short rigid rhinoscope (see Fig. 18.1) attached to a good light source – of specific help in the examination of the ostial regions – or a short flexible rhinoscope, which is also useful for examining the posterior parts of the nasal cavity, as well as permitting examination of the epipharynx and larynx.

Rhinoscopic Findings

The following should be noted: any structural deformities, the amount and the condition of nasal surface

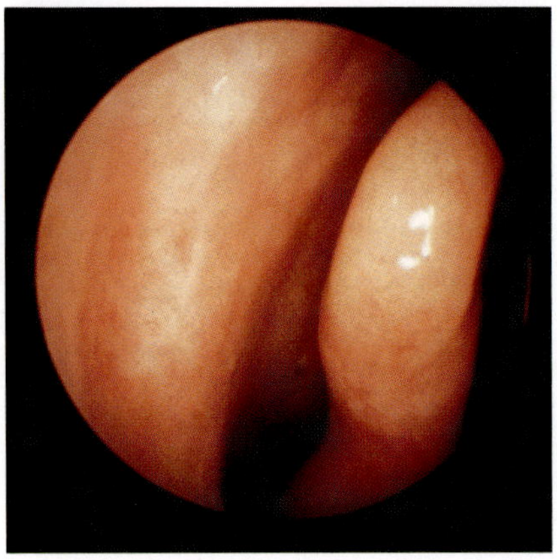

Fig. 18.1 A rigid rhinoscopic examination of a normal nose. The interior of the right nasal cavity is shown, with a straight nasal septum to the right and the middle turbinate on the left. (Courtesy of Jan Kumlien, MD.)

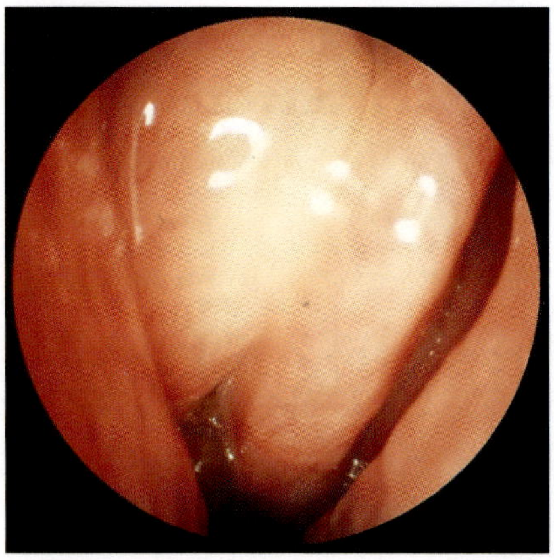

Fig. 18.2 A rigid rhinoscopic examination from a patient with a small nasal polyp in the right nasal cavity, immediately below the middle turbinate. (Courtesy of Jan Kumlien, MD.)

liquids, and the condition of the mucous membranes. Unilateral nasal obstruction may indicate a foreign body. Structural deformities such as septal deviations should be noted, and their site specified. The presence or absence of polyps should be noted (Fig. 18.2). The amount and character of the surface liquid might be useful when it comes to differentiating infection from other conditions. Is there any watery fluid, mucoid fluid, or pus? The condition of the mucous membrane should be evaluated. The colour, texture, and signs of scars or lesions should be specifically evaluated. An allergic condition might be indicated by the traditional bluish tint. Since there are several causes for nasal symptoms (Fig. 18.3), these steps are essential.

Examination of Extranasal Regions

Other regions which should be assessed are the eyes, ears and the dermal costume.

- In the eyes, the presence or absence of conjunctivitis or watering with conjuctival injection and oedema should be noted.
- Since otitis media and middle ear effusions may occur with increased frequency in children with allergic rhinitis, the ears should be examined, looking especially for any middle ear pathology. This is best done using the otomicroscope. Tympanometric examination is also helpful.
- Atopic skin diseases also may occur with increased frequency, so the physician should check for urticaria or eczematous lesions.

Causes of Nasal Symptoms	
Mechanical factors	**Infections**
Septal deviation Nasal polyps Nasopharyngeal tumours Nasal tumours Sinusal tumours Congenital choanal atresia Meningocele	Viral infection Bacterial infection Adenoiditis Sinusitis Leprosy Immunodeficiency
Allergy	**Miscellaneous**
Seasonal allergic rhinitis Perennial allergic rhinitis	Vasomotor rhinitis Rhinitis medicamentosa Pregnancy Kartagener's syndrome Antihypertensives Wegener's granulomatosis Cystic fibrosis Liquorrhoea nasalis Atrophic rhinitis Ozaenae

Fig. 18.3 Causes of nasal symptoms.

Test Procedures

The history and physical examination should be supplemented with an allergen reactivity test.

Skin Tests

The routine test for allergy of the upper airways is the skin prick test (SPT). It should be carried out when there are no other obvious reasons for the nasal symptoms (Fig 18.4). A clear-cut history of seasonal allergic rhinitis in an adult patient who responds favourably to symptomatic treatment does not necessarily require confirmation by an SPT. The SPT panel should include a positive and a negative control and the major airborne allergens for the area in question.

The intracutaneous test is seldom used for the work-up of patients with upper airway problems and should be reserved for specific occasions, as indicated elsewhere.

Blood Tests

The traditional test for allergy has been the determination of blood eosinophilia. High numbers indicate that atopy is present. To some degree the eosinophilia is dependent upon the size of the diseased organ and therefore the usefulness of this test for rhinitis is limited. The same applies to the determination of total IgE. This procedure cannot be used as a screening procedure for the presence of an allergic condition.

An alternative procedure, a multi-RAST, which indicates the presence of a specific IgE to any of the commonest airborne allergens, is useful for screening, however. This could be of value when there are no facilities for performing an SPT. The value of RAST procedures is discussed in Chapter 11. RAST is indicated when it comes to testing for the specific allergens which are not available for skin tests or when an SPT cannot be performed because a patient is taking treatment, e.g. histamine H_1-antagonists, which

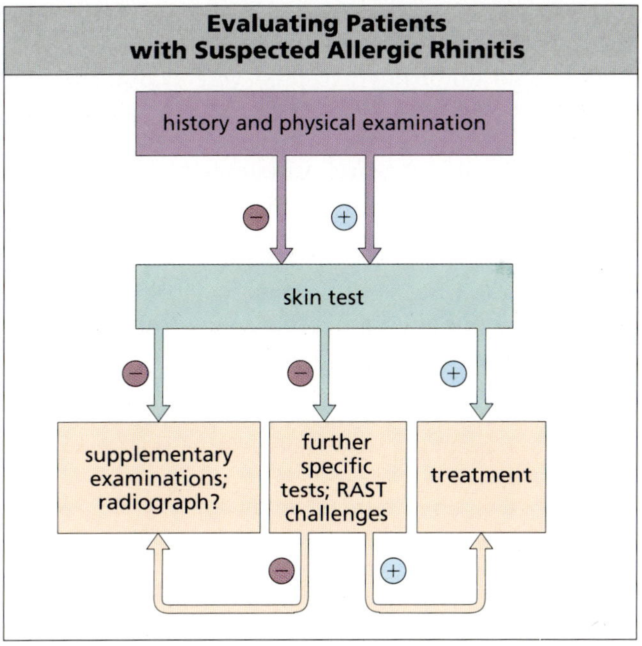

Fig. 18.4 A simplified scheme for evaluating patients with upper airway problems which are suspected of being allergic in origin. If the skin prick test confirms the history, treatment can be instituted. Otherwise, further examinations and tests are indicated.

suppress the cutaneous response. The specific value of other procedures such as the basophil histamine release test is still uncertain.

Nasal Challenge

A nasal challenge can be used to test for specific as well as non-specific reactivity. Non-specific reactivity may be tested using methacholine and histamine as the challenge agents. The test for specific reactivity involves the application of the specific allergens to the nasal mucosa. Some of the tests used to monitor the changes in the challenge situation (Fig. 18.5) may also be used to monitor the progression of disease.

Test for non-specific reactivity

The overlap in the upper airways between normals and 'hyperreactive' patients is greater than in the lower airways and the clinical usefulness of such tests for the assessment of the degree of non-specific reactivity is therefore limited. Methacholine, when given locally in the nasal cavity in the dose range of 0.1–10 mg, will generally produce a monosymptomatic secretory response. A simple way to determine the volume of the rhinorrhoea is to have the subject in a head-forwards position and collect the delivered volume of secretion in a funnel. Alternatively, preweighed tampons may be inserted into the nose to absorb exudate fluid which may be quantified by weighing.

Histamine has also been used to assess the degree of non-specific reactivity. When given locally in the dose-range of 0.1–10 mg, histamine will produce all the nasal symptoms relevant to allergic rhinitis. The evaluation of this response is therefore more complex and may involve the same techniques that are used for the determination of specific reactivity. The clinical usefulness of the histamine challenge is similar to that of methacholine challenge.

Test for specific reactivity

There are some clinical situations that may call for a nasal allergen challenge. These include confirmation or rejection of a suspected allergen where the history and skin test are not completely in agreement. Furthermore, it may sometimes be of interest to see whether a local allergy is present. The bulk of nasal allergen challenges have, however, been performed primarily for research purposes in order to understand nasal pathophysiology and to test potentially beneficial drugs.

There is no generally accepted technique for performing a nasal allergen challenge or for monitoring the clinical response. In the clinical setting, a simple sneeze count and a score for the other symptoms may well be sufficient, but if a graded (quantitative) response is required for research purposes, more complicated techniques are needed. The risks involved in the nasal challenges are minimal and, even if total nasal blockage occurs, other organs are seldom affected.

Challenge of the nasal mucosa

The allergens used should be well characterized and standardized. An aqueous solution is the easiest way of introducing them into the nasal cavity. A widespread distribution of the allergens is obtained using a mechanical pump spray.

Monitoring the nasal reaction

The reaction to allergen comprises three main symptoms: sneezing, nasal blockage, and nasal secretions. All three are relevant and should be monitored.

Sneezing is the result of a central reflex elicited in the sensory nerve endings in the nasal mucosa. It is easy to grade by counting and is the most reproducible of the nasal symptoms in the challenge procedure.

Methods for Monitoring Nasal Symptoms During Active Disease or After Challenge

Sneezes	Blockage	Secretion	Itching
counting symptom score	symptom score nasal peak flow rhinomanometry acoustic rhinometry	symptom score volume measurement weight measurement nasal lavage	symptom score

Fig. 18.5 Methods for monitoring nasal symptoms during active disease or after challenge.

Nasal blockage is the result of the pooling of blood in the capacitance vessels of the mucosa, and to some degree the result of tissue oedema. Nasal blockage can be assessed subjectively by means of symptom scoring; there are several objective techniques which can be used for assessing the degree of nasal blockage: rhinomanometry, which is the determination of nasal airflow/pressure relationships (Fig. 18.6); nasal peak flow determination (Fig. 18.7) and the recently introduced acoustic rhinometry see (Fig. 18.8). Of the rhinomanometric procedures, the active anterior technique is preferred. In this technique, the patient's normal nasal breathing is assessed and the nasal cavities are assessed separately. The presence of a nasal cycle (alternating baseline nasal congestion and decongestion) may, however, give rise to problems in the interpretation of the results obtained. There is no uniformly accepted way of determining when a change in any of these parameters should be considered as positive, and they must still be considered to be mainly research instruments. The recently introduced acoustic rhinometry uses the reflection of sound to determine the cross-sectional area of the nasal cavity over its entire length. This is a promising technique which will permit the determination of the cross-sectional area in order to determine the site of a mucosal swelling, for example.

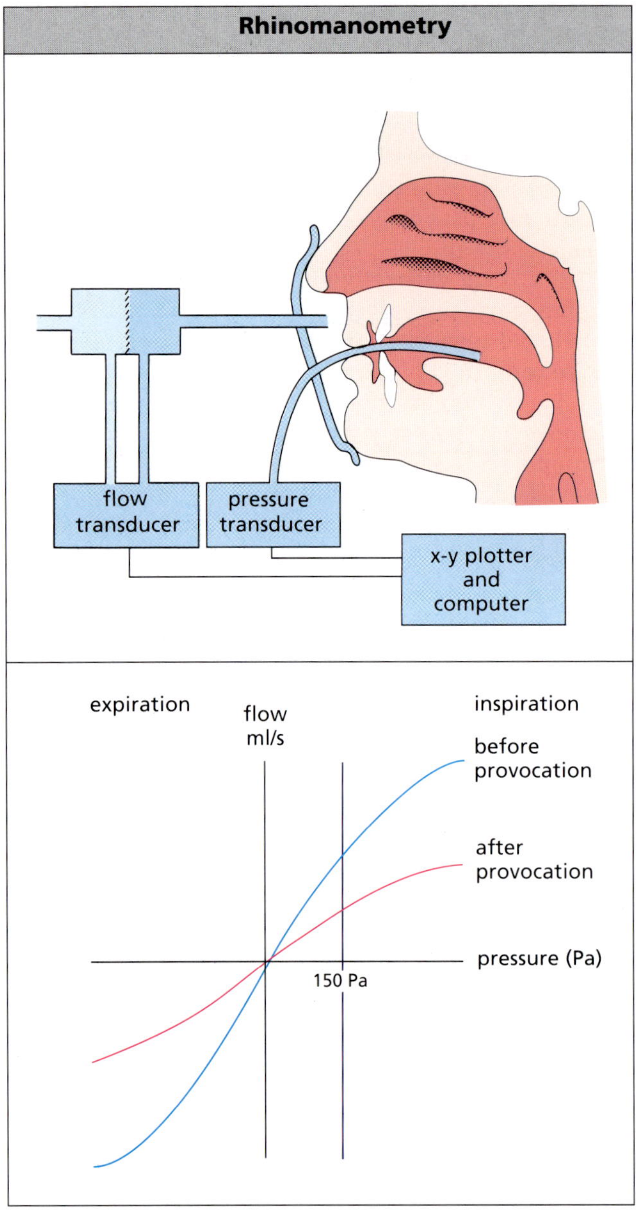

Fig. 18.6. The rhinomanometric examination. [top] The subject breathes through the nose via an anaesthetic mask to which a flow transducer is attached. A further tube is introduced into the mouth and held tightly between the lips. This is attached to a pressure transducer to measure mouth pressure. [below] Pressure and flow are plotted on an x–y plotter. Resistance may be calculated by reading flow at a constant pressure, 150 Pa in this example.

Increase in nasal surface liquid or nasal secretions is the third main symptom. Weighing the blown secretion is a simple way to determine the amount of liquid produced.

It may also be of interest to assess any changes in the specific composition of the nasal surface liquid. Lavage of the nasal cavity with saline solution before and after challenge with allergen and the subsequent analysis of various markers of specific cell activation have been performed (Fig. 18.9). It is important to wash out the nasal cavity at fixed time intervals, and a thorough cleansing of the nasal cavity is sometimes necessary before the lavage/challenge procedure. As described in Chapter 17, histamine or tryptase may be used as markers of mast cell activation, and eosinophil cationic protein (ECP), major basic protein (MBP), and eosinophil-derived neurotoxin (EDN) are markers of eosinophil activation. In addition, IgA and lysozyme may be used as functional markers for glandular secretion, and albumin/fibrinogen for plasma leakage. At present, these techniques are primarily useful for research and have contributed to our knowledge of the pathophysiology of upper airway allergic reactions. Their application to the clinical setting has still not been defined. The lavage technique has, however, also been used successfully to monitor the allergic inflammation of the upper airways during natural allergen exposure as well as the effect of therapeutic intervention. Increases similar to those seen in the challenge situation, namely increased surface levels of TAME-esterase, bradykinin, albumin, and ECP, have also been demonstrated during clinical disease.

Monitoring the Home Allergen Exposure

By using a specific device adapted to a vacuum cleaner, a sample of house dust can be obtained can then be assessed for its content of mite allergens. Symptoms of upper airway allergy can thus be related to the degree of home exposure to this allergen.

Morphological Examination

To assess the severity of the disease, or to elucidate whether the upper airway disease is of allergic origin, a morphological evaluation of the upper airways mucosa is required. Several techniques are available for demonstrating or monitoring cellular changes within and on the surface of the nasal mucosa (Fig 18.10). The various cytological techniques are relatively easy to perform, without major discomfort or risk to the patient. Biopsy should only be undertaken

Nasal Peak Flow Determination

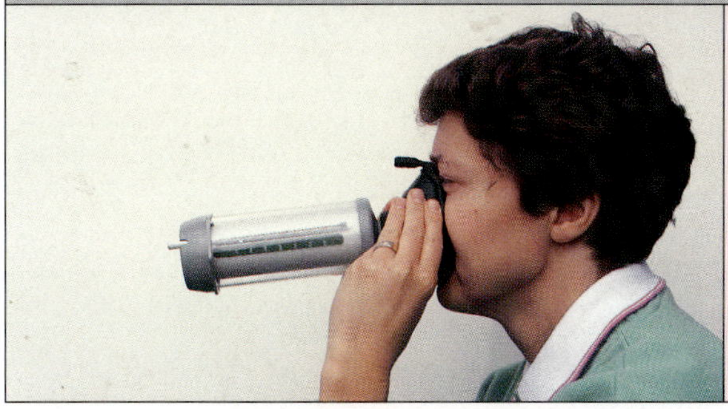

Before provocation

352 ml/sec

367 ml/sec ⇨ relevant number

342 ml/sec

After provocation

252 ml/sec

240 ml/sec

260 ml/sec ⇨ relevant number

Fig. 18.7 A nasal peak flow determination which can be made on expiration or inspiration. A maximum nasal breath is performed with the mask fitted tightly around the nose without influencing the nasal alii. The peak flow is determined at least three times and the highest value is noted. After an allergen challenge, lower values may be obtained.

Acoustic Rhinometry

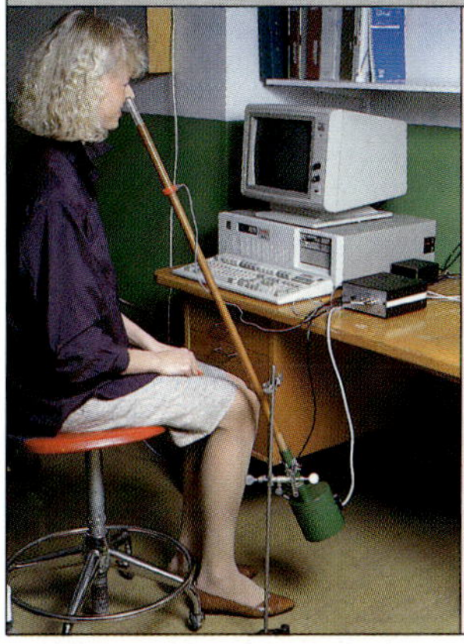

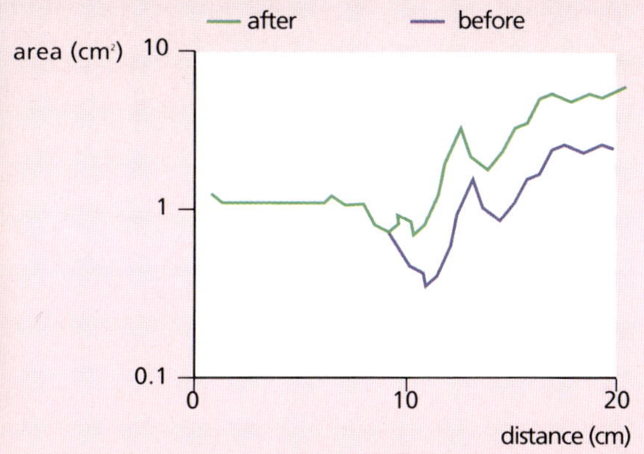

Fig. 18.8 [left] The determination of the nasal geometry using acoustic rhinometry. The spark sound is led to the nasal cavity through the long tube where a microphone is fitted some distance from the nosepiece. The difference in the time and intensity of the sound is monitored and this information is used to compute the nasal geometry with the aid of the computer. [right] Allergen challenge will induce a mucosal thickening, which can be determined using this method.

Nasal Lavage

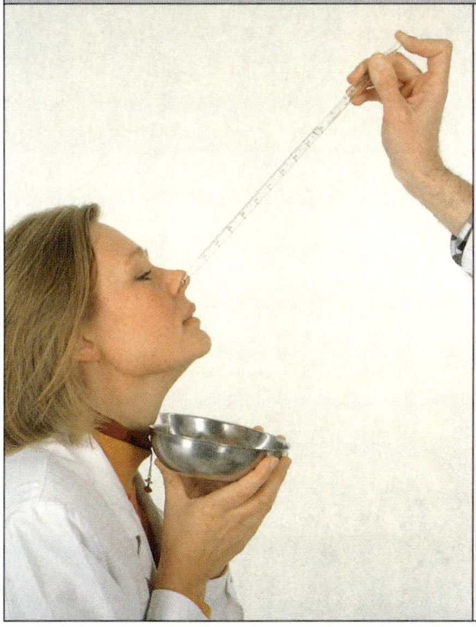

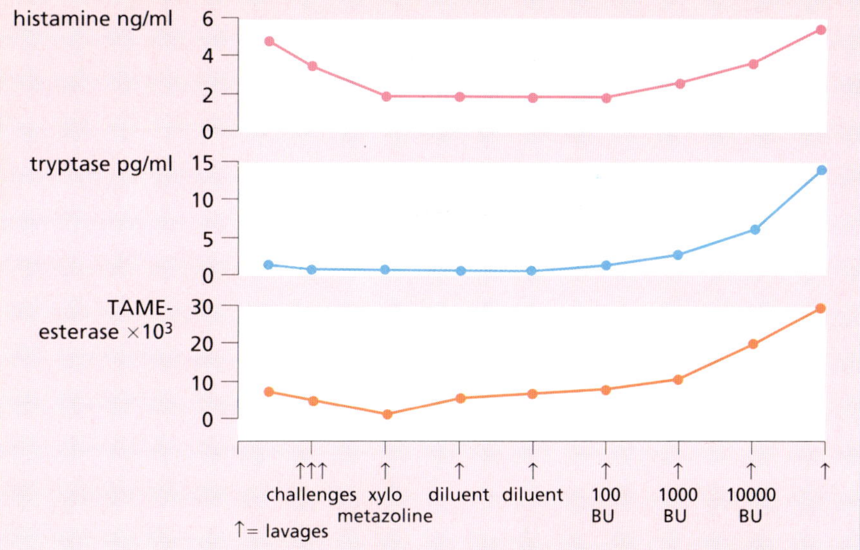

Fig. 18.9 A nasal lavage can be performed by administering normal saline solution (approximately 5 ml/nasal cavity) whilst simultaneously closing the epipharynx. A nasal allergen challenge can be performed during a series of repeated lavages at a fixed time interval. [right] Increasing doses of allergen in an allergic individual will produce increasing quantities of markers of mast-cell activation such as histamine, tryptase, TAME esterase and plasma proteins.

Sampling Cellular Material from the Nasal Cavity

	Smears	Blown secretions	Imprint	Lavage	Scraping	Biopsy
quantitative	no	no	yes	yes	yes	yes
secretions included	yes	yes	yes	no	no	no
electron microscopy	no	no	no	yes	yes	yes
biochemistry	no	no	no	yes	yes	yes
easiness in handling	+++	++	++	++	++	++

Fig. 18.10. Methods of obtaining cellular material from the nasal cavity, showing the usefulness of the different methods.

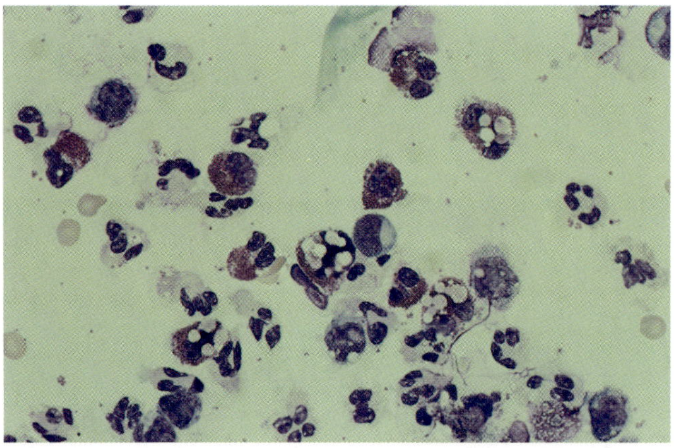

Fig. 18.11 Brush sample from a patient with seasonal allergic rhinitis during natural allergen exposure, showing a few neutrophils, some epithelial cells and several eosinophils, some with vacuoles indicating ongoing secretory activity (Giemsa stain x 400).

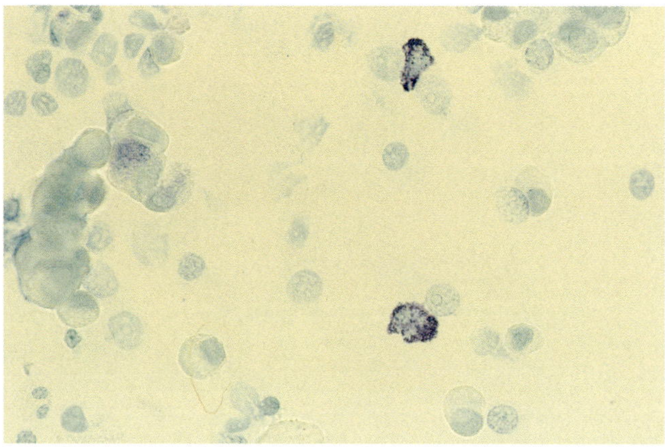

Fig. 18.12 Brush sample from a patient with seasonal allergic rhinitis during natural allergen exposure. A toluidine blue stain is used for the specific visualization of mast cells. Two granulated mast cells against a virtually unstained background are shown (x 400).

by someone who is very familiar with the nasal anatomy, and who is prepared to deal with the frequently profuse post-biopsy bleeding. Until now, the main focus has been to demonstrate the presence or absence of eosinophils (Fig. 18.11). The density of the mast cells or basophils is also of interest (Fig. 18.12). The presence of eosinophils is a sign of active inflammatory disease of allergic origin. It has also been taken as a sign of susceptibility to topical glucocorticoid therapy. In seasonal allergic rhinitis there is a strong correlation between seasonal exposure to allergen and the local eosinophil density. The presence and density of mast cells on the mucosa or within the epithelium indicates the severity of the disease.

Supplementary Investigations

Radiology

It has been suggested that sinus disease is often associated with upper airway allergy but the predisposing factors are unclear. There are no specific studies which demonstrate an increase in acute sinusitis in patients with seasonal allergic rhinitis. On the other hand, it has also been claimed that there is an increase in the frequency of upper airway allergy in patients with 'chronic sinusitis'. As the diagnosis is mainly based on radiographic examination, a plain radiograph of the sinus regions may be useful (Fig. 18.13). Better visualization of the nasal cavity and the sinus region is obtained using a CT scan specifically directed towards the ethmoidal and ostial regions where pathology is often present (Fig. 18.14). A minor degree of mucosal swelling in the maxillary sinuses in conjunction with the allergic ailment is not indicative of sinusitis, but should instead be interpreted as part of the overall allergic condition and not treated specifically. Nevertheless, the presence of fluid in one or more of the sinuses, or their complete opacification, needs to be further evaluated by either sinus puncture or sinuscopy (Fig. 18.15).

Ultrasound

This is another technique which can be used to detect air-fluid levels in the maxillary and frontal sinuses. It is easy to perform, but requires a good deal of training in order to obtain reproducible results and to grade the pathology.

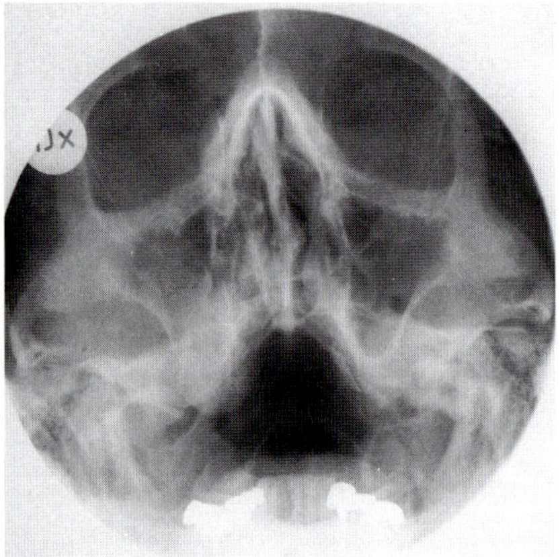

Fig. 18.13 Plain radiograph of the sinuses. A mucosal thickening specifically in the maxillary sinuses is shown (Courtesy of Olof Kalm, MD.)

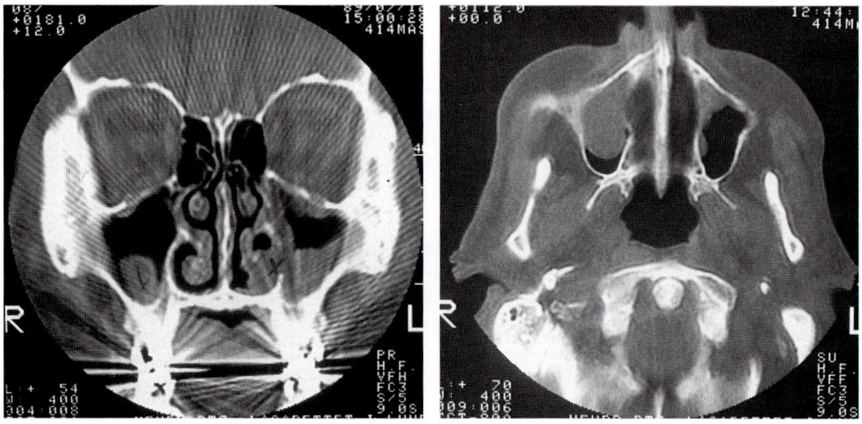

Fig. 18.14 CT scan of the sinus regions from the same patient as in Fig. 18.13 showing mucosal thickening not only in the maxillary sinus region but also in the ethmoidal region (Courtesy of Olof Kalm, MD.)

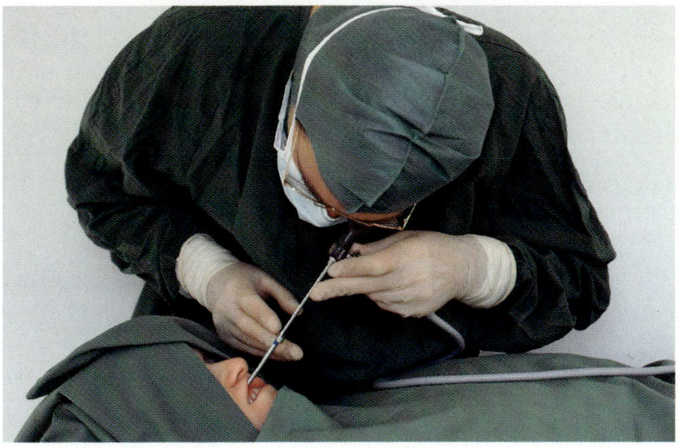

Fig. 18.15 Sinuscopy using a rigid endoscope. A puncture is performed in the fossa canina under local anaesthesia and the sinuses can be visualized. (Courtesy of Jan Kumlien, MD).

Efficacy of Various Drugs in Treatment of Rhinitis			
Drug	**Sympton**		
	sneezes	blockage	secretions
α– stimulant	–	++	–
SCG	+	+	+
anti-histamines	++	–	+
topical glucocorticoids	++	++	++
anticholinergic	–	–	++

Fig. 18.16 Efficacy profile of the drugs used to treat allergic rhinitis. Some of the drugs inhibit only one nasal symptom, e.g. α-agonist on nasal blockage, while others have a more widespread activity, e.g. topical glucocorticoids.

Treatment

Information

The most important element in the treatment is information to the patient. If the patient is a child, the parent should be the target for the information. It cannot be stressed sufficiently that successful treatment depends on the patient understanding the nature of the disease, and that it may be a lifelong ailment in which the symptoms can often be treated successfully but the success rate is largely dependent on the co-operation of the patient. Books or pamphlets can often be helpful.

Allergen Avoidance

Avoidance regimens improve symptoms by decreasing the exposure to allergen which trigger the allergic reactions. This approach is usually successful, and should be strictly enforced when there is an allergic reaction to foods, drugs, or animals. Because seasonal pollens and moulds have a widespread airborne distribution, complete avoidance of these allergens is difficult if not impossible. Sometimes a total change of environment might be of value.

Measures designed try to reduce the degree of mite exposure in the home include covering mattresses, boxsprings, and pillows in vinyl or synthetic materials. More extreme measures include the removal of upholstered furniture, stuffed animals, carpeting, and wall hangings to eliminate dust traps. However, the cost:benefit ratio of taking more drastic measures such as major house renovation is doubtful. Careful and regular cleaning with a wet mop is important. The benefit of local air filtration is limited, and calls for careful maintenance of the filters if it is to be useful.

In the case of mould allergy, the local environment should be kept dry and dense vegetation around the house eliminated. It might also be useful to avoid raking leaves and other similar activities.

It is also important to try to eliminate other local irritants as much as possible. The importance of a non-smoking environment cannot be stressed enough.

Drug Treatment

Several pharmacological agents are available for the treatment of hay fever symptoms, most of which have different efficacy profiles as is shown in Fig. 18.16. A combination of drugs with different effect profiles can be productive. The conjunctivitis which is often present, and as troublesome as the nasal symptoms, should also be treated.

α-stimulants (decongestants)

Vasoconstrictors are used by millions of hay-fever sufferers, both as topical preparations and as tablets. All the nasal vasoconstrictors which are available commercially possess α-adrenoceptor stimulant properties to a greater or lesser degree (Fig. 18.17) and cause contraction of the smooth muscle of the venous erectile tissue, thereby increasing reactive hyperaemia

Effects of Sympathomimetics				
	Vasoconstrictor activity	**Duration of action**	**Rapidity of action**	**Lack of reactive hyperaemia**
epinephrine	+	++	+	+
noradrenaline	+	+	++	+
adrenaline	++	+	+++	+
xylometazoline	++	+++	+	+++
oxymetazoline	++	+++	+	+++
naphazoline	++	++	++	++

Fig. 18.17 Profiles of α-adrenergic stimulants used in the nasal cavity.

and rebound congestion. The most popular topical preparations contain xylometazoline or oxymetazoline. Their duration of action is long, and they remain effective after prolonged use with little risk of rebound congestion. They can be recommended for occasional limited use for up to two weeks. The risk of rhinitis medicamentosa, in which nasal obstruction becomes unresponsive to venoconstrictive agents, is even lower when the decongestant is administered orally. However this route of administration is associated with several disturbing and undesirable side-effects including bladder dysfunction, restlessness, nausea, vomiting, insomnia, headache, tachycardia, dysrythmias, hypertension, and angina, and is contra-indicated in patients with cardiovascular disease, thyrotoxicosis, glaucoma and in those taking monoamine oxidase inhibitors. As many of these receptor-blocking drugs are available without prescription, patients at risk should be warned of their possible harmful effects.

Antihistamines

The development of histamine antagonists began 60 years ago at the Pasteur Institute. The first compound to be used successfully in humans was phenbenzamine. Since then many drugs with antihistaminic activity have been introduced into clinical practice (Fig. 18.18). These include chlorpheniramine, triprolidine and promethazine. Whilst all of them exhibit competitive H_1-receptor antagonism, their therapeutic index is low, and the large doses needed for therapeutic efficacy lead to the unwanted effects of sedation and blockade of cholinergic and α-adrenergic receptors. The more recent introduction of antihistamines, such as terfenadine, astemizole, loratadine, and cetirizine, which have little or no sedative or anticholinergic effect, has reawakened interest in the use of antihistamines in the treatment of hay fever. The increased potency of these newer antihistamines, together with their lack of sedation resulting from their relative inability to cross the blood–brain barrier, allows the administration of doses with good therapeutic benefit. Their greatest therapeutic benefit is on rhinorrhoea, and they also have a beneficial effect on sneezing and itching, but little or no effect on nasal blockage.

The side-effects of antihistamines may be minimized by administering them as nasal sprays, as has been suggested for one of the newer drugs, levocabastine. Although the putative sensitizing effect of topically applied antihistamines has been questioned, the risk of such unwanted effects appears to be minimal when it comes to application on to mucous membranes.

Since the effect of antihistamines on nasal obstruction is limited, a logical step would therefore be to combine these drugs with an α-adrenoceptor agonist which only affects nasal obstruction. These combinations, which are now being introduced with the newer non-sedating antihistamines, represent an alternative therapy. However, these combinations also carry the side-effects and precautions associated with the oral vasoconstrictor agents. The combination of H_1- and H_2-receptor antagonists has also been suggested to be more effective than H_1-blockers alone in reducing nasal congestion, suggesting that H_2-receptors may be present on nasal blood vessels. However histamine H_2-receptor blockade in isolation has no demonstrable therapeutic value.

Effects of Antihistamines

	Duration	Specificity	Effects on cognitive function
triprolidine	a few hours	+	+
terfenadine azatadine cetirizine	up to 9-10 hours	++ ++ ++	– – –
hydroxyzine chlorphenir-amine	20-25 hours	+ +	+ ++
astemizole	19-20 days	++	–

Fig. 18.18 Major features of antihistamines used to treat upper airway allergic diseases.

Anticholinergics

From a theoretical point of view, atropine ought to be of considerable benefit in the control of the symptom of watery rhinorrhea and virus-induced rhinitis. The basis of this assumption is the fact that the rhinorrhoea is primarily the result of glandular hypersecretion. However, its presumed efficacy has only been tested to a limited degree largely because of the undesirable anticholinergic effects occurring in other organs, such as dryness of the mouth and blurred vision. Topical administration would be of interest but, since atropine is readily absorbed, it is likely to carry systemic effects prior to any topical efficacy. However, an atropine derivative, ipratropium bromide, is poorly absorbed from mucous membranes, and patients whose predominant symptom is that of profuse nasal discharge may well benefit from this drug. This is also relevant for patients with a perennial non-allergic, vasomotor rhinitis in which the main symptom is watery hypersecretion.

Anti-inflammatory agents

Sodium cromoglycate (SCG) was introduced in the 1960s. Despite intensive study, its mode of action remains controversial. Traditionally, it is considered to act by stabilizing mast cells and, if this were indeed a mode of action, this drug would be particularly useful for the treatment of allergic rhinitis. Its clinical efficacy in allergic rhinitis is less than that of the topical glucocorticoids, but more or less equal to that of antihistamines. Recent evidence suggests additional mechanisms of action pertinent to mucosal inflammation, including inhibitory effects on eosinophils, platelets, and macrophages. SCG is also especially useful for the treatment of ocular problems which often accompany rhinitis. The administration of SCG is safe, and minimal or no side-effects have been reported. Patient compliance is hampered by its short duration of action, necessitating topical administration up to six times daily.

Nedocromil sodium is a recent addition to the family of anti-allergic drugs of which SCG is the prototype. While being somewhat more potent than SCG, there is little evidence that nedocromil sodium provides great therapeutic benefit over its predecessor. Its potential anti-inflammtaory effects are evident from its ability to reduce the accumulation of mast cells in the nasal mucosa during the pollen season. Like SCG, nedocromil sodium has an excellent safety profile, making it particularly popular amongst paediatricians.

Corticosteroids

Topical treatment. The introduction in the 1970s of topical glucocorticoids for nasal use has provided several effective treatment alternatives for allergic rhinitis, including beclomethasone dipropionate, budesonide, triamcinolone acetonide, flunisolone acetonide and fluticasone propionate. They are more efficacious than antihistamines and SCG, and can be administered conveniently once or twice daily. It should, however, be explained clearly to patients that the maximal benefit of glucocorticoids is not immediate but may take a several days. Furthermore, it should be explained that if the drugs are to be effective they must reach the target organ. This means that if symptoms are already present it may be necesary to open up the nasal cavity with a topical decongestant prior to glucocorticoid aerosol administration. Sometimes a short course of oral glucocorticoids may be necessary to open up the nasal cavity.

The use of topical glucocorticoids during the last decade has provided us with a great deal of information about their safety. They have limited local and systemic side-effects and may be used even for long-term treatment in adults. In the case of long-term treatment, rhinoscopy is recommended once or twice a year. One should not hesitate to use topical glucocorticoids for seasonal disease in children as long as the nozzle fits into the nasal opening. Long-term treatment should not be instituted without careful individual evaluation, as is the case with all drugs. Some patients may suffer from local irritation from the nozzle, with blood spottings. Septal perforations is an infrequent side effect.

Systemic treatment. When given systemically, glucocorticoids are highly effective in all forms of rhinitis. However, they all have systemic side-effects, whether given as depot-injections or orally, and the benefit:risk ratio should be considered. Depot-injection are simple but have been linked to disfiguring muscle atrophy after repeated injection. In cases of severe seasonal allergic disease, the administration of oral prednisolone or prednisone to cover some peak days may be considered. If, however, more regular treatment fails then specific hyposensitization should be considered.

Hyposensitization

This is an alternative which should be considered if patients do not respond to any allergen avoidance measures combined with traditional pharmacological therapy. Before it is started, a careful explanation must be given to the patient outlining the details and commitment required. It is a long-term programme involving frequent injections with increasing quantities of allergenic extracts in the build-up phase, and then maintenance treatment with the allergen for at least three years. The treatment has been shown to be effective in allergic rhinoconjunctivitis to clear-cut allergens like pollens, mites, and animal dander. Hyposensitization carries with it the risk of a systemic anaphylactic reaction should an allergen penetrate directly into the blood stream. Consequently, facilities for resuscitation must be available, and procedures using highly potent allergens should be avoided. Because of the possible risks of immunotherapy, some countries have introduced guidelines to govern the use of this form of therapy.

Relationships to Other Organs

In any of the treatment programmes for upper airway allergy, the ocular symptoms must not be neglected since they may well be just as severe as the nasal symptoms. The eye should, therefore, also be treated either locally with a vasoconstrictor or antihistamine or systemically with antihistamines.

Upper–Lower Airway Interaction

One of the main organs that may be affected indirectly by upper airway disease or by the dysfunction of the upper airways is the lung. It has been suggested that the failure of the upper airways to humidify and clean the inspired air effectively might precipitate or aggravate asthma. Asthma is often associated with upper airway disease. Up to 80 per cent of the adult population with asthma also suffers from upper airway symptoms. These symptoms often precede the onset of asthma. It is not known whether early intervention in terms of the nasal symptoms will affect the onset of lower airway problems. However, since asthma is considered to be a more serious disease, the frequently associated upper airway problems are often overlooked and undertreated. The active and successful treatment of the upper airways may therefore not only reduce nasal symptoms but will also benefit the lower airways.

Sinus–Ear Interaction

Sinus afflictions are common among asthmatic hay fever sufferers and should generally be considered to be part of the airways disease and treated as such. A careful diagnostic examination is necessary. The possibility of polyps, possibly provoked by non-steroidal anti-inflammatory drugs (NSAIDs), should also be considered. The sinus disease may well call for surgical intervention which may include a functional endoscopic surgical (FES) procedure. Ear disease has been linked to allergy in children in particular but, as no direct causal relationship has been demonstrated, the treatment should be directed primarily towards the ear disease as such.

Nasal Polyps

Nasal polyps have sometimes been linked to allergic disease, partly because they often contain eosinophils. The clinical finding is often one of musosal bags filled with fluid lying in the nasal cavity (see Fig. 18.2). There is however very little evidence of a clear-cut allergic origin for these polyps. When lower airway problems are present, the link to NSAID-sensitivity should be considered. Smaller polyps may shrink on topical glucocorticoid treatment, while larger polyps may require surgical intervention. The endoscopic approach may be productive. In such cases, topical glucocorticoids decrease the recurrence rate.

Differential Diagnosis

The most common differential diagnosis is perennial non-allergic rhinitis (see Fig. 18.3). The clinical relevance of dividing this group into subgroups is limited except perhaps for the demonstration of cytological changes such as the presence of eosinophils. However, the more common problems which the physician sees are endocrine disturbances, such as nasal congestion as a complication of pregnancy, oral contraceptives, or hypothyroidism, giving rise to a thickened and oedematous nasal mucosa. Rhinitis medicamentosa with a rebound vasodilatation, (side-effects of terbutaline and reserpine) often produce an oedematous and red nasal mucosa which should not be confused with true rhinitis.

Further Reading

Bierrnan CW, Pierson WE, Donaldson JA, eds. International symposium on allergy and associated disorders in otolaryngology. *J Allergy Clinical Immunol* 1988; **81**:939.

Fireman P. Otitis media and nasal disease: A role for allergy. *J Allergy Clinical Immunol* 1988; **82**:917.

Mygind N, Dahl R, Pipkorn U. *Rhinitis and Asthma. Similarities and Differences*. Copenhagen: Munksgaard, 1990.

Mygind N, Pipkorn U. *Allergic and Vasomotor Rhinitis; Pathophysiological Aspects*. Copenhagen: Munksgaard, 1987.

Naclerio RM, Meier HL, Kagey-Sobotka A, Adkinson NF Jr, Meyers DA, Norman PS, Lichtenstein LM. Mediator release after nasal airway challenge with allergen. *Am Rev Respir Dis* 1983; **128**:597.

Pipkorn U, Proud D, Lichtenstein LM, Kagey-Sobotka A, Norman PS, Naclerio RM. Inhibition of mediator release in allergic rhinitis by pretreatment with topical glucocorticosteroids. *New Engl J Med* 1987; **316**:1506.

Chapter 19

Conjunctivitis – Pathophysiology

Introduction

The term conjunctivitis, in its literal meaning of inflammation of the conjunctiva, covers a broad spectrum of disease processes. This chapter aims to outline the pathophysiology of the conjunctival disorders which are thought to have an allergic basis.

In the mildest form of allergic conjunctival disorders, the conjunctiva becomes swollen and inflamed in response to an acute allergic insult, such as pollen. This is a seasonal disorder which, although unpleasant, is not sight threatening. When the antigen occurs all the time, e.g. house dust mite, the conjunctiva can become persistently inflamed (perennial allergic conjunctivitis) but again, sight-threatening complications do not occur. At the other end of the spectrum are disorders such as vernal keratoconjunctivitis and atopic keratoconjunctivitis which do have blinding complications when the cornea becomes involved and for which current therapeutic agents are, at best, only partially effective.

In order to understand the pathophysiology of these disorders, the anatomy, including the histology, and immunology of the normal conjunctiva must be understood.

The Normal Conjunctiva

Anatomy

Structure

The three major zones of the conjunctiva – the tarsal and bulbar conjunctiva, and the fornices (upper and lower) – are shown in Fig. 19.1.

Histology

The normal conjunctiva consists of an epithelial covering of stratified columnar cells, two to five cell layers thick, resting on the lamina propria which is composed of loose connective tissue (Fig. 19.2). The conjunctival epithelium is continuous with the stratified squamous epithelium of the cornea and with the keratinized stratified squamous epithelium of the epidermis of the skin at the lid margin, along the posterior margin of the openings of the tarsal glands.

Goblet cells are scattered along the surface of the conjunctiva. Their secretion is important in lowering the surface tension of the tear film, to preserve its stability.

Scattered in the connective tissue of the conjunctiva are the conjunctival glands, which are similar to the lacrimal glands. Their ducts open directly on to

Structure of Normal Eyelids and Conjunctiva

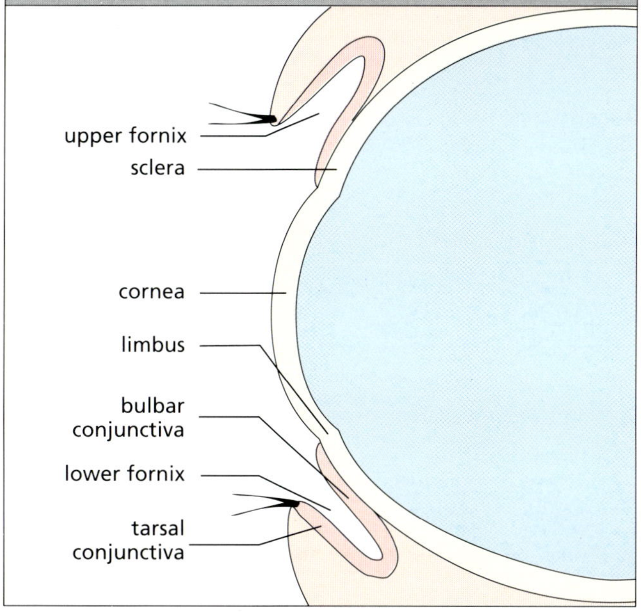

Fig. 19.1 The eyelids and conjunctiva.

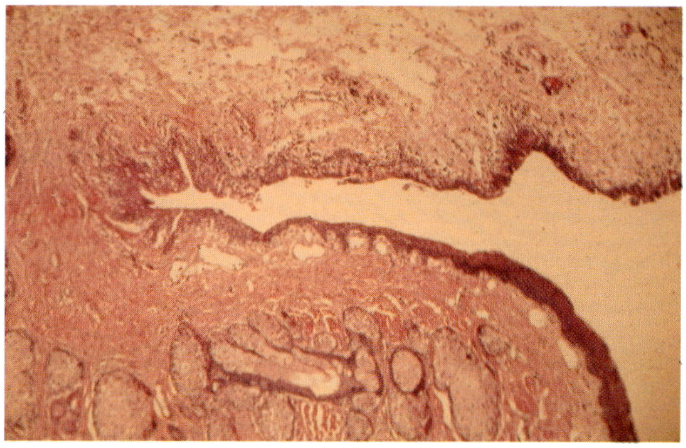

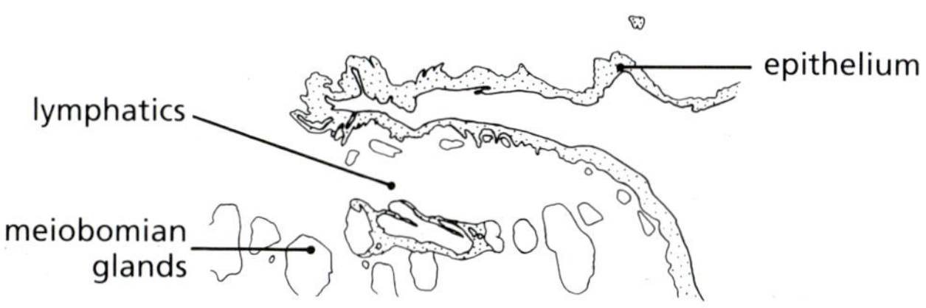

Fig. 19.2 Normal histology of conjunctiva showing goblet cells within the epithelium lymphatics in the submucosa and the sebaceous Meiobomian glands. Haematoxylin and eosin (H&E) (× 16).

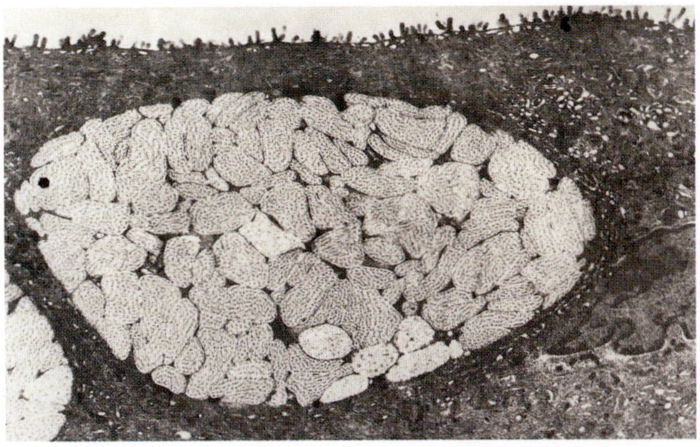

Fig. 19.3 Transmission electron micrograph showing microvillae of conjunctival epithelium above a goblet cell. (× 12,500).

the free surface of the conjunctiva. The goblet cells produce mucin which keeps the conjunctival surface smooth, enabling moisturization of the hydrophobic corneal surface by the aqueous layer of the tear film.

At the ultrastructural level, the surface conjunctival cells are hexagonal and completely covered in microvilli, which can be seen by transmission electron microscopy (Fig. 19.3). These microvilli are thought to enlarge the resorbent area of the epithelium and to stabilize and anchor the tear film.

In the submucosa, collections of lymphocytes are found superficially, whereas fibrous tissue, blood vessels, nerves, smooth muscle and conjunctival glands are found in the deeper parts. These lymphocytes are part of the lymphoid system known as the mucosal-associated lymphoid tissue (MALT) and are not present in the conjunctiva of the newborn infant (this is also true for macrophages) but are acquired, presumably on exposure to air-borne antigens.

Blood supply

The arterial supply of the conjunctiva is provided by the anterior and posterior conjunctival arteries and the anterior ciliary artery. The veins accompany the arteries and drain into the palpebral veins or directly into the superior and inferior ophthalmic veins. The conjunctiva is a very vascular organ with all areas having an extensive vascular bed.

Nerve supply

The sensory innervation of the conjunctiva is mostly from the nasociliary (via the long ciliary nerves) frontal and lacrimal branches of the ophthalmic

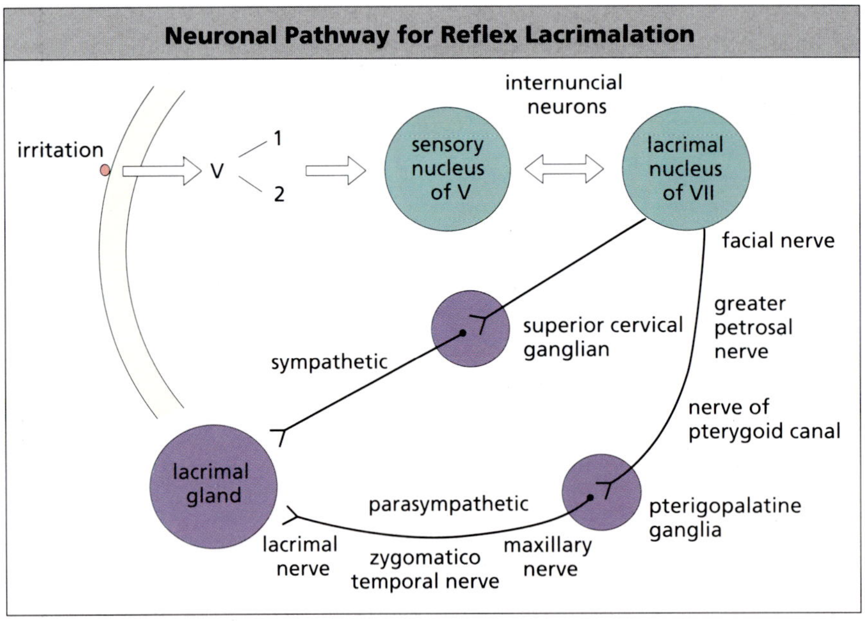

Fig. 19.4 The neuronal pathway for reflex lacrimation.

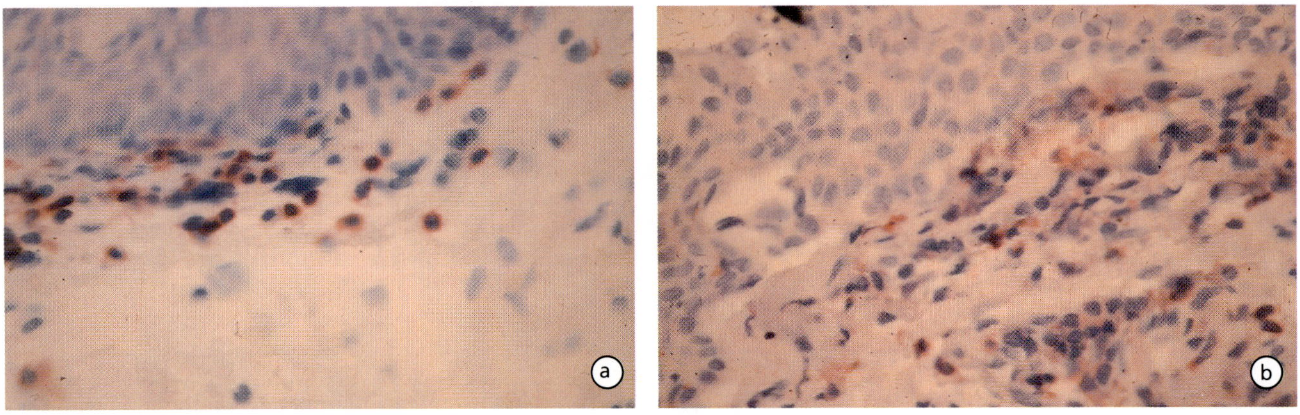

Fig. 19.5 Submucosal T and B cells stained immunohistochemically using monoclonal antibodies UCHL1. (a) (T cells), (b) L26 (B cells). (× 100).

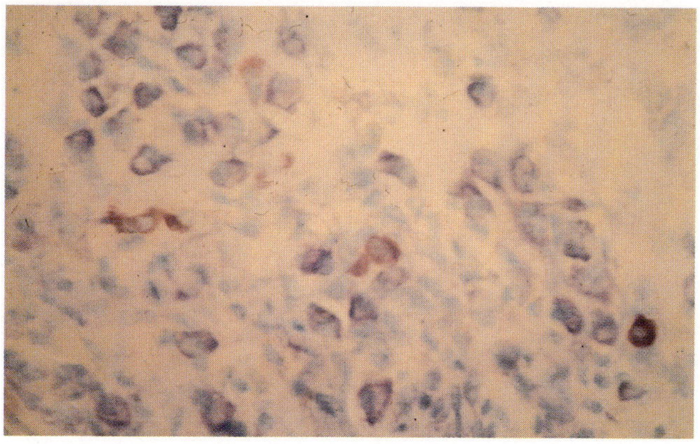

Fig. 19.6 Toluidine blue metachromatic staining of mast cells in submucosa. (× 100).

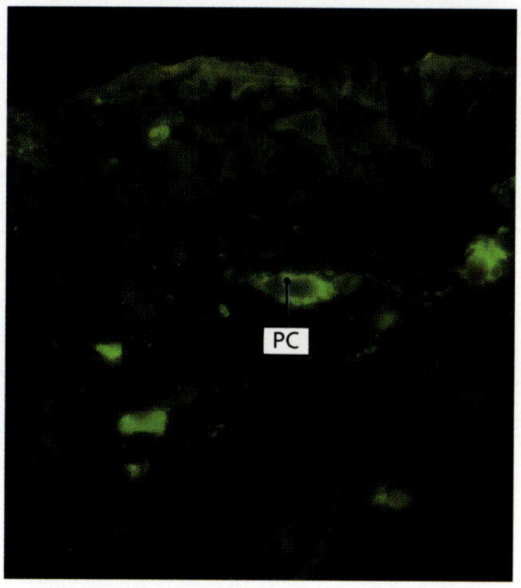

Fig. 19.7 Immunofluorescent staining of IgA-producing plasma cells (pc) in epithelium and submucosa. (× 100).

division of the trigeminal nerve. Reflex lacrimation secondary to irritation or inflammation of the cornea and conjunctiva occurs due to the connections of the sensory nucleus of the Vth cranial nerve (trigeminal nerve) with the lacrimal nucleus of the VIIth cranial nerve (facial nerve) in the brainstem (Fig. 19.4). Lacrimal secretion occurs as a consequence of stimulation of the autonomic nerves which supply the lacrimal gland.

Immune Function

Both T and B lymphocytes are present in the submucosa (Fig. 19.5), comprising the MALT, although T cells predominate. Their numbers vary greatly between different regions of the conjunctiva and with the age of the individual. In addition, macrophages and large numbers of mast cells are present, the latter particularly in relation to blood vessels and lymphatics (Fig. 19.6). Dendritic cells in the epithelium and macrophages in the stroma express class II HLA antigens and probably act as local antigen-presenting cells for activation of T lymphocytes. The macrophages and lymphocytes serve as a second line of defence to deal with antigens which have escaped binding by the surface IgA and have breached the conjunctival epithelium. Recent studies on the conjunctival mast cells have shown them to be predominantly of the connective tissue rather than mucosal subtype. The mast cells contain both the neutral proteases tryptase and chymase in their secretory granules; normally they are confined to the submucosa and not present in the epithelium.

In the normal conjunctiva, there are six times as many IgA-secreting plasma cells as those secreting IgE. IgA is secreted by plasma cells in the submucosa (Fig. 19.7) and has to be transported across the epithelial cells to reach the outer surface. The epithelial cells make the secretory component which is thought to facilitate the transport of IgA into the tears and also protect it from degradation by enzymes present in the tears (Fig. 19.8). The main function of IgA on the conjunctival surface is to prevent micro-organisms adhering to and penetrating the conjunctival surface.

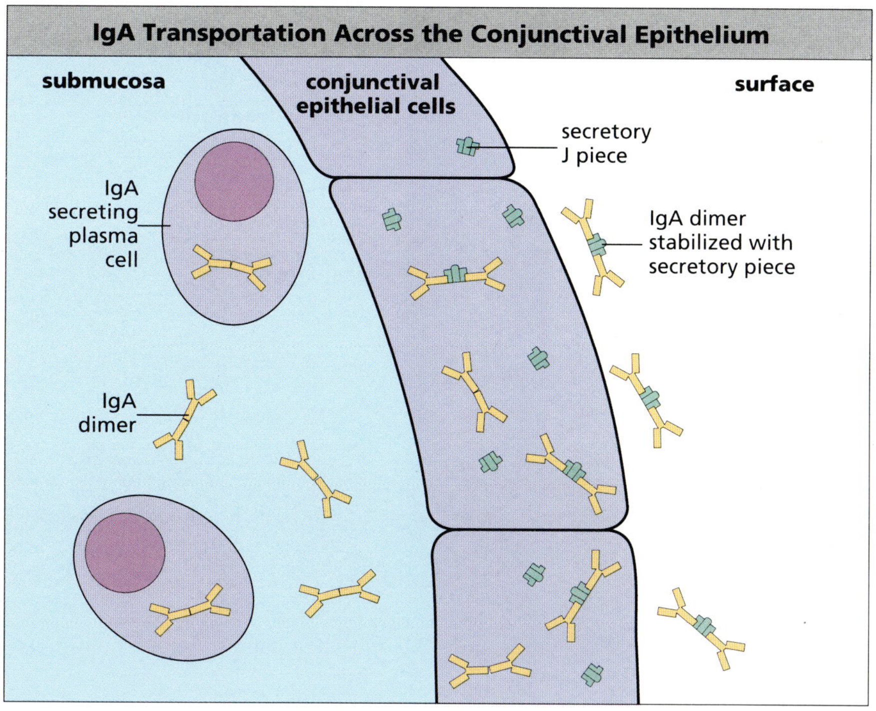

Fig. 19.8 Transport of IgA across the conjunctival epithelium.

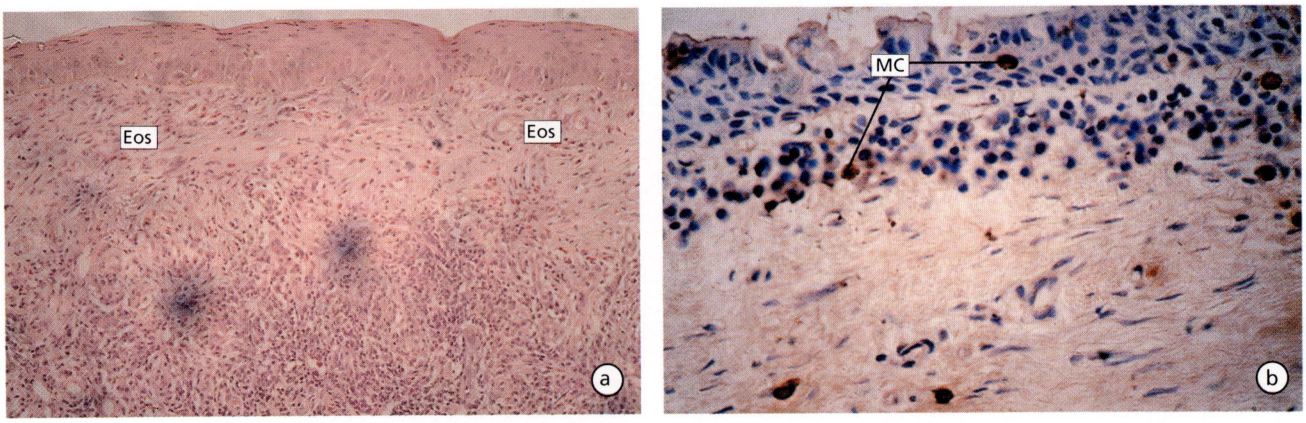

Fig. 19.9 (a) Seasonal acute conjunctivitis (SAC) with large numbers of eosinophilic leucocytes (Eos) present in the oedematous submucosa. Plasma cells are seen in a deep chronic inflammatory cell infiltrate. H&E (×40).

(b) Mast cells (MC) demonstrated immunohistochemically in the epithelium and submucosa in perennial allergic conjunctivitis (PAC). (×100). (Courtesy of Mr Stephen Morgan.)

Pathophysiology of Allergic Conjunctival Disorders

Features of all types of allergic conjunctivitis are redness, itching and swelling of the conjunctiva. The redness occurs as a result of dilatation of the vascular bed, itching from sensory nerve stimulation, and oedema from altered post-capillary venule permeability. In the inflammatory process, the arteriolar blood flow increases which results in extravasation of plasma in areas of increased vascular leakiness.

Seasonal Allergic and Perennial Allergic Conjunctivitis

These disorders are similar except in their time course. Pollen is a common cause of seasonal allergic conjunctivitis (SAC), rhinitis and asthma. Since pollen is present in the air for a relatively short length of time, the symptoms are confined to the period of exposure. In perennial allergic conjunctivitis (PAC), the allergen is present most of the time, as are the symptoms. House-dust mite and animal dander are common causes. The clinical picture of PAC is less dramatic than in the acute episode of SAC and, on examination, inflammation may appear to be very mild.

The histology of the conjunctiva from each of these disorders is shown in Fig. 19.9. The major finding is an increase in mast-cell numbers. Previous exposure to the allergen results in local IgE production at the allergen entry site, e.g. the conjunctival surface. IgE production by B cells involves digestion and presentation of the allergen to T cells by macrophages and dendritic cells, followed by T-cell help and stimulation and maturation of B cells to plasma cells. The locally-produced IgE binds to mast cells; some enters the circulation and binds to receptors on circulating basophils and mast cells in other tissues.

Re-exposure to the allergen results in binding of the allergen by the mast-cell bound IgE, and degranulation of the mast cells occurs secondary to cross-linking the IgE (see Chapter 4). The pathological features are thought to be a direct result of the mediators, both preformed and newly synthetized, which are secreted by activated mast cells. Histamine release results in vasodilatation and increased vascular permeability which facilitates tissue deposition of plasma components. Tryptase is a proteolytic enzyme capable of activating C3 and the complement cascade. Prostaglandins, particularly PGD2, increase vascular permeability and potentiate the vasodilator effect of bradykinin. Kinins also have a direct vasodilating effect and these effects, together with those of the sulphidopeptide leukotrienes, result in conjunctival oedema.

Since mast cells seem to be responsible for the inflammatory response seen in SAC and PAC, treatment is directed at preventing mast-cell degranulation with sodium cromoglycate. Both SAC and PAC are helped considerably by topical application of this drug.

Atopic Keratoconjunctivitis

Patients with atopic dermatitis, who often have other atopic disease such as asthma, may develop atopic keratoconjunctivitis (AKC). It usually affects older patients rather than children. Histologically the conjunctiva is hyperaemic and oedematous and is infiltrated by lymphocytes, plasma cells and eosinophils (Fig. 19.10). The epithelium can become hyperplastic with increased numbers of goblet cells. The limbal

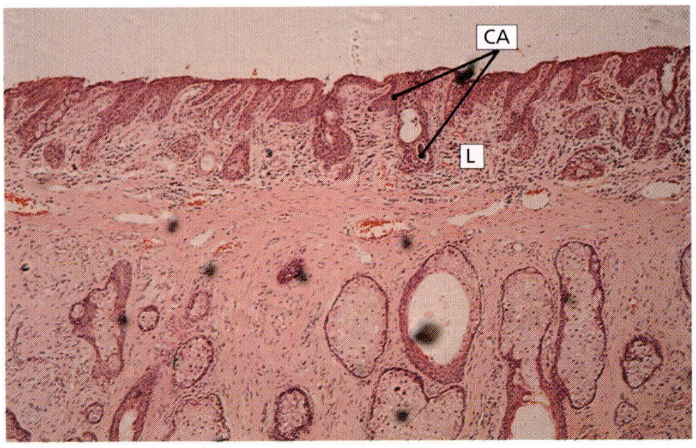

Fig. 19.10 Atopic keratoconjunctivitis. Crypt abscesses (CA) are present in the epithelium and there is a band-like lymphocytic infiltrate (L). H&E (× 40).

portion of the cornea can also become infiltrated with inflammatory cells, particularly eosinophils, and vascularization follows. Linear or stellate scars can form on the tarsal conjunctiva.

Patients with atopic eczema also have an increased incidence of keratoconus. There are many theories why this should be, but obvious inflammation in the cornea does not occur.

Serum levels of IgE are usually elevated while those of IgA, IgM and IgD are normal. Peripheral blood lymphocytes appear to be functionally depressed and reduced in number, but this may be due to recruitment into affected areas of skin. An eosinophilia is common.

The mechanisms of damage to the conjunctiva in AKC are unclear. Infection is often superimposed, particularly by staphylococci. Why scarring occurs is unknown, but further work on the immunopathology should allow a greater understanding of the cellular interactions in the conjunctiva and cornea which result in this sight-threatening disorder.

Vernal Keratoconjunctivitis

In the UK, vernal keratoconjunctivitis (VKC) is usually seasonal, occurring mainly in the spring in children and young adults, many of whom are atopic. In other countries, such as Israel and Africa, it is often a continuous inflammatory process occurring at any time of the year, and atopy is not a consistent finding. Itching is a predominant feature and visual loss can occur from associated corneal problems.

Increased levels of histamine, pollen-specific IgE and IgG antibodies, C3, C3a, factor B and proteins derived from eosinophils have been described in the active stages of VKC. Raised numbers of both IgA-producing and IgE-producing plasma cells in the conjunctiva have been reported. In one study, 76 per cent of VKC patients had specific IgE antibodies to pollen antigens in tears, which had been produced locally in the conjunctiva. Both local and systemic eosinophilia occurs.

The main histological features of VKC are shown in Figs 19.11–13. The major immunological feature differentiating it from SAC and PAC is the large number of T cells, particularly of the $CD4^+$ type, in the stroma (Fig. 19.11). Mast cells, eosinophils and plasma cells are also a feature and are commonly found in the epithelium (Fig. 19.12). Swelling and death of the blood vessel endothelial cells can occur, with increased permeability demonstrated by extravasation of erythrocytes and fibrin. Thickening of both the conjunctival epithelium and stroma occurs, the latter being due to extensive deposition of collagen. Mast cell and eosinophil granules are seen free in the tissues (Fig. 19.13). In limbal lesions, many B cells accumulate in addition to T cells, of which the $CD8^+$ subtype predominates.

Many plasma cells are seen, with most being IgA^+ and IgG^+. IgE^+ plasma cells are rarely seen, suggesting that IgE in the tears may come from local degranulated mast cells and is not produced by local plasma cells. In the stroma, extensive deposition of collagen can occur. As this disease process is only partially affected by sodium cromoglycate, it is likely that cells other than mast cells are involved in the inflammatory response. Activated $CD4^+$ T cells can secrete interleukins, such as IL-3 and IL-5, which *in vitro* can act as growth factors for mast cells. In addition, these lymphokines can activate eosinophils and result in their degranulation, with eosinophil major

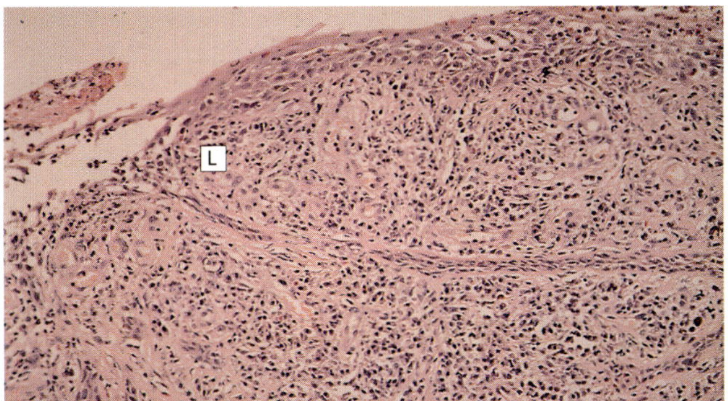

Fig. 19.11 Vernal keratoconjunctivitis (VKC) showing massive lymphoid infiltration (L) (which can be shown by immunohistochemistry to consist predominantly of T cells) in the submucosa. H&E (× 40).

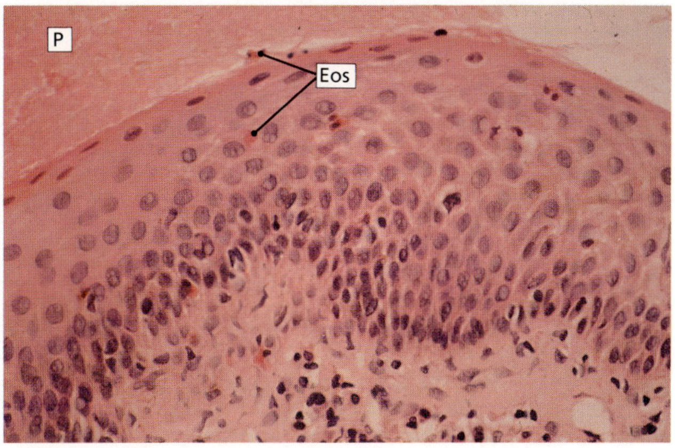

Fig. 19.12 Plaque (P) lying on surface of conjunctival epithelium infiltrated by eosinophils (Eos) in VKC. H&E (× 100).

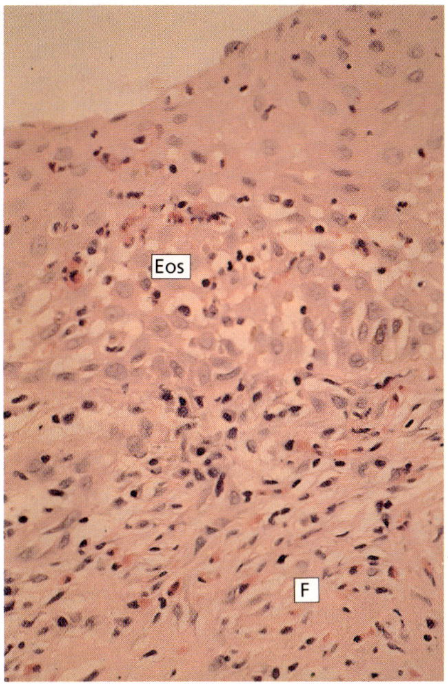

Fig. 19.13 Eosinophil (Eos) and mast cell debris in epithelium and increased fibroblastic (F) activity in submucosa in VKC. H&E (× 100).

Fig. 19.14 Transmission electron micrograph showing alternating bands of fibrinous debris from corneal vernal plaque. (× 3,000).

basic protein (MBP) being released into the tissues. This protein is cytotoxic to epithelial cells and may also be a mast cell activator.

Corneal abnormalities occurring in VKC can threaten sight. Collections of eosinophils can be found at the limbus (Trantas dots) and plaque-like deposits occur in the anterior cornea which contain mucus or stratified layers of epithelial cells (Fig. 19.14). A diffuse epithelial keratitis can also occur which is thought to be the result of MBP release. In patients with VKC who are neither atopic nor have seasonal disease, sodium cromoglycate is much less effective, suggesting that the mast cells in these patients may not be so important in the pathophysiology of this condition.

Some patients with VKC have been helped by topical cyclosporin treatment. This drug works by

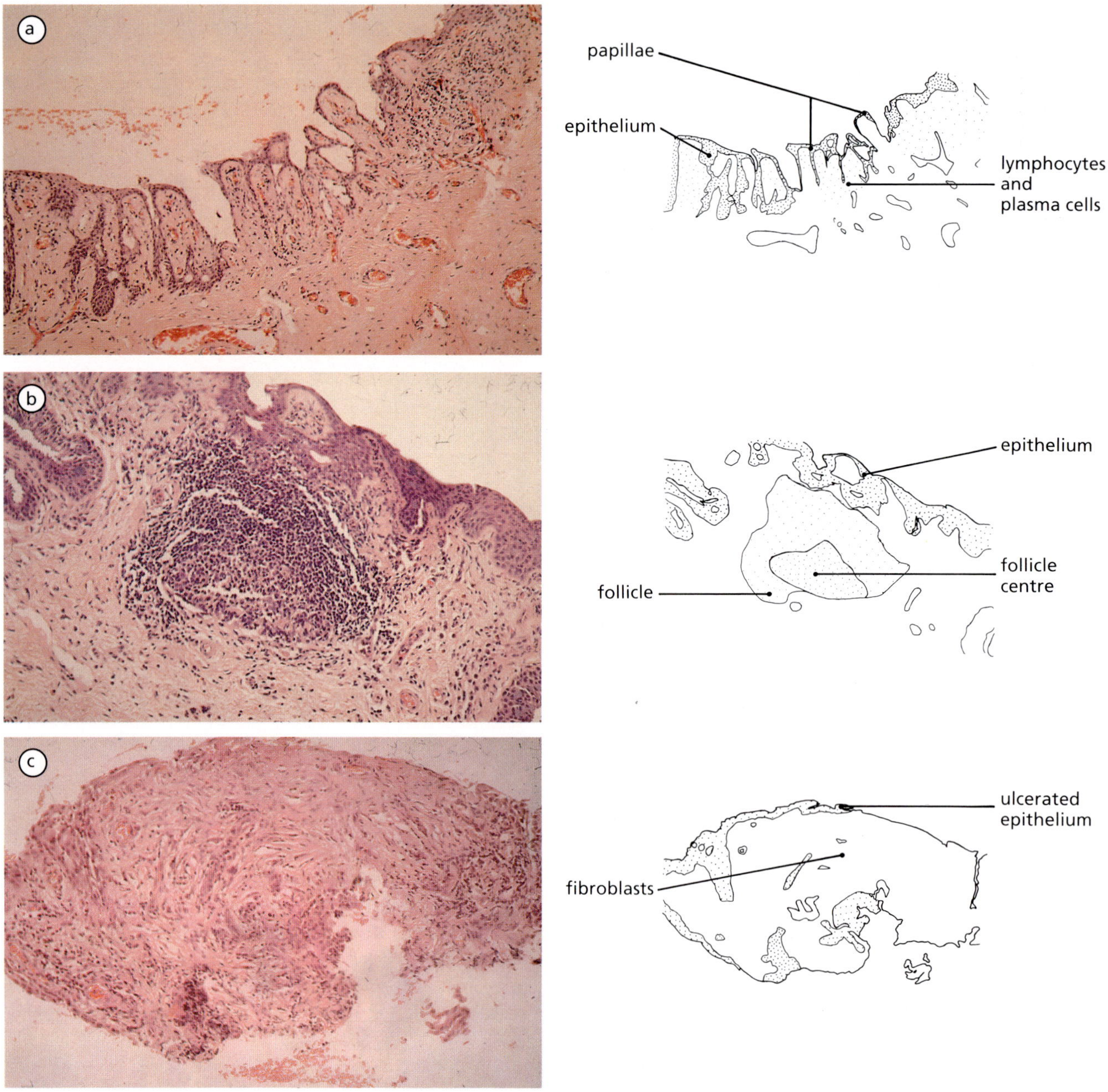

Fig. 19.15 (a) Giant papillae and subepithelial lymphocytic infiltrate in giant capillary conjunctivitis. H&E (× 40). (b). Lymphoid follicle in submucosa with follicle centre in GPC. H&E (× 65). (c) Ulcerated epithelium above fibroblastic proliferation in submucosa of patients with GPC. H&E (× 40).

inhibiting the release of lymphokines (such as IL-2 and interferon-gamma) secreted by activated T cells; its usefulness may reflect the role these cells play in the pathogenesis of this disorder.

It is likely that lymphocyte/mast-cell/eosinophil interactions occur in this disease and until more is known about the interactions *in vivo*, a more successful therapeutic approach will be difficult.

Giant Papillary Conjunctivitis

This disorder occurs in contact-lens wearers (hard, soft and gas permeable) and has many histological similarities to VKC, but does not involve the cornea. Itching is less of a feature than in VKC and tear histamine levels are lower or normal. Giant papillary conjunctivitis (GPC) may be associated with atopy, has no seasonal variation and occurs in both sexes and all ages. Other causes, apart from contact lenses, are exposed corneal sutures, plastic ocular prostheses, extruded scleral buckles and cyanoacrylate glue. Asymptomatic soft contact-lens wearers have been shown to have a traumatized conjunctival surface, and on electron microscopy more branched microvilli are found. However, there is no abnormal cellular infiltrate in the conjunctiva. Patients with GPC also do not have a delayed (Type IV) hypersensitivity response on skin testing with the chemical preservatives, making allergy to these compounds unlikely.

Irregular conjunctival epithelium, elevated into papillae, is found, with infiltration by mast cells, eosinophils, basophils, neutrophils and occasional lymphocytes (Fig. 19.15a), and follicle formation can occur. The stroma is similarly infiltrated but fewer eosinophils and basophils are seen compared to VKC, and lymphoid follicles may be present (Fig. 19.15b). Abnormal collagen outgrowths occur which flatten and push aside the normal micropapillae, and ulceration of the conjunctival surface can occur (Fig. 19.15c). Decreased amounts of lactoferrin have been found in tears of GPC patients and it has been suggested that this could contribute to increased coating of the contact lens with bacteria and their products, thereby initiating an ocular inflammatory response. Lactoferrin inhibits activation of the classical complement pathway by preventing formation of the C3 convertase. Increased local production of IgE, IgG and IgM has also been detected in the tears.

In contrast to VKC, levels of both histamine and eosinophil MBP in the tears are normal. Deposits on soft contact lenses are a constant feature but not all patients with deposits progress to GPC. It has been suggested that a combination of an allergic response to the deposits and trauma may contribute to the pathology.

Conclusions

The mast cell has been considered to be the major effector cell type in all the conjunctival diseases described. While this is likely to be true in the milder forms of allergic conjunctival disease, both the clinical response to inhibitors of mast cell degranulation and the immunopathology provide evidence for the involvement of other cell types. Both eosinophils and lymphocytes are present in large numbers in the more severe VKC and AKC, suggesting a role in pathogenesis. Activated lymphocytes can secrete lymphokines known to stimulate mast cells and eosinophils *in vitro*. In addition, both mast cells and eosinophils can produce lymphokines, including tumour necrosis factor (TNF-α), *in vitro*. It is possible to hypothesize that the lymphokines secreted by the lymphocytes could activate both the mast cells and eosinophils. These cells then start to secrete other lymphokines which have damaging effects on the tissues.

Whether the *in vitro* situation can also occur *in vivo* remains to be seen. Significant therapeutic developments for AKC and VKC will depend on finding the effector cells involved and the mechanisms of tissue damage. Both the eosinophil and the lymphocyte are likely to be involved, as well as the mast cell, and a greater understanding of interactions between these cell types is very timely.

Further Reading

Abelson MB, Madiwale N, Weston JH. Conjunctival eosinophils in allergic ocular disease. *Arch Ophthalmol* 1983; **101**: 555–556.

Allansmith MR, Baird RS, Greiner JV. Vernal conjunctivitis and contact lens-associated giant papillary conjunctivitis compared and contrasted. *Am J Ophthalmol* 1979; **87**: 544–555.

Allansmith MR, Ross RN. Giant papillary conjunctivitis. *International Ophthalmology Clinics* 1988, **28** (4): 309–316

Barishak Y, Zavaro A, Samra Z, Sompolinsky D. An immunological study of papillary conjunctivitis due to contact lenses. *Current Eye Res* 1984; **3** (10): 1161–1168.

Baryishak YR, Zavaro A, Monselise M., Samra Z, Sompolinsky D. Vernal keratoconjunctivitis in an Israeli group of patients and its treatment with sodium cromoglycate. *Br J Ophthalmol* 1982; **66**: 118–122.

Befus AD, Bienenstock J, Denburg JA, eds. *Mast cell differentiation and heterogeneity*. New York: Raven Press, 1986.

Denburg JA, Dolovich J, Harnish D. Basophil, mast cell and eosinophil growth and differentiation factors in human allergic disease. *Clin Exp Allergy* 1989; **19**: 249–254.

El-Asrar AMA, Geboes K, Misotten L, Emarah MH., Maudgal PC, Desmet, V. Cytological and immunohistochemical study of the limbal form of vernal keratoconjunctivitis by the replica technique. *Br J Ophthalmol* 1987; **71**: 867–872

El-Asrar AMA, Van den Oord JJ, Geboes K, Missotten Luc, Emarah MH, Desmet V. Immunopathological study of vernal keratoconjunctivitis. *Graefe's Archive Clin Exp Ophthalmol* 1989; **227**: 374–379.

Galli SJ, Austen KF, eds. *Mast cell and basophil differentiation and function in health and disease*. New York: Raven Press, 1989.

Gleich GJ, Frigas E, Loegering DA, Wassom DL, Steinmuller D. Cytotoxic properties of the eosinophil major basic protein. *J. Immunol* 1979; **123** (6): 2925–2927

Morgan SJ, Williams J, Walls AF, Church MK, Holgate ST, McGill JI. Mast cell numbers and staining characteristics in the normal and allergic conjunctiva. 1991; **87**: 111–116.

Sompolinsky D, Samra Z, Zavaro A, Barishak R. A contribution to the immunopathology of vernal keratoconjunctivitis. *Documenta Ophthalmologica* 1982; **53**: 61–92

Chapter 20

Conjunctivitis – Diagnosis and Treatment

Introduction

The conjunctiva is a mucous membrane whose entire surface – including the part beneath the eyelids – is connected with the air of the environment by the tear film. It can be involved in allergic reactions similar to those that affect other body surfaces. Such reactions liberate noxious substances into the tear film; some of these erode the surface of the cornea, thereby threatening vision. The allergic diseases of the eye surface have distinct clinical patterns.

History Taking

The history is a vital component of the diagnosis of allergic eye disease.

Atopic diathesis
Most patients have a personal or family history of other atopic diseases such as asthma, eczema, or hay fever. Because the allergic eye diseases, apart from seasonal conjunctivitis, are much rarer than these other atopic conditions, they are unlikely to feature in the family history.

Age of onset
Allergic eye disease appears before the age of 30 years in more than 80 per cent of patients.

Symptoms
Characteristic symptom complexes are usual. Itching is very common, and causes much distress. Eye rubbing may be severe, and it has been suggested that it may play a part in the development of keratoconus, in which the cornea thins and steepens, a disease commoner in atopic than in non-atopic people. Tearing is universal in active allergic eye disease.

Mucus accumulation and discharge are often troublesome. The mucus is unlike normal conjunctival mucus, being profuse, tacky, and stringy. Photphobia usually indicates corneal involvement. Blepharospasm accompanies photophobia. Conjunctival oedema and hyperaemia cause the bulbar surface to take on a 'glassy' appearance, with dilated blood vessels. 'Morning misery' – the author's term – is characteristic of vernal keratoconjunctivitis: the child is unable to open the eyes on awaking, because of a combination of sticky mucus, photophobia, and blepharospasm. Attempts to open and clear the eyes often take an hour or more, so that the child arrives late for school.

Timing
Aeroallergens predominate in allergic eye disease, and seasonal allergens produce seasonal disease. Thus seasonal allergic conjunctivitis will appear at the same time as its causative pollen or mould, whereas perennial allergens such as *Dermatophagoides* provoke perennial disease, which however usually shows seasonal variations.

Location
Allergic eye diseases can be as sensitive to geographical location as are other manifestation of the atopic state. Parents of children with vernal keratoconjunctivitis usually know of locations where the symptoms improve and others which can be relied upon to worsen them.

Provoking factors
Non-specific ocular irritants such as smoke may aggravate the symptoms of allergic eye disease, as may exposure to reactive chemicals such as isocyanates, and to other environmental or occupational factors. Certain food and food additives, such as tartrazine, occasionally exacerbate ocular allergies.

Examination

Examination of the Ocular Surfaces

Before a diagnosis of allergic eye disease can be entertained the surfaces of the eye must be examined. This can be done with the naked eye, using a bright pen torch for illumination, although a magnifying glass, a watchmaker's eyeglass, or a pair of spectacle loupes will help. (Ophthalmologists use a slit lamp biomicroscope which provides a range of illuminations – slits, spots, broad beams – at variable intensity, and can magnify the surface of the eye up to 40-fold.)

The lids and lid margins
The lids are under observation as soon as eye contact is made with the patient. Swelling or discolouration, indicative of inflammation, should be noticed, as should whether the upper lids droop – known as ptosis and, in allergic eye conditions, a sign of possible active disease. Also observe whether blinking is regular and complete. 'Flick blinking' – incomplete closure of the lids – is quite often seen in contact lens wearers.

Blepharospasm – spasm of the orbicularis oculi muscles – occurs in corneal and conjunctival inflammation and is often accompanied by photophobia.

The anterior lid margins can be examined with the pen torch. Observe the lashes and note whether they are normal or whether the lash bases are cuffed or the lid margins are crusted. These signs, and redness and swelling of the anterior lid margin, indicate anterior marginal blepharitis.

The posterior lid margins are brought into view if the lid is partially everted by gentle finger pressure on the skin adjacent to them. The openings of the Meibomian glands, between 20 and 25 to each lid margin, are seen near the poterior border. Observe whether the posterior lid margins are squared (normal) or rounded (indicating chronic disease). Note whether the Meibomian gland orifices are small and even, which is normal, or unevenly dilated as in chronic marginal disease. Attempt to express the Meibomian secretion by gently squeezing the lid against the eyeball with the finger. The secretion is normally clear and fluid, but may be yellow and semisolid, or even a solid wax, in chronic lid margin disease. The mucocutaneous junction should be just behind the Meibomian orifices; if in front of them this may indicate chronic inflammation with shrinkage.

The conjunctival surfaces

The conjunctiva lines the underside of the eyelids and is reflected on to the anterior surface of the eyeball, blending with the corneal epithelium at the limbus. The surface markings of the conjunctiva are shown in Fig. 20.1. The part lining the tarsal plates is the tarsal conjunctiva; that beyond the tarsal plates in the fornices of the conjunctival sac is the forniceal conjunctiva; and that part on the eyeball surface is the bulbar conjunctiva. All of these parts are continuous and all can be involved in inflammatory processes, but in allergic conjunctivitis it is the tarsal conjunctiva in particular that is involved. It has not been satisfactorily explained why the forniceal and bulbar surfaces often appear clinically normal when obvious tarsal conjunctival disease is present.

The bulbar conjunctiva is examined by looking directly at the eye. If the patient is asked to look up and then down while first the lower lid and then the upper lid is gently retracted with the finger, the whole of the bulbar surface can be seen.

The tarsal conjunctiva is examined by everting the lids. The lower tarsal surface is seen when the lower lid is drawn downwards by a finger placed near the lid margin. It usually helps if the patient looks up. The upper tarsal surface is seen when the upper lid is everted over a cotton bud, a glass rod, or other narrow object (Fig. 20.2). The eyelashes can be grasped to produce the eversion. This will not hurt if the patient looks down and continues to do so.

The lower forniceal conjunctiva can be seen if the lid is retracted more forcibly than when the lower tarsus is being examined. It is continuous with the lower tarsal conjunctiva and no junction is visible. The upper forniceal conjunctiva can only be examined with the aid of a retractor such as Desmarre's (Fig. 20.3). The patient should look as far down as possible. The manoeuvre often causes discomfort. Nevertheless it is important to examine this area where, for example, the follicles typical of viral and chlamydial infection are commonly seen.

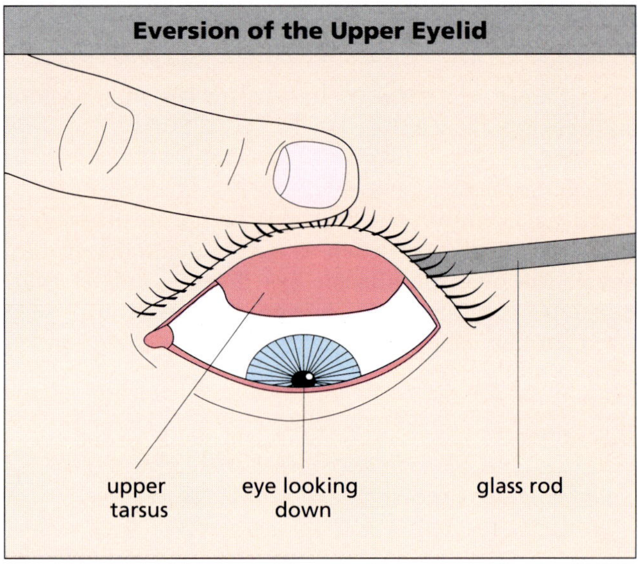

Fig. 20.2 Eversion of the upper lid to allow examination of the upper tarsal conjunctiva.

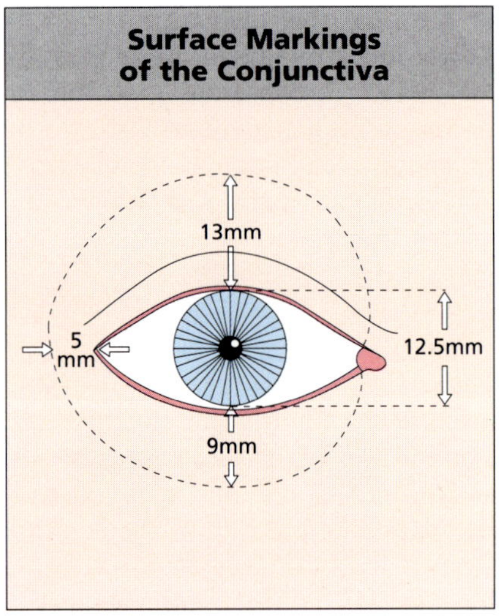

Fig. 20.1 The surface markings of the conjunctival fornices.

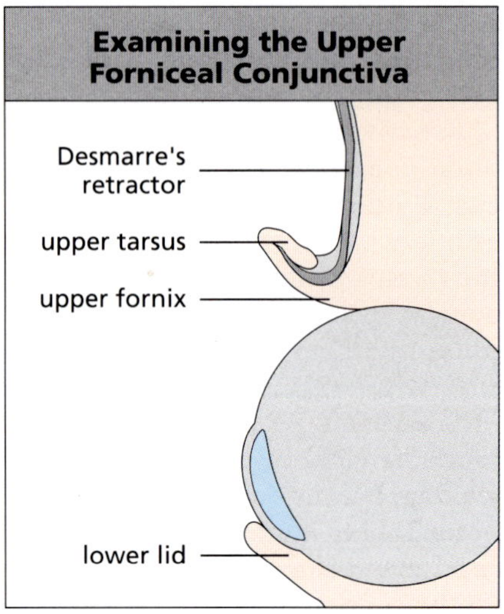

Fig. 20.3 Eversion of the upper lid using a Desmarre's retractor.

Tissues Involved in Allergic Eye Disorders	Tarsal Conjunctiva	Limbus	Cornea	Lid Margin
Seasonal allergic conjunctivitis	+	–	–	–
Perennial allergic conjunctivitis	+	–	–	–
Vernal keratoconjunctivitis	++	++	++	±
Atopic keratoconjunctivitis	++	+	++	++
Giant papillary conjunctivitis	++	±	–	–

Fig. 20.4 Summary of the clinical signs of five allergic eye diseases.

When examining the conjunctiva, which is normally smooth and transparent, the following points should be checked. Hyperaemia shows as an enhanced pinkness or redness of the surfaces. Oedema produces a filmy or glassy appearance and an apparently jelly-like consistency. If the surfaces are infiltrated, it will generally be impossible to see the normal vascular pattern through the conjunctiva. Follicles and papillae show as elevations of the tarsal conjunctival surface; if they are pale and glistening they are probably follicles; if flat and pink with a central vessel they are likely to be papillae. Micropapillae, up to 0.3 mm in diameter, occur in the normal eye. If they are larger than 0.3 mm in diameter (macropapillae) or larger than 1 mm in diameter (giant papillae) they are abnormal. Scarring shows as pallor of the surface in reticular, linear, or sheet pattern. Cicatrization (shrinkage) of the conjunctival surface produces shortening of the tarsal surfaces and entropion (inturning) of the lid margins. A thin string of mucus in the lower fornix is normal; a larger quantity, and flecks of mucus in the tear film, are abnormal.

The cornea and limbus

The cornea and limbus are best examined with the slit lamp biomicroscope. However some features can be seen with the naked eye.

The cornea should be perfectly smooth and transparent and have a spherical profile at its centre, flattening gently towards its edges. Any imperfection on its surface will be shown as a disturbance of the normal bright (specular) reflex of a light source such as a pen torch. Surface lesions are seen more easily if a little fluorescein is placed in the tear film (by dipping the end of a manufactured impregnated paper strip into the marginal tear meniscus) and the cornea is examined with a cobalt blue light. (Medical pen torches are often supplied with a blue filter that can be placed over the beam.) It should be possible to decide whether the corneal surface appears perfectly clear, as is normal, or whether there are opacities which may be either infiltrates or scars. The quality of any surface disturbance should be noted: if it is finely dusted this indicates punctate epithelial keratitis; if there is a localized epithelial defect this is a macroerosion or an ulcer; and if the surface disturbance is white or yellowish and dry in appearance, corneal plaque may be present. Mucus adherent to the corneal surface is always pathological.

The limbus is the zone immediately surrounding the cornea and is normally invisible to the naked eye, but when it is inflamed it becomes visible; it may appear pale or pink, and swollen in an annular pattern. Discrete swellings may indicate limbal vegetations. The presence of small white dots (Trantas' dots) is diagnostic of vernal keratoconjunctivitis.

Fig. 20.4 shows the particular tissues involved in five allergic eye diseases.

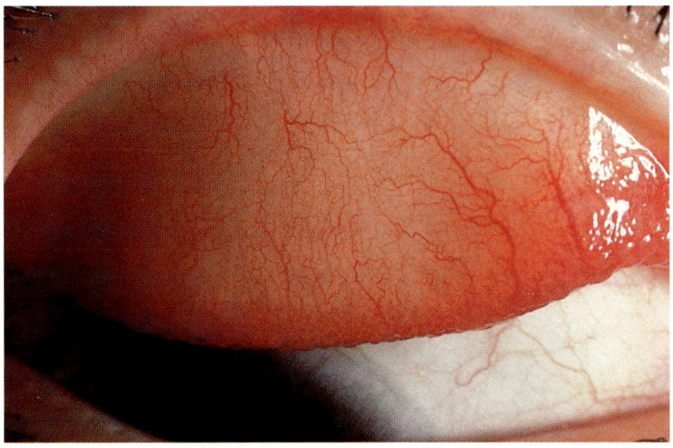

Fig. 20.5 The upper tarsal surface in SAC.

Allergic Conjunctivitis – the Clinical Conditions

Season Allergic Conjuntivitis (SAC) (Hay Fever Conjunctivitis)

SAC is the commonest form of allergic conjunctivitis, for it affects nearly every hay fever sufferer to some degree. There is no threat to sight. In the hay fever season the eyes become itchy, pink, and watery. There is no visual disturbance except that caused by the excessive tearing.

The characteristic clinical finding is of minimal or no signs. The tarsal surfaces are slightly hyperaemic and oedematous and small papillae may be seen (Fig. 20.5). There may also be minimal hyperaemia and oedema of the bulbar conjunctiva. The lids, cornea, and limbus are not affected.

In man, the conjunctival response to histamine appears to be mediated entirely by H-receptors; H_2-antagonists such as cimetidine have no effect on this response. However the conjunctival microvascular permeability response caused by mast cell activation comprises both histaminergic and non-histaminergic components, the latter involving PGD_2, leukotrienes, and kinins.

Treatment consists of avoiding or minimizing exposure to the allergen(s). If this is not possible, systemic antihistamines (often prescribed for nasal symptoms) are usually effective in controlling the symptoms. Topical antihistamine preparations have a minor role to play; the antihistamine is usually combined with a vasocontrictor to reduce conjunctival injection. Prolonged use of these preparations can cause contact conjunctivitis. Drops of sodium cromoglycate 2 per cent solution are effective when applied four or more times daily to both eyes. Some patients derive additional benefit from sodium cromoglycate 4 per cent ointment placed in both eyes at bedtime. Topical steroid preparations are strictly contraindicated in this mild, non-sight-threatening disease because their posiible side-effects, such as glaucoma, cataract, and potentiation of corneal infection, are sight-threatening.

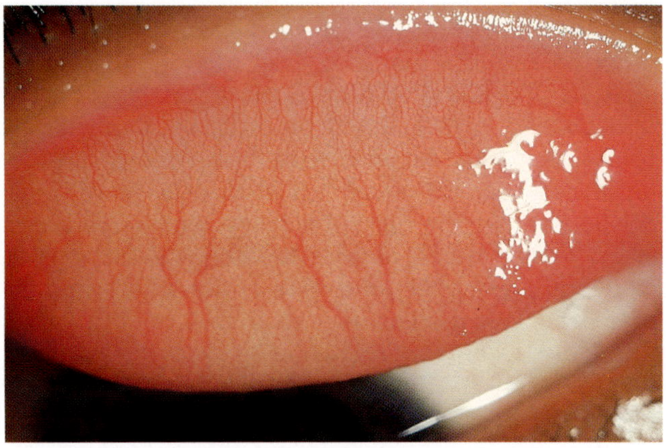

Fig. 20.6 The upper tarsal surface in PAC.

Contact lens users may find that their lens tolerance decreases while the condition is active.

Perennial Allergic Conjunctivitis (PAC)
PAC can be thought of as the perennial equivalent of SAC. There is evidence to suggest that in temperate climates it may represent a response to house dust mite which is perennially present. The symptoms and signs are exactly as for SAC, except that both tend to be milder (Fig. 20.6). Treatment is along the same lines as for SAC. Hyposensitization therapy has not proved reliably effective in either condition. PAC may preclude or limit successful contact lens wear.

Vernal Keratoconjunctivitis (VKC)
In the United Kingdom, VKC is a rare, self-limiting, often seasonal ocular allergy that affects young children, especially boys, who usually have a personal or family history of atopy (Fig. 20.7). The condition is a common and serious cause of ocular morbidity in

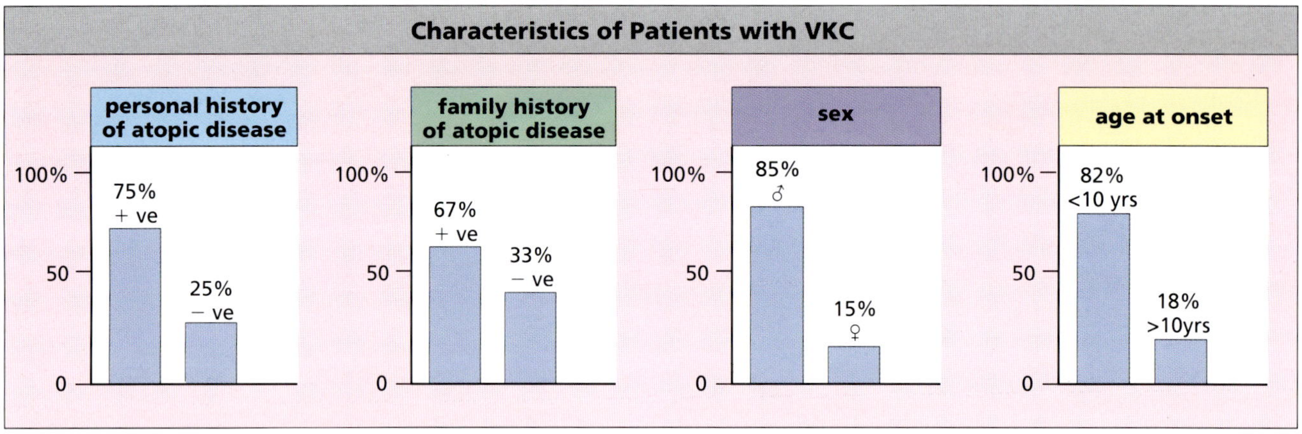

Fig. 20.7 The characteristics of VKC patients from a series of 100. (Data modified from Buckley RJ. Long-term experience with sodium cromoglycate in the management of vernal keratoconjunctivitis. In: Pepys J, Edwards AM. *The Mast Cell*. London: Pitman Medical, 1980: 518–523.

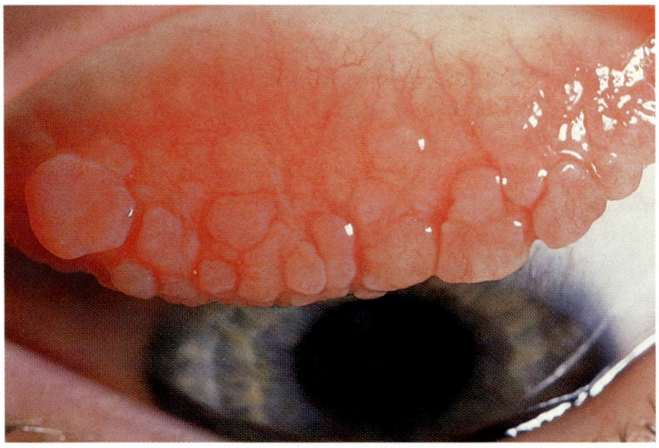

Fig. 20.8 The upper tarsal surface in VKC showing giant papillae.

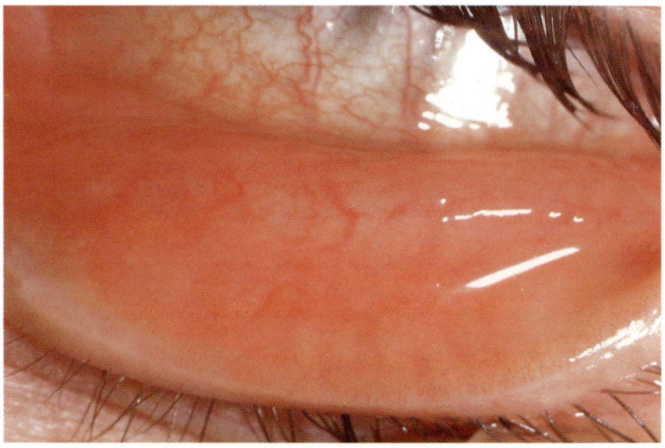

Fig. 20.9 The lower tarsal surface in VKC showing non-specific inflammation.

parts of the Mediterranean basin, the Middle East, the Far East, Africa, and South America.

The symptoms are itching, photophobia, blepharospasm, blurred vision, and 'morning misery' – an inability to open the eyes in the morning. There is often discomfort associated with the stringy inflammatory exudate.

The most characteristic sign of VKC is the development of giant papillae (over 1 mm diameter), also known as cobblestone papillae, on the upper tarsal conjunctiva (Fig. 20.8). Other conjunctival areas show less specific signs of inflammation (Fig. 20.9). In the later stages, fine sub-epithelial scarring is seen also. When the disease is active, the conjunctival surfaces are hyperaemic, oedematous, and infiltrated, and a tenacious mucus is present (Fig. 20.10). The limbus may show hyperaemia and infiltration, and discrete swellings known as vegetations may be present (Fig. 20.11). Small white dots, first described by Trantas, are typical of vernal limbitis (Fig. 20.12).

The most serious aspect of the condition is the corneal involvement. At its mildest, there is a punctate disturbance of the epithelium (Fig. 20.13). If not treated the lesions coalesce to form a macroerosion (Fig. 20.14); deposition of mucus and fibrin can then result in the formation of plaque (Fig. 20.15).

In VKC the signs can be remarkably different in severity between the two eyes. This phenomenon has not been satisfactorily explained.

Treatment is generally in the hands of the ophthalmologist, because 80 per cent of cases require topical corticosteroids. For the majority, however,

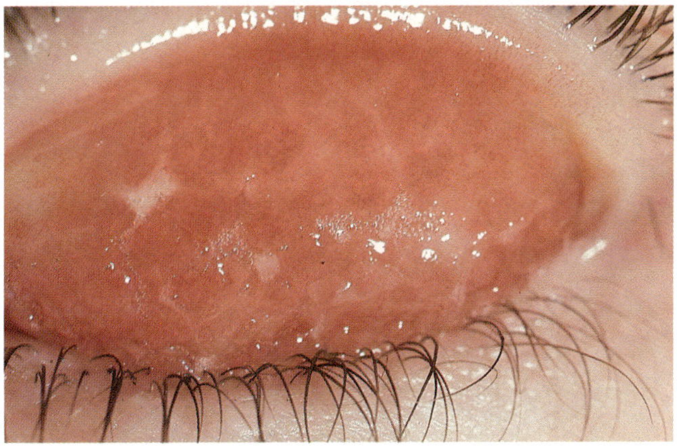

Fig. 20.10 Active vernal conjunctivitis.

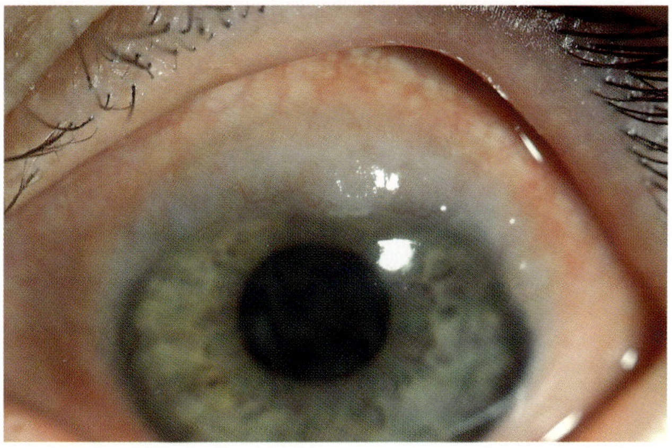

Fig. 20.11 Limbal vegetations in VKC.

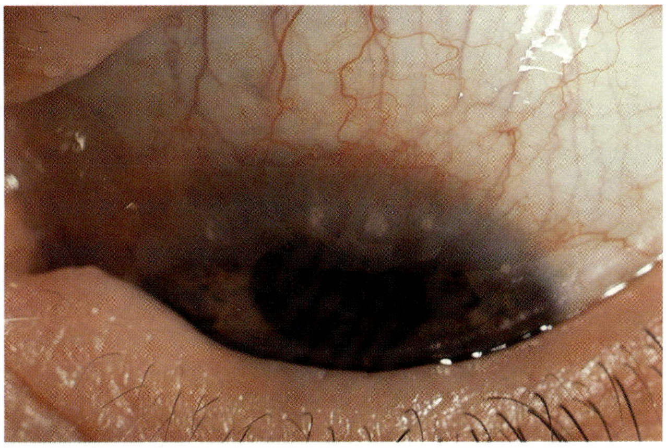

Fig. 20.12 Trantas' dots at the limbus in VKC.

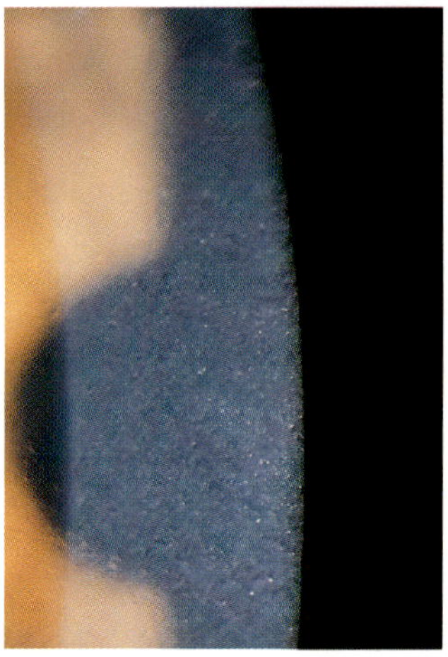

Fig. 20.13 Punctate epithelial keratitis in VKC.

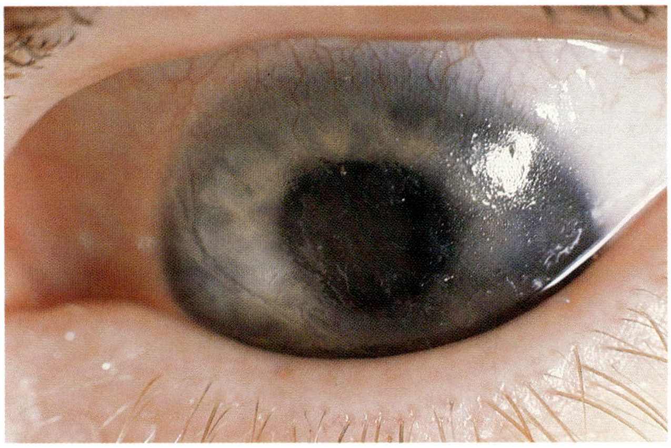

Fig. 20.14 Macroerosion in VKC.

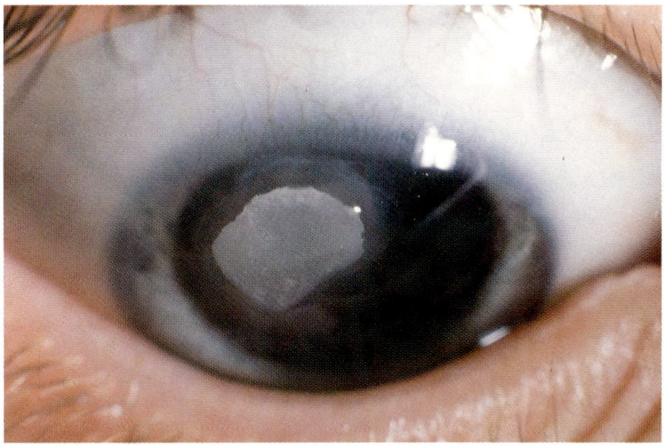

Fig. 20.15 Corneal plaque in VKC.

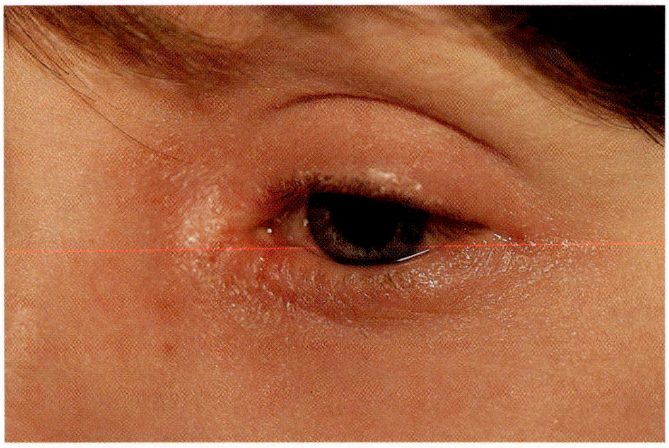

Fig. 20.16 The lids in AKC.

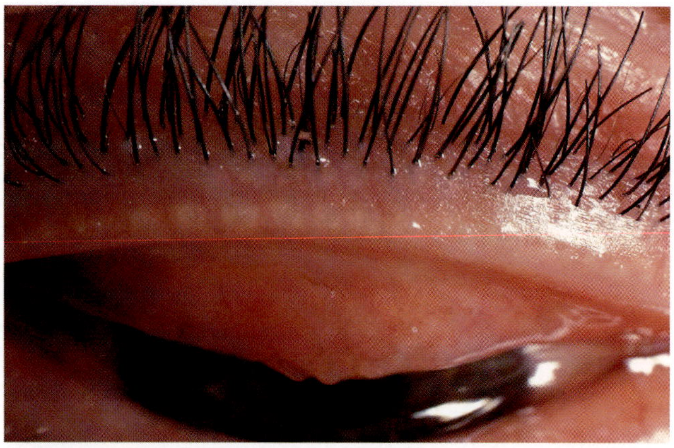

Fig. 20.17 The upper tarsal surface in AKC.

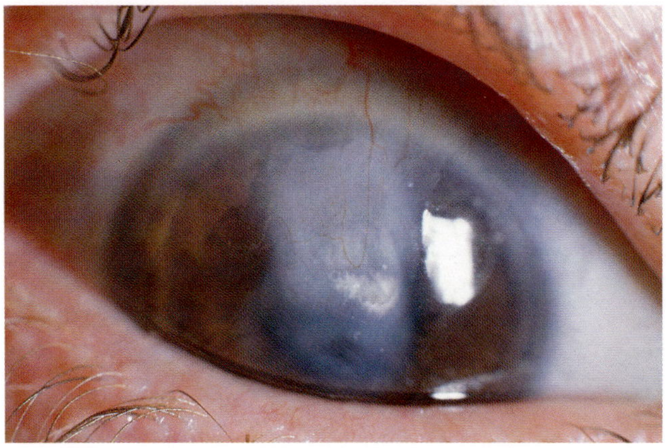

Fig. 20.18 Corneal scarring and neovascularization in AKC.

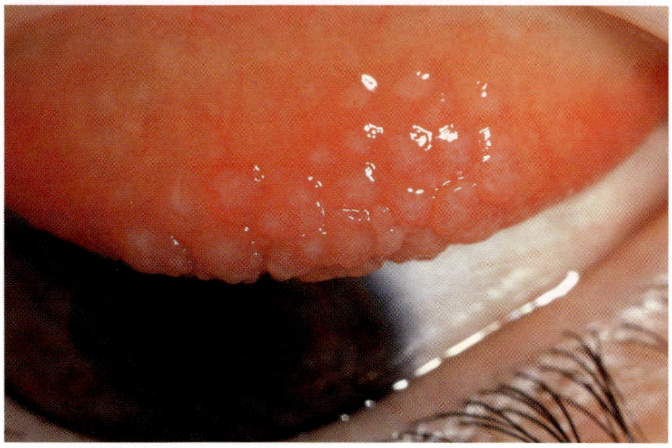

Fig. 20.19 The upper tarsal surface in GPC.

some benefit is obtained from sodium cromoglycate, as 2 per cent drops and/or 4 per cent ointment, which also reduces the need for corticosteroids. In an acute case, strong topical steroid preparations (eg prednisolone 1 per cent or dexamethasone 0.1 per cent) are given frequently, up to once hourly. As the condition comes under control the dose is reduced in frequency and strength. Additional relief is provided by mucolytic drops which dissolve the symptom-producing abnormal mucus. One such is acetyl cysteine 5, 10, or 20 per cent. When the corneal epithelium is breached by a macroerosion or by plaque topical antibiotic drops, such as chloramphenicol 0.5 per cent, are often prescribed as antibacterial prophylaxis.

When corneal plaque is present, medical therapy is aimed at quietening the conjunctival inflammation as rapidly as possible. The plaque is then surgically removed by lamellar dissection using the operating microscope. General anaesthetic is usually required, as most patients are children. Re-epithelialization usually takes place in a few days after this procedure.

VKC usually resolves spontaneously at or after puberty; but it may metamorphose into atopic keratoconjunctivitis.

Atopic Keratoconjunctivitis (AKC)

This condition can be thought of as an adult equivalent of VKC. It is a rare sight-threatening lifelong disease of young atopic adults, predominantly males. The lid margins and facial skin are conspicuously involved in this condition.

The lid margins are thickened, posteriorly rounded, and often keratinized, and are chronically infected, usually with *Staphylococcus epidermidis* or *S. aureus*. There is usually facial eczema involving the eyelids (Fig. 20.16). The conjunctiva shows a chronic intense infiltration, papillae, and often shrinkage (Fig. 20.17). There is limbal inflammation. The cornea is subject to epithelial defects progressive scarring and neovascularization (Fig. 20.18). Corneal plaque similar to that of VKC is sometimes seen, as is spontaneous corneal perforation. Associations have been recorded with eye rubbing, keratoconus, atopic cataract, and retinal detachment.

The management of AKC is difficult, and afflicted patients can never be cured. It is important to control the lid margin disease with sodium bicarbonate lotion applied daily, topical antibiotic ointment, and systemic antibiotic in long-term low-dose regime such as doxycycline 100 mg daily for three to six months. The facial eczema should be treated with topical medications. Corticosteroid ophthalmic preparations are likely to be necessary; the ophthalmologist will have to exercise much care in order to avoid unwanted side-effects. Sodium cromoglycate has been reported to be effective, most particularly in corticosteroid-sparing.

Giant Papillary Conjunctivitis (GPC)

Foreign body-associated giant papillary conjunctivitis, as it should properly be called, was first reported in wearers of soft contact lenses in 1974. It is now recognized that it occurs in wearers of all types of

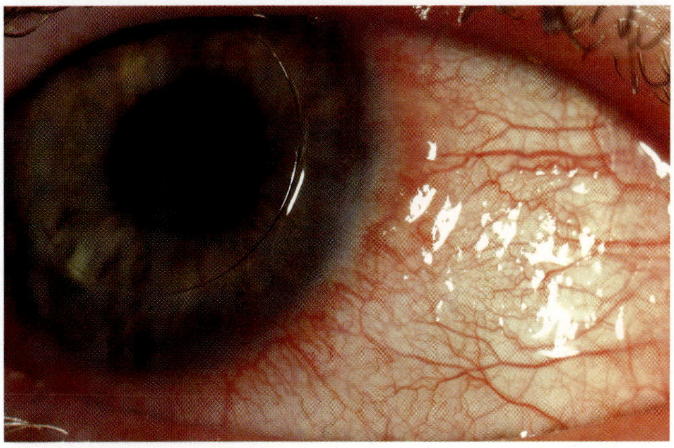

Fig. 20.20 Limbal inflammation in GPC.

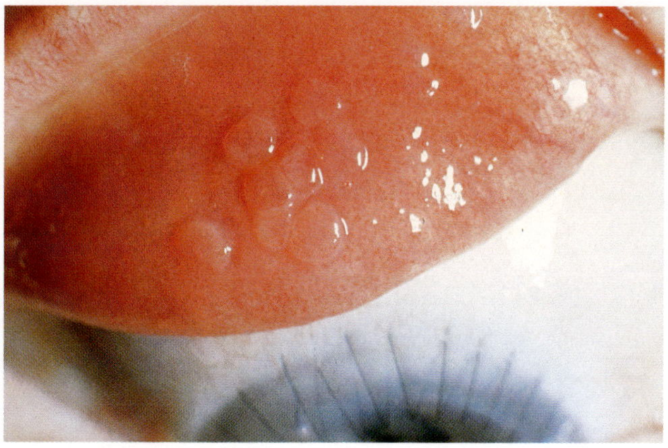

Fig. 20.21 Suture-induced GPC: the offending corneal sutures and the tarsal surface showing giant papillae.

lenses and ocular prostheses and in association with other foreign bodies such as protruding sutures on the ocular surface.

While giant papillae are defined as having a diameter of 1 mm or more, there is a further category of papillae, namely macropapillae of 0.3 mm to 1 mm in diameter, whose presence in macropapillary conjunctivitis (MPC) may be considered to be a mild developmental or *forme fruste* version of GPC.

The onset of symptoms occurs a few weeks to many months after contact lens or prosthesis wear has begun. There is discomfort and a tendency for mucus to accumulate on the lens. Patients complain of ocular itching when the lens is removed. The tolerance of the lens, as measured by the daily wearing time, is reduced. There is a tendency for the lens to displace upwards under the upper lid. The patient may notice that the symptoms are alleviated if a brand new lens is worn.

The signs on the upper tarsal conjunctiva are very similar to those of VKC (Fig. 20.19), but the lower tarsus is less often involved. In severe cases there may be limbal inflammation as well (Fig. 20.20) resembling but milder than that seen in VKC. The cornea, however, is not involved.

GPC is managed by careful attention to lens hygiene, by improvement of the fit and surface quality of the lenses or prosthesis, by minimizing the wearing time, and as a last resort by drugs. There may be a place for the use of disposable contact lenses worn on a daily basis. Suture GPC (Fig. 20.21) is usually cured by removal of the offending suture(s). Sodium cromoglycate has been shown to be effective in the management of GPC. Topical steroid preparations should not be used as they are very much more sight-threatening than the condition itself, except in the case of prosthesis wearers.

Conclusion

The allergic eye diseases and their treatment with topical steroids can be sight-threatening. Allergists should be aware of the threat to the ocular tissues of their patients. Furthermore, they should recognize that they are in a position to manage the less serious conditions, and that cases of VKC, AKC, and GPC should be referred to an ophthalmologist with an interest in the external eye.

Further Reading

Allansmith MR. *The Eye and Immunology*. St. Louis: CV Mosby, 1982.

Bailey CS. Allergic conjunctivitis and contact lens wear. *Journal of the British Contact Lens Association* 1991; **14**: 219–221.

Buckley RJ. Vernal keratoconjunctivitis. *International Ophthalmology Clinic* 1989; **29**: 303–308.

Dart JKG, Buckley RJ, Monnickendam M, Prasad J. Perennial allergic conjunctivitis: definition, clinical characteristics and prevalence. A comparison with seasonal conjuntivitis. *Transactions of the Ophthalmological Societies of the United Kingdom* 1986; **105**: 513–520.

Foster CS, Rice BA, Dutt JE. Immunopathology of atopic conjunctivitis. *Ophthalmology* 1991; **98**: 1190–1196.

Tuft SJ, Kemeny MD, Dart JKG, Buckley RJ. Clinical features of atopic keratoconjunctivitis. *Ophthalmology* 1991; **98**: 150–158.

Chapter 21

Urticaria – Pathophysiology

Introduction

The urticarias are a heterogeneous group of disorders. Many triggers and mechanisms can lead into a final common pathway involving the degranulation of mast cells and the production of the raised, red, and itchy, but transient weals of variable duration which are characteristic of urticaria (Fig. 21.1). When deeper tissues with more capacity for oedema swell, angioedema results (Fig. 21.2). Despite the variability of the urticarias, all types have many factors in common, such as histamine release. Thus, evidence obtained from one type of urticaria can often assist in the understanding of other types.

The urticarial response might be considered physiologically as a defence mechanism against unwanted intrusion: for example, the response to an insect bite, which gives rise to scratching to remove the insect, and vasodilatation to facilitate clearance of toxic material. Urticaria can occur because of a disturbance anywhere in the response pathway, from the provoking stimulus to the chemical response (Fig. 21.3). Thus, the reaction could be firing in error in the absence of a trigger, or there might be a deficiency in the downregulation of the response.

Complex interactions between mast cells and other cells extend the area of interest to the regulatory effects of cytokines and the release of chemotactic factors, which in turn attract neutrophils and eosinophils. The cellular responses lead to activation of chemical pathways involving ecosanoids, neuropeptides, complement, and fibrinolytic and kinin pathways. These might amplify the response or play a part in triggering the degranulation of mast cells.

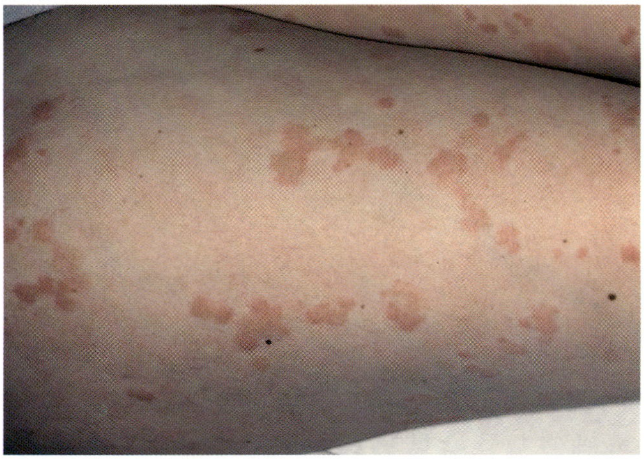

Fig. 21.1 Typical appearance of urticaria.

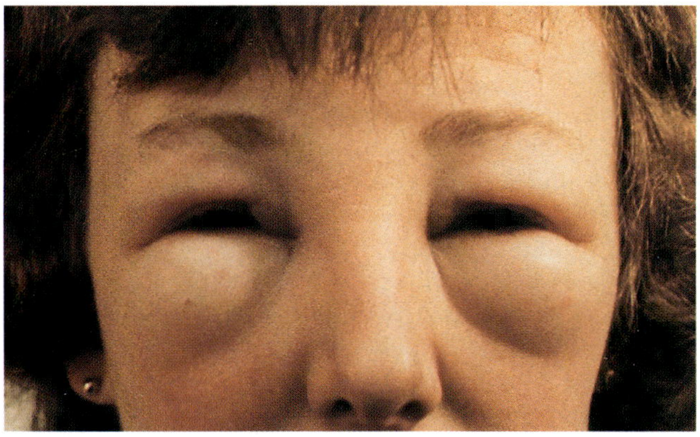

Fig. 21.2 Angioedema.

Pathophysiology of Urticaria

Histopathology

The principal histological finding in most forms of urticaria is dermal oedema, which in the case of angioedema extends into the subcutaneous tissues. There is a variable cellular infiltrate around vessels, in which lymphocytes usually predominate; they are

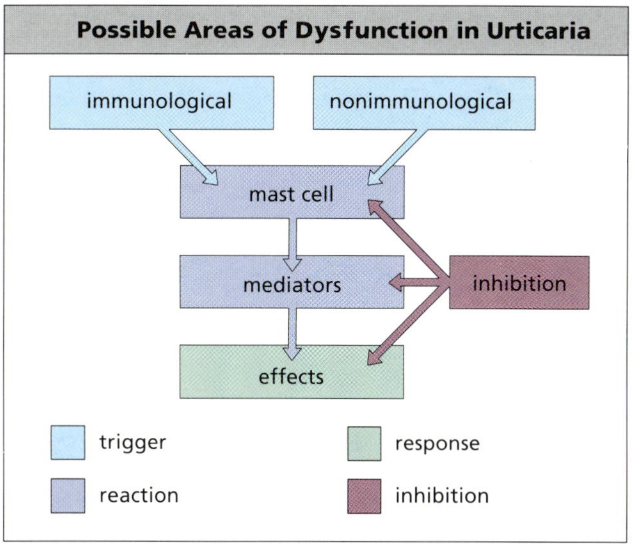

Fig. 21.3 An overview of possible areas of dysfunction in urticaria arising from a defect in triggering, reaction, response, inhibition, or a combination of these factors.

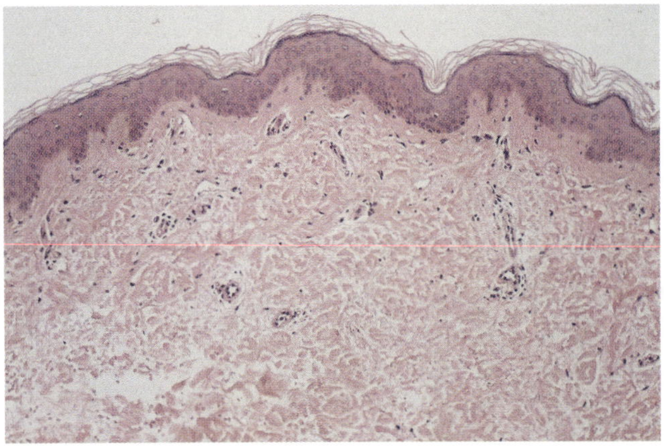

Fig. 21.4 Histology of chronic idiopathic urticaria showing dermal collagen separated by oedema and a sparse, perivascular inflammatory cell infiltrate. (× 10).

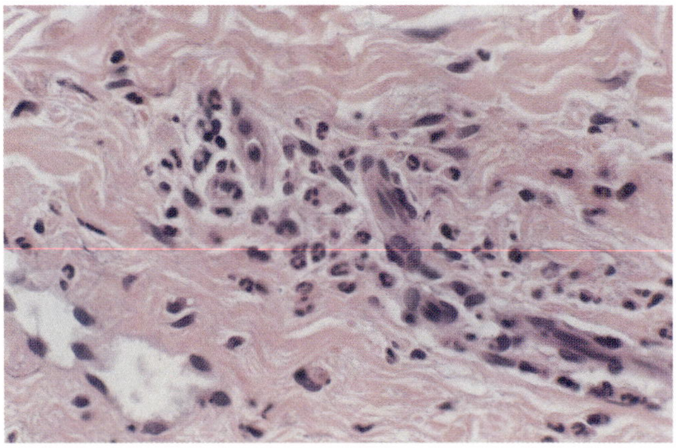

Fig. 21.5 Histology of urticarial vasculitis showing a predominantly neutrophil polymorphonuclear cell infiltrate with swelling of endothelial cells, vessel thickening. However, fibrinoid necrosis and nuclear dust are not seen. (× 40).

accompanied by neutrophil and eosinophil polymorphs (Fig. 21.4). With the use of electron microscopy, degranulating mast cells can be seen, and they may be accompanied by activated and degranulating eosinophils which deposit major basic protein. An electron microscopic study of cold-induced urticarial vasculitis revealed clumping of platelets.

On the other hand, in the syndrome of urticarial vasculitis, there may be evidence of a leucocytoclastic vasculitis with endothelial cell swelling, retraction, or necrosis, and a mixed but predominantly neutrophil infiltrate in the walls of venules, accompanied by a variable degree of deposition of fibrinoid material and nuclear dust formation (Fig. 21.5). However, the degree of vasculitis is variable and endothelial cell necrosis is not always seen. Russell-Jones and colleagues in London have described a continuum of histological change between these two extremes, and this has led to problems of definition in the urticarial vasculitis syndrome.

The presence of polymorphs in the vessel wall has been extensively studied by Winkelmann, who found that this phenomenon was more frequent in patients with physical urticarias, particularly dermographism, although it is also seen in cold and cholinergic urticaria. As neutrophil and eosinophil infiltration precedes that of mononuclear cells, the timing of the biopsy in relation to the onset of the lesion is important and will influence the histopathological picture. Among the physical urticarias, delayed pressure urticaria has an unusual time course with a delay of several hours between elicitation and response. In the first five hours after a pressure stimulus, neutrophils and eosinophils predominate (Fig. 21.6a) whilst in later lesions lymphocytes and eosinophils are seen (Fig. 21.6b). These lymphocytes are predominantly activated T helper cells. The delayed wealing response probably results from the activity of the infiltrating cells.

Activated T helper cells also form an important part of the infiltrate in chronic idiopathic urticaria, accounting for up to 70 per cent of the cells present, and their role is considered below. Another important finding which needs to be substantiated is the tenfold increase in mast cell numbers reported by Natbony and co-workers.

Triggering Factors

The simple model for urticaria is the type I anaphylactic response. In this response, antigen crosslinks to antigen-specific IgE which is bound to mast cell membranes, and so initiates the complex series of biochemical events which lead to the release of preformed mediators and the generation of newly formed mediators. Such mechanisms are commoner in atopic patients; in patients with a known allergen, the urticaria is consequently short-lived. Although IgE serum levels are usually normal, this may not reflect tissue-bound IgE. An enzyme-linked immuno-sorbent assay (ELISA) revealed antibodies to milk, ovalbumin, and gliadin in 60 per cent of sera from patients with chronic idiopathic urticaria, but these antibodies were predominantly of the IgG4 type and suggested a state of chronic antigenic stimulation.

Although allergic mechanisms are not demonstrable in all types of urticaria, this mechanism is involved in many of the acute allergic reactions to ingested food or drugs. Curiously such reactions do not always resolve quickly after elimination of the allergen. For example, dermographism can develop after penicillin allergy, penicillin therapy for syphilis, and treatment of scabies. After a generalized reaction to griseofulvin a personal patient developed cold urticaria. From such clinical evidence, it seems that an immunological stimulus can alter the host's reactivity, rendering him responsive to stimuli other than the allergen; the mast cells become 'irritable' and degranulate more easily.

Patients with chronic urticaria release more histamine than do controls, both spontaneously and with the mast-cell degranulating agents compound 48/80 and codeine. Some findings conflict with this view, particularly where histamine release by basophils is examined. This may be because of the exhaustion of histamine stores by the urticaria itself, or because of a state of desensitization arising

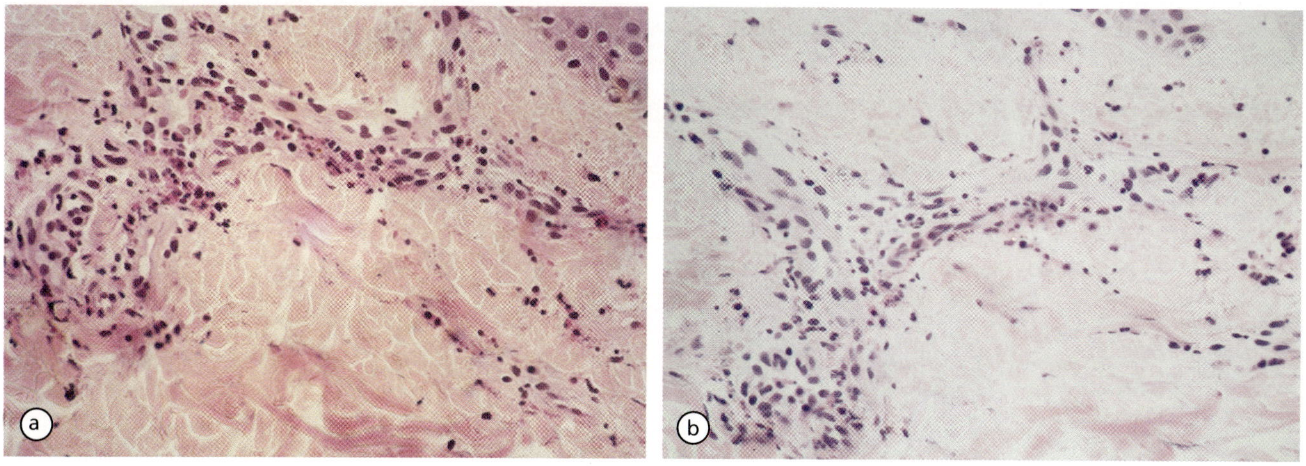

Fig. 21.6 Histology of delayed pressure urticaria showing (a) a predominance of neutrophils and eosinophils at six hours; and (b) a predominance of lymphocytes after 24 hours. (× 25). (Courtesy of Dr A Kobza Black, St John's Centre, St Thomas's Hospital.)

from chronic antigen exposure. Alternatively histamine itself may act through H_2 receptors to inhibit basophil activation.

Degranulation of mast cells in human skin may be stimulated by immunological mechanisms and various non-immunological stimuli such as the anaphylatoxins C3a and C5a, lymphokines, opioid analgesics, histamine releasing factors (HRFs), and neuropeptides such as substance P (see Fig. 21.7). Other chemicals act to release histamine by mechanisms which are uncertain; these include dextran, aspirin, and food additives such as tartrazine and benzoates. It is conceivable that mast cells are 'irritable' because of their chemical milieu, and numerous factors may have an additive effect on the equilibrium to favour degranulation.

This may help to explain some of the inconsistencies relating to reactions to food additives where evidence of IgE-mediated sensitivity is scanty. Patients showing a reaction on provocation with tartrazine during the active phase of chronic urticaria fail to react when the urticaria spontaneously remits. Thus it would seem likely that a pharmacological mechanism is involved. This is supported by the observations of Murdoch and colleagues who demonstrated asymptomatic histamine release in normal volunteers challenged with tartrazine. In cases with consistent responses to food additives they also showed reproducible mediator release by mast cells with azo food dyes.

Some of the cross reactivity of food additives may be explained by their metabolic fate. Azo dyes undergo a reductive cleavage in the gut to form sulphanilic acid and a pyrazolone; these can form sulphophenylhydrazine, which resembles aminopyrine anti-inflammatory drugs. Benzoates, which are used as preservatives in food, have a structure which is similar to aspirin. One possible mode of activity for these substances is through interference in the cyclooxygenase pathway of prostaglandin synthesis. Likewise, the more frequent and important non-specific exacerbation of chronic urticaria caused by aspirin in up to 40 per cent of patients is thought to have a pharmacological basis, perhaps acting through the inhibition of cyclooxygenase and thereby increasing the substrate and production of the lipoxygenase products, leukotrienes and mono-HETEs.

Infection can trigger urticaria in hepatitis B where the mechanism may be an immune complex vasculitis. More commonly, viral infections cause an exacerbation of pre-existing urticaria, possibly by means of interferon acting either to enhance release of mediator from mast cells or to decrease the number of T-suppressor lymphocytes. Infection can precipitate cold urticaria, perhaps through cross-sensitivity between the virus and an epitope revealed in the skin on cold challenge.

In about 50 per cent of patients with active chronic idiopathic urticaria, an unknown serum factor of molecular weight of more than 30kDa produces a weal and flare, which closely mimics the response to compound 48/80 (a mast-cell degranulating agent), and serum retains this activity when the patient is challenged after remission. The nature of this unknown circulating urticariogen remains speculative, but it may be a cytokine, a histamine releasing factor, an anti-IgE, or even an antigen which might vary between patients. The view that the factor may be an autoantibody is supported by the observed association of urticaria with autoimmune thyroid disease, Kaplan having recently found IgG and IgM autoantibodies directed against IgE in five out of nine patients with cold urticaria, and in three out of six patients both with urticarial vasculitis and chronic urticaria.

Mediators

Mast cell degranulation releases preformed granule-associated mediators and new mediators generated from membrane phospholipids. In some urticarias the effects of these mediators may be amplified and prolonged by the activation of kinin and complement and by the release of further mediators from infiltrating cells

Histamine has a central role as a mediator and, when injected alone, it reproduces the appearance of

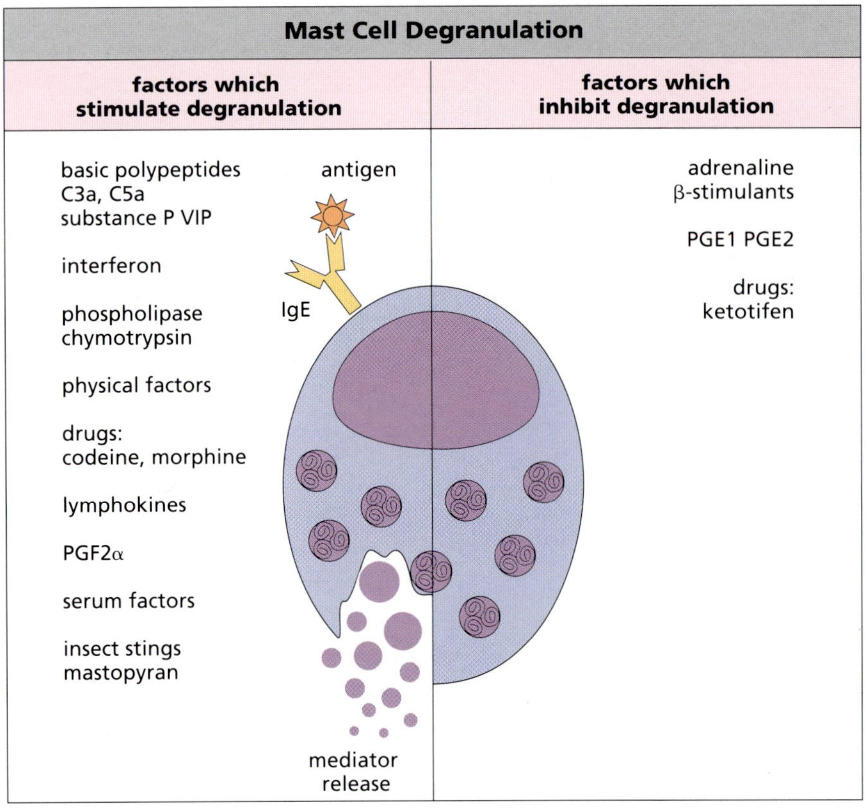

Fig. 21.7 Factors exciting and inhibiting mast cell degranulation.

urticaria with a transient, red, raised, and itchy weal, and sometimes causes systemic effects (Fig. 21.8). Frequently demonstrated in the physical urticarias, its importance is reflected in the beneficial effects of H_1 antihistamines.

Equally, however, the incomplete blockade of urticaria by these drugs serves as an indicator of the importance of other mediators in urticaria. During severe episodes, or where the stimulus to a physical urticaria has been great, systemic effects can result; for example, bronchospasm accompanying cholinergic urticaria, or headaches accompanying cold urticaria. In such situations experimental induction of urticaria is accompanied by significant elevation of histamine levels in the blood. Histamine levels are increased both in the lesions and the normal skin of patients with chronic urticaria. The responsiveness of the skin to histamine is also slightly increased in patients with urticaria.

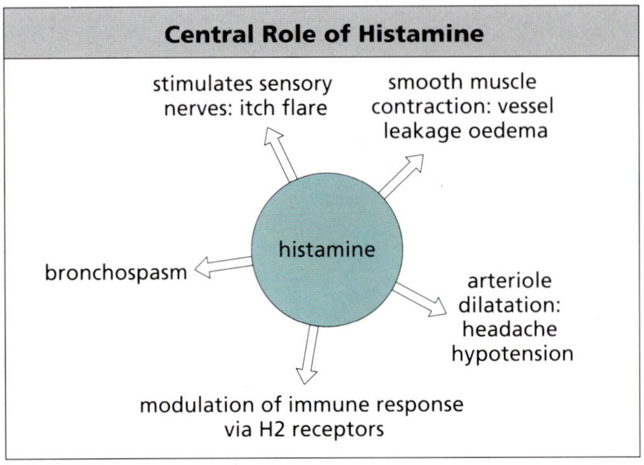

Fig. 21.8 Histamine has a central role in producing the urticarial response and the accompanying signs.

The newly formed phospholipid mediators are rapidly metabolized and are therefore difficult to demonstrate in experimental urticaria. Prostaglandin D_2 is the most frequently demonstrated of this group and yet the quantity released is insufficient to have a significant role in the production of weals, except in mastocytosis where higher levels resulting from increased numbers of mast cells contribute to flushing and hypotension. These are relieved by cyclooxygenase inhibitors. Prostaglandin D_2 may also play a part in the anaphylactic response to bee stings.

Leukotriene release has been sought in many of the urticarias, but evidence for their involvement is restricted to one study in delayed pressure-induced urticaria which implicated LTB_4, and a recent study by Lawlor and colleagues in which LTC_4 rose, though this was not statistically significant. The metabolic product LTE_4, to which LTC_4 is rapidly metabolized, has been demonstrated in cold urticaria. Release of platelet activating factor (PAF) like lipid was found in one study of cold urticaria, and was inhibited by doxepin which was also found to modulate the clinical response. Electron microscopy of intense cold urticaria has also shown platelet clumping which might be indirect evidence of its release in urticaria. However, markers of platelet activation (platelet factor 4 and β-thromboglobulin) are not increased in blood after induction of cold urticaria

Although PAF and leukotriene are chemotactic factors, there are other incompletely characterized neutrophil chemotactic factors of high molecular weight released in cold, heat, solar, and cholinergic urticaria. Eosinophil chemotactic factors are released from human mast cells after antigen challenge, and have been demonstrated after challenge testing in cold urticaria.

Mast cell-derived proteases tryptase, chymase, and carboxypeptidase are also important, as they can induce further mast cell degranulation and activate complement, kinins, and Hageman factor, thereby amplifying the reaction. They might also partially digest collagen and ground substance to facilitate the movement of phagocytic cells through the skin and enhance vascular permeability. In high concentrations, chymase may also lead to blister formation by allowing local detachment of the epidermis. Levels of proteases are elevated in lesions of mastocytosis. Other evidence for their involvement is indirect (see inhibitory factors). Enzymes may also take part in the destruction of mediators.

Kinins

Kinins are oligopeptides released from larger kininogen proteins by the action of kinogenases or kallikrein. Three kinins present in man are bradykinin, kallidin and methionyl-lysyl-bradykinin. As well as being potent vasodilators they relate closely to the coagulation and fibrinolytic systems, with high molecular weight kininogen augmenting the activation of factor XII (Hageman factor). This in turn activates kallikrein. As well as producing kinins, kallikrein produces fibrinolytic plasmin from its precursor (Fig. 21.9).

Bradykinin and kallidin are partially converted to inactive peptides by angiotensin converting enzymes (ACE) and this is thought to be the mechanism of the angioedema reported with the ACE-inhibiting drugs captopril and enalapril. Because of impaired inhibition, the effects of kinins are exaggerated and increased levels of bradykinin have been reported in this type of angioedema.

Because C1 esterase inhibitor, which is deficient in cases of hereditary angioedema, inhibits kallikrein, it is likely that kinins have a role in this disorder (see below). The release of kinins has also been demonstrated in dermographism.

Complement

Complement may be activated in several ways in urticaria. In urticarial vasculitis, complement is activated via the classical pathway by IgG and IgM in immune complexes, and the same mechanism could be active to a variable degree in other forms of urticaria. Alternative pathway activation might result from venoms, antigens, IgA, or radiological contrast media but the mechanism of its activation in some physical urticarias is not well understood. Furthermore, trypsin derived from mast cells cleaves C3 to form C3a and C3b. Once activated, complement C3a, C4a, and C5a anaphylatoxins have the capacity to induce histamine release from cutaneous mast cells and, therefore, are possible mediators of urticaria. In addition, C5a is a potent neutrophil chemotactic agent. These peptides also contract smooth muscle independently of histamine although this action may be mediated by the ecosanoids. When injected intradermally they cause a weal and flare reaction, and pruritus.

Classical or alternative pathway activation of complement have been described in between 0 and 30 per cent of patients with chronic idiopathic urticaria, but earlier studies may have included some patients with urticarial vasculitis. C4 and C2 deficiency have been reported in isolated cases of cold urticaria, and in two cases of localized heat-induced urticaria levels of C3 and factor B fell, indicating activation of the alternative pathway.

Neuropeptides

Neuropeptides are a large family of potent mediators secreted by nerves; in the skin the principal secretors are the sensory neurons. Substance P, calcitonin gene-related peptide (CGRP), and neurokinin A (NKA) have received the most attention and can be

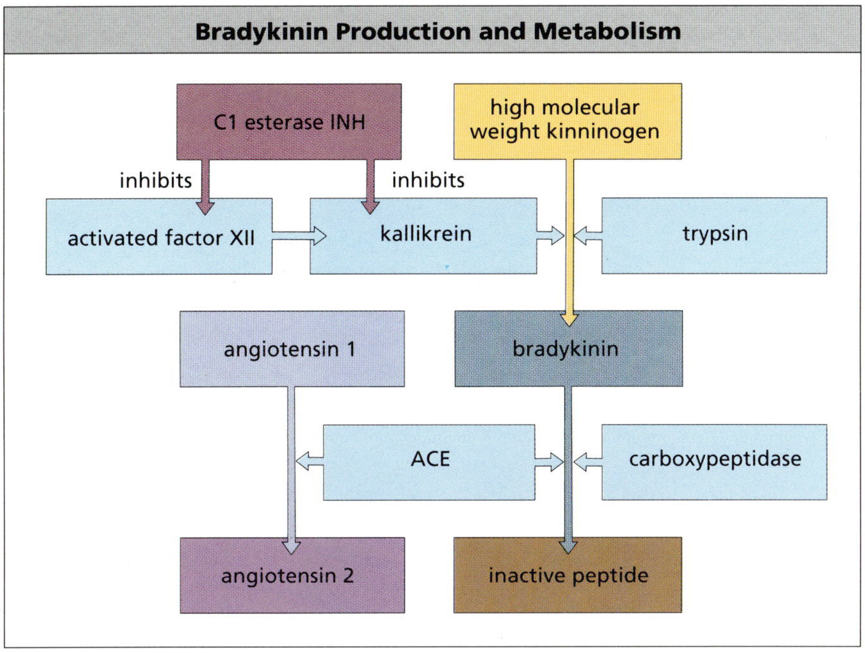

Fig. 21.9 Production and metabolism of bradykinin. Inhibitors of angiotensin converting enzyme (ACE) induce angioedema by inhibiting bradykinin metabolism. In hereditary angioedema down-regulation of kinin formation is deficient.

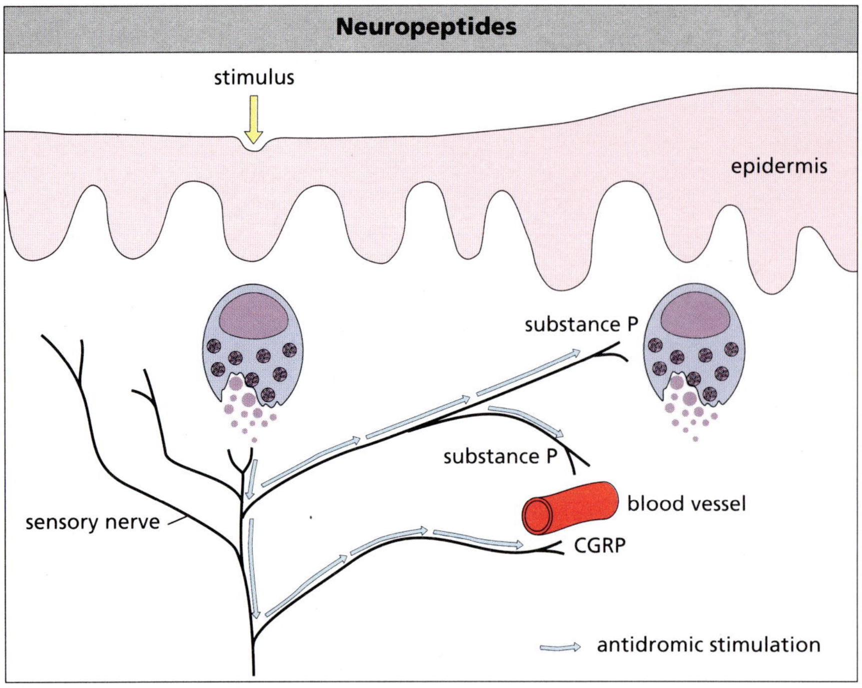

Fig. 21.10 Following a stimulus such as friction, mast-cell derived mediators initiate an axon reflex, which releases neuropeptides by antidromic stimulation, thereby propagating flare and amplifying the response.

demonstrated by immunohistochemistry within sensory neurons, around blood vessels, eccrine sweat glands, and sometimes within the same nerve. Substance P, CGRP, and NKA are all thought to participate in the axon reflex flare which follows firm stroking of the skin or injection of histamine (Fig. 21.10). Substance P produces erythema mainly by activating mast cells which then release histamine , but it produces oedema by a direct effect on blood vessels; CGRP and NKA act directly on blood vessels. Unlike other mediators, the potent vasodilatory effect of CGRP lasts for six to 24 hours after intradermal injection, and the affected skin is surrounded by an area of pallor. The metabolites of CGRP are chemotactic for eosinophils.

Evidence for the involvement of these substances and the related compound vasoactive intestinal peptide (VIP) come from direct measurements or indirect evidence whereby nerves are depleted of neuropeptides using topical capsaicin prior to provocation. Substance P and VIP are increased in the lesional and non-lesional skin of patients with cold urticaria and dermographism compared to controls, and it is possible they potentiate the reaction. Eight cases of cold and localized heat urticaria are reported to have been blocked by pre-treatment with capsaicin. The neuropeptides, particularly VIP and atrial natriuretic peptide, which are both implicated in the regulation of sweating, are also strong candidates for involvement in cholinergic urticaria where the stimulus is neurogenic.

Because codeine and morphine degranulate mast cells it is possible that the endogenous opioid peptides exert a similar effect, thereby forming another link between central nervous events and the skin. Dynorphin, β-endorphin and α-neoendorphin can all induce histamine release at low concentrations by non-immunological mechanisms similar to basic polypeptides (see Chapter 5).

Protease Inhibitor Abnormalities

Abnormality	Condition
reduced α1-antitrypsin (α1-AT)	cold urticaria idiopathic angioedema
reduced total antitrypsin (TAT)	cold urticaria
reduced α1-antichymotrypsin (ACT)	cold urticaria cholinergic urticaria
reduced inter-α-trysin inhibitor (IαTI)	chronic urticaria angioedema
increased α1-AT and TAT	delayed pressure urticaria chronic idiopathic urticaria

Fig. 21.11 Examples of urticarias associated with protease inhibitor abnormalities.

Inhibitory factors

Once triggered, reactions are terminated by destruction of the mediators, and application of 'brakes' to pathways of secondary activation such as complement and kinin formation. Some mediators are inactivated by becoming bound to heparin; others are removed by granulocytes and macrophages. The effects of mediators of urticaria are likely to be accentuated if the natural inhibitors of those mediators are deficient. It can also be postulated that recurrent and excessive mediator release consumes the inhibitors, after which further mediator release is unopposed.

The protease inhibitors exert a controlling influence over the protease enzymes released from mast cells and leucocytes, but they also inhibit enzyme activity in the complement cascade, kinin, clotting, and fibrinolytic systems. This group of enzymes overlaps considerably in specificity and comprises αl-antitrypsin (αlAT), αl-antichymotrypsin (ACT), inter-α-trypsin inhibitor (IαTI), α2 macroglobulin antithrombin III, and C1 esterase inhibitor (C1-INH).

Deficiencies or increases in levels of protease inhibitors have been demonstrated in association with urticaria. Some of these are listed in Fig. 21.11. However, it should be emphasized that estimates of protease levels differ between studies, and that some patients have urticaria with normal levels of protease. Some of the variability may arise as a result of the consumption of protease inhibitors which are suicidal. These protease inhibitors form soluble complexes with the enzyme which are then removed. However, there may be a subgroup of patients who are genetically predisposed to cold urticaria and angioedema because of protease deficiency.

Whether protease deficiency is causal or not, boosting inhibitors offers an alternative treatment. Treatment of patients with chronic urticaria using Trasylol, a protease inhibitor particularly active against kallikrein, has been found to be effective in some patients with chronic urticaria, and danazol has been used to correct the deficiency of ACT in cholinergic urticaria with good results. This drug is also anecdotally effective in some patients with chronic urticaria and pressure-induced urticaria.

Endothelial Cells and Fibrinolysis

The wealing response in urticaria results from the effects of mediators on vessels. Histamine is a potent releaser of plasminogen activator, which in turn initiates fibrinolysis and removes fibrin from the endothelium. This allows serum to pass through and in turn activates complement, kinins, and mast cells. Thus fibrinolytic activity is increased after intracutaneous injection of histamine or substance P, and also in normocomplimentaemic urticaria. In urticarial vasculitis cutaneous fibrinolytic activity is reduced, possibly by exhaustion of available plasminogen activator.

Endothelium is also an important gate through which leucocytes must pass. The attraction of cells to sites of inflammation is influenced by the expression of intercellular adhesion molecules on the surface of endothelial cells. Endothelial cells produce cytokines,and respond to cytokines. Interleukin-l (IL-1), derived from mononuclear phagocytes and epidermal cells, stimulates the production of prostacyclin by endothelium, so producing vasodilator and anti-platelet effects. It also increases PAF production by endothelium and adhesion molecule expression. By producing the cytokines IL-l and IL-6, endothelial cells might also participate in lymphocyte activation at the site of inflammation. The involvement of these mechanisms in urticaria have not been studied.

Role of Lymphocytes and other Leucocytes

The lack of infiltrate in early lesions of urticaria rules against an initiating role for other inflammatory cells. However, after the release of chemotactic factors, neutrophils, eosinophils, and macrophages (all of which can in turn generate mediators) are attracted to the lesion to prolong the reaction. Eosinophil-derived major basic protein has been demonstrated in pressure, solar, and chronic urticarias. It releases histamine from basophils and induces a weal and flare reaction when injected intradermally. This suggests an active role for eosinophils in these types of urticaria. Polymorphs and macrophages may also play a part in removing antigen and mediators and therefore in terminating the reaction.

T lymphocytes are important in immunoregulation of the sensitizing phase of type I IgE-mediated hypersensitivity, but the increase of activated T helper cells in urticarial lesions suggests an active role for these cells. An incompletely characterized factor derived from antigen-stimulated mononuclear cells can release histamine, IL-3,and GM-CSF, which have some histamine-releasing activity. Activated T cells produce the mast cell growth factor IL-3 and also release an antigen specific factor which, like IgE, can arm mast cells to react to that antigen.

Mast cells produce several factors that are chemotactic for lymphocytes. Once activated, mast cells can themselves produce IL-3 and IL-4 (which stimulates B cells). It is therefore conceivable that mast cell degranulation could initiate a chain of events leading to an expanded population of reactive mast cells (Fig. 21.12). At the time of writing, none of these

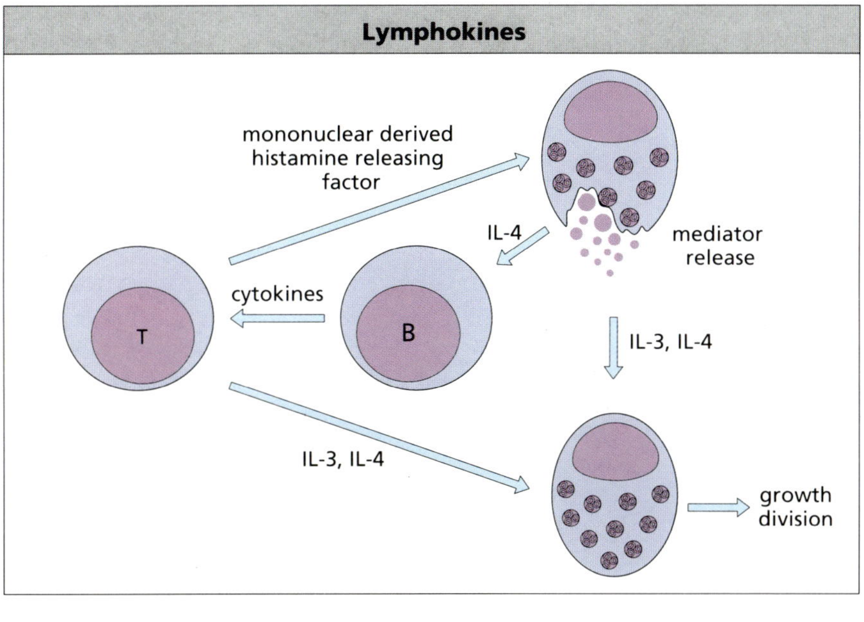

Fig. 21.12 T cell/mast cell interactions of possible importance in chronic urticaria, pressure urticaria, and mast cell hyperproliferation.

Physical Urticaria		
Urticaria	**Stimulus**	**Mediators**
dermographism	friction	histamine, kinin, substance P
cholinergic	nervous stimulus to sweating	histamine, eosinophil chemotactic factors, neutrophil chemotactic factors
cold	cold contact	histamine, prostaglandin D2 neutrophil chemotactic factors eosinophil chemotactic factors platelet activating factor-like lipid, LTE_4
delayed pressure	pressure	histamine, LTB_4 (?), LTC_4 (?)
heat contact	heat contact	histamine, neutrophil chemotactic factors, complement activation
solar	light	histamine, eosinophil chemotactic factors, neutrophil chemotactic factors
vibratory	vibration	histamine

Fig. 21.13 Types of physical urticaria.

lymphokines has been demonstrated in urticaria, but their involvement is suggested by the finding of migration inhibitory factor (a macrophage activating factor produced by endothelial and mononuclear cells) in endothelial cells and dermal dendrocytes of patients with acute and chronic urticaria and urticaria pigmentosa.

Clinical Manifestations of Urticaria

Physical Urticarias

In the physical urticarias, specific physical stimuli trigger mast cell degranulation, with the release of mediators (Fig. 21.13). With the exception of delayed pressure urticaria, the weals tend to be short-lived and may not represent the same pathological process as in idiopathic urticaria. However, these conditions lend themselves to laboratory investigation because of the ability to reproduce the reaction under controlled conditions and much of the current understanding of mediators in urticaria is based on this type of experiment. Common ways of examining the production of mediators are: sampling of fluid from suction blisters overlying the reaction; sampling of blood draining the area of induction (e.g. the antecubital fossa of an arm immersed in cold water for cold urticaria); and performing an abrasion to remove the epidermis and applying a fluid-filled receptor cell for mediators diffusing from the underlying dermis. As these are all invasive techniques which can release mediators themselves, control experiments are important.

In many of the physical urticarias there is evidence of a passively transferable reactivity, which presumably involves IgE recognizing a molecule released or conformationally altered by the appropriate physical stimulus. However, within each class of physical urticaria there is heterogeneity, accounting for variable findings, and frequently there is overlap with patients displaying more than one type of physical urticaria, suggesting a predisposition or defect in recognition of self-antigens.

Dermographism

In symptomatic dermographism, passive transfer has frequently been reported, predominantly with IgE, although IgM- and IgA-mediated, passively transferable dermographism are also recorded. The response is mast cell dependent and blocked by prior degranulation of mast cells. Histamine is involved in weal production, and reflex axon transmission via substance P produces the flare. In cases lacking a detectable IgE-mediated reaction it is plausible that mechanical trauma directly activates mast cells as it does in urticaria pigmentosa. In some cases an anergic cofactor is required in order to render the skin dermographic.

Cold urticaria

There are several variants of cold urticaria (Fig. 21.14) which is frequently transferable and IgE mediated (25–50 per cent), although rarely it can be mediated by other immunoglobulins, cryoglobulins, and cryofibrinogen. Because it is well suited to investigation, many mediators have been isolated (Fig. 21.13). Histamine is the most important of these mediators and can produce systemic effects (see Fig. 21.8). Protease inhibitors may be deficient, in some patients complement may be activated, and there is sometimes evidence of vasculitis. Often the onset of

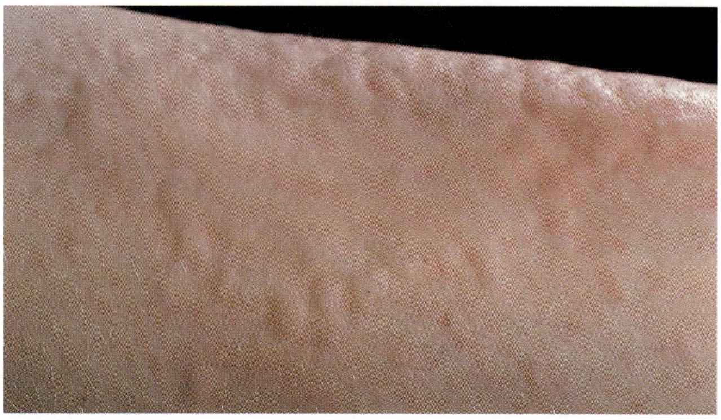

Fig. 21.14 Urticarial wealing reaction following contact with an ice cube for 10 minutes in a patient with cold urticaria.

the urticaria can be traced back to some antigenic trigger such as viral infection, syphilis, infestation, or allergies to drugs including penicillin and griseofulvin. When patients with cold urticaria are exposed repeatedly to cold, a state of tolerance can be induced in which the mast cells and mediators are intact. This suggests a state of unresponsiveness of mast cells, perhaps from blockade of binding sites or depletion of the cold-related antigen.

Cholinergic urticaria

In cholinergic urticaria, the reaction is not to heat; rather it is triggered by the nervous stimulus to sweating. Acetylcholine released from nerves is important but, as results of from trials involving the intracutaneous administration of acetylcholine are variable, there are probably other important mediators involved. It is possible to block the reaction with local anaesthetics or high doses of anticholinergic drugs, although this is not practical in therapy. Histamine release has been repeatedly shown; this possibly contributes to the bronchoconstriction which can occur. Chemotactic factors are released, leading to a neutrophil infiltrate. A deficiency of the inhibitor α1-antichymotryptase has also been noted; if this deficiency is treated, there is some improvement in the clinical condition. Only rarely has an IgE response been identified in this type of urticaria.

Delayed pressure urticaria

Delayed pressure urticaria requires intact mast cells for its induction, and experimental degranulation of mast cells using compound 48/80 causes a response similar to that elicited by pressure testing in these patients. Both stimuli are followed by a delay of four to eight hours before producing the response.

Delayed pressure urticaria differs from other types of urticaria in that it frequently accompanies ordinary chronic urticaria and the lesions are deeper and more persistent. The lack of response to antihistamines suggests that histamine is less important here than in other types of urticaria. Other mediators in delayed pressure urticaria include kinins, the chemotactic factor LTB-$_4$ in one study, and a statistically insignificant rise in LTC-$_4$/D-$_4$/E-$_4$ in six patients. Products of the chemotactically recruited polymorphs and lymphocytes (see Fig. 21.6) are likely to be more important. The delay in the development of this response is likely to be due to the time taken to for these cells to be recruited, lymphokines and eosinophil major basic protein being likely initiators of the response.

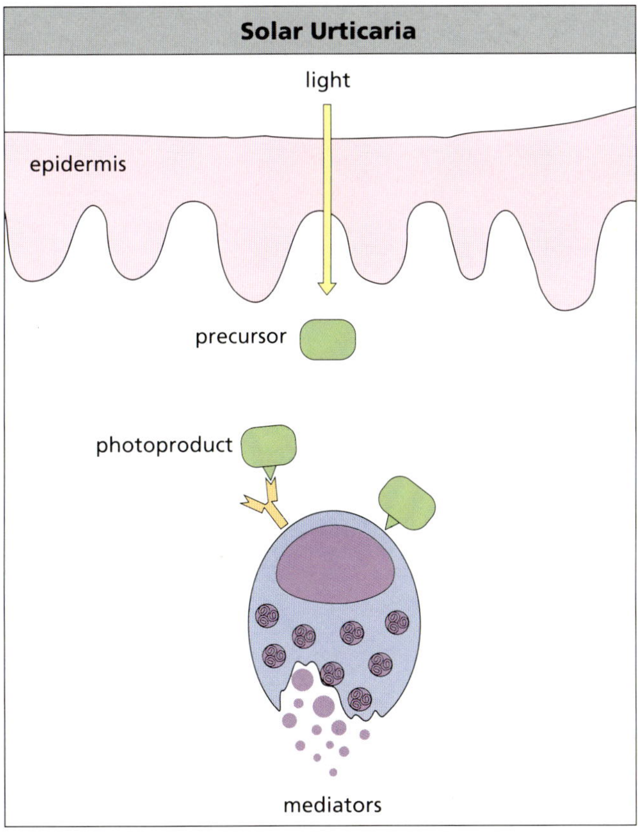

Fig. 21.15 Mechanisms of solar urticaria.

Solar urticaria

Solar urticarias are also of mixed aetiology; causes include porphyria, lupus erythematosus, and drugs. The eliciting light can be in the spectrum of visible light, UVB, or UVA. A precursor is converted to an antigenic photoproduct which triggers IgE-mediated release. In type 1 the antigen is unique to patients with the disorder, whilst in type 2 the antigen is present in normal irradiated skin but only causes a response in those affected. The precursor can sometimes be demonstrated in the patient's serum and its removal by plasma exchange prevents the response. Passive transfer is complicated, since IgE, precursor, or photoproduct may be transferred. This explains reverse passive transfer in type 2 solar urticaria, whereby irradiation of the skin produces a photoproduct but no reaction until serum from a type 2 patient, containing IgE directed against the photoproduct, is injected. Prior irradiation with different wavelengths of light can alter the precursor, and so inhibit or augment its subsequent activity. The mechanisms of solar urticaria are shown in Fig. 21.15.

There are also thought to be two types of localized heat urticaria, one in which histamine is released from mast cells, and another in which mast cells are not required but complement is activated by either pathway.

In the rare vibratory angioedema, histamine release and endothelial cell swelling have been described in the absence of mast cell degranulation, suggesting possible release of histamine from endothelium.

Urticarial Vasculitis

The syndrome of urticarial vasculitis usually includes other systemic manifestations – most commonly arthralgia, but also general malaise, glomerulonephritis, obstructive pulmonary disease, or ophthalmic, gastrointestinal or central nervous vasculitis. The skin lesions are the most frequent manifestation. Compared to other forms of urticaria, they are often more prolonged, lasting for more than 24 hours, often feel firmer to the touch, and often leave some pigmentation, scaling, or faint purpura even after they have resolved.

The pathogenesis is that of an immune complex vasculitis similar to the arthus reaction. This leads to a neutrophil infiltrate and leucocytoclastic vasculitis of variable degree (see histology). The antigen involved is unknown in most cases, although some cases of systemic lupus erythematosus, serum sickness, and hepatitis B can present with an identical clinical picture. Frequently there is evidence of complement activation and consumption, usually via the classical pathway, but sometimes via the alternative pathway. Complement factors Cl, C3, C4, and properdin, along with IgM, IgG, and fibrin are often demonstrated in blood vessel cells and along the basement membrane using direct immunofluorescence. However, the pattern is not specific to this condition. Immune complexes have been demonstrated in the serum of many patients with urticarial vasculitis using the Clq assay, and there are several reports of a 7S protein containing IgG which precipitates with Clq but which is not specific for this disorder.

With complement activation there is release of C3a and C5a which are chemotactic and cause mast cell degranulation. LTB_4 probably also contributes to the chemotactic attraction of neutrophils which release lysosomal enzymes and generate superoxides. Platelet activation and aggregation together with activation of fibrinolysis (above) could also contribute, resulting in vasodilatation, increased permeability, and a variable degree of damage to endothelial cells which may swell, undergo fibrinoid necrosis, or shrink and retract. Whether immune complexes from the circulation initiate the vasculitis, arise as a result of tissue damage, or accumulate because of defective mechanisms for clearance is not understood.

Hereditary Angiodema

The syndrome of hereditary angioedema is characterized by painless, non-pruritic swellings which are not erythematous and which predominantly affect the extremities and the face. These persist for two to three days and are precipitated by emotion and trauma. There may be an accompanying mottling of skin but there is no urticaria. Oedema in the gut gives rise to episodic, severe, colicky abdominal pain and vomiting. It is important to recognize this, because swelling in the pharynx and larynx can lead to asphyxiation. Inherited in an autosomal dominant fashion, there are two forms of the disease. In the commonest (Type 1), occurring in 85 per cent, Cl-INH protein is present in low amounts (5-31 per cent of normal) due to decreased synthesis and increased metabolism. In type 2, an antigenically similar protein is present in normal amounts but, because of point mutations in the reactive centre, it is functionally impaired. The exact protein mutation varies between different families. The normal Cl-INH gene has recently been characterized by genomic cloning, and in type 1 families repetitive sequences in this gene lead to deletion or repetition of sequences at the site of mutation. Although the exact locus of the

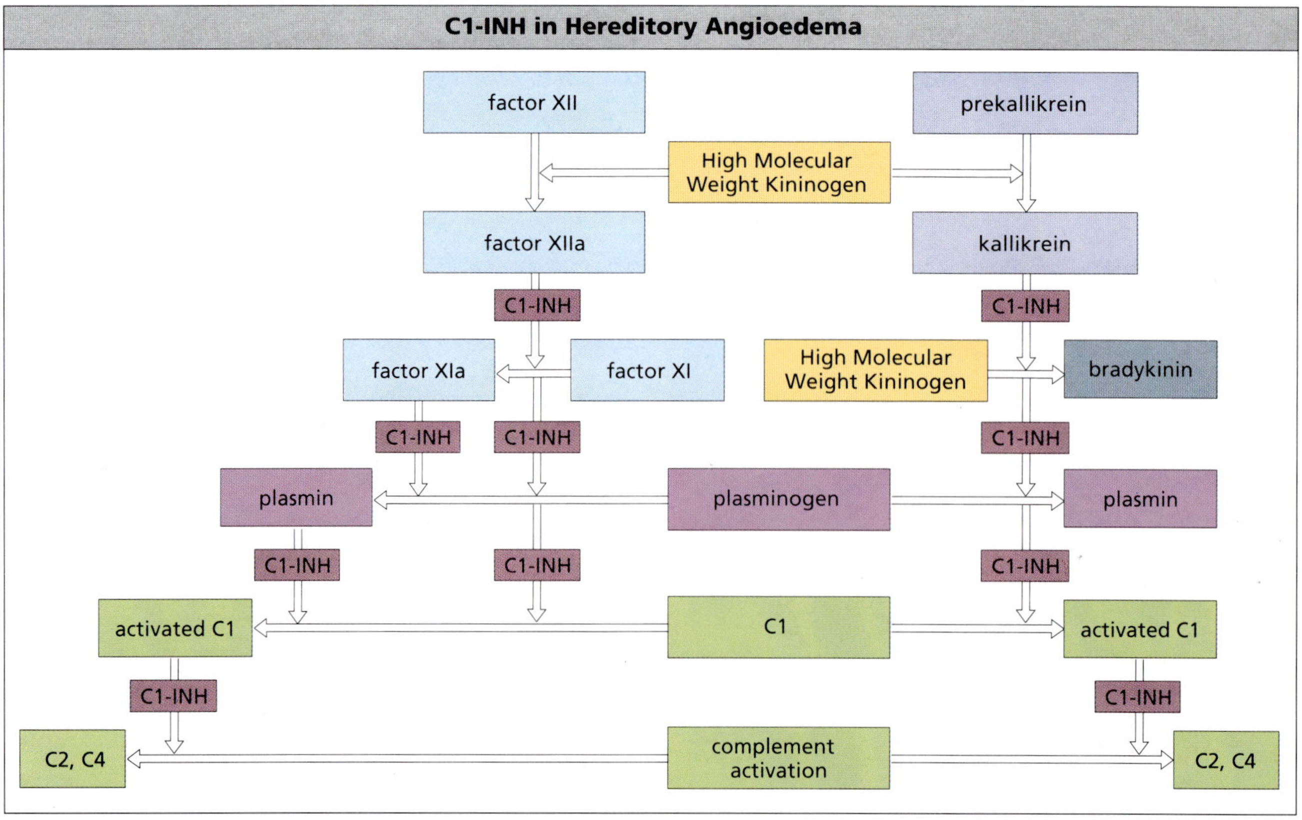

Fig. 21.16 The role of C1 esterase inhibitor (C1-INH) in hereditary angioedema. The enzyme inhibits complement activation, kinins, fibrinolysis, and thrombosis; therefore its deficiency in hereditary angioedema means that these pathways are potentiated. Adapted from Kerr and Yeung-Laiwah (1987).

mutation varies between families, it is now technically feasible to diagnose at birth the DNA defect in these families.

Cl-INH is the only inhibitor which inactivates activated Clr and Cls, which are the initial enzymes of classical complement activation. If deficient, complement activation is facilitated with consumption of C4 and C2. Levels of Cls rise during an attack and can reproduce lesions when injected into Cl-INH deficient patients but the suggested role for a C2 kinin released by C2 is now doubted. Cl-INH also inhibits kallikrein, plasmin and activated Hageman factor (Fig. 21.16). Evidence for major participation of fibrinolytic or coagulation pathways is lacking and it seems likely that bradykinin plays the major role in increasing permeability, as evidenced by low levels of HMWK and increased levels of kallikrein.

In addition to the familial forms of this disorder there are two acquired forms with similar clinical features. Primarily in patients with B cell lymphoproliferative disorders there is a two- to three-fold increase in Cl-INH metabolism, possibly arising from continuous activation of Cl by anti-idiotype antibodies directed against the abnormal B cells, which leads to Cl-INH complex formation and removal. The angioedema can, however, precede the clinical manifestations of the malignancy. A rarer mechanism in acquired Cl-INH deficiency is the auto-immune development of anti Cl-INH antibodies which predispose the protein to cleavage.

Urticaria Pigmentosa/Mastocytosis

This spectrum of disease is characterized by an accumulation of mast cells in different sites of the body. It almost always involves the skin (Fig. 21.17). The extent ranges from a solitary mastocytoma, through to the spontaneously resolving lesions of childhood urticaria pigmentosa, and the more progressive adult forms which lead to accumulation of mast cells in the viscera, bones and marrow, and a very rare leukaemia of mast cells.

In all forms of cutaneous involvement, rubbing the lesion brings about wealing (Fig. 21.18), and with extensive involvement the level of histamine in the blood is increased, as are the levels in the urine of its metabolites, methyl-imidazole acetic acid and methyl histamine. Prostaglandin D2 is also significantly raised to levels which contribute to the systemic symptoms of flushing, headache, wheeze, diarrhoea, and syncope.

Derived from stem cells in the marrow, mast cells bear many markers and characteristics in common with macrophages and monocytes which in disease states accumulate in the histiocytosis X spectrum. Mast cells depend on cytokines (Fig. 21.12) particularly IL3 and IL4 for growth and in adult patients with widespread involvement, the author and coworkers have shown an increase in circulating activated T helper cells which may be playing a part in driving cell proliferation. Mast cells themselves have recently been shown to synthesize IL3, IL4 and G-CSF and could be involved in maintaining the state of proliferation. Mast cells in mastocytosis differ from normal mast cells morphologically being larger with larger granules and nuclei but retain normal functional integrity and surface markers (Fig. 21.19). The increased melanin pigmentation over skin lesions is thought to result from chronic stimulation of melanocytes by mast-cell-derived heparin and by glycosaminoglycans.

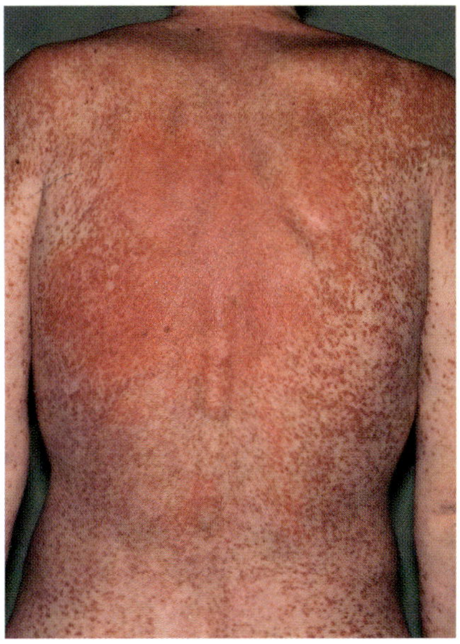

Fig. 21.18 Clinical appearance of a patient with systemic mastocytosis. The extensive skin lesions urticate on rubbing (Darier's sign).

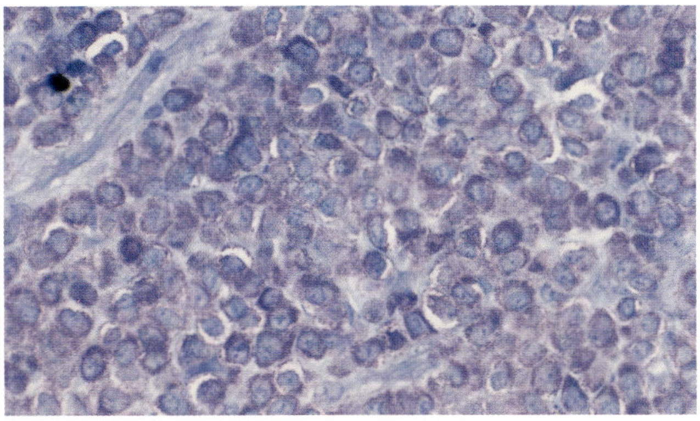

Fig. 21.17 Histology of mastocytosis showing accumulation of tightly packed aggregates of mast cells with nuclei becoming cuboidal rather than spindle shaped. Cell borders are prominent and the cytoplasm is filled with metachromatically staining granules. Toluidine blue (× 40).

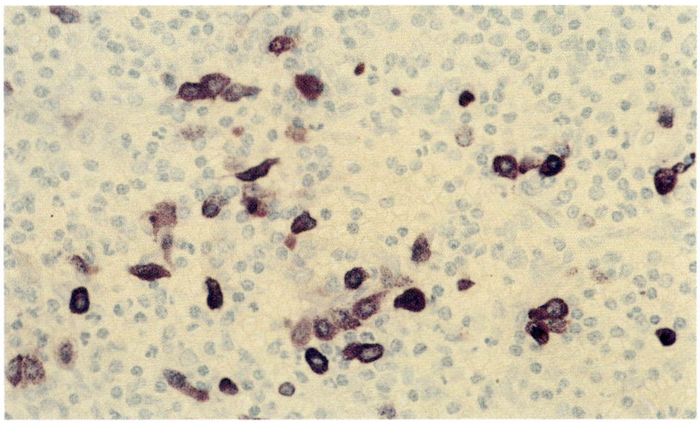

Fig. 21.19 Spleen from patient with systemic mastocytosis stained with toluidine blue demonstrating extensive mast cell infiltration.

Further Reading

Champion RH, Greaves M W, Kobza Black A, Pye RJ, eds. *The Urticarias*. Edinburgh: Churchill Livingstone, 1985.

Czarnetzki BM. Urticaria. In: *Immune Mechanisms in Cutaneous Disease* Ed: D A Norris. New York: Dekker, 1989.

Czarnetzki BM. *Urticaria*. Berlin: Springer-Verlag, 1986.

Grattan CEH, Hamon CGB, Cowan MA, Leeming RJ. Preliminary identification of a low molecular weight serological mediator in chronic idiopathic urticaria. *Brit J Derm*. 1988; **119**:179–183.

Gruber LB, Baeza ML, Marchese MJ, Agnello V, Kaplan AP. Prevalence and functional role of anti-IgE autoantibodies in urticarial syndromes. *J Invest Derm*. 1988; **90**:213–217.

Kerr MA, Yeung-Laiwah. Cl-Inhibitor Deficiency and Angioedema. In: *Complement in Health and Disease* Ed: K Whaley. Lancaster: MTP Press, 1987.

Lawlor F, Barr R, Kobza Black A, Cromwell 0, Isaacs J, Greaves MW. Arachidonic acid transformation is not stimulated in delayed pressure urticaria. *Brit J Derm* 1989; **121**:317–321.

Leenutaphong B, Holzle E, Plewig G. Pathogenesis and classification of solar urticaria, a new concept. *J Am Acad Derm*.1989; **21**:237–240.

Lewis-Jones MS, Barnes,RMR, Macfarlane AW, Curley RK, Johnstone FM, Finn R. Frequency and isotope distribution of serum antibodies reactive with dietary proteins in adults with chronic urticaria. *Clin & Exp Derm*.1987; **12**:419–423.

Maltby NH, Ind PW, Causon RC, Fuller RW, Taylor GW. Leukotriene E4 release in cold urticaria. *Clin & Exp All* 1989; **19**,:33–36.

Murdoch RD, Pollock I, Young E, Lessof MH. Food additive induced urticaria, studies of mediator release during provocation tests. *J Royal Coll Phys* 1987; **21**:262–266.

Natbony SF, Phillips ME, Elias JM, Godfrey HP, Kaplan AP. Histologic studies of chronic idiopathic urticaria *J Allergy Clin Immun* 1983; **71**:177–183.

Ormerod AD, Herriot R, Davidson RJL, Sewell H. Adult mastocytosis: an immunophenotypic and flow cytometric investigation. *Brit J Derm* 1990; **122**:737–744.

Rosenstreich DL. Chronic urticaria, activated T cells and mast cell releasability. *J Allergy Clin Immun* 1986; **78**:1099–1102.

Russell-Jones R, Bhogal B, Dash A, Schifferli J. Urticaria and vasculitis, a continuum of histological and immunopathological changes. *Brit J Derm* 1983; **108**:695–703.

Shanahan F, Lee TDG, Bienenstock J, Befus AD. The influence of endorphins on peritoneal and mucosal mast cell secretion. *J Allergy Clin Immun* 1984; **74**:499–504.

Wasserman SI. Mediators of immediate hypersensitivity. *J Allergy Clin Immun* 1983; **72**:101–115.

Wodnar-Filipowicz A, Heusser CH, Moroni C. Production of the haemopoietic growth factors GM-CSF and interleukin-3 by mast cells in response to IgE receptor mediated activation. *Nature* 1989; **339**:150–152.

Chapter 22

Urticaria – Diagnosis and Treatment

Introduction

Urticaria appears on the skin as multiple, short-lived and itchy erythematous and wealing lesions. Each individual lesion generally lasts less than 24 hours, with the exception of particular variants of the disease which will be described later. At any instant the morphology varies from blotchy erythematous macules to annular erythematous lesions (Fig. 22.1) with or without concurrent wealing (Fig. 22.2). Individual weals may be as small as 1–2 mm in diameter, but they can reach several centimetres.

Angioedema is characterized by deeper swelling of the skin and mucous membranes caused by oedema of the skin, mucous membranes and subcutaneous tissues. It is not itchy and swellings may reach several centimetres in diameter. Erythema and pain do not necessarily occur. The swelling is sudden in onset and generally short lived, disappearing to leave completely normal skin within 24 to 72 hours. Oedema of the respiratory or gastrointestinal tracts may be a serious complication in the hereditary form, but is rarely of major importance in other forms. Although often solitary, over 45 per cent of cases of angioedema are associated with urticaria.

While in a few patients any of several causes may be responsible for the development of urticaria and angioedema, the majority of patients do not have an identifiable underlying cause for their disease.

Classification

It is traditional to divide urticaria and angioedema into acute and chronic forms. Any urticaria with a short-lived history, e.g. present for less than six to 12 weeks, can arbitrarily be assigned to the acute form, while eruptions of longer duration are placed in the chronic category. The diagnosis of acute urticaria is generally retrospective, whereas that of chronic urticaria has further implications. For a clinical classification of urticaria, see Fig. 22.3.

Diagnosis

Taking a comprehensive history from the patient is the single most important diagnostic procedure which can be performed. The relevant information, which usually emerges during the first interview, should include the duration of the disorder, the presence or absence of systemic symptoms and the time course of each lesion. Information about all potential physical provoking factors including heat, cold, exercise, local pressure, friction, and sunlight should be sought (see Fig. 22.4). Enquiries about an association with food and drugs should be made, although this is rare in chronic urticaria. A detailed description of the morphology of the lesions should be obtained, including information about their size, colour, shape and location. Any tendency to develop purpura should also be noted. Symptoms associated with the eruption – itching, pain, burning, or tingling – may be present. If angioedema is prominent, enquiry about any difficulty in swallowing, and shortness of breath or wheezing should be made. Many patients with urticaria also have associated systemic symptoms including headache, dizziness, syncope, wheezing, vomiting, abdominal pain, diarrhoea, or general malaise.

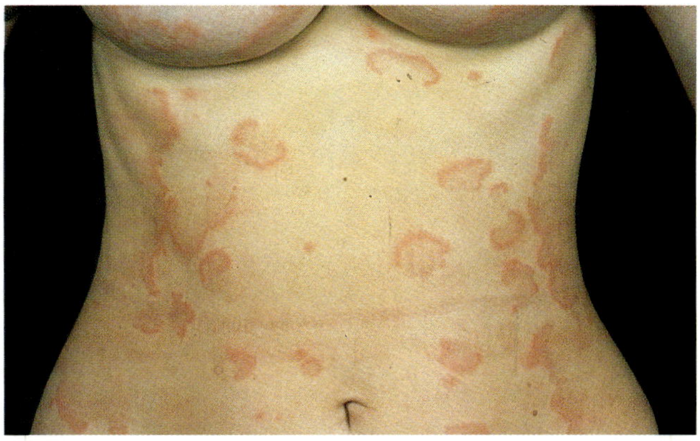

Fig. 22.1 Annular urticarial lesions. (Courtesy of Mr S Robertson, Institute of Dermatology, St John's Dermatology Centre, London.)

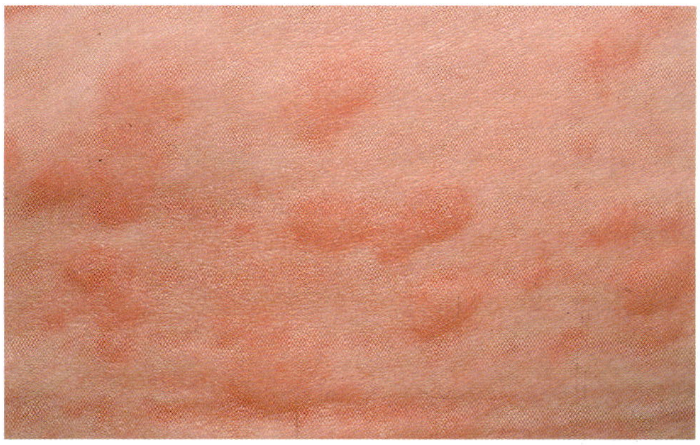

Fig. 22.2 Urticarial weals. (Courtesy of Mr S Robertson, Institute of Dermatology, St John's Dermatology Centre, London.)

The Urticarias – Causes and Investigations		
Type of Urticaria	**Causes**	**Clinical Investigations**
acute idiopathic	not known	1. history and examination if patient is well, no investigations are mandatory
IgE-mediated	food drugs	1. history – often a medical emergency 2. possible RAST testing 3. possible oral challenge
pseudo-allergic	drugs, especially cyclooxygenase inhibitors radiocontrast media food preservatives/colourings	1. history 2. occasionally skin prick testing 3. possible oral challenge
serum sickness	foods certain drugs radiocontrast media	1. history and examination 2. assessment of other system involvement - joints, haematological, respiratory, gastrointestinal
contact	foods (especially immunological contact urticaria) chemicals, metals (especially non-immunological contact urticaria)	1. history 2. skin testing with suspected substance
chronic idiopathic	not known	1. history and examination 2. diagnostic testing generally not indicated
the physical urticarias	mechanical stimuli changes in temperature water, light	1. history 2. specific challenge 3. skin biopsy in certain conditions
hereditary angioedema	autosomal dominant inheritance	1. history 2. serum levels of C1 inhibitor, C2, and C4
acquired C1 inhibitor deficiency	associated with lymphoproliferative or auto immune disease	1. history 2. serum levels of C1 inhibitor and C1
urticarial vasculitis	not known	1. history and examination 2. skin biopsy for histology 3. assessment

Fig. 22.3 A summary of the causes and appropriate clinical investigations of the various types of urticaria.

Physical Agents Which Cause Urticaria
friction
cold
pressure
heat
water
sunlight
contact substances

Fig. 22.4 Physical factors which can cause urticaria.

Acute Reactions

Acute Idiopathic Urticaria

There are no data documenting the prevalence of this condition.

As described above, weals vary in size: they may be only 2 to 5 mm in diameter; or they may involve very large areas, up to 30 cm or more in diameter and occur together with various patterns of macular and papular erythema. The lesions often itch, but this is not invariable. They are generally present for less than 24 hours. In approximately half the patients, angioedema occurs during the same period of time. Of the mucous membranes which become swollen, the eyelids are the most common (69 per cent), followed by the lips (65 per cent), tongue (21 per cent) and then swelling of any other part of the body including the face, the ears, under the chin, the genitalia, hands, feet, trunk, and arms. In idiopathic urticaria the skin is completely normal afterwards except for the occasional appearance of purpura, especially on the legs, which may be caused by scratching of the itchy lesions.

Acute Allergic Urticaria

The most dramatic IgE-mediated allergic reaction is associated with systemic anaphylaxis (see Chapter 27), which develops rapidly over five to 30 minutes. Prodromal symptoms include itching and tingling affecting the palms and soles, external ear, soft palate, or genital area. This is followed by nausea, vomiting, a feeling of pressure under the sternum, and shortness of breath. If the reaction proceeds, then hypotension, visual disturbance, itching, bronchoconstriction, urticaria, angioedema, laryngeal oedema, and cardiac arrhythmias may occur. A minor IgE-mediated reaction will cause urticaria without proceeding to systemic anaphylaxis.

Excluding drug reactions and insect stings, acute allergic urticaria comprises between 2 and 5 per cent of the total number of cases of urticaria seen at a dermatology clinic.

Agents Which Frequently Cause IgE-Mediated Anaphylaxis And Urticaria	
bee stings	milk
wasp stings	nuts
penicillin	beans
transfusion of blood and/or blood products	potatoes
	celery
fish	parsley
shellfish	spices

Fig. 22.5 Common agents which can cause IgE-mediated skin reactions.

Frequently Implicated Causes Of Non-Immunologic Reactions	
Acetylsalicylic Acid (aspirin)	Naproxen
Diclofenac	Paracetamol (Acetominophen)
Fenoprofen	Phenylbutazone
Ibuprofen	Tolmetin
Indomethacin	radiocontrast media
Ketoprofen	plasma expanders
Mefenamic Acid	local anaesthetics
Metamizol	

Fig. 22.6 Chemicals which can cause pseudo-allergic urticarial reactions.

Some of the more common agents which cause IgE-mediated skin reactions are listed in Fig. 22.5.

Pseudo-Allergic Urticarial Reactions

Pseudo-allergic or non-immunological urticarial reactions, sometimes referred to as idiosyncratic, intolerance or anaphylactoid reactions, do not have an immunological basis. As a consequence they may be precipitated on first exposure to the inducing chemicals. Some of these chemicals are listed in Fig. 22.6. Furthermore, reactions are not substance-specific, and unrelated compounds have the ability to induce a similar reaction in the same individual.

The incidence and severity of reactions are related to the dose of compound and they always resolve with removal of the drug and sometimes disappear spontaneously. Psuedo-allergic urticarial reactions occur most commonly after ingestion of aspirin or other cyclooxygenase inhibitors, suggesting an aberration in arachidonic acid metabolism (see Chapter 28). In up to 75 per cent of urticaria patients, aspirin may aggravate the condition, but severe reactions are much less common. Radiocontrast media, plasma expanders, including high and low molecular weight dextran, and local anaesthetics may also be precipitants. Although the contribution of preservatives, dyes and colourings to the pathogenesis of urticaria is controversial, tartrazine in orange colouring and other dyes, including ponceau (red), sunset yellow, amaranta (red), brilliant blue, eryth rosine (red), and indigotine (blue) may cause an anaphylactoid reaction. The preservatives which are most commonly implicated are benzoic acid, salicyclates, ascorbic acid, parabens, sulphites, and antioxidants.

Any clinical reaction may vary from urticaria and angioedema to an attack consisting of diffuse erythema of the skin, urticaria, angioedema, hoarseness, nasal congestion, lacrimation, wheezing, faintness and hypotension. If untreated a severe attack may lead to death.

Another cause of non-immunological reactions are agents which cause mast cells to release histamine. The release of histamine by cutaneous mast cells causes weal formation locally and systemic symptoms in more severe cases due to overspill of histamines into the circulation. This reaction is generally considered to be distinct from the pseudo-allergic reactions described above. Some of the more common agents which induce mast cell histamine release include morphine, codeine, and turbocurarine.

The angiotensin converting enzyme (ACE) inhibitors, captopril and enalapril, may cause angioedema and urticaria in susceptible individuals. The skin reaction starts within a few days of commencing therapy and may be severe. The most likely mechanism of action of these drugs is inhibition of peptidase enzymes which degrade bradykinin into inactive products.

Serum Sickness

Serum sickness, in the form of a Type III hypersensitivity response, may occur in individuals injected with foreign serum or other foreign antigens. If the antigen is present in the circulation for sufficient time, IgG and IgM form antigen/antibody complexes with the offending antigen. These complexes may then precipitate in the tissues, including the skin. Serum sickness may occur after ingestion of many drugs, particularly penicillin, sulphonamides, thiouracil, and dephenylhydantoin. It may also occur after intravenous radiocontrast media.

The onset of serum sickness is between six and 12 days after administration of the antigen, or sooner if there has been previous exposure. The clinical illness varies from mild to severe. Locally, there is usually a skin eruption which spreads from the injection site, and systemically the individual may experience fever, arthralgia, arthritis, lymphadenopathy, cough and wheeze, headache, malaise, and gastrointestinal disturbance. Nephritis and neurological abnormalities may also occur. Routine haematological examination may demonstrate a leucocytosis with a moderate eosinophilia, an elevated ESR, and evidence for activation of the complement pathway. The illness may last for days or even weeks and occasionally it may be fatal.

Diagnostic Testing

Diagnostic Testing in IgE-Mediated Allergic Reactions

Individuals who have life-threatening reactions to a single well-defined agent should avoid the offending substance and should not be investigated further. In most other cases the cause of the reaction is not clear, usually because more than one agent is ingested at the same time, or because an episode may represent an 'idiopathic' exacerbation of their condition. Investigation rarely provides a clear answer although with certain well-defined allergens, such as milk proteins in infants or peanut lectins in adults, a search for a specific IgE is worthwhile.

Laboratory measurement of total IgE levels is usually of little or no help in the diagnosis of allergic urticaria. In a certain limited number of patients, determination of the allergen-specific IgE antibody by radioallergosorbent test (RAST) may be helpful as it quantifies serum antigen-specific IgE, not that which is bound to mast cells and basophils. The RAST test is positive in those individuals whose degree of sensitization is considerable. An outline of the RAST test is shown in Fig. 22.7 and discussed in Chapter 28. RAST testing is generally not performed routinely in urticaria, as the role of IgE antibody is dubious in most cases, but circumstances in which it might be undertaken include: a suspicion that a specific allergen has caused a severe reaction so that skin testing would be dangerous; a discrepancy between the patient's history and skin test results; to follow the course of desensitization; and for the purposes of clinical research.

Diagnostic Testing in Non-Immunological Urticarial Reactions

Skin prick testing does not correlate well with either subjective symptoms or objective exacerbations of non-immunological reactions. Because false positive prick tests do occur, the results should be considered in conjunction with the patient's history before deciding that a specific agent is responsible.

Prick testing is performed on the flexor aspect of the forearm. A drop of each test substance is placed on the patient's skin and the skin is then pricked through the drop using a lancet. The lancet needs only to be wiped clear between different test substances. If the patient is sensitive, a severe reaction may occur. Reactions are evaluated semiquantitatively in relation to a control substance.

Oral provocation tests may correlate more exactly with exacerbating factors but their interpretation is difficult, both because of the variability of urticaria itself, and because some patients react to placebo. Some authorities insist that the patient is free from symptoms without any drug treatment if oral challenge testing is to be used. Patients are admitted to hospital, placed on a restrictive diet, and the test substances in gelatin capsules are introduced at specific times over each 24-hour period. Often investigators give a challenge battery to outpatients who are instructed to continue their normal diet and to take regular low dose antihistamine therapy throughout the test period. During oral challenge testing, a positive response may occur at any time during the 24 hours following ingestion of the challenge agent. If a positive response does occur, the patient is instructed not to continue with testing until the reaction has disappeared. All possible positive responses need to be checked by repeating part or all of the oral challenge battery. If a similar response occurs on two occasions to a single agent, then the challenge should be considered positive.

While in the past many exacerbations were attributed to ingested food substances, the pattern of urticaria does not always change following elimination of substances which have given positive oral challenge test results. For this reason, in the United Kingdom at least, oral challenge testing is not part of the routine investigation of urticaria although it is frequently undertaken if the patient so wishes. A suggested oral challenge battery is shown in Fig. 22.8.

Diagnostic Testing in Penicillin Allergy

Laboratory investigations should be confined to RAST testing if an anaphylactic reaction has occurred. If a rash of indefinite aetiology is being investigated, then intracutaneous skin testing is an option to consider. The disadvantages are that mediator release from the skin test itself may cause a severe systemic reaction, and that skin testing is falsely negative in 50 per cent of cases in which there is a positive history. The antigenic determinants used are benzylpenicilloyl-polylysine and benzylpenicillin, and testing should begin using very low concentrations, and slowly increased only if no reaction occurs. It is suggested that epicutaneous testing should be

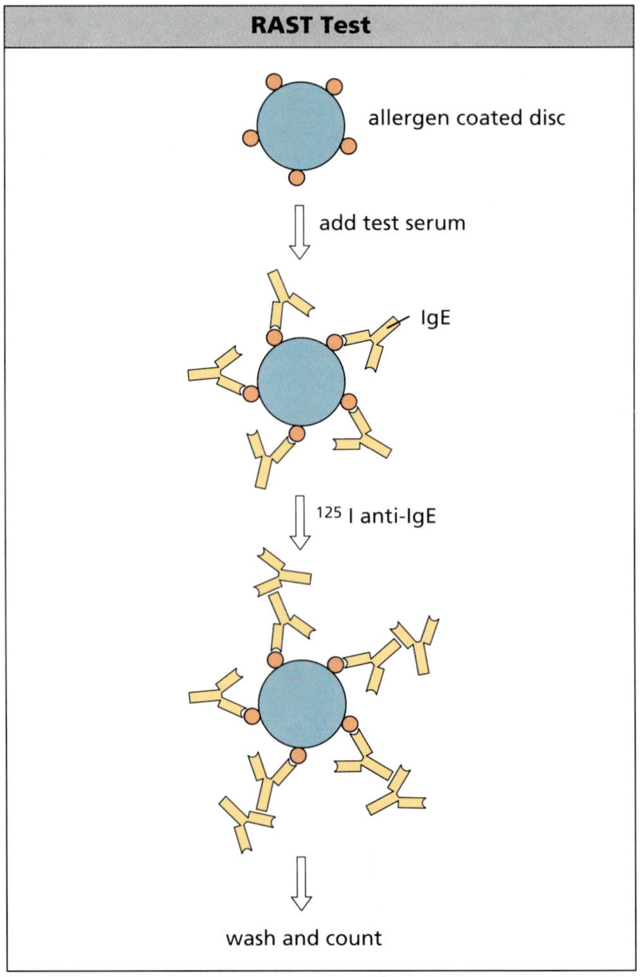

Fig. 22.7 Schematic Representation of RAST test

performed first. If this is negative, prick testing should be performed; if this is negative, prick testing in increasing concentrations may be undertaken.

Contact Urticaria

Immediate contact reactions appear between a few minutes and one hour after exposure to the offending substance. They usually disappear within 24 hours. The reactions vary in severity:

- the weakest reactions are characterized by itching, tingling, or burning and are accompanied by erythema
- the prototype reaction is a weal and flare
- a severe reaction is characterized by generalized urticaria with systemic symptoms; this phenomenon is known as the contact urticaria syndrome.

Other types of reaction include protein contact dermatitis, in which itching, erythema, swelling, or tiny vesicles occur in patients with dermatitis of the hand, and a reaction which occurs after eating certain foods such as milk, eggs, shrimps, and peanuts; this causes itching, tingling, and oedema of the oropharynx.

Contact urticaria may be considered in two main groups: immunological and non-immunological contact urticaria.

Immunological Contact Urticaria

Immunological contact urticaria is commoner in atopic subjects than in those who have no obvious atopy. Initial sensitization usually occurs through the respiratory or gastrointestinal tracts, although sensitization through the skin may also occur. Patients often give a history of swelling of the lips or buccal mucous membranes following the ingestion of certain foods such as eggs, fish, nuts, milk, meat, seafood, or vegetables. However, this reaction may also occur after exposure to a wide spectrum of animal or plant products, metals, fragrances, or medications.

Non-Immunological Contact Urticaria

This is the commoner form of contact urticaria, and it occurs in healthy asymptomatic people who often have no history of previous exposure. The triggering substances are frequently of low molecular weight. Substances known to produce this kind of reaction include ammonia, persulphate, demethyl sulphoxide, cinnamic aldehyde, and benzoic acid. Like immunological contact urticaria, animal and plant products (including nettles and primula), metals, preservatives, and disinfectants may also be responsible.

Investigation of Contact Urticaria

The diagnosis should be based on a full history, and on skin testing with the suspected substance.

The simplest test is the 'rub test' in which the suspected substance is rubbed gently on normal or slightly affected skin. The test site is inspected for signs of a reaction at 60 minutes.

The 'use test' is a further investigation in which the patient handles the suspected provoking agent in precisely the same way as when the symptoms appeared.

In an open patch test, 0.1 ml of the test substance is spread on a 3×3cm area of the skin of the upper back or the on extensor aspect of the upper arm. The test should first be performed on unaffected skin, and, if negative, performed on previously affected or currently affected skin. A positive reation may appear within 15 to 60 minutes, and consists of a weal and flare reaction or pinpoint vesiculation indistinguishable from eczema.

Occlusive patch testing may be more sensitive than the open application. Patches should be left on for 15 to 20 minutes and a positive reaction will occur within 45 minutes after application.

Scratch-patch testing may also be performed, in which the scratch made through the suspected agent is covered by a Finn Chamber (Epitest Ltd, Finland) for 15 minutes. The area is observed five minutes after the removal of the test chamber for a weal and flare reaction.

Drug and Diet Challenge Test Schedule Used at St John's Dermatology Centre

1. Control
2. Tartrazine 10mg*
3. Control
4. Sodium Benzoate 500ng*
5. Control
6. 4-Hydroxybenzoic Acid 200mg
7. Control
8. Yeast Extract 0.6g
9. Control
10. Penicillin 0.5mg
    (not to be given if history of asthma or severe penicillin reaction)
11. Control
12. Aspirin 100mg
13. Aspirin 500mg
    (not to be given if history of asthma or severe aspirin reaction)
    Add the following instruction to the label:
    'Omit today's dose if the weals were increased by the previous test.'
14. Control
15. New Coccine 10mg*
16. Control
17. Canthaxathine 100 mg*
18. Control
19. Sunset Yellow 10mg*
20. Control
21. Annatto 10mg
22. Control
23. Butylhydroxytoluene 50mg
24. Control
25. Butylhydroxyanisol 50mg
26. Control
27. Ascorbic Acid 600mg
28. Control
29. Sodium Nitrate 100mg
30. Control
31. Quinoline Yellow 10mg
32. Control
33. Sodium Gluamate 200mg

* One tenth of the dose to be given if a child is under 10 years or if there is a history of asthma.

Fig. 22.8 A suggested oral challenge battery, used as a diagnostic test in non-immunological urticarial reactions.

Testing for specific antibody by RAST is seldom used in the investigation of contact urticarial reactions but may be positive in patients with immunological allergy. As systemic reactions have been reported, this danger should be borne in mind.

Chronic Idiopathic Urticaria

The morphology of the eruption of chronic urticaria is similar to that of acute urticaria. The diagnosis is made when the urticaria or angioedema has been present either daily or episodically for an arbitrary period of longer than six to 12 weeks. This group of patients is the largest subgroup of those suffering from urticaria seen at dermatology clinics, and 70 per cent of all urticaria patients have chronic idiopathic urticaria. The association between chronic idiopathic urticaria and the physical urticarias, especially delayed pressure urticaria, requires that the possible co-existence of one or more of the physical urticarias should be considered in all patients with chronic idiopathic urticaria.

Many underlying diseases have been noted in patients with chronic urticaria but in the vast majority there is no underlying related disease. Thus laboratory investigations in those patients who are otherwise well at their first visit are not indicated. By making the diagnosis of chronic urticaria we are, for practical purposes, labelling the disorder 'idiopathic' (hence the term chronic idiopathic urticaria). However it is reasonable to bear in mind that a patient with an acute illness such as hepatitis or brucellosis may have urticaria, and that there is a higher incidence of immune thyroid disease in those with chronic idiopathic urticaria, although this is not usually overt. It is extremely rare for focal sepsis, candida, dermatophyte infection, or parasitic infestation of the gastrointestinal tract to have any effect on the course of chronic idiopathic urticaria, and searching for the above infections or infestations is not mandatory. If food additives have any part to play in the pathogenesis of chronic idiopathic urticaria, then they should be considered as non-immunological urticarial reactions and diagnostic testing performed as described above.

When the diagnosis of chronic idiopathic urticaria is made, it is vital for the patient to realize that laboratory tests and 'allergy' tests are not usefully performed in this disease and that chronic idiopathic urticaria is not a manifestation of an 'allergy' as we normally understand it.

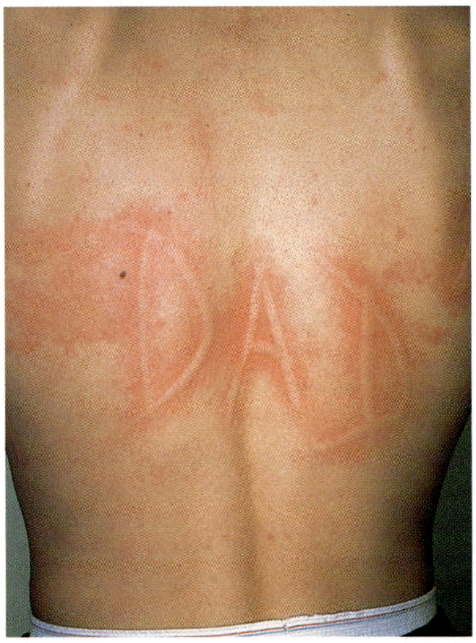

Fig. 22.9 Symptomatic dermographism. This weal and flare reaction is produced by lightly stroking the skin. (Courtesy of Professor M Greaves, Institute of Dermatology, United Medical and Dental School, University of London.)

The Physical Urticarias

The physical urticarias are those in which reproducible wealing occurs in response to a specific physical stimulus. These physical urticarias comprise approximately 20 per cent of all cases of urticaria referred to dermatology clinics, and make up the largest group of patients apart from those with chronic idiopathic urticaria.

As two or more physical urticarias are frequently present in the same person (a phenomenon known as 'clustering'), a battery of physical urticaria tests should be performed in anyone in whom a physical urticaria is suspected. Rarely, certain physical urticarias can be transmitted genetically, but most appear to be acquired. The eliciting physical stimuli are divided into mechanical trauma, temperature change, light, and water. The main physical urticarias will be reviewed briefly.

Cutaneous Responses to Mechanical Stimuli

Simple dermographism
In this condition, a weal and flare reaction without itching occurs after stroking the skin with moderate

Dermographometer

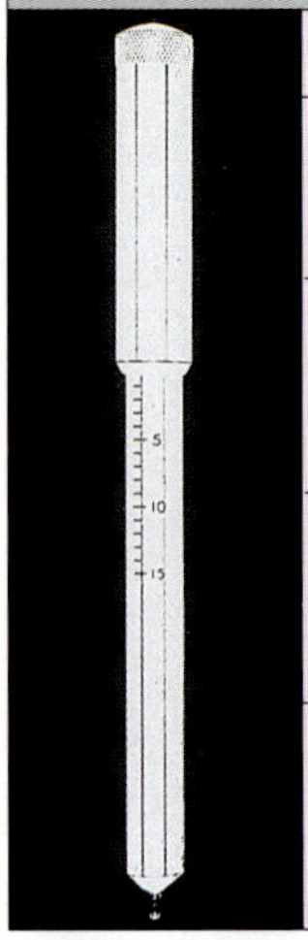

Marking	Presure Equivalent
0	2.0×10^5Pa (20.4 g/mm^2)
5	5.87×10^5Pa (59.9 g/mm^2)
10	9.75×10^5Pa (99.4 g/mm^2)
15	14.12×10^5Pa (144.0 g/mm^2)

Fig. 22.10 A calibrated dermographometer. This instrument is stroked longitudinally at the pressures shown to demonstrate symptomatic dermographism. An itchy weal and flare response which occurs at a pressure of 3.6g/mm^2 (3.5×10^5 Pa) confirms the diagnosis. The same instrument is used to confirm the diagnosis of delayed pressure urticaria. In this condition it is set at 9.75×10^5 Pa and is held perpendicularly and firmly against the skin of the back for varying numbers of seconds. A positive response consists of a papule which appears at least 30 minutes after the stimulus is applied.

pressure. This occurs in about 5 per cent of the normal population, and may be regarded as physiological.

Symptomatic dermographism
Symptomatic dermographism is distinguished from simple dermographism by the presence of itching associated with a weal and flare reaction, occurring within minutes of gentle stroking of the skin (Fig. 22.9). Patients complain of itching which often seems out of proportion to the visible wealing. Symptoms occur at sites of minor frictional stimuli, such as the areas around collars and cuffs, from shower jets, and after towelling and hair combing.

The diagnosis is most easily confirmed using a calibrated dermographometer, an instrument consisting of a stylus attached to a spring (Fig. 22.10). The pressure on the spring can be easily adjusted and the corresponding pressures are read from a scale on the side of the instrument. An itchy wealing response occurs when the stylus is stroked longitudinally on the upper back. A positive response occurring at a stroking pressure of $3.6 g/mm^2$ or less confirms the diagnosis.

Other less common forms of dermographism include delayed dermographism, localized dermographism, cholinergic dermographism, transient dermographism, and dermographism associated with cutaneous mastocytosis.

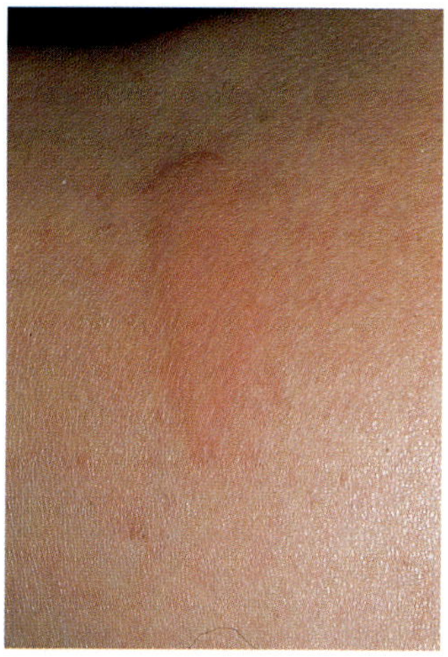

Fig. 22.11 Delayed pressure urticaria. This delayed swelling is produced by a bra strap. (Courtesy of Professor M Greaves, Institute of Dermatology, United Medical and Dental School, University of London.)

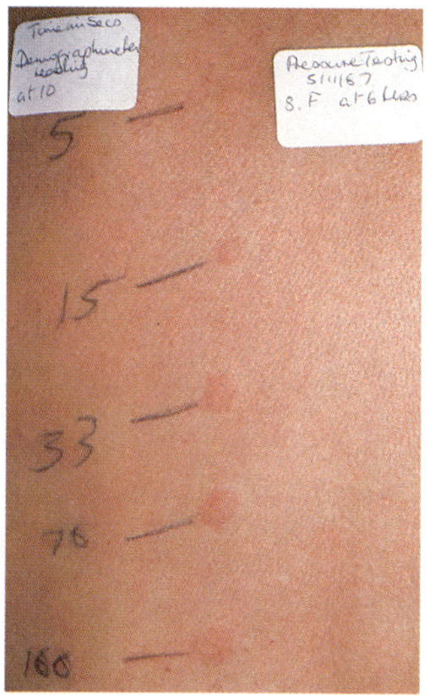

Fig. 22.12 Dermographometer pressure testing; positive pressure tests seen at six hours. (Courtesy of Professor M Greaves, Institute of Dermatology, United Medical and Dental School, University of London.)

Delayed pressure urticaria
In delayed pressure urticaria, constant perpendicular pressure applied to the skin causes delayed cutaneous erythema, dermal oedema, and subcutaneous oedema. Reactions develop slowly, becoming obvious between 30 minutes and nine hours after the pressure stimulus has been applied. The lesions are itchy and painful and may last up to 48 hours. Patients develop lesions under bra straps, watches, belts, and shoes (Fig. 22.11), or after leaning against furniture, crossing legs, or resting elbows on a desk. Swelling of the hands and feet occur after manual activity such as using a screw driver, and on the soles of the feet after walking, jogging, and climbing ladders. This swelling is difficult to distinguish from chronic idiopathic angioedema.

The diagnosis is suspected from the history and may be confirmed by the application of perpendicular pressure to the skin which shows a palpable lesion if inspected six hours later. In practice, the most reproducible way to confirm the diagnosis is to use a calibrated dermographometer (see Fig. 22.10). The dermographometer, set at a pressure of 9.75×10^5 Pa is held perpendicularly and firmly against the skin of the back, lateral to the spine at positions approximately 5cm apart, for five, 15, 33, 70 and 100 seconds. A positive pressure test is indicated by a palpable lesion at test sites when inspected six hours later (Fig. 22.12).

If a dermographometer is not available, a 7kg weight can be suspended in a crepe bandage from the shoulder or thigh for 15 minutes. However, this semiquantitative method is less reliable, and false negative responses are more common.

Vibratory angioedema
This condition is rare. Local erythema and oedema of the skin and subcutaneous tissue occur in response to repeated repetitive high frequency stretching of the skin (Fig. 22.13). If the stimulus is sufficiently intense, a systemic reaction may occur. The disorder is more commonly transmitted as an autosomal dominant condition, although sporadic cases have been reported. Preliminary testing to confirm the diagnosis may be performed using a laboratory whirl mixer

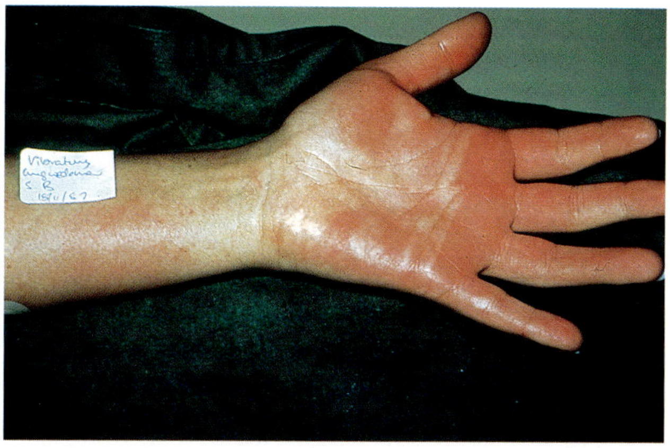

Fig. 22.13 Vibratory angioedema. Vibration induced swelling of the palm and forearm. (Courtesy of Professor M Greaves, Institute of Dermatology, United Medical and Dental School, University of London.)

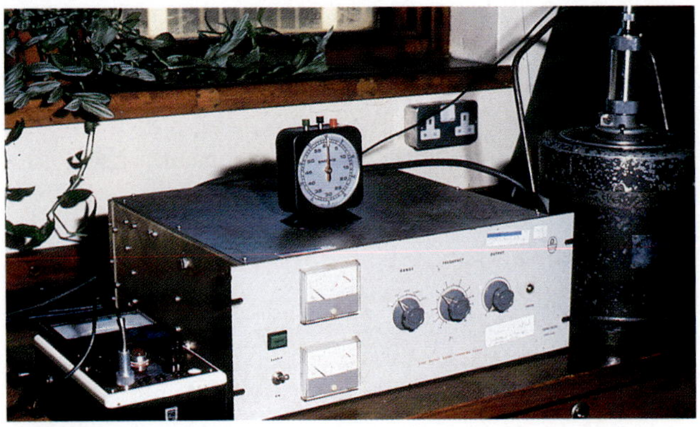

Fig. 22.14 The instrument constructed to provoke vibratory angioedema. The patient grasped the vibrator bar, showed on the left, which was attached to a pwer amplifier and a vibration meter. (Courtesy of Professor M Greaves, Institute of Dermatology, United Medical and Dental School, University of London.)

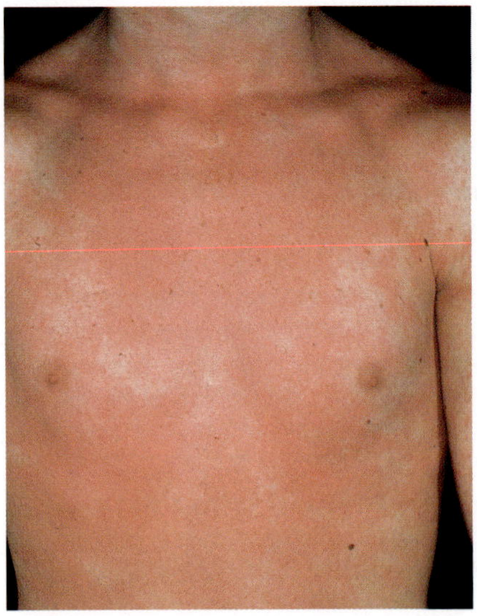

Fig. 22.15 Cholinergic urticaria: wealing occurring after exercise. (Courtesy of Mr S Robertson, Institute of Dermatology, St John's Dermatology Centre, London.)

applied to the skin. If oedema and erythema occur, then a calibrated vibration appratus may be set up (Fig. 22.14).

Cutaneous Reactions to Changes in Temperature

Cholinergic urticaria

In cholinergic urticaria, extensive wealing develops in response to taking exercise, a hot bath or shower, intense transient emotional stimuli, or after ingestion of spicy food (Fig. 22.15). Individual lesions consist of pinhead-sized weals with a bright red flare. These may become confluent to form larger weals. In many patients, the lesions are confined to the upper half of the body, and in some, wealing is associated with angioedema.

The diagnosis is made by the reproduction of the eruption by exercise or by passively raising the body temperature. To reproduce the eruption, exercise must be continued until the patient is semi-exhausted and sweating. Patients may jog on the spot, run up and down stairs, cycle on an exercise bicycle, or even run on a treadmill wearing an occlusive suit. The body temperature may be raised passively by immersion in a bath kept at 42°C for 10 to 15 minutes. The weals can be blocked by topical pre-treatment of the skin with a 6 per cent hyoscine solution.

Rarer variants of cholinergic urticaria include persistent erythema, exercise-induced anaphylaxis, and food-dependent, exercise-induced urticaria.

Localized heat urticaria

This rare condition is one which oedema and erythema occur after the local application of heat to the skin. In experimental situations the temperature necessary to produce lesions varies between 38°C and 49°C. Symptoms may last up to two hours. The condition is distinct from cholinergic urticaria in that it cannot be suppressed by pre-treatment with topical hyoscine.

Cold urticaria

Most wealing reactions to cold are idiopathic (essential, primary), and usually occur on the limbs when they are exposed to cold weather. Wealing reactions to cold which are secondary to systemic disease with associated serum abnormalities are extraordinarily

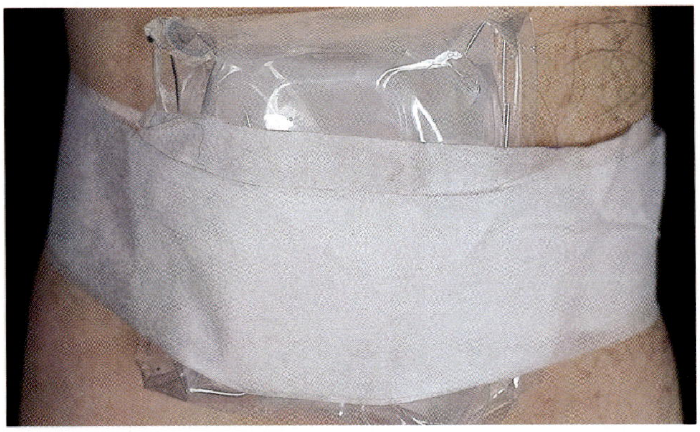

Fig. 22.16 To demonstrate cold urticaria, an ice cube (at 1°C) covered in polythene is taped to the patient's forearm and kept in place for 20 minutes. A positive response will occur between five and seven minutes after removal of the ice. (Courtesy of Professor M Greaves, Institute of Dermatology, United Medical and Dental School, University of London.)

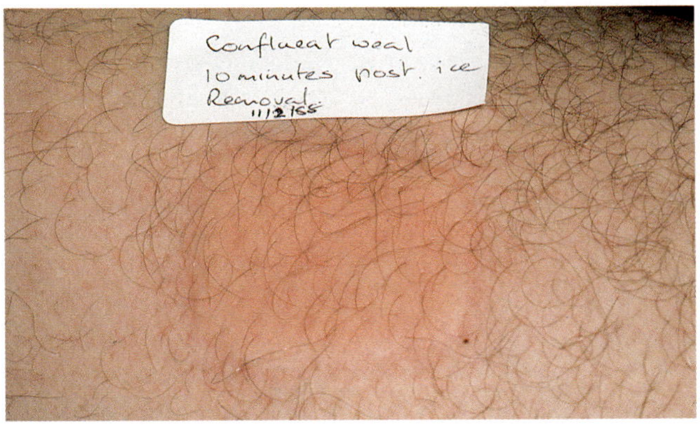

Fig. 22.17 Cold urticaria: a positive ice cube test. (Courtesy of Professor M Greaves, Institute of Dermatology, United Medical and Dental School, University of London.)

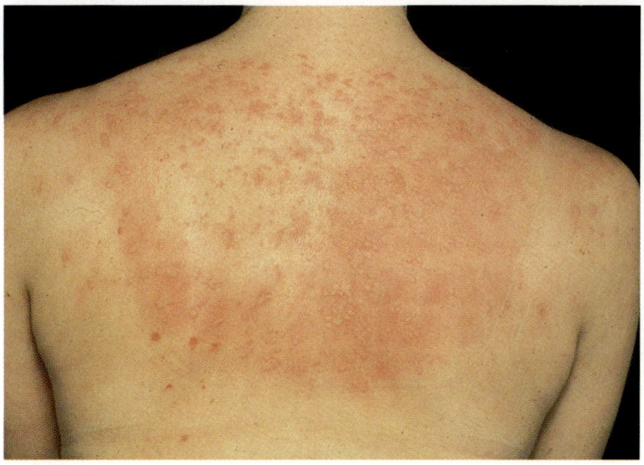

Fig. 22.18 The eruption in solar urticaria is confined to the area exposed. (Courtesy of Dr J Hawk, Photobiology Department, St John's Dermatology Centre, London.)

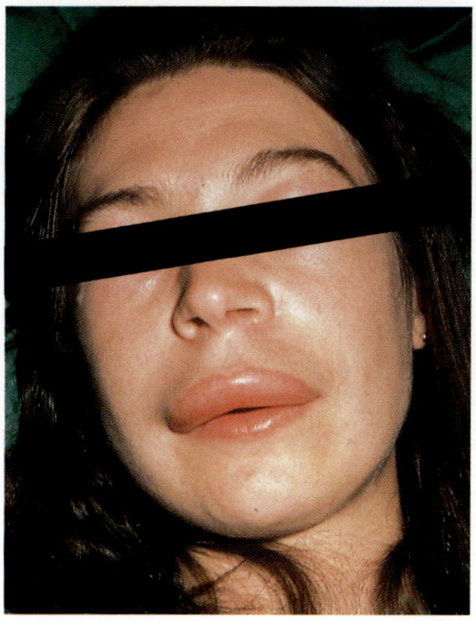

Fig. 22.19 Swelling of the lips in herediatry angioedema. The appearance may be identical in acute angioedema. (Courtesy of Dr Susan Parker, St John's Dermatology Centre, London.)

rare. Secondary cold urticaria with associated cryoglobulin and cryofibrinogen in the serum does occur but is rarely encountered in practice.

Idiopathic acquired immediate cold contact urticaria is the most common form of cold urticaria. Itching, burning, erythema, and wealing occur after removal of cold stimulus from the skin. Patients experience symptoms on exposed sites during cold weather or if exposed to a cold wind or to cold rain. Removing cold objects from the freezer or leaning against something cold may also cause symptoms. The reaction occurs on rewarming the skin. If the cold stimulus is of sufficient intensity, then dizziness, headache and syncope may occur because of the high systemic levels of histamine and other mast cell products. Cold water bathing should be forbidden because of the risk of drowning caused by dizziness and stiffening of the limbs.

The diagnosis is confirmed by placing a melting ice cube at 1°C in a polythene glove and fixing it to the forearm with micropore tape for 20 minutes. A patient with active disease will weal at the test site within 10 minutes of removal of the ice cube (Figs 22.16 and 22.17). With a more generalized response elicited by immersion of the whole forearm in cold water, high levels of histamine may be detected in venous blood draining from the arm.

Aquagenic Urticaria

Aquagenic urticaria is a cutaneous reaction to water. It presents as itching and wealing at sites of contact with water independent of its temperature. Lesions occur more frequently on the upper part of the body, reach their maximum size and intensity 30 minutes after exposure to water and decrease after 30-60 minutes. Morphologically the weals of aquagenic urticaria resemble those of cholinergic urticaria, but they are not caused by heat, exercise, or emotional stimuli. To confirm the diagnosis, a tepid shower for 15 minutes will generally reproduce the lesions.

Solar Urticaria

The cutaneous reaction to light in patients with solar urticaria presents as diffuse cutaneous erythema and intense wealing occurring particularly in areas of the skin which are not normally exposed. The reaction is rapid, developing between 30 seconds and three minutes after exposure, and it is limited exactly to the area of exposure (Fig. 22.18). Lesions are described as itchy, pricking, tingling, or burning and they disappear within an hour. If larger areas of the body are involved then systemic symptoms may occur.

Tests to confirm the diagnosis are generally carried out in a photobiology unit using a monochromator or a solar simulator. The response is immediate in those patients who have the disorder, thus distinguishing it from the much more common polymorphic light eruption, which is not a form of urticaria and which appears hours, rather than minutes, after exposure to light.

Hereditary Angioedema

Hereditary angioedema must be considered in a patient who has suffered from intermittent attacks of severe skin or mucosal oedema since childhood. Clinically, the swellings are often proceeded by local trauma, such as dental extraction. A major attack is frequently preceeded by a prodromal rash which consists of annular erythema and weals. Involvement of the gastrointestinal tract and upper respiratory tract is common (Fig. 22.19). In severe cases, gastrointestinal involvement can simulate an acute surgical emergency with severe abdominal pain and vomiting, and in the respiratory tract, laryngeal involvement may lead to respiratory obstruction and death. The swellings may appear after prodromal feelings of anxiety and cause little or no pain or itch. They are not erythematous and last for up to three days before fading away to leave a normal appearing skin.

Hereditary angioedema is inherited as an autosomal dominant trait which is expressed in heterozygotes. This condition exists in two forms: Type I, which accounts for 80–85 per cent of cases, where there is a quantitative deficiency of C1 esterase inhibitor (C1-inhibitor); and Type II where there is a functional abnormality of the inhibitor due to aberrant gene coding (Fig. 22.20). In both cases angioedema results from the unopposed actions of proteases which lead to the production of mediators capable of increasing vascular permeability to produce oedema. Diagnosis of both may be made by a functional assay for C1-inhibitor, and they may be distinguished by concomitant use of an immunological assay which will detect the level of the dysfunctional enzyme (Type II) as normal.

Using immunological assays, a plasma level of less than 100mg/ml of C1-inhibitor is indicative of the Type I form of the disease. In addition, C4 levels, and C2 levels, are reduced in both Type I and Type II whereas C1 and C3 levels are normal. C2 levels maybe reduced between attacks. C4 levels maybe reduced during remissions in patients with Type I disease.

Acquired C1-inhibitor deficiency

A group of patients have been identified who have an identical chemical picture to that of hereditary angioedema, including laboratory evidence of C1-inhibitor deficiency, but who have no family history of the disease. These patients have acquired C1-inhibitor deficiency, characterized by low levels of C1. This is in contrast to the hereditary form, in which C1 levels are usually normal. Some patients also have lymphoproliferative disease, while others have auto-immune diseases such as SLE.

Urticarial Vasculitis

Urticarial vasculitis is a disorder which presents clinically as an urticarial eruption, but which histopathologically shows a picture of vasculitis. There are some diagnostically useful clinical differences between 'classical' urticaria and urticarial vasculitis. In urticarial vasculitis the lesions are present for a longer duration – often between three and seven days. In contrast to the predominant symptom of itching in urticaria, patients with urticarial vasculitis also describe burning and sometimes painful lesions. Urticarial vasculitis may present as purpuric or frankly vasculitic lesions in addition to urticarial lesions and, rarely, bullae may occur. When clearing, the urticarial lesions may leave residual erythema, scaling, or purpura. Urticarial vasculitis may also present as angioedema which may also leave a residual bruised appearance with scaling or purpura. Since treatment with H_1-antihistamines is generally ineffective in controlling symptoms, urticarial vasculitis should be considered in patients with apparently unremarkable urticaria who do not respond to antihistamines.

The incidence of systemic involvement in urticarial vasculitis follows the pattern of involvement in systemic vasculitis. Joint involvement occurs in up to 75 per cent of patients, renal involvement in 30 per cent, gastrointestinal involvement in 25 per cent, pulmonary involvement in 20 per cent and opthalmic involvement in 10 per cent. Joint problems may range from flitting arthalgia to full-blown arthritis. Microscopic haematuria and proteinuria are present if the kidneys are involved, but impairment of renal function is rare. Abdominal pain, nausea, vomiting, and diarrhoea may occur, and pulmonary problems include chronic obstructive airways disease, asthma or pleural effusions. Neurological involvement may simulate a tumour or cause optic atrophy. Conjunctivitis, uveitis and episcleritis can occur.

Laboratory abnormalities are common but not invariable. A raised ESR is perhaps the most common abnormality while other abnormalities are those associated with vasculitis or immune complex disease. Hypocomplementaemia, when it occurs, frequently correlates well with systemic disease. Other abnormalities occasionally found include antinuclear antibodies in low titre, elevated immunoglobins, false positive syphilis serology, the presency of cryoglobulins, and a positive rheumatoid factor. Specific histopathological findings are vital to an accurate diagnosis of urticarial vasculitis as is described in the following section.

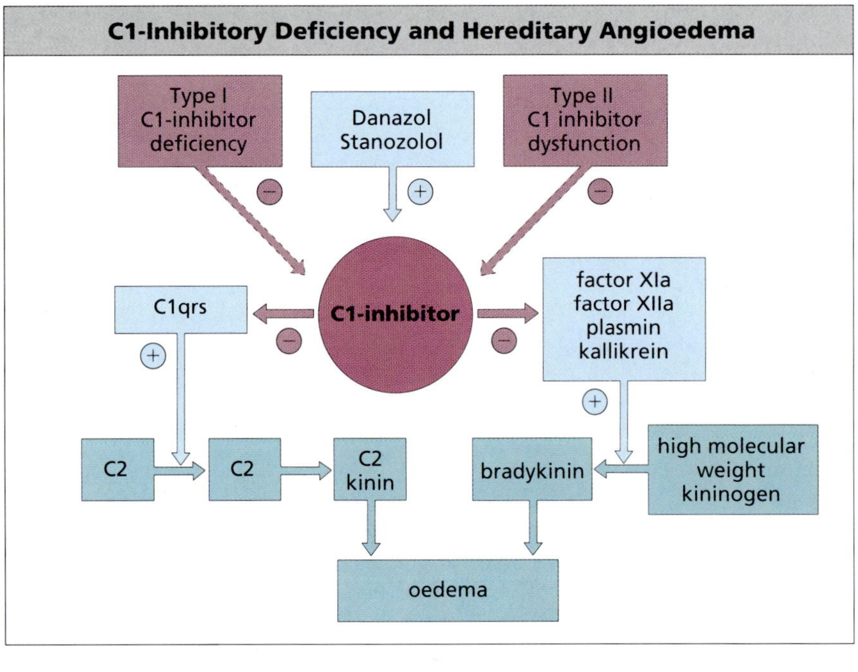

Fig. 22.20 The role of C1 esterase inhibitor (C1-inhibitor) in hereditary angiooedema. C1-inhibitor deficiency (Type I) or dysfunction (Type II) allows unregulated action of plasma enzymes which cause oedema forming enzymes. The modified androgens, danazol and stanozolol stimulate the liver to synthesize greater amounts of C1-inhibitor.

Histopathology of the Urticarias

The histopathological picture in most forms of urticaria is non-specific. A skin biopsy is generally performed only if urticarial vasculitis or delayed pressure urticaria is suspected, as the histopathological appearances are more specific in these conditions. In most forms of urticaria, dermal oedema with a sparse peri-vascular lymphocytic infiltrate is seen under the light microscope. Rarely, the lymphocytic infiltrate may be prominent. Eosinophils may also be present.

The histopathological features of urticarial vasculitis are those of a cutaneous vasculitis. An infiltrate consisting mainly of neutrophils is visible both in and around the blood vessel walls (Fig. 22.21). Varying numbers of eosinophils and mononuclear cells are present and scattered nuclear fragments, known as 'nuclear dust', may be found within the dermis. The blood vessel walls appear abnormal because of oedema and deposition of fibrin within them. In delayed pressure urticaria there is no vasculitis but the cellular infiltrate is heavy and may extend into the subcutaneous fat. Earlier lesions show an infiltrate composed of neutrophils and eosinophils (Fig. 22.22) while later lesions show an infiltrate composed of mononuclear cells and eosinophils (Fig. 22.23).

Treatment of Urticaria

The primary treatment of urticaria, whether acute idiopathic urticaria, IgE-mediated allergic serum sickness, or chronic urticaria is with H_1-antihistamines. These drugs are effective in most cases if given in adequate dosage. In general the lesions are controlled more effectively with a continuous dosage, as it takes approximately three days for maximum saturation to be reached. The question of tolerance to antihistamines has not been completely clarified but should it occur, then cross-tolerance to other antihistamines would be expected. Temporary cessation of treatment is the only way to restore sensitivity to the drugs. A β-adrenoceptor stimulant, such as salbutamol or terbutaline, may be given during the H_1-antihistamine-free period, but control will generally not be as good. In patients who are difficult to control, a tricyclic antidepressant drug, for example doxepin which also possesses H_1 and H_2 antihistaminic activity may be used. H_2 receptors blocking drugs are not effective on their own and do not add therapeutic benefit in the conditions listed above. If a severe anaphylactoid reaction occurs, prompt subcutaneous administration of adrenaline, intramuscular or intravenous adminstration of H_1-antihistamines, and intravenous hydrocortisone is mandatory. Intubation may be necessary if airway obstruction occurs.

For treatment of serum sickness, systemic corticosteroids may be added to the antihistamine therapy.

The Physical Urticarias

Symptomatic dermographism is normally well controlled using H_1-receptor blocking antihistamines. This is also the only urticaria in which addition of an H_2 blocker confers useful therapeutic benefit.

Cold urticaria responds moderately well to H_1-antihistamines, particularly the newer more potent and minimally sedating variety. Although cyproheptadine has been described as being particularly effective, it is not a suitable long-term treatment because of its side effects of drowsiness and weight gain. Furthermore, it is doubtful if cyproheptadine would in fact confer more benefit than the newer antihistamines. 'Desensitization' or tolerance treatment, by repeated exposure of the skin to cold until it becomes refractory to challenge, is of value in strongly motivated patients.

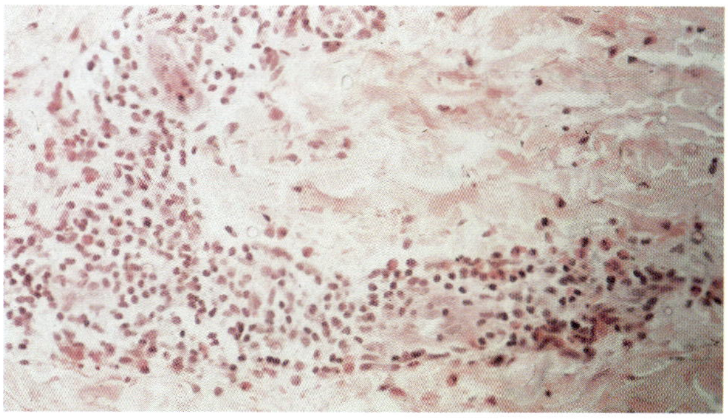

Fig. 22.21 Urticarial vasculitis: the blood vessel is obliterated by the infiltrate. (Courtesy of Professor M Greaves, Institute of Dermatology, United Medical and Dental School, University of London.)

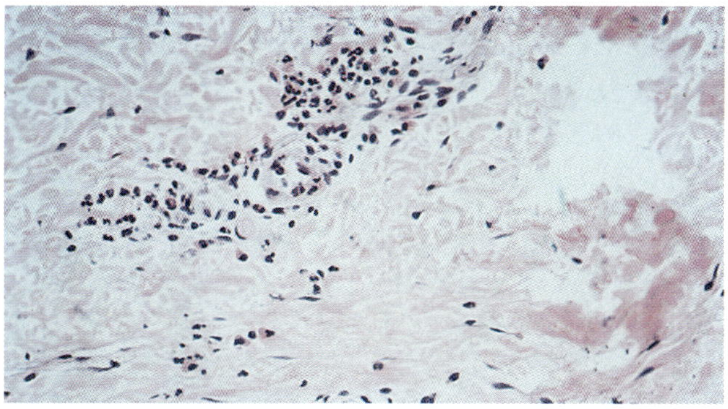

Fig. 22.22 Delayed pressure urticaria: An early lesion showing a collection of neutrophils and eosinophils. (Courtesy of Professor M Greaves, Institute of Dermatology, United Medical and Dental School, University of London.)

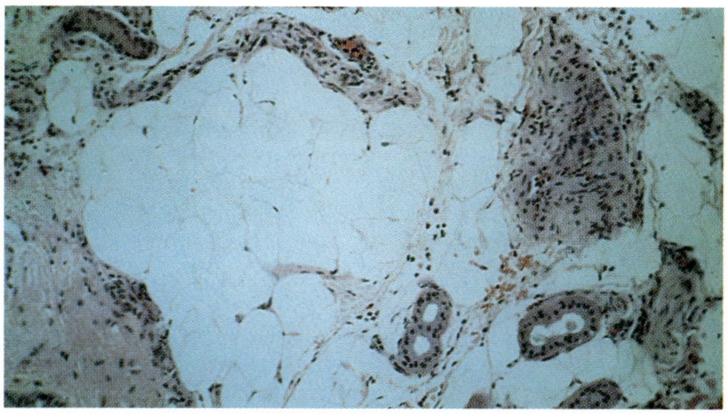

Fig. 22.23 Delayed pressure urticaria: A later lesion in which the infiltrate composed mainly of mononuclear cells and eosinophils is seen. (Courtesy of Professor M Greaves, Institute of Dermatology, United Medical and Dental School, University of London.)

Delayed pressure urticaria is a therapeutic problem. Explanation, avoidance of pressure to the skin as far as possible, and treatment of associated chronic urticaria with H_1-antihistamines is important. Non-steroidal anti-inflammatory drugs have not been shown to be effective and may make the chronic urticaria worse. Colchicine is not effective. Systemic corticosteroids in large doses are effective in some patients but, due to the side effects, are not recommended unless the disability is very severe.

The response of cholinergic urticaria to H_1-antihistamine therapy is variable and therapy generally raises the level of the stimulus threshold but does not achieve control. In those patients who are severely affected, danazol may be used. The recommended dose of danazol of 600mg per day has produced a significant improvement over a four-week period. The side effects of danazol, which include hepatic dysfunction and virilization, may limit its use. Interval treatment is a possible alternative.

Aquagenic urticaria has a rather poor response to H_1-antihistamine therapy but since no more effective treatment is available, potent H_1-antihistamines with minimal sedative properties eg terfenadine, cetirizine, or loratidine should be used.

In solar urticaria, traditional H_1-antihistamine therapy is only partially effective. Of the newer minimally sedating antihistamines terfenadine 240mg per day has been evaluated and is effective.

Hereditary Angioedema

In acute attacks of hereditary angioedema, the treatment of choice is C1-inhibitor concentrate in a dose of 24,000–36,000 units. This can be administered by the patient if necessary and the onset of action is within one hour. Alternatively, fresh frozen plasma can be used but this is less convenient, as it requires hospital attendance, carries the risk of infection and, at least theoretically, could in fact make the angioedema worse because it contains C1-esterase and C1 as well as C1-inhibitor.

Tranexamic acid may also be used in an acute attack in a dose of 1g two hourly as a treatment, or as an adjunct to replacement theraphy. A 2 per cent ephedrine spray or subcutaneous adrenaline can be used to relieve oropharyngeal oedema.

In patients suffering infrequent mild attacks, prophylaxis on a continuous basis may not be justifiable because of the risk of side effects. In these patients use of C1-inhibitor inhibitor concentrate administered when necessary is the preferred management. The most satisfactory prophylactic drugs are the attenuated androgens danazol and stanozolol which raise the circulating levels of C1-inhibitor, although these never reach normal. A suggested dose regime is shown in Fig. 22.24. As patients with hereditary angioedema often improve spontaneously the possibility of stopping the drug should be investigated regularly. Tranexamic acid has been used as a prophylaxis in a dose of 1g three times daily but this carries the risk of thromboembolism.

Urticarial Vasculitis

There is no single effective treatment for this condition. H_1-antihistamines are usually poorly effective, and non-steroidal anti-inflammatory drugs give mixed results. Hydroxychloroquine, dapsone, and colchicine have been reported to be effective in certain patients. Sulphasalazine and gold have also been used successfully on occasion. Systemic steroids may be the most consistently effective treatment but all other modalities should be explored first because treatment may need to be long term.

Hereditary Angioedema		
Drug	**Dose**	**Regime**
Danazol	200–600mg daily	Daily for 1 month, then 5 days on, 5 days off.
Stanozolol	1–2mg daily	Daily for 1 month, then 5 days on, 5 days off.

Fig. 22.24 Prophylactic treatment of hereditary angioedema by oral attenuated androgens.

Further Reading

Warin RP, Champion RH. *Urticaria*. London: WB Saunders Ltd, 1974.

Czarnetzki BM. *Urticaria*. Berlin: Springer-Verlag, 1986.

James J, Warin RP. An assessment of the Role of Candida Albicans and Food Yeasts in Chronic Urticaria. *Br J Derm* 1971; **84**:227–237.

Juhlin L. Recurrent Urticaria: Clinical Investigation of 300 Patients. *Br J Derm* 1981; **104**:369–382.

Warin RP, Smith RP. Challenge Test Battery in Chronic Urticaria. *Br J Derm* 1976; **94**:401–406.

Champion RH, Greaves MW, Kobza Black A, Pye RJ. *The Urticarias*. Edinburgh: Churchill Livingstone, 1985.

Juhlin L, ed. Urticaria. *Seminars in Dermatology*: 1987; 6:4.

Chapter 23

Eczema and Contact Dermatitis – Pathophysiology

Introduction

The terms 'eczema' and 'dermatitis' are generally used synonymously, and for the purpose of this chapter the term dermatitis will be used to describe all forms of disease which involve the eczematous process. By far the greatest amount of research has been performed on allergic contact dermatitis which is a form of delayed hypersensitivity reaction, and the mechanisms involved have been reasonably well worked out. Whether delayed hypersensitivity plays a role in the other kinds of dermatitis remains an open question.

Dermatitis is generally classified as being exogenous, implying an external causation, or endogenous (which might be better named 'non-exogenous') where no external cause is evident (Fig. 23.1). The only two types of dermatitis where hypersensitivity mechanisms are likely to be of major importance are allergic contact dermatitis and atopic dermatitis, but there is evidence that delayed hypersensitivity to ingested nickel may cause pompholyx. Allergic contact dermatitis to Compositae is common in photosensitivity dermatitis, and irritant contact dermatitis is common in atopic dermatitis, which suggests that the various types of dermatitis are more closely related than has been previously thought. Most of this chapter will describe allergic contact dermatitis and atopic dermatitis, but the other causes of dermatitis will be discussed briefly.

Classification of Dermatitis	
Exogenous	**Non-exogenous**
allergic contact irritant contact photosensivity	atopic seborrhoeic nummular (discoid) asteatotic varicose pompholyx

Fig. 23.1 Classification of dermatitis

Exogenous Dermatitis

Allergic Contact Dermatitis

Allergic contact dermatitis is a common dermatological problem which is widely considered to be a form of delayed hypersensitivity. Thus if the relevant allergen, usually a hapten, is applied to the skin of a sensitive patient an eczematous reaction resembling the disease will be elicited over a period of one to three days.

Clinically the patient will present with dermatitis which is localized to the area of the hypersensitivity response (Fig. 23.2a). Common allergens include:

- metals such as nickel and cobalt in buckles, zippers, fasteners, jean studs, etc;
- chromium salts in cement, tanned leather, green textile dyes;
- paraphenylenediamine (a black dye);
- medicaments such as neomycin and synthetic local anaesthetics;
- rubber accelerators, resins such as colophony and epoxy resins, fragrances in soaps and toiletries, and cream and ointment bases containing wool alcohols and parabens.

In many parts of the world nickel is the most common offending allergen, being more common in women due to the custom of ear piercing, and the wearing of non-gold ear-rings which cause sensitization. Experimental work has shown that ingested nickel will also cause a dermatitis in skin which has

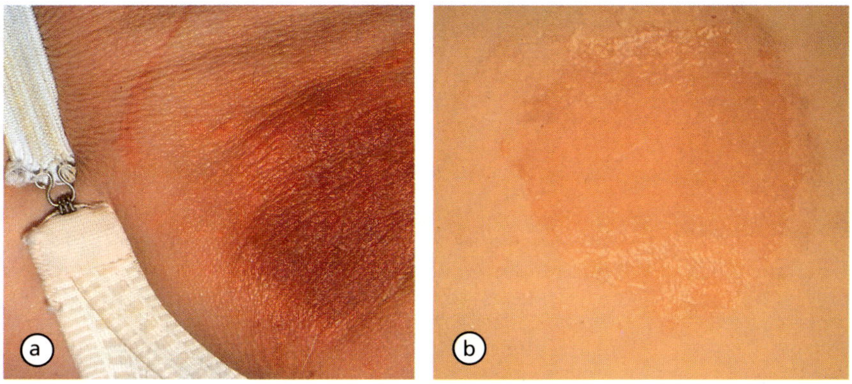

Fig. 23.2 Allergic contact dermatitis due to a nickel brassiere clip. The diagnosis is confirmed by a positive patch test to 5 per cent nickel sulphate in petrolatum.

previously been in contact with nickel, causing a pompholyx-like picture. In North America, plants – particularly poison oak and poison ivy – are a common cause of allergic contact dermatitis. A battery of common allergens has been defined in several parts of the world, and they differ from continent to continent.

The cause of allergic contact dermatitis may be immediately apparent, or it may take considerable expertise to define, especially when it is caused by industrial processes at work. The diagnosis is confirmed by applying the suspected causative chemical in a petrolatum base for 48 to 72 hours, after which a positive patch test with an eczematous reaction will be elicited (Fig. 23.2b).

Immunological components of normal skin
Normal skin contains the necessary cell types for most immune responses. Antigen presentation is the key event in delayed (type IV) hypersensitivity; Langerhans' cells in the epidermis form an extensive network to trap and process epicutaneously applied antigens (Fig. 23.3). Langerhans' cells are bone-marrow-derived dendritic cells which are closely related to macrophages. They are characterized by having the cortical thymocyte antigen CD1, and by containing a unique organelle, the Birbeck granule, on electromicroscopic examination. In the dermis, dermal dendrocytes, other 'indeterminate' cells, and certain types of macrophage are all available for antigen presentation.

The skin also contains other 'resident' cells with immune potential. Mast cells are moderately numerous in the dermis and relatively fixed in number, although the numbers may increase under certain conditions. Several cell types not previously considered to have a role in immunity are now known to

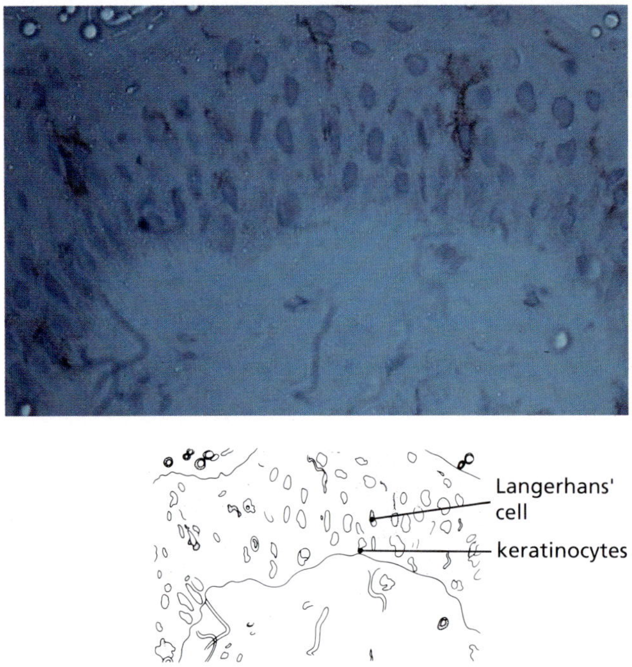

Fig. 23.3 Langerhans' cells in a skin section stained using a monoclonal antibody to CD1a. These dendritic cells comprise 3 per cent of epidermal cells (×312).

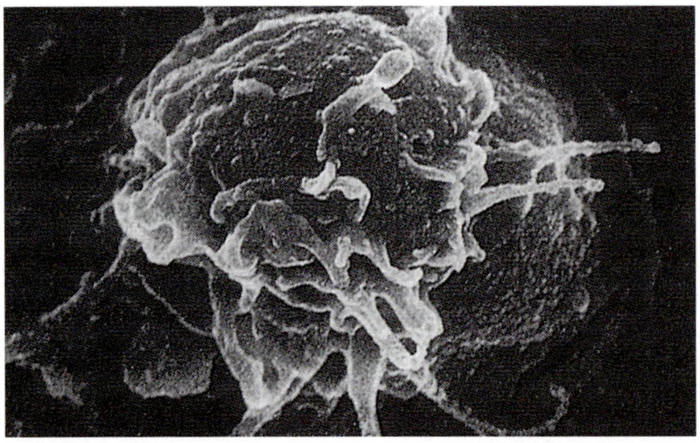

Fig. 23.4 Veiled cells (courtesy of Dr Ian Kimber and reproduced from *International Archives Allergy App Immun*, 1989; **89**:202 by permission of S Karger AG, Basle.

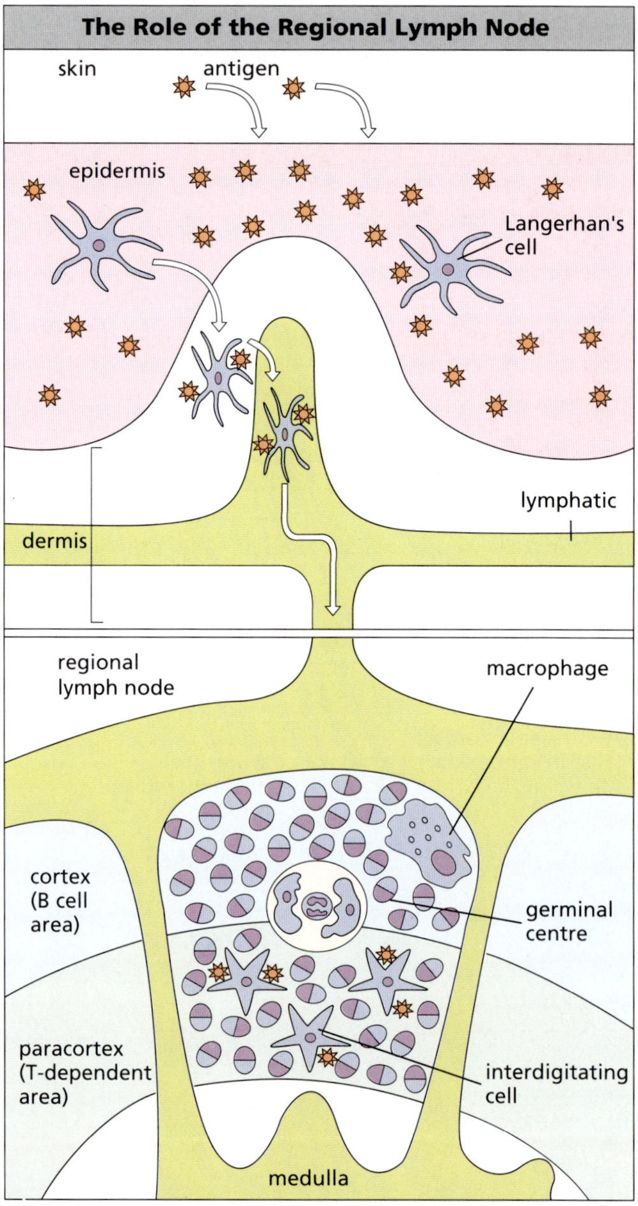

Fig. 23.5 Antigen-bearing Langerhans' cells migrate, via the lymphatics, to the regional lymph nodes. In the paracortical area they interdigitate with $CD4^+$ T lymphocytes resulting in the generation of antigen-specific memory T cells.

take part in some immune responses. For example, keratinocytes and endothelial cells express MHC class II antigens and adhesion molecules, and can play a role in immune responses. T lymphocytes are continually circulating through the skin. A special sub-group, which represent a minority of circulating lymphocytes, home in on the epidermis and are known as intra-epithelial lymphocytes. These T cells are $CD3^+$ and T cell antigen receptor $(TCR)1^+$, but are $CD4^-$ and $CD8^-$. They probably have a primitive cytotoxic function.

The integration of resident skin immune cells, circulating lymphocytes, and the regional lymph nodes has led to the concept of the 'skin-associated lymphoid tissue', much as similar systems have been described for the gut and other 'mucosa-associated lymphoid tissue'. Adhesion molecules and MHC class II antigens can be expressed by keratinocytes and endothelial cells, and Langerhans' cells can express class II antigens. Adhesion molecules and class II antigens take part in skin immune reactions. Cytokines and eicosanoids are produced by several types of cell found in the skin.

The nature of contact allergens

Contact allergens are usually simple chemicals that are haptens and need to link with proteins in the skin before they become antigenic. Under normal circumstances the skin can only be penetrated by molecules that have a molecular weight of less than 1 kDa. Thus haptens may be readily absorbed transcutaneously whereas larger protein allergens may not. For example, dinitrochlorbenzene (DNCB) can be shown to penetrate the epidermis within 30 minutes of its epicutaneous application. Once in the extravascular spaces, most haptens bind in a covalent fashion to their carrier protein – usually serum proteins or the cell membranes of keratinocytes or Langerhan's cells. Metals such as nickel and cobalt are an exception, as they may form complexes with their carrier proteins.

Sensitization and tolerance

For most allergens the development of contact hypersensitivity occurs in only a minority of exposed people. Usually tolerance, a state of specific unresponsiveness to the antigen, is produced. However, certain allergens have a high likelihood of inducing sensitivity. One example is dinitrochlorbenzene, which will sensitize over 90 per cent of normal individuals.

Sensitization takes about 10 to 14 days to develop and become demonstrable in man after the epicutaneous application of an allergen such as dinitrochlorbenzene. If examined prospectively, it is characterized clinically on about the 10th day by an eczematous flare reaction at the site of the sensitizing application. Histologically, an influx of $CD4^+$ lymphocytes is seen and the keratinocytes express MHC class II antigens.

Epicutaneously applied allergen attaches to the Langerhans' cell membrane and is then internalized. Some of the fragments which result from the processing of the antigen are expressed on the surface of the Langerhans' cell in association with MHC class II molecules. The Langerhans' cell then moves out of the epidermis into the dermis and from there into the draining lymphatics and on to the regional lymph nodes. Dermal dendritic cells may also carry antigen.

The antigen-bearing Langerhans' cells, which arrive via the afferent lymphatics where they appear as 'veiled' cells (Fig. 23.4), congregate in the paracortical areas of the regional lymph nodes. Here they take the form of interdigitating cells and have the opportunity to present the processed antigen (associated with MHC class II molecules) to a large number of T lymphocytes (Fig. 23.5). It is this act of antigen presentation (see Chapter 7) and the cells and factors that regulate it which determines the development of type IV hypersensitivity. If sensitization develops, a population of antigen-specific sensitized $CD4^+$ T lymphocytes is produced.

Elicitation phase of allergic contact dermatitis

Antigen presentation. Fig. 23.6 illustrates that an antigen applied epicutaneously to the epidermis is again haptenized and taken up by the Langerhans' cells, which process it and express it on their cell surface in association with class II molecule. As with sensitization, the Langerhans' cells migrate quite rapidly – certainly within 24 hours – from the epidermis to the dermal lymphatics and then to the paracortical

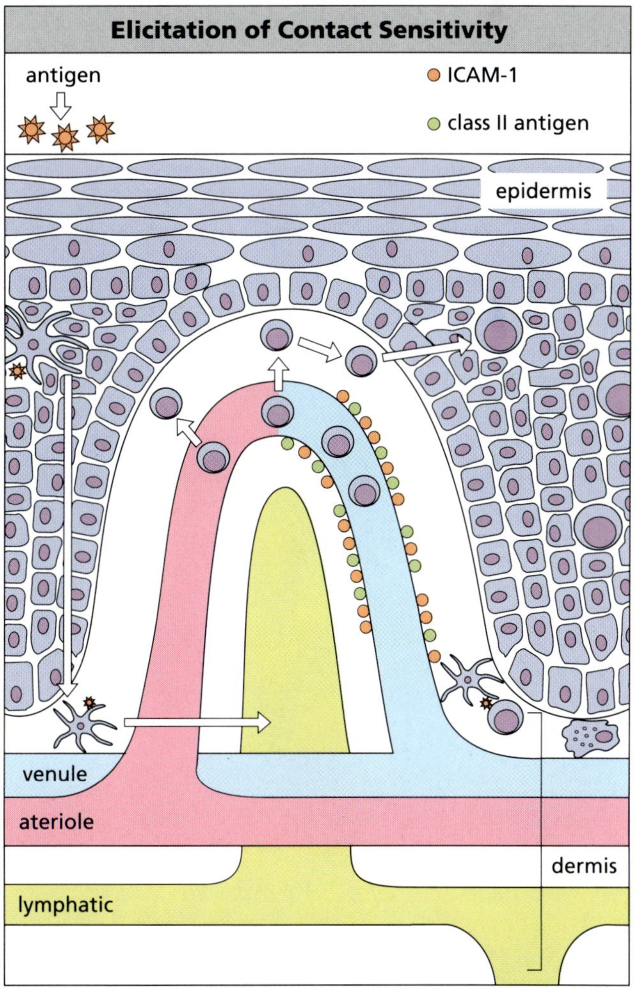

Fig. 23.6 The presentation by Langerhans' cells of processed antigen to T cells results in a cascade of events leading to the influx of mononuclear cells into the dermis and epidermis and the development of dermatitis.

regions of the regional lymph nodes. In the lymph nodes and, as recent work suggests, in the dermis itself, processed antigen is presented to specifically sensitized 'memory' T lymphocytes which have the phenotype $CD4^+$, $CD45RO^+$, $CD29^-$, $CD45RA^-$. This 'secondary response' results in the increased production of antigen-specific effector $CD4^+$ T cells which eventually migrate to the challenged skin site.

Looked at in more detail (Fig. 23.7) antigen presentation requires that the antigen-presenting cell (a Langerhans' cell in this context) express the antigen in association with MHC class II molecules (HLA-DR) to a $CD4^+$ T cell which has a T-cell receptor capable of recognizing the MHC class II molecules/antigen complex. The CD4 and CD3 surface markers are involved with this process. Interleukin-1 (IL-1) is produced by the Langerhans' cell, which stimulates the T cell in several ways. The T cell will itself become activated to produce a number of cytokines, including IL-2 and interferon-γ (IFN-γ), which characterize cell-mediated immunity. The T cell will also express more IL-2 receptors on its surface membrane, and it is induced to proliferate.

Recruitment and retention. The production of cytokines by activated T cells results, through a variety of mechanisms, in the accumulation of antigen-specific and non-antigen-specific 'effector' T cells in the skin. The local production of IFN-γ induces the expression by keratinocytes firstly of intercellular adhesion molecule-1 (ICAM-1), and later of MHC class II molecules. It also up-regulates the MHC class II expression by Langerhans' cells. Such expression occurs within 24 to 48 hours of antigen challenge and has the effect of allowing T cells to bind to the keratinocytes displaying these molecules (Fig. 23.8). Cytokines are also responsible for attracting mononuclear cells to the epidermis and dermis in a non-antigenic-specific manner. Probably less than 10 per cent of T cells in an allergenic contact dermatitis site are allergen-specific.

Mast cells are found to be activated early in the response, possibly due to the effect of cytokines released by T cells, and they amplify the reaction by dilating capillaries and encouraging the migration of mononuclear cells from the circulation.

Endothelial cells themselves are stimulated by IFN-γ to express ICAM-1 and class II molecules which leads to the 'preferential migration' of mononuclear cells to the skin. Circulating T lymphocytes, through their expression of leucocyte function antigens (LFA), recognize adhesion molecules (such as ICAM-1, recognized by its ligand LFA-1) on the surface membranes of endothelial cells and keratinocytes, and can bind to these cells. This further increases the trafficking of mononuclear cells through the skin.

Production of dermatitis. Cytokines such as IL-1, IL-2, and IFN-γ are integrally involved in the initiation and promotion of the type IV contact hypersensitivity responses. Cytokines – most of which are not antigen specific and which are produced by the

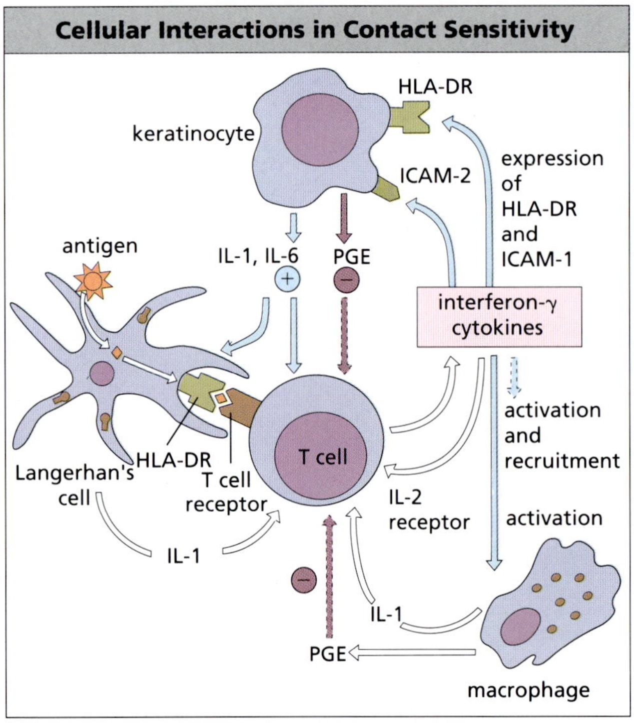

Fig. 23.7 Cytokines and eicosanoids are important in the regulation of the reaction.

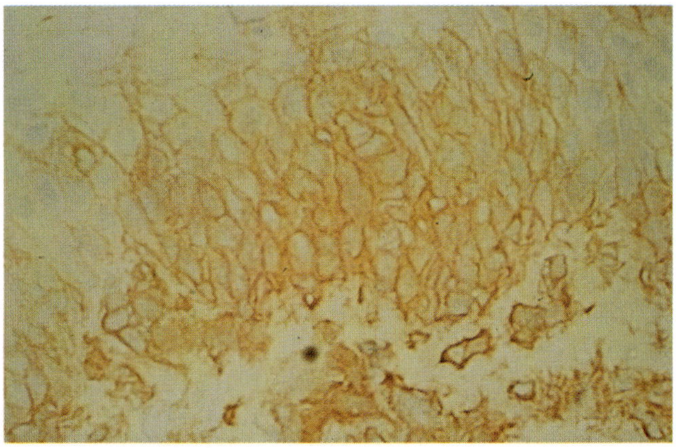

Fig. 23.8 MHC class II antigen expression by keratinocytes in allergic contact dermatitis (×400).

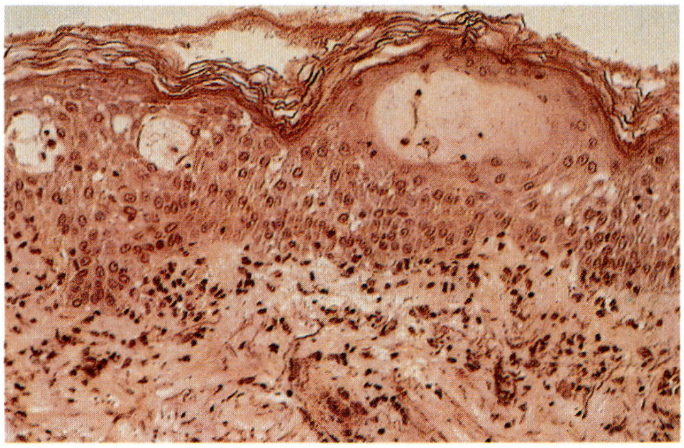

Fig. 23.9 Histological appearance of allergic contact dermatitis. The epidermis is odematous with microvesicle formation and mononuclear cells have infiltrated the dermis and epidermis (×130).

mononuclear cells that are attracted to the site – are largely responsible for the inflammation and dermatitis that results. Eicosanoids, leukotrienes and other lipid mediators, are produced in the epidermis in allergic contact dermatitis. They may contribute towards 'inflammation' but could also down-regulate the reaction. Keratinocytes expressing class II antigens are believed to act as target cells for activated effector T lymphocytes.

Immunohistopathology. Allergic contact dermatitis is characterized histologically by:

- oedema and spongiosis of the epidermis;
- oedema of the papillary dermis; and
- a mononuclear infiltrate in the dermis which extends into the epidermis (Fig. 23.9).

The earliest histological change, seen about four hours after epicutaneous challenge with an antigen, is a peri-appendageal and perivascular mononuclear cell infiltrate. By eight hours, mononuclear cells have begun to infiltrate the epidermis. The infiltrates increase to a maximum at about 48 to 72 hours (by which time there is oedema of the epidermis, after which the reaction subsides. The majority of infiltrating cells are $CD4^+$ (Fig. 23.10), with smaller numbers of $CD8^+$ cells also being found. The numbers of Langerhans' cells are increased in the epidermis at 24 to 48 hours, and $CD1a^+$ cells are seen in the dermal infiltrate. Macrophages invade the dermis (and epidermis) at 48 hours. Basophils have been observed in the infiltrate in some reactions.

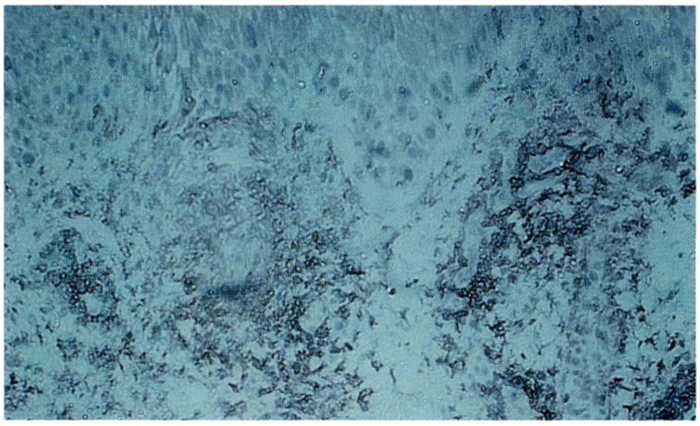

Fig. 23.10 $CD4^+$ lymphocytes in an allergic contact reaction. The majority of T cells infiltrating this 96 hours allergic patch test are of the CD4 phenotype.

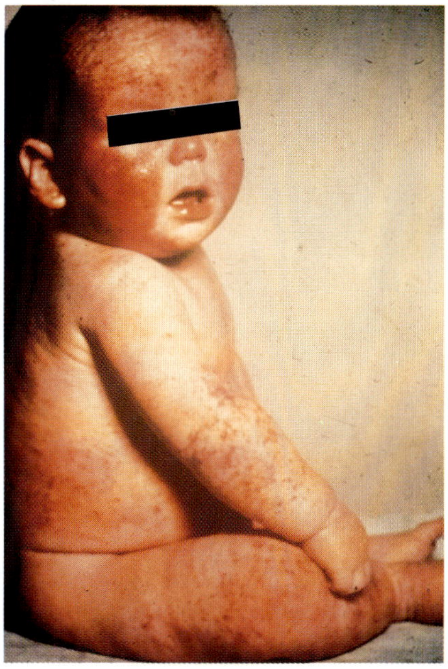

Fig. 23.11 Child with widespread atopic dermatitis.

Down-regulation of the response

The reaction begins to wane after 48 to 72 hours. Down-regulation results from a number of mechanisms. Macrophages, which have infiltrated the site after 48 hours, produce prostaglandins (principally of the E series) which inhibit both the production of IL-1 and IL-2, and also natural killer cell activity. Other eicosanoids, such as leukotriene B4, may induce $CD8^+$ suppressor cells which dampen down the reaction. Destruction of the antigen, by enzymatic or cellular degradation, leads to a tailing off in the response.

Keratinocytes are thought to be capable of down-regulating the response in three main ways:

(1) if T-cell binding to MHC class II antigen-positive keratinocytes is strong, this can lead to unresponsiveness and halt the inflammation (MHC class II positive keratinocytes might, contrariwise, enhance epidermal T-cell proliferation through the release of cytokines, if the T cells bind predominantly to Langerhans' cells);

(2) the keratinocytes which express MHC class II antigen could induce specific suppressor cells which can modify the reaction; and

(3) keratinocytes can produce eicosanoids such as prostaglandins of the E series which inhibit effector lymphocytes (Fig. 23.7).

Irritant Contact Dermatitis

This usually occurs on the hands, and is due to contact with irritant substances such as detergents and oils. It is not a hypersensitivity reaction, as no sensitization is required and patch testing will produce only a non-eczematous irritant reaction in almost all patients. It is therefore a chemical irritant effect on the skin which may occur in anyone who is in contact with detergents and oils or other irritants, but is particularly common in patients with atopic dermatitis.

Photosensitivity Dermatitis

This is an extremely complex condition which represents a spectrum of disease rather than a single disease. Sometimes known as the photosensitivity dermatitis/actinic reticuloid syndrome, it occurs almost exclusively in males and is characterized by severe photosensitivy. A number of patients have a demonstrable history of contact dermatitis due to plants of the Compositae family, but the reason or significance of this association is at present unclear.

Non-exogenous Dermatitis

Atopic Dermatitis

Atopic dermatitis (Fig. 23.11) is an enigma. Whereas the other manifestations of atopy such as asthma, allergic rhinitis, allergic conjunctivitis, and IgE-mediated food allergy involve IgE-mediated mechanisms, this does not appear to be the case in atopic dermatitis. Histological examination of the skin in acute atopic dermatitis reveals a picture similar to that of atopic dermatitis, with microvesication in the epidermis and a lymphohistiocytic infiltrate in the dermis, without obvious mast cell degranulation or eosinophil infiltration. Despite this, major basic protein has been demonstrated in the dermis of patients with atopic dermatitis, which suggests that eosinophils may be involved initially.

IgE-mediated allergy

Atopic dermatitis presents with a wide spectrum of severity. At the mild end of the spectrum, the patient has minimal atopic dermatitis affecting only the flexures, notably the cubital and popliteal fossae (Fig. 23.12); these patients often have no other atopic manifestations and tend to have normal total serum IgE concentrations with negative skin prick tests and RAST to common inhaled and food allergens.

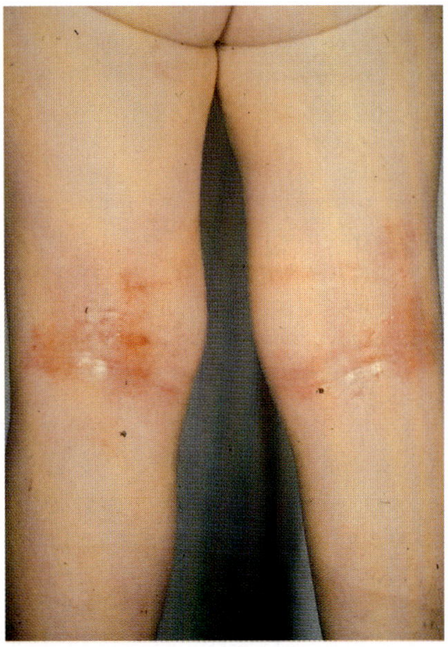

Fig. 23.12 Child with flexural (mild) atopic dermatitis.

At the other end of the spectrum, patients with severe generalized atopic dermatitis tend to have allergic asthma, seasonal and perennial rhinitis, allergic conjunctivitis, and sometimes IgE-mediated food allergy and IgE-mediated drug allergy. These patients tend to have very high total serum IgE concentrations (up to 200 000IU/ml), and produce high concentrations of IgE to common inhalants and occasionally also to foods. The IgE concentrations in 45 patients with severe atopic dermatitis are shown in Fig. 23.13. It has also been observed that atopic dermatitis patients have IgE bound to Langerhans' cells in the skin. The functional significance of this is unclear.

The role of IgE-mediated allergy in atopic dermatitis is controversial. The fact that 20 per cent of patients with atopic dermatitis have normal serum IgE concentrations and no positive allergy tests argues against IgE mechanisms being of central importance in the intrinsic pathogenesis of the disease. However it is probable that IgE allergy is an important complicating factor. Patients with atopic dermatitis produce high concentrations of IgE against inhalants, and many patients say that their atopic dermatitis becomes worse when in close contact with dogs or cats to which they know they are allergic because they also develop allergic rhinitis and asthma. Also, some atopic dermatitis patients develop eczema around the eyes and nose during the pollen season which accompanies their allergic conjunctivitis and rhinitis (Fig. 23.14). In these cases it seems likely that mast cell degranulation in the skin and mucous membranes leads to the eczematous reaction.

House dust mite allergy

The relationship between atopic dermatitis and house dust mite is also controversial. Approximately 75 per cent of patients with severe atopic dermatitis

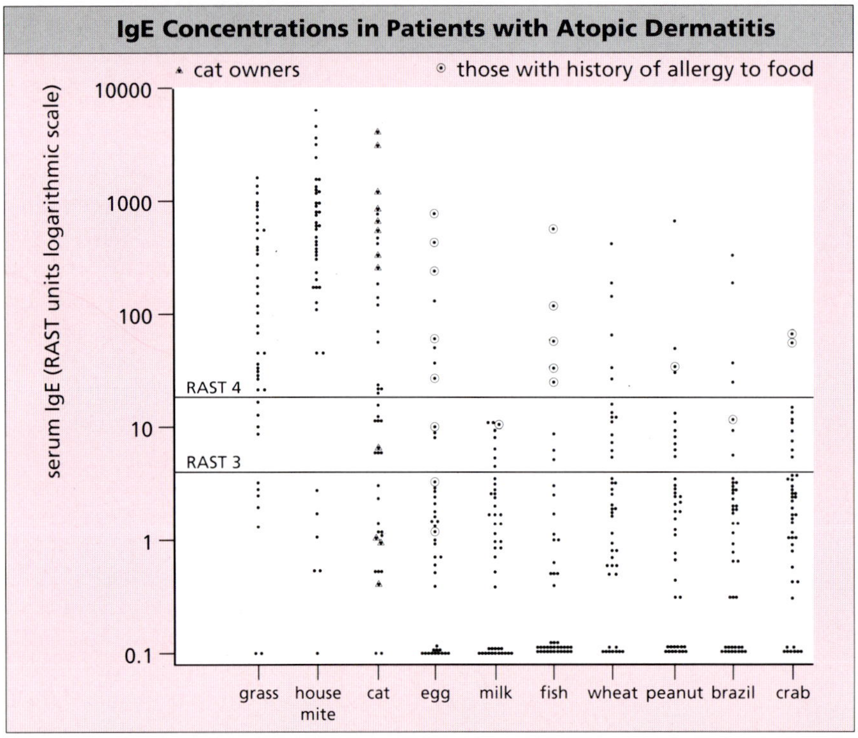

Fig. 23.13 Specific IgE concentrations (1 RAST unit = 1 IU total IgE) in 45 subjects with atopic dermatitis to 3 inhalants and seven foods.

produce very high concentrations of IgE to mite allergens (Fig. 23.13). It has also been shown that a majority of atopic dermatitis patients have high lymphoproliferative responses to the house dust mite, which confirms that such patients can produce a delayed hypersensitivity reaction to the mite in addition to an immediate response. Furthermore, patch tests to mite allergens produce an erythematous response, although the infiltrate in the dermis consists largely of eosinophils and basophils, which is unlike the histological picture in patch tests to allergens such as nickel or dinotrochlorobenzene. There is evidence to suggest that mite allergen, when applied to eczematous skin, will exacerbate the eczema in atopic dermatitis patients with house dust mite allergy, indicating that this is a complicating factor in patients with severe atopic dermatitis. Further evidence that mite allergen is implicated derives from the observations that patients scratch most in bed at night where there is a high mite density, and tend to improve in the relatively mite-free environment of hospital, even when not under specific treament. Also, removal of the carpet and curtains from the bedroom, and covering the pillows and mattress with plastic may sometimes be helpful for patients with severe atopic dermatitis.

Food allergy

Food intolerance may also be important as a complicating factor in some atopic dermatitis patients. Roughly 25 per cent of patients with severe atopic dermatitis have IgE-mediated food allergy to common foods such as eggs, milk, wheat, nuts, fish and shellfish, to which they produce high serum concentrations of IgE (Fig. 23.13). The symptoms include angioedema of the mouth and face, contact urticaria of the face where the food is in contact with the mucous membranes and skin, generalized itch and urticaria, with wheeze and systemic anaphylaxis (associated particularly with nuts) following absorption of food allergens. Many of these symptoms are immediate, occurring within 15 minutes of food ingestion, but patients may also describe late symptoms, such as pruritus and worsening of the eczema occuring eight to 24 hours later. In some patients the late symptoms follow directly on from the immediate manifestations, e.g. angioedema of the face leading to eczema of the face, a situation analagous to the dual reaction in asthma (Fig. 23.15).

Adults are usually aware of the fact that they have food allergy, and avoid that food assiduously. However, in those allergic to hen's eggs, which may be present in small quantities in foods such as sauces, a strict egg-free diet, even though difficult to observe, may be helpful in ameliorating their atopic dermatitis. IgE-mediated allergy is much commoner in children, who usually acquire it during the first year of life after being weaned from breast milk. Although most outgrow it by the age of five, the elimination of the offending food, and its substitution with milk substitutes such as soya milk or Pregestemil can cause a dramatic improvement of their atopic dermatitis. As most children develop food allergy and eczema during the first year of life, it is not surprising that some paediatricians believe that atopic dermatitis is solely due to food allergy. It is still unknown why children first develop food allergy and atopic dermatitis, then become sensitive to house dust mites and animal dander, often concurrently developing asthma which improves around puberty, and then finally progress to grass-pollen allergy, which often presents as seasonal rhinitis and continues into adulthood (see Fig. 23.16).

Food intolerance

In atopic dermatitis, IgE-mediated food allergy is not the whole story as far as food intolerance is concerned. Many adult patients assert that alcoholic beverages (particularly in excess!), food colourings such as tartrazine, and highly spiced foods cause worsening of the eczema on the day after ingestion. This pattern is not consistent with an IgE mechanism. Furthermore, in the case of cow's milk and wheat, a considerable number of patients do not have

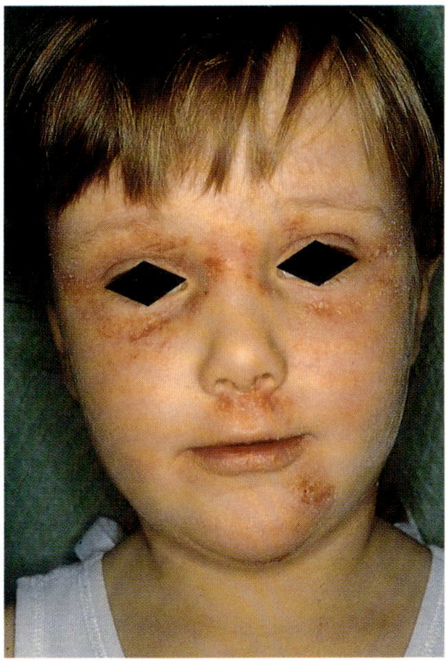

Fig. 23.14 Child with atopic dermatitis related to allergic rhinitis and conjunctivitis during the pollen season.

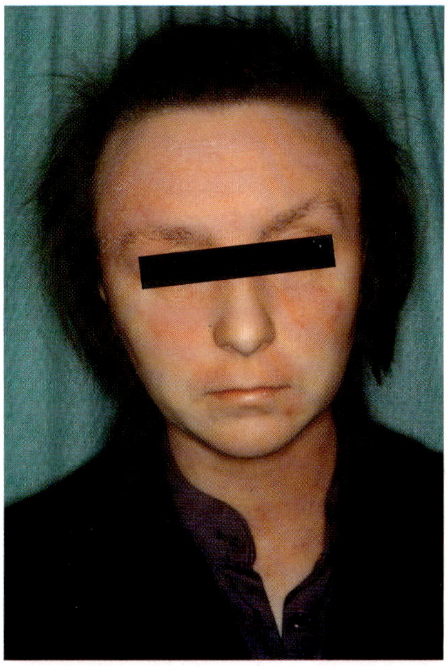

Fig. 23.15 Milk-allergic patient with atopic dermatitis of face which has developed 24 hours after angioedema induced by milk ingestion.

demonstrable IgE-mediated allergy to these food allergens, but still react with worsening of the eczema on food challenge. This suggests that mechanisms unrelated to IgE-mediated hypersensitivity must also be involved, but what these are is at present unclear. However, in both food allergy and food intolerance it seems likely that mast cell degranulation is the initiating factor, followed by neutrophil and eosinophil infiltration and second-phase leukotriene release, which leads on to exacerbation of the atopic dermatitis. The T lymphocyte is also receiving much attention today as a possible orchestrating cell for hypersensitivity responses.

It thus seems that inhalant allergy, food allergy, and food intolerance (due to non-immunological mechanisms) are all complicating factors in atopic dermatitis. These factors vie with other precipitating factors such as stress, secondary infection of the skin, and contact with skin irritants to cause worsening of the eczema (Fig. 23.17). The possible relationship between immediate and delayed hypersensitivity to inhalant and food allergens and the skin is summarized in Fig. 23.18.

Anergy in atopic dermatitis
In contrast to allergy which is so common in atopic dermatitis patients, many also have evidence of anergy or immunosuppression. It has been shown that these patients have:
- diminished delayed type hypersensitivity skin responses to dinitrochlorbenzene, to candidal antigens and to streptokinase/streptodornase
- reduced lymphocytic transformation responses to PPD, herpes simplex virus and *Staphylococcus aureus*
- reduced numbers of circulating T helper cells
- reduced antibody dependent cytotoxicity
- reduced NK cell activity.

This may result from feedback inhibition by cytokines from one T-cell subtype on the development and function of another, the complexities of which are only now being unravelled. This makes patients with atopic dermatitis unduly susceptible to infections, particularly virus infections, leading to eczema herpeticum (generalized herpes simplex infection) (Fig. 23.19) and eczema vaccinatum (generalized vaccinia virus infection), two important and at times lethal complications of atopic dermatitis. Fortunately this anergy is temporary, being worse when the atopic dermatitis is severe, and returning to normality when the atopic dermatitis is in a good phase. This may be confirmed by lymphocyte transformation responses to *Staphylococcus aureus*, which are very low in severe atopic dermatitis patients but return to within the normal range after treatment of the atopic dermatitis (Fig. 23.2).

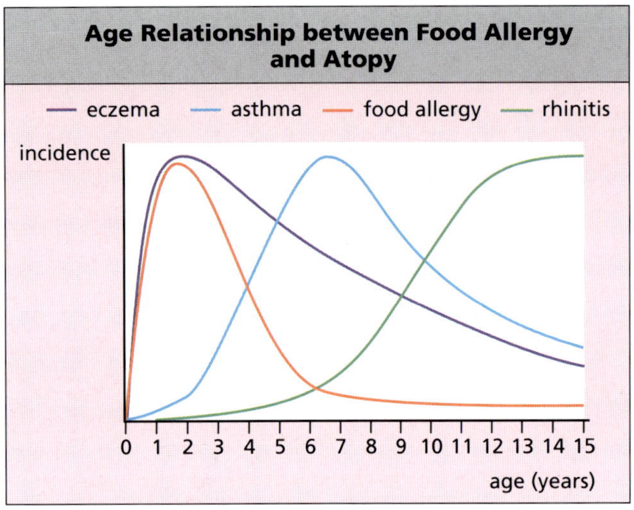

Fig. 23.16 Typical time course of diseases in the atopic syndrome. atopic dermatitis usually presents during the first year of life, and is often outgrown by the age of 14. Food allergy also usually presents in the first year of life, and is outgrown by the age of five. Asthma develops later, usually between the ages of three and seven, and is often outgrown by the age of 14. Allergic rhinitis presents later still, around the age of seven, and continues into adulthood.

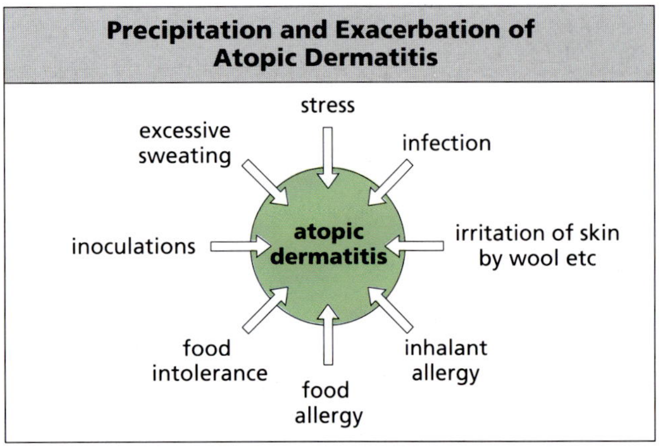

Fig. 23.17 Complicating factors in atopic dermatitis.

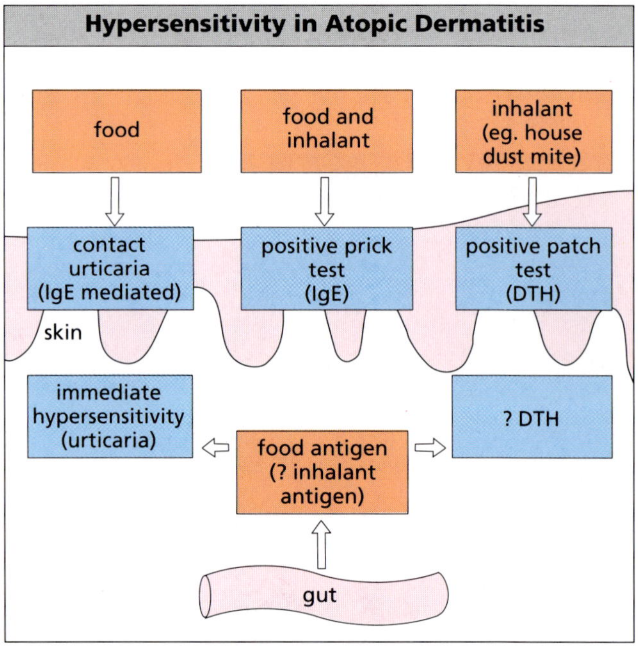

Fig. 23.18 The relationship between immediate and delayed hypersensitivity to inhalant and food allergens, and the skin.

Seborrhoeic Dermatitis

This common disease may present either in infancy or adulthood. As it tends to occur in areas where there is greatest sebaceous activity, it has been postulated that sebaceous gland secretions may be involved in the pathogenesis. There is also evidence that *Pityrosporum furfur* is implicated, particularly as anti-yeast preparations may ameliorate the seborrhoeic dermatitis.

Infantile seborrhoeic dermatitis occurs during the first six months of life, possibly resulting from maternal androgen influence on the sebaceous glands. The condition is relatively common after puberty and tends to affect areas of marked sebaceous activity, particularly the hair-bearing areas, the face, the flexures, chest and back. In both groups, differentiation from atopic dermatitis may be difficult, though in seborrhoeic dermatitis serum IgE concentrations are usually normal.

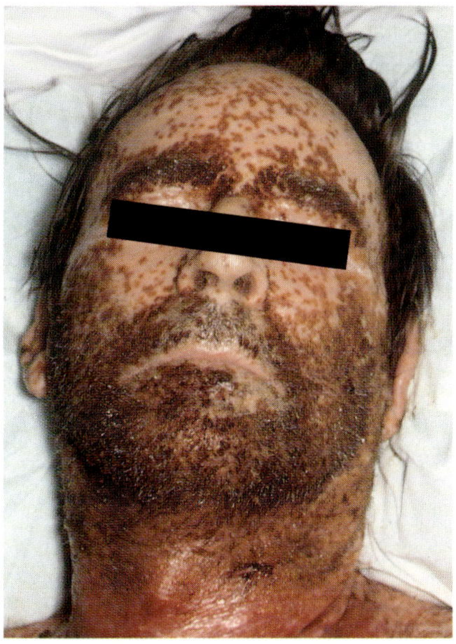

Fig. 23.19 Adult patient with severe eczema herpeticum.

Nummular Dermatitis (discoid eczema)

This is also relatively common and is characterized by the development of coin-shaped areas on the trunk and limbs. It is debatable whether it is a single entity, and certainly some patients with atopic dermatitis may present with discoid lesions. Its pathogenesis is unknown.

Asteatotic Dermatitis

This occurs on the limbs and trunk of elderly patients. The skin is dry and scaly, probably because of increased water loss through the skin due to diminished integrity of the horny layer of the epidermis, coupled with decreased lipid secretion in the sebum, and hormonal changes. The dryness leads to eczema, which may be extensive. The problem may be compounded by the over-enthusiastic use of soap and by diuretics. It may also be the presenting sign in hypothyroidism.

Varicose Dermatitis (stasis eczema)

This occurs on the ankles of patients with varicose veins. The pathogenesis is debatable.

Pompholyx

This presents in a characteristic pattern with large blisters on the palms and soles. Its pathogenesis is unknown, but experimental work has shown that nickel-allergic patients develop a pompholyx-like picture when given reasonably large quantities of nickel by mouth. The ingestion of other haptens which cause allergic contact dermatitis may also cause pompholyx.

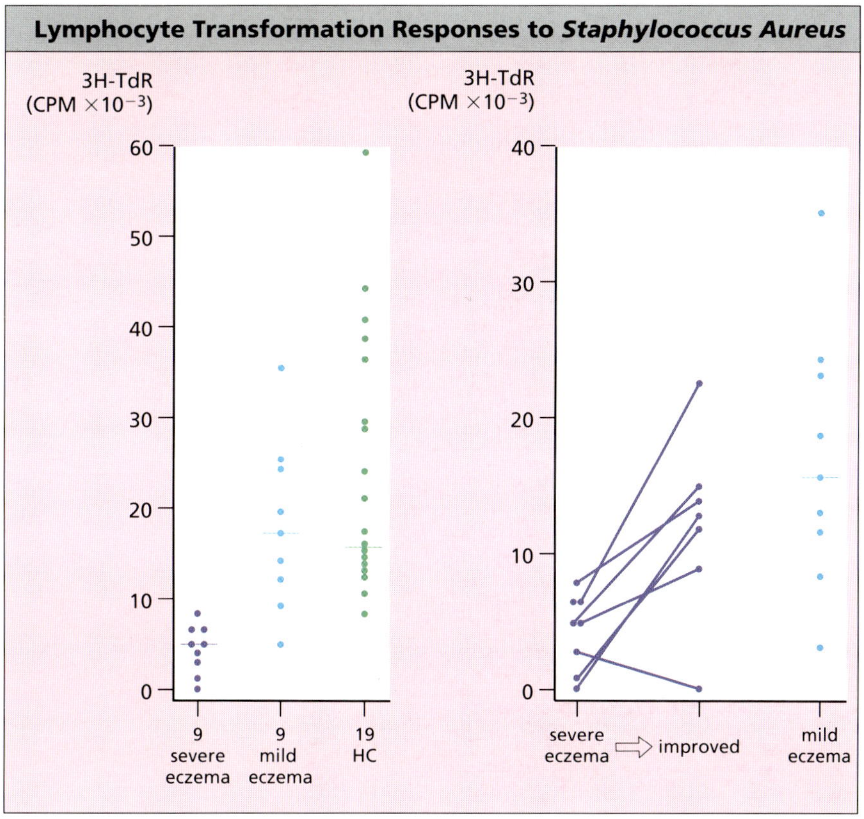

Fig. 23.20 [left] Lymphocyte transformation (LT) responses to *Staphylococcus aureus* (which is found on the skin of almost 100 per cent of patients with severe atopic dermatitis) comparing groups with severe atopic dermatitis, mild atopic dermatitis, and healthy controls (HC). [right] LT responses to *Staphylococcus aureus* in patients with severe atopic dermatitis before and after treatment. The responses return to normal when the atopic dermatitis is treated effectively.

Conclusions

Eczematous reactions thus represent a heterogenous group of conditions which share a delayed onset and relative chronicity amongst their characteristics. Most are associated with an extrinsic allergenic trigger and yet the symptoms of an immediate allergic reaction are either absent or a prelude to the more delayed eczematous reaction. Histological examination of eczematous lesions illustrates the accumulation of $CD4^+$ T lymphocytes as a characteristic feature. As described in Chapter 9, much the same picture is observed with the more chronic phases of immediate hypersensitivity reactions.

So what could be the reason for the differences? A clue is now begining to emerge from detailed studies of cytokine production from $CD4^+$ lymphocytes. In mice, two distinct and mutually exclusive subsets of T-helper (TH) lymphocytes have been described: TH_1 which secrete IL-2, IFN-γ, and TNF-β, and which are generally associated with delayed or cell-mediated hypersensitivity response;, and TH_2 which produce IL-4, IL-5, IL-6 and IL-10 and which are associated with immediate IgE-mediated allergic responses. Recent studies have demonstrated that analogous human Th cells may be induced in tissue culture and sub-cultured from tissues undergoing allergic reactions. It would seem likely then that the dominant T cell in eczematous tissues would be the TH_1 cell and the cytokine production from this cell would co-ordinate the chronic reactions which are seen with allergen exposure.

Further Reading

Barnetson RStC, Atherton DJ. Clinical aspects of the endogenous eczemas. *Med International* 1983; **27**:1255–1260.

Barnetson RStC, Wright AL, Benton EC. IgE mediated allergy in adults with severe atopic eczema. *Clin Exp Allergy* 1989;**19**:321–325.

Gawkrodger DJ, McVittie E, Carr MM, Ross JA, Hunter JAA. Phenotypic characterization of the early cellular responses in allergic and irritant contact dermatitis. *Clin Exp Immun* 1986;**66**:590–598.

Gawkrodger DJ, Carr MM, McVittie E, Guy K, Hunter JAA. Keratinocyte expression of MHC class II antigens in allergic sensitization and challenge reactions and in irritant contact dermatitis. *J Invest Derm* 1987;**88**:11–16.

Nickologg B J (1988). Role of interferon-gamma in cutaneous trafficking of lymphocytes with emphasis on molecular and cellular adhesion events. *Arch Derm* 1988;**124**:1835–1843.

Norris PG, Schofield O, Camp RDR. A study of the role of house dust mite in atopic dermatitis. *Brit J Derm* 1988;**118**:435–440.

Rawle FC, Mitchell EB, Platts Mills TAE. T cell response to the major allergens from the house dust mite *Dermatophagoides pteronyssinus*, antigen P1: comparison of patients with asthma, atopic dermatitis and perennial rhinitis. *J Immun* 1984;**133**:195–201.

Sauder DN. Allergic contact dermatitis. In: Thiers BH, Dobson RL, eds. *Pathogenesis of skin disease*. New York: Churchill Livingstone,.1986:3–12.

Threstrup-Pedersen K, Larsen CG, Ronnevig J. The immunology of contact dermatitis. *Contact Derm* 1989;**20**:81–92.

Chapter 24

Eczema and Contact Dermatitis – Diagnosis and Treatment

Allergic Contact Dermatitis

As detailed in the previous chapter, allergic contact dermatitis is a delayed-type hypersensitivity reaction, mediated largely by previously sensitized lymphocytes, that causes inflammation and oedema in the skin. It is estimated that 80 per cent of all dermatitic problems on the hands and forearms are due to allergic contact dermatitis, which is therefore responsible for a very large amount of time lost from work. In this type of dermatitis, prior exposure to the responsible allergen is necessary, either briefly or over many years. This last point is often difficult for patients to understand.

Pathological Features

The pathology of allergic contact dermatitis is non-specific and similar to that of dermatitis in general. It may be acute, subacute or chronic. Features of acute dermatitis are oedema and spongiosis in the epidermis, with the presence of lymphocytes, and with a few eosinophils and other cells in the dermis. In subacute dermatitis the epidermal oedema is less striking, and there is usually a greater cellular infiltrate, occasionally with some early thickening of the epidermis. This sign is called acanthosis. Chronic dermatitis, which does not develop until the allergen has been present and causing the problem for several months, is characterized by an obvious thickening or acanthosis of the epidermis and a relatively mild infiltrate. Oedema is usually absent.

Clinical Features

Females present more commonly than males with allergic contact dermatitis, and there is an increase in incidence with advancing age. The clinical features of allergic contact dermatitis will depend on the type of allergen responsible (Fig. 24.1). In general, however, nickel dermatitis is characterized by erythema, scaling and induration, causing pruritus

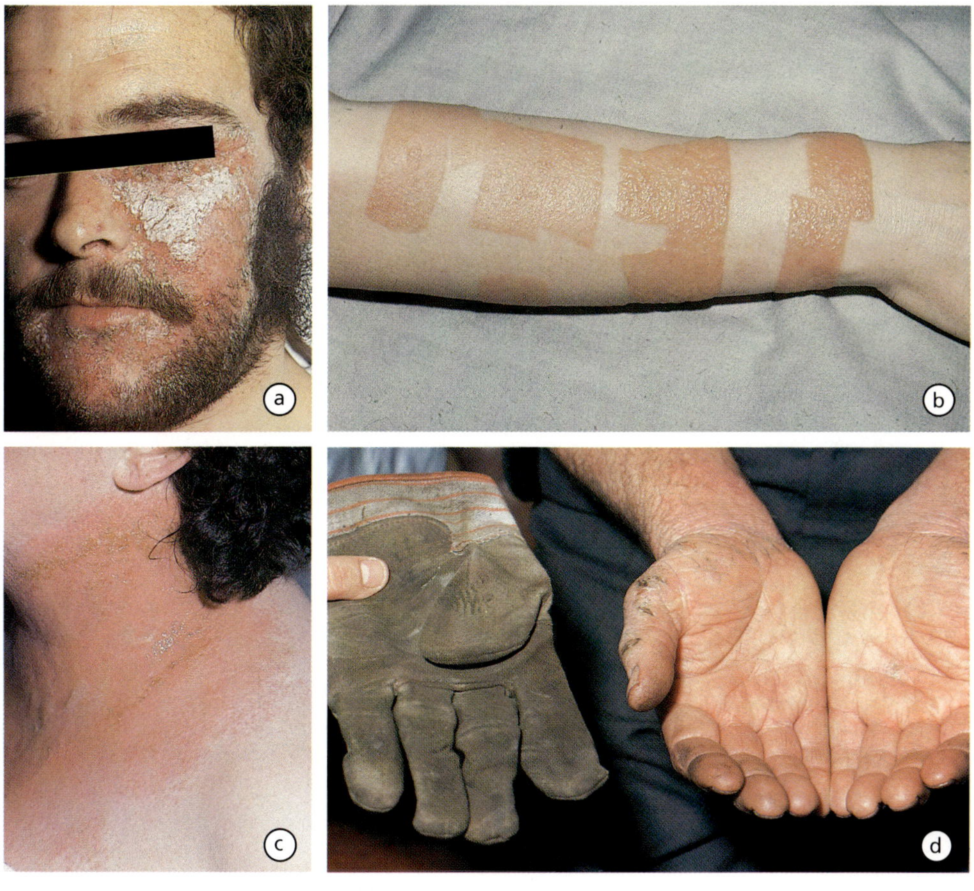

Fig. 24.1 (a) Contact dermatitis caused by eyedrops containing neomycin.
(b) Contact dermatitis to elastoplast.
(c) Contact dermatitis to perfume spray.
(d) Contact dermatitis to industrial gloves.

at sites of contact with metal, such as jewellery, watch straps and metal studs or buttons in jeans. Contact dermatitis caused by material found in articles of footwear is commonly found on the dorsum of the feet, which is an important point in differentiation from fungal infection of the feet (Fig. 24.2). Airborne allergic contact dermatitis causes striking facial oedema and erythema.

The important points in the clinical identification and management of allergic contact dermatitis are listed in Fig. 24.3. In taking the patient's history, it is important to consider occupational, household and recreational exposure to possible allergens. Common sources of allergens in Europe and North America are shown in Fig. 24.4. For legal reasons, many sufferers are keen to incriminate an allergen handled in the course of their employment, but frequently contact allergic dermatitis arises from sources in the home. It is therefore important to take a clear history of materials handled in the course of work, domestic activities, hobbies and sporting activities, and of any other part of the patient's life that is possibly relevant. Many patients find it difficult to understand that material handled for many years can suddenly give rise to an allergic contact dermatitis; similarly, allergy to a regular cosmetic or washing powder may not be regarded by the patient as a possible cause of their problems. In such cases it must be remembered that new, improved formulations are introduced and also that it is often the preservative, rather than the main ingredient of such preparations, which gives rise to problems.

Contact dermatitis caused by an allergy to airborne material may be difficult to identify, but this can occur, for example, with plants or with fine particles of rubber dust in cars. In clinical diagnosis, this condition is often confused with photosensitive dermatitis.

Nickel dermatitis

Obvious areas of involvement are under rings, watches, bracelets and other sites of direct contact with metal, such as jean studs (Figs 24.5 and 24.6). Less obvious areas are the eyelids and the nape of the neck. Nickel dermatitis is extremely common in women, and in Scandinavia is said to affect 10 per cent of the female population. A high proportion of patients with allergic contact dermatitis first develop their problem after ear-piercing. The frequency of nickel dermatitis is currently increasing in incidence in the male population, and this may be due to greater popularity of ear-piercing in this group. Other sites of contact with metal which may give problems are spectacle frames, coins in pockets, and household utensils containing nickel. To determine whether a metal contains nickel, a spot test can be carried out using diamethylglyoxime. This gives rise to a pink colour if nickel is present in the material tested. There is continuing controversy as to whether the nickel content of a normal diet can provoke or aggravate pre-existing nickel dermatitis.

Chromate dermatitis

Dermatitis of the hands and forearms is commonly caused by chromate. Hexavalent metal salts of chromate are among the most important causes of contact reactions. They are found in cement, detergent, bleaches and match heads and are used in tanning leather. They produce a dry lichenified hand dermatitis (Fig. 24.7).

Formaldehyde

Formaldehyde is found in cosmetics, cigarettes, newsprints, fabric softener and coating for wrinkle-resistant fabrics, such as drip-dry shirts. Preservatives such as Bromopol, Dowicil 200 and Germal also contain formaldehyde. Shampoo contains many formaldehyde releasers.

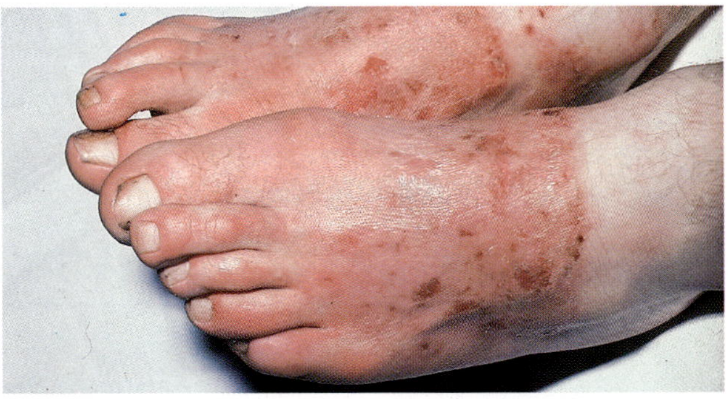

Fig. 24.2 Contact dermatitis to footwear.

Steps in Diagnosis and Management of Allergic Contact Dermatitis	
taking an accurate history initial treatment of skin protection from suspected allergen	patch testing good communication of results allergen avoidance

Fig. 24.3 Major points in identification and management of allergic contact dermatitis.

Common Allergen Sources in Allergic Contact Dermatitis	
nickel	clothing clasps, earrings, spectacle frames, jewellery, coins, household utensils
chromate	leather, bleaches, matches, cement
formaldehyde	preservatives, cosmetics, cigarettes, newsprint, fabric softeners, wrinkle-resistant clothes
ethylenediamine	preservatives in creams, aminophylline, paints, cross-reaction with antihistamines (e.g. hydroxyzine)
mercaptobenzothiazole	rubber products (especially boots and gloves), catheters
thiurams	rubber products, fungicide in paint and soap, paraphenylenediamine hair dye, clothing dye, stockings and tights
plants	*Primula obconica* (Europe), *Rhus* (poison ivy – North America)

Fig. 24.4 Common agents causing allergic contact dermatitis and their sources.

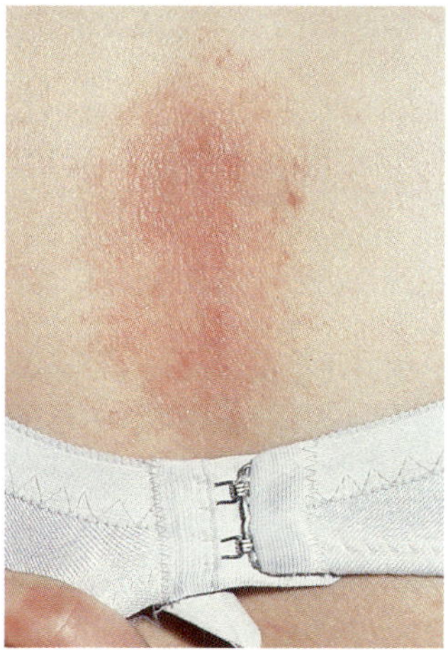

Fig 24.5 Nickel sensitivity to metal clips in underwear.

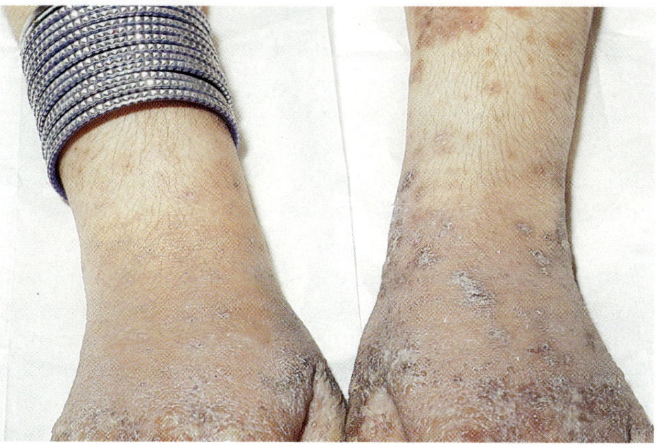

Fig. 24.6 Nickel sensitivity to bracelets.

Ethylenediamine
Ethylenediamine is widely used, for example as a preservative in some topical medications; as a substance complexed with theophylline to make the water-soluble aminophylline and as a catalyst in some rapid-drying polymer paints. Sensitive patients may also cross-react with some antihistimaines, such as hydroxyzine and promethazine.

Mercaptobenzothiazole
Mercaptobenzothiazole (MBT) is an accelerator used in the manufacture of both natural and synthetic rubber. It is responsible for footwear dermatitis, particularly to rubber boots; 'toe puff' dermatitis, which is caused by the insert of rubber or synthetic rubber material used to preserve the appearance of shoes; and dermatitis to rubber gloves. It may also cause allergic contact dermatitis to catheters.

Thiurams
Thiurams are rubber accelerators and are also found as fungicides in paints and soap. Users of rubber gloves may be allergic to thiurams.

Paraphenylenediamine
Paraphenylenediamine (PPD) is the main component of most hair dyes and is also used in dyeing stockings and tights. Allergic contact dermatitis after application of a hair dye or on the legs of women is commonly due to PPD.

Plant dermatitis
Plant allergy is a common cause of dermatitis in those who handle plants professionally, such as florists. In the UK, P*rimula obconica* is a common cause of problems (Fig. 24.8). The allergen involved is primin which is airborne and which can cause an acute reaction. In the USA, *Rhus* ivy causes an extremely severe allergic contact dermatitis, often with linear vesicles. Other plants which can cause allergic contact dermatitis include the Compositae family, such as dahlias and chrysanthemums. Tulip bulb handlers may also develop a problem with a dry cracked dermatitis on the finger tips, caused by handling bulbs.

Diagnosis
Once the possible major allergen has been identified by taking a good history, the initial management of all types of suspected allergic contact dermatitis consists of a period of 3–4 weeks' protection from that allergen and the use of an appropriate potency topical steroid to return skin to a normal state. Thereafter, there should ideally be a 3–4 week period with use of only an emollient, as topical steroids may partly suppress the patch test response, and the use of systemic steroids in doses of 20 mg of prednisone or greater daily will certainly do so. Without this preparation for patch testing, both false-positive and false-negative results may be obtained.

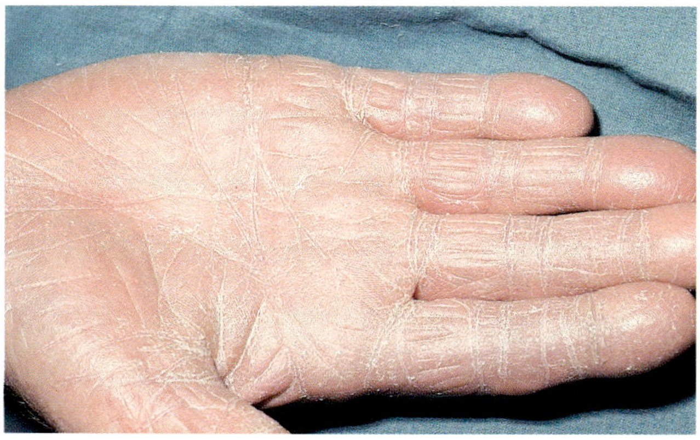

Fig. 24.7 Hand dermatitis caused by chromates.

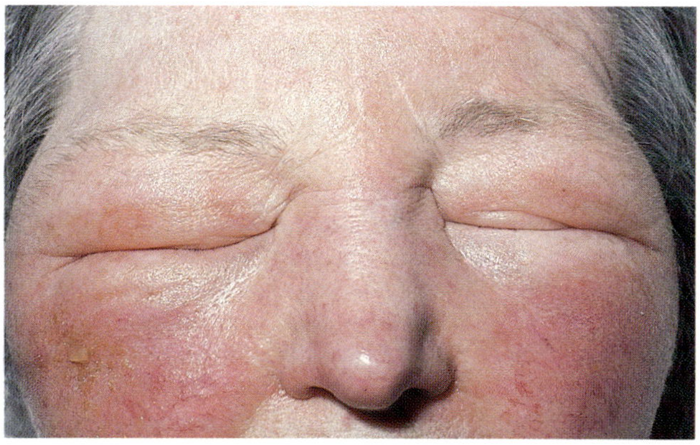

Fig. 24.8 Plant dermatitis. Facial dermatitis eruption caused by *Primula obconica.*

Patch testing

The technique of patch testing is deceptively simple. The European standard battery of allergens, shown in Fig. 24.9, is a collection of of the commonest known allergens. A similar battery is available for North America. The allergens are prepared in appropriate concentrations in an appropriate diluent, which is usually white soft paraffin, and are applied to the skin on inert metal discs, such as Finn chambers (Fig. 24.10). Sets of ready-prepared allergens on an appropriate backing, which simplify the process and facilitate its use in general practice, are now commercially available. After 48 hours, the battery of chambers is removed and areas of erythema or induration noted (Fig. 24.11). A similar reading takes place 48 hours after removal of the chambers (i.e. 96 hours after first application of the material).

Interpretation of patch tests requires skill and experience. A well-demarcated, red, raised area is almost certainly not due to an allergic contact dermatitis but to an irritant reaction. False-positive reactions may be due to patch testing too soon after treatment of acute dermatitis and false-negatives may be due to prior use of topical steroids. Adverse reactions during patch testing include a severe irritant reaction which may cause blistering, sensitization to material which the patient has not previously met, anaphylaxis which is rare but recorded, the development of a Koebner reaction if the patient has a tendency to psoriasis or lichen planus, and a flare of pre-existing dermatitis.

It is common on patch testing to identify not just one but several possible allergens which show positive reactions. Interpretation of such a set of readings requires common sense and a knowledge of the patient's history of exposure to the materials in question. Cronin has estimated that 64 per cent of positive results can be accurately predicted on the basis of the clinical history, and Veien in Scandinavia has found that overall 17 per cent of all patch tests, both negative and positive, are clinically relevant. It must also be remembered that in the normal healthy population, with no skin disease at the time of testing, around 9 per cent will have unexpected, apparently irrelevant, positive results.

In addition to the European standard battery, additional batteries are available for certain body sites and for certain occupations. Specific sets available include a footwear battery, a battery for hand problems, and a battery for testing hairdressers for allergens commonly handled in the course of their employment. Very often it is these subsidiary tests which give clinically meaningful results. It is of course essential to have a comprehensive knowledge of the substances which contain the identified allergens.

European Standard Contact Dermatitis Testing Battery

potassium dichromate	0.50%	mercapto mix	2.00%
neomycin sulphate	20.00%	epoxy resin	1.00%
thiurams mix	1.00%	paraben mix	15.00%
paraphenylenediamine free base	1.00%	paratertiarybutylphenol formaldehyde resin (BPF resin)	1.00%
cobalt chloride	1.00%	fragrance mix	8.00%
benzocaine	5.00%	ethylenediamine dihydrochloride	1.00%
formaldehyde	1.00%	Dowicil 200	1.00%
colophony	20.00%	nickel sulphate	5.00%
quinoline mix	6.00%	Kathon	0.01%
balsam of Peru	25.00%	mercaptobenzolthiazone	2.00%
PPD-black rubber mix	0.60%	primin	0.01%
wool alcohols	30.00%		

All agents are prepared in a white soft paraffin base with the exception of nickel, which is in aqueous solution.

Fig. 24.9 This panel of common allergens has been indentified by the European Contact Dermatitis group. Batteries from North America and other major geographical zones have minor differences.

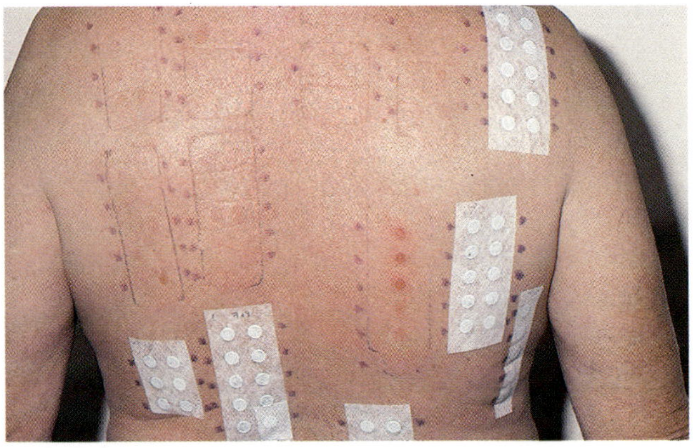

Fig. 24.10 Patch testing. General view showing number of allergens which can be tested for at any one time.

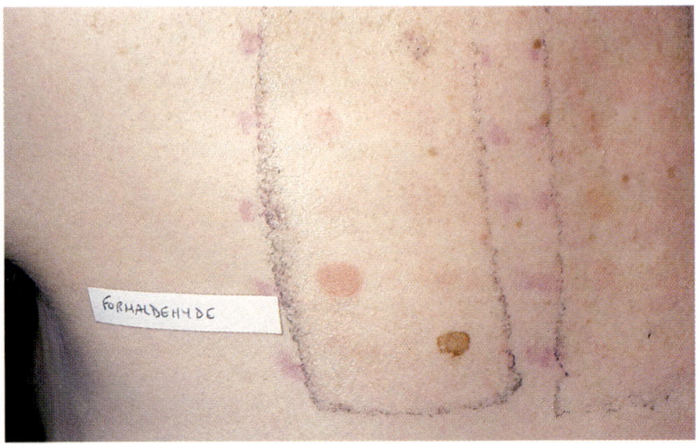

Fig. 24.11 Patch testing showing 48 hours positive reaction to formaldehyde.

Patch testing variations. In the case of many potential allergens, the classic 48-hour closed patch test is inappropriate as it does not give a true reflection of the contact with the allergen in normal daily life. Consequently a number of alternatives have been introduced, for example the open patch test, the repeated open application test, prick tests and, on occasion, intradermal tests. In particular situations, such as a suspected cosmetic allergy, one of these tests may give more meaningful results than the conventional patch test.

In vitro *identification of allergens*
It will be seen from the above that patch testing is a mixture of an art and a science. For many years there have been efforts to develop a more sensitive *in vitro* test. Most attention has been paid to the use of lymphocyte transformation and macrophage migration inhibition to predict cell-mediated hypersensitivity. At the time of writing, the success rate of these tests is around 60 per cent, similar to that of a good clinician on taking an accurate history. It is anticipated that *in vitro* techniques will be developed in the near future so that their predictive value will increase significantly.

Management
Once the likely causes of the patient's dermatological problems have been determined by patch testing, it is very important to communicate this information to the patient in a way that he or she can easily understand. This involves careful explanation of the material or materials which contain the offending allergen. In situations such as nickel dermatitis, this involves a very long list of items handled every day. Many contact dermatitis clinics have a small display of materials which contain the incriminating allergens and, for the patient to keep, written advice on what to avoid as well as on possible alternatives. This information must also be given to the primary care physician as his or her support will be needed.

It is particularly important to spend time with patients who have been found to have an allergic contact dermatitis to a material handled for many years. The usual reaction to this information is one of disbelief, and patients must be persuaded to try to avoid the substance in question and to chart the subsequent change in their dermatitis. In many centres, a liaison health care visitor or district nurse can be of great value in visiting the home to point out materials which contain the responsible allergen. This is extremely helpful, for example with, rubber dermatitis in detecting sources of rubber in furniture, bedding, etc.

In the case of an allergen which is handled at work, a factory visit, and liaison with the factory medical officer, is of great importance to try to ensure that the individual can be maintained in employment but is not exposed to the offending allergen during the daily routine. Frequently this can be achieved by a change of job within the factory, and every effort should be made to achieve this. Avoidance, even of the major allergen, is not always totally effective. For example, Fregert has reported that while relevant positive patch tests may have been obtained and reasonable avoiding action taken by the patient, some 70 per cent of such patients will still have some degree of dermatitis. This probably reflects the difficulty of complete avoidance of many allergens.

As with many other areas of medicine, medicolegal aspects of allergic contact dermatitis are becoming more prominent. This is particularly so where allergens encountered at the place of employment are incriminated. Patients should be warned, however, that trying to prove conclusively that allergic contact dermatitis was contracted solely through their employment can result in lengthy proceedings, often with a disappointing financial outcome. In cases where the extent of the problem is such that a large proportion of the workforce is at risk, government legislation may intervene. For example, in Scandinavia, chromate was removed from cement because of its association with contact dermatitis. Government legislation may also be introduced to protect the population at large. For example, in Scandinavia, it is illegal to sell earrings or other items of jewellery which contain nickel.

Conclusion and Future Prospects
At present there is no standard method of desensitizing patients to a recognized contact allergen. It is possible that, with greater advances in our understanding of the interaction between sensitized lymphocytes and Langerhans' cells, the induction of tolerance may become the standard management. However this therapeutic option is not currently open to the practitioner.

Atopic Dermatitis

Atopic dermatitis is a chronic relapsing and remitting form of dermatitis which is characterized by a tendency to develop IgE antibodies to a wide variety of materials. As with contact dermatitis, it may present clinically as an acute, subacute or chronic disease.

Pathological Features
The pathology is that of a dermatitis reaction in which the predominant cell involved is the lymphocyte rather than the mast cell or the eosinophil. Thus, the morphological presentation of a biopsy from a patient with atopic dermatitis is that of a type IV rather than of a type I allergic reaction. There is no specific diagnostic pathology of atopic dermatitis and biopsy is therefore not a recommended method of confirming a diagnosis.

Clinical Features
Patients with atopic dermatitis usually present within the first 2 years of life. The typical presentation is that of a fretful, irritable infant aged 3–6 months, who is clearly uncomfortable and who attempts to rub his skin or scratch, once the scratch reflex is fully developed. In the young infant, the trunk and cheeks are frequently involved and, as the

infant develops, the limbs also become involved. A high proportion of infants with the condition have a positive family history of atopic dermatitis, asthma or allergic rhinitis in one or both parents. A small proportion of patients present with atopic dermatitis before the age of 6 months. At this age it is important to exclude the more common dermatological problem of infantile seborrhoeic dermatitis. Clinical differentiation between infantile atopic and infantile seborrhoeic dermatitis can be extremely difficult and is frequently not possible. In this situation, the clinician is wise to defer a definitive diagnosis until the child is aged 9–12 months, when the clinical picture will be clearer and laboratory investigations will be more likely to give a meaningful result.

The infant with atopic dermatitis has erythematous oozing lesions, predominantly on the cheeks. As the child grows, the affected sites tend to be the hands, the neck area and feet, particularly under straps of footwear. The older child has predominant involvement behind the knees (Fig. 24.12) in the elbow folds, and frequently also on the face. The adult with atopic dermatitis has a more generalized distribution, commonly with diffuse involvement on the trunk and upper thigh area. Individual lesions are erythematous, excoriated and frequently oozing, with some degree of secondary bacterial infection. With continual rubbing and excoriation, the skin becomes lichenified and develops a thickened coarse appearance.

The facial appearance of a patient with chronic atopic dermatitis is characteristic, with premature small wrinkles underneath both eyes – Dennie-Morgan folds – and frequently loss of the outer third of the eyebrow through rubbing of the face on the pillow while sleeping. This is referred to as Hertoghes' sign. The characteristic white dermographism of the atopic patient gives rise to an unhealthy pallor. Although most patients with atopic dermatitis are encouraged to keep their nails cut very short to avoid excoriation of the skin by scratching, many patients buff or rub at their skin using the flat surface of the nail which gives rise to a striking shine on the nail.

A proportion of children with atopic dermatitis, usually between the ages of 4 and 12 years of age, develop striking involvement of the soles of the feet (Fig. 24.13). These tend to be active children who enjoy sporting activities and the cutaneous lesions are of a smooth shiny plantar surface of the soles of the feet and the balls of the toes with, on occasion, painful hacks. This appearance is termed juvenile plantar dermatosis, and although it may be found in the absence of atopic dermatitis, it is more common in atopic children. It tends to be self-limiting and is unusual in older teenage children and adults.

Some children with atopic dermatitis have a so-called inverse pattern of involvement with more striking involvement of the extensor aspects of the limbs than of the flexor aspects. This pattern is associated with a poorer prognosis for eventual clearance.

A minority of patients with atopic dermatitis do not develop their first lesions until later childhood, teenage years or even when young adults. This is unusual, and there is evidence from long-term studies to suggest that this later onset of atopic dermatitis carries a poorer prognosis for clearance. Interesting individual case reports are recorded of patients who develop atopic dermatitis for the first time after acute intercurrent infection, such as infectious mononucleosis, and after successful marrow transplantation for leukaemia.

There are conflicting reports of the association between atopic dermatitis and respiratory symptoms. In many patients there is an inverse relationship, with skin symptoms which tend to be least troublesome when the respiratory symptoms are maximal and vice-versa, while in other patients both skin and respiratory symptoms may flare together. Individual patients tend to have a specific pattern which both they and their families know well. Similarly individual patients tend to show a variation in the seasonal severity of their problems, with some patients tending to flare in the autumn and winter months while others flare in the spring and summer. Once again the individual patient tends to know his or her own pattern.

A large proportion of patients with chronic atopic dermatitis have an associated dry skin. In the past this has been considered by many dermatologists to be a variant of autosomal dominant ichthyosis, but recent work has suggested that the dry skin of atopic dermatitis is a distinct entity. Dry skin is frequently hypersensitive and mildly pruritic, and its control may do much to control the pruritus of atopic dermatitis.

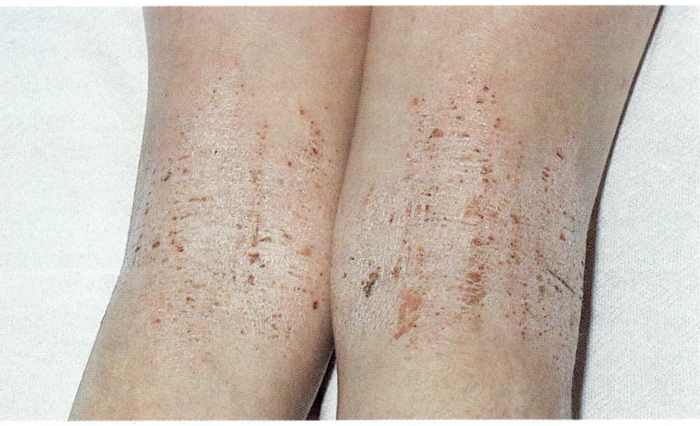

Fig. 24.12 Atopic dermatitis. View of thickened and excoriated skin on the backs of knees.

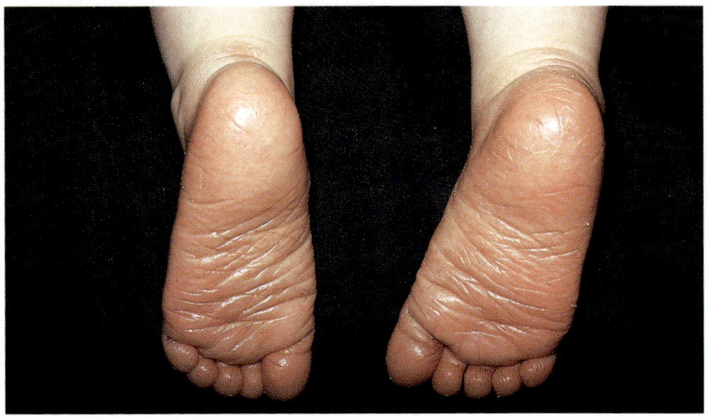

Fig. 24.13 Juvenile plantar dermatosis.

Dermatological Presentations

Nipple dermatitis.
Young women with atopic dermatitis may develop persistent and at times severe dermatitis which involves the nipple and periareolar area (Fig. 24.14). This may be the first sign of an atopic tendency, or may occur in a patient who has had problems in infancy which then cleared through the teenage years.

Nummular dermatitis
As its name suggests, nummular dermatitis is characterized by the presence of coin-shaped, usually moist, excoriated lesions, found predominantly on the limbs (Fig. 24.15). It is also associated in many patients with an atopic tendency, and is commonest in young adults where it may occur as the first sign of an atopic tendency. As with nipple dermatitis, nummular dermatitis may be a problem which declares itself in adult life in a patient who has had atopic dermatitis in infancy.

Hand dermatitis
A proportion of patients with hand dermatitis have an associated atopic tendency. This should be considered particularly with regard to hairdressers, nurses and others whose work involves persistent exposure of the skin to detergents, soaps and other 'degreasing' material.

Light-sensitive dermatitis
Some patients who have light-sensitive dermatitis are also atopic, a factor which should be borne in mind in the diagnosis of their disease.

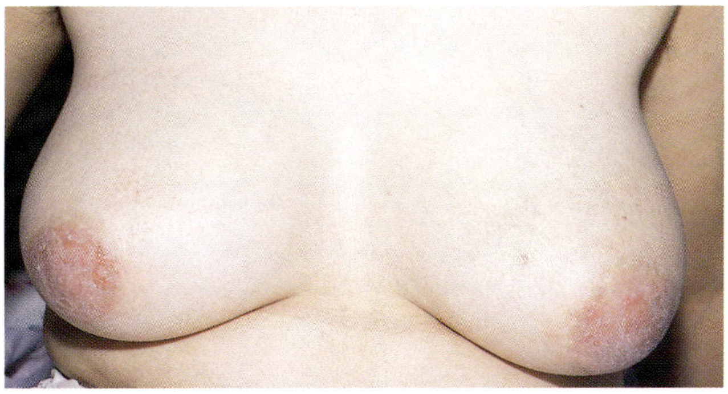

Fig. 24.14 Nipple dermatitis.

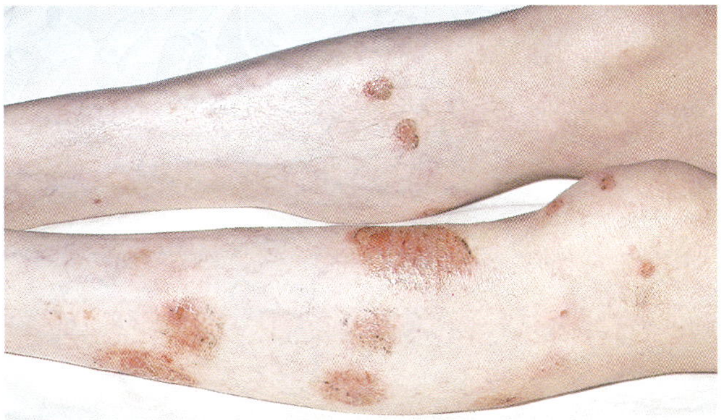

Fig. 24.15 Nummular dermatitis.

Infection and Atopic Dermatitis

Patients with atopic dermatitis are unusually susceptible to certain cutaneous viral and bacterial infections. Of these, colonization with *Staphyloccocus aureus* is most common (Fig. 24.16); indeed *S. aureus* may be found on the skin of children and adults with atopic dermatitis, despite there being no clinical evidence of infection. This finding appears to be relatively specific for the atopic state, as patients with other types of dermatitis do not have large quantities of *S. aureus* on their skin. Furthermore there is some evidence of a causative relationship between *S. aureus* colonization and the severity of disease, as increased numbers of bacteria are associated with more severe disease and treatment of the staphylococcal colonization of the skin is associated with an improvement in the symptoms of atopic dermatitis.

Patients with atopic dermatitis have a higher than expected incidence of warts caused by the human papilloma virus, and of cutaneous fungal infections. They are also susceptible to severe infection when exposed to the herpes simplex type 1 virus, which causes a complication of the atopic state called eczema herpeticum or Kaposi's varicelliform eruption (Fig. 24.17). The susceptibility to infection is so great that even after fleeting exposure to the herpes simplex virus, for example a light kiss from a relative with a cold sore on the lip, the affected patient may develop a widespread and disseminated vesicular eruption. In a patient with severe excoriations caused by pre-existing dermatitis, it may be difficult to identify these new vesicles.

Herpes simplex infection is an important and at times severe complication of atopic dermatitis, with a possibility of lethality if this is not identified and treated appropriately with speed. All parents of children with atopic dermatitis and all adult patients must be aware of the importance of protecting their children, as well as themselves, from the herpes simplex virus.

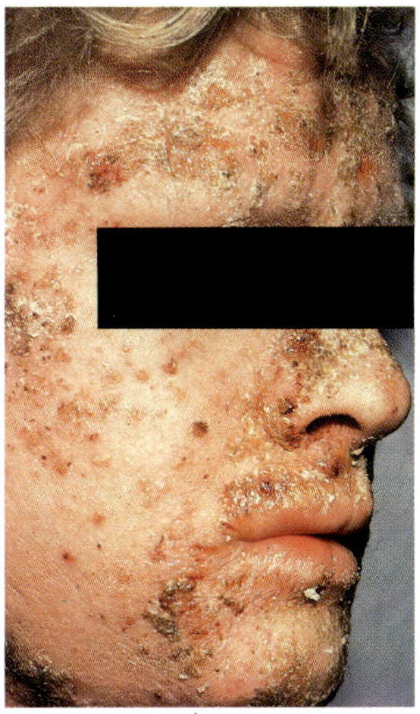

Fig. 24.16 Atopic dermatitis with obvious secondary infection and impetiginization on face.

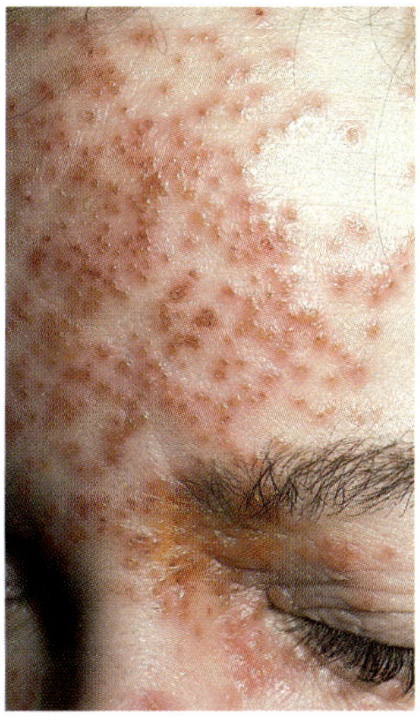

Fig. 24.17 Eczema herpeticum (Kaposi's varicelliform eruption).

Food Allergy and Atopic Dermatitis

This is a controversial and confusing area, particularly as there is a tendency in the literature to confuse true food allergy with food intolerance. A number of patients, particularly infants with atopic dermatitis, appear to have a temporary intolerance to certain ingested foodstuffs, particularly cows' milk, and other dairy products. When mixed feeding is introduced, this intolerance is frequently noticed by parents as vomiting after feeds of cows' milk together with, on occasion, clear evidence of erythema and deterioration of the dermatitis lesions around the area of the mouth. Some parents also notice a flare in the general condition of their child's skin 24–48 hours later, as a result of the systemic delivery of the offending food allergens to the skin. A high proportion of children with this type of food intolerance will outgrow the problem, and reintroduction of the previously offending foodstuffs 6–12 months after the first problem will not be associated with further deterioration. However, in about 10 per cent of older patients with severe atopic dermatitis, there does appear to be a true association between ingestion of some foodstuffs, commonly proteins, and deterioration of their atopic dermatitis lesions.

Diagnosis

Patients with atopic dermatitis frequently have eosinophilia, but this is of neither sufficient frequency nor magnitude to be of diagnostic value. In the atopic patient, prick-testing to allergens will produce a large number of positive results, many of which, while demonstrating allergy *per se,* will not necessarily have clinical relevance. Thus, it is seldom of therapeutic value to the patient to note these allergens, or to take appropriate avoiding action.

Estimation of total circulating IgE level using the PRIST technique demonstrates that approximately 80 per cent of patients with atopic dermatitis have an abnormally high level of this antibody. The highest levels are recorded in those with additional respiratory symptoms and in those with apparently associated food allergy or intolerance. Estimation of total circulating levels of serum IgE is not reliable under the age of 1 year as, before this time, a number of infants who have transient seborrhoeic dermatitis will have elevated levels. It should also be borne in mind that up to 15 per cent of the normal population have serum IgE levels above the normal range and that very high levels may be recorded in helminthic infestation. Thus total serum IgE levels are neither completely sensitive nor totally specific markers of the atopic dermatitis patient

The RAST test to identify IgE levels specific to allergens is now widely used in the diagnosis of atopic dermatitis. The most common allergens identified are illustrated in Fig. 24.18. In the young child, the bulk of the IgE is directed against ingested foodstuffs; but at about 2 years of age this pattern changes and, in the older child and adult, inhaled allergens, particularly the house dust mite, appear to be responsible for a large proportion of the IgE. A positive RAST test to the allergens mentioned in Fig. 24.18 will help in confirming a diagnosis of atopic dermatitis, but repeated tests are of little clinical value or relevance. As patients improve spontaneously, total and specific IgE levels tend to fall, but this is usually several months after observed clinical changes.

Management

Management of atopic dermatitis can be divided into general management of the skin, specific use of anti-inflammatory agents and antihistamines (Fig. 24.19), and experimental therapy.

General management

General management of atopic patients usually begins with control of the commonly associated dry skin. If this is treated, the need for topical steroid therapy will be greatly reduced. Most patients benefit from an emollient, either added to the bath, used after the bath or applied continuously to the skin. The use of soap should be restricted, and an emollient preparation, such as emulsifying ointment BP, substituted. Most patients will learn well by trial and error which specific emollient preparations best suit their skin.

Patients with atopic dermatitis should avoid materials which irritate the skin. These frequently include both natural products, such as wool, and synthetic fibres. Pure cotton is usually the most comfortable clothing for the majority of patients with atopic dermatitis. Patients with atopic dermatitis should also endeavour not to move rapidly from one environmental extreme to another as large changes in ambient temperature, particularly from cold to hot, and changes in humidity are also associated with deterioration of their condition.

Common Allergens in Atopic Dermatitis	
infants	ingested allergens: milk, fish, eggs
older children and adults	airborne allergens: house dust mite, pollens, cat and dog hair and dander

Fig. 24.18 Common allergens associated with atopic dermatitis.

Steps in Standard Management of Atopic Dermatitis	
general management	use emollient avoid sudden environmental change in temperature and humidity avoid allergen sources
anti-inflammatory treatment	topical corticosteroids as appropriate – avoid high-potency combinations systemic antihistamines topical bacteriostat or antibiotic

Fig. 24.19 Major points in the standard management of atopic dermatitis.

Patients should take reasonable steps to reduce their environmental exposure to allergens. This can be difficult with some allergens, but with others the precautions are obvious, for example households with a severely atopic child should not keep a cat or dog. Although the house dust mite is ubiquitous and difficult to control, every effort should be made to reduce the prevalence of the mite in the environment, particularly in the sleeping environment. A non-permeable mattress cover will be of some value, as high mite counts are usually found in mattresses. The avoidance of fitted carpets and substitution of venetian blinds for curtains are also useful measures in controlling house dust mite exposure.

Anti-inflammatory agents
The mainstay of control in atopic dermatitis is the appropriate use of topical corticosteroid creams and ointments. These must be handled with care and under regular supervision since topical steroids are absorbed through the skin and the inappropriate use of high potency steroids, may lead to unwanted topical and systemic effects, including hypothalamopituitary-adrenal (HPA) suppression, particularly in young children in whom growth and development may be retarded. It is normal dermatological practice to use a steroid no more potent than topical hydrocortisone on the face and only moderately potent steroids on other body sites (Fig. 24.20). Topical steroids are divided into four increasing potency ranges from grade I, containing hydrocortisone, to grade IV. As preparations vary widely throughout the world, current national formularies should be consulted.

Systemic corticosteriods will benefit severe chronic atopic dermatitis, but must be reserved for exceptionally stubborn cases in view of their side effects. Many dermatologists find that the addition of a topical antibacterial agent to the steroid preparation will apparently improve the atopic dermatitis and for many this is routine practice. Others prefer to use intermittent short courses of systemic antibiotics. The most useful antibiotics are those which have a specific antistaphylococcal action, such as flucloxacillin.

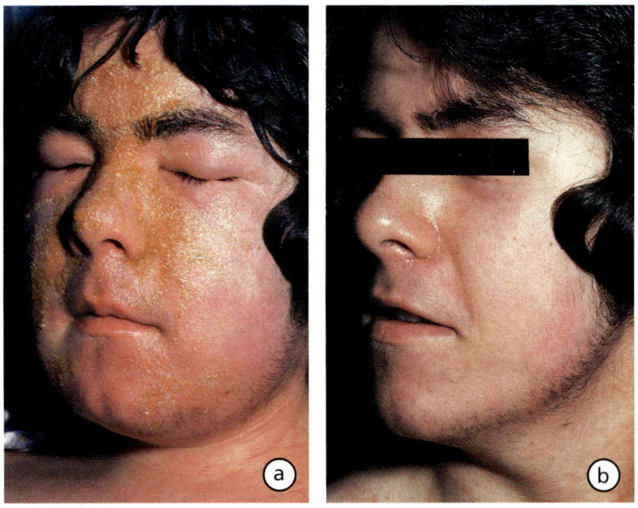

Fig. 24.20 Acute contact dermatitis of the face caused by topical antibiotic, (a) at presentation and (b) 72 hours after application of a topical steroid.

Management of eczema vaccinatum requires systemic acyclovir. After virological confirmation of the presence of the herpes simplex virus, the patient should be given either oral or intravenous acyclovir depending on the severity of the exacerbation and on the need to obtain a rapid response. Topical acyclovir is of relatively little value.

Although messy, topical coal tar preparations still have a place in the management of atopic dermatitis. Tar has a mild anti-inflammatory action, and can be of particular value in treating thickened lichenified skin.

Antihistamines
Systemic histamine H_1-receptor antagonists are frequently prescribed for patients with atopic dermatitis, but their value is disputed. It is found that initially these antihistamines are of some benefit to individual patients, particularly with regard to pruritus at night and loss of sleep. However patients appear to become quickly habituated to a specific antihistamine, and it will be found that steady increases in the dose of the chosen preparation are required. Newer non-sedating histamine H_1-antagonists are suitable for daytime use, but most patients with chronic severe atopic dermatitis will find the older antihistamines of more value, possibly because of the sedative action rather than the specific antihistaminic actions of the drugs. There is no evidence that histamine H_2-antagonists are of value in atopic dermatitis as single agents, although there are one or two studies which suggest that the addition of an H_2-blocker to an H_1-blocker may be of some additive value.

Experimental therapy
Experimental techniques in atopic dermatitis currently under review fall into four main categories: the use of dietary measures, of photochemotherapy, of immunosuppressants (such as azathioprine and more recently cyclosporin) and of unsaturated fatty acids (such as evening primrose oil).

Dietary measures can be divided into preventative and curative approaches. The preventative approach involves the delayed introduction of mixed feeding, and the exclusive breast-feeding of infants known to be at high risk in eczema families. Clear evidence of a beneficial effect is difficult to obtain in individual cases, but a recent study of feeding patterns in premature infants does suggest that in this infant group the incidence of atopic dermatitis at 18 months is lower in exclusively breast-fed babies. There is no comparable convincing study for normal birth weight infants.

The curative approach concerns dietary control of established disease. This may be either by exclusion of an item of food which the patient or parent has specifically noticed to exacerbate the disease, or by non-specific exclusion of foods, particularly dairy foods and other proteins. The first approach is obviously logical, but identification of provoking foods can be difficult, particularly if there is a 48-hour gap between ingestion and the flaring of symptoms.

Exclusion of dairy products is a very popular move with parents of affected children, but this must be done with supervision, preferably of a trained dietitian, as there is a very real risk of the child becoming calcium-depleted. Of those patients who use dietary manoeuvres to control their skin lesions, about 10 per cent notice benefit. A very small number of patients with severe and intractable disease derive benefit from an elemental diet.

Photochemotherapy, or PUVA, has been used as a therapeutic dermatological tool since the mid-1970s. The principal of the therapy is the ingestion of an oral photosensitizing drug, psoralens, followed 2 hours later, when circulating levels of the drug are maximum, by exposure of the skin to long-wave ultraviolet light (UVA). This routine is of established value in the control of other dermatological problems, such as psoriasis and cutaneous lymphoma, and its value has recently been recorded in a small number of older children with severe and persistent atopic dermatitis. The exact mechanism of action in atopic dermatitis is not established, but ultraviolet light is known to have an immunosuppressive effect on the epidermal Langerhans' cells, and also on a subset of circulating T lymphocytes, and it is postulated that this is the mode of action.

PUVA therapy is not without side effects, and high cumulative doses are associated with the development of non-melanoma skin cancer, and pre-cancerous changes on the skin. In view of the fact that atopic dermatitis is a chronic condition, and that many sufferers are young patients, use of PUVA therapy other than in strictly controlled circumstances is not recommended. Natural sunlight or artificial UVB therapy has for many years been used as supportive therapy in some centres but there are no controlled clinical trials of its value.

Immunosuppressants. The use of immunosuppressive agents in atopic dermatitis is also limited to patients with severe disease and should not be considered in children. There are a number of anecdotal reports of the benefit of azathioprine in atopic dermatitis, but no good controlled clinical trial. The immunosuppressive agent cyclosporin has recently been used in clinical studies, particularly by Voorhees and colleagues. With oral cyclosporin, doses of 2–5 mg/kg/day have produced striking improvements in atopic dermatitis patients. The drug is known to have a specific effect on T-helper cell function, and it is possible that this is the mode of action in atopic dermatitis.

As with other forms of immunosuppression, cyclosporin therapy is associated with side effects, including hypertension, renal damage, growth of facial hair and an increased risk of developing lymphoma. At present, cyclosporin should therefore only be used in a clinical trial setting, in patients with severe and intractable atopic dermatitis.

Unsaturated fatty acids. Oral ingestion of unsaturated fatty acids, such as evening primrose oil, has been recorded in open studies to benefit some aspects of atopic dermatitis in adults. No such benefit has yet been recorded in children. The postulated mode of action is by raising levels of dihomogammalinoleic acid, thus bypassing a defect in δ-6-desaturase activity. This theoretical mode of action has not yet been proven, and not all studies of the use of evening primrose oil are positive.

Conclusion and Future Prospects

At present the exact aetiology of atopic dermatitis is not well established, in spite of a wealth of studies on related pharmacological and immunological abnormalities. It is to be hoped that further research will integrate some of these observations, and lead to more logical approaches to both prevention and cure

Further Reading

Adams RM. *Occupational Skin Disease,* 2nd Ed. CV Mosby: St Louis, 1989.

Cronin E. *Contact Dermatitis.* Churchill Livingstone: Edinburgh, 1980.

Fisher, AA. *Contact Dermatitis*, 3rd Ed. Lea & Febiger: Philadelphia, 1986.

Rajka G. *Essential Aspects of Atopic Dermatitis*. Springer-Verlag: Berlin, 1989.

MacKie RM, Cochran REI, Cobb S, Thomson, J. Total and specific IgE levels in patients with atopic dermatitis. *Clin Exp Dermatol* 1979; **4**:187–195.

Yates VM, Kerr REI, MacKie RM. Early diagnosis of infantile seborrhoeic dermatitis and atopic dermatitis – clinical features. *Br J Dermatol* 1983;**108**: 633–638 .

Yates VM, Kerr REI, Frier K, Cobb SJ, MacKie RM. Early diagnosis of infantile seborrhoeic dermatitis and atopic dermatitis – total and specific IgE levels. *Br J Dermatol* 1983;**108**:639–645.

Chapter 25

Gastrointestinal Allergic Disease – Pathophysiology

Introduction

The gastrointestinal tract is exposed to an enormous load of potentially antigenic foreign material, and it is a measure of the efficient exclusion and handling of these antigens that damaging reactions to food are so uncommon. However, this is a controversial area and little is known for certain about the mechanisms of gastrointestinal allergic diseases in man. For example, the best studied and most frequently encountered food allergy in children is a sensitivity to cows' milk, yet the immunopathogenesis remains unclear. Similarly, in coeliac disease (gluten enteropathy) it is not clear whether the abnormal immunological phenomena demonstrated are of primary importance or are secondary to a more fundamental biochemical abnormality.

The oesophagus, stomach and colon are impervious to macromolecules and are protected by non-immune means from local allergic reactions. The highly absorptive and permeable small intestine is the site of interest .

Role of the Gastrointestinal Epithelium as a Mucosal Barrier

The average diet contains many potential antigens and yet in health the great majority of these are excluded by a combination of non-immune and immune means. Non-immune factors are those acting entirely within the lumen of the gastrointestinal tract, including normal gastric function, where acid and pepsin digestion limit the presentation of antigens to the small intestine and where peristalsis reduces the time available for absorption of an antigen through the mucosal barrier. On the mucosal surface, the mucus acts as an effective molecular sieve, preventing contact of molecules greater than approximately 17 kDa with the mucosal surface. This layer may be up to 600 μm in depth and excludes proteolytic enzymes and intact food proteins, but allows through polypeptides and the products of digestion. The mucus layer maintains a hydrogen ion gradient in the stomach and the duodenum, ensuring that the mucosal cells are in contact with fluid at a near neutral pH. As the luminal surface of the mucus layer becomes degraded, it is replaced by synthesis from goblet cells, resulting in a steady flow of mucus which tends to counteract penetration by food antigens.

Increased exposure of the mucosa to bacterial products, lectins or food antigens stimulates the secretion of mucus. As mucus interacts with potentially toxic substances, peristalsis results in their removal from the surface of the mucosal layer. The composition of the intestinal cell membrane is of importance in determining whether bacteria or toxins bind to a mucosal cell and this changes markedly as the cell migrates up the villus. The adult microvillus membranes bind less antigen than immature cells. Immature epithelial cells have the ability to ingest macromolecules directly by endocytosis and to transport them to the portal circulation. This property is important in the absorption of maternal immunoglobulins, but diminishes at about the age of three months, when intestinal closure is said to occur.

Mucosal Immunity

The intestinal mucosa acts as a major barrier limiting foreign antigen access to the body. For many years it has been realised that non-epithelial cells also exist in profusion within the intestinal epithelium and comprise macrophages, mast cells, lymphocytes, eosinophils and neutrophils, while plasma cells occur mainly in the lamina propria.

Mucosal antibodies of the IgA class can be stimulated independently from the systemic immune system. There are highly specialized membranous epithelial cells (M cell, microfold cell) present in clusters, particularly in the distal small bowel, which overlie collections of gut-associated lymphoid tissue (GALT). These cells have few microvilli, a poorly developed overlying mucus layer and absent lysosomal organelles. This specialized structure allows macromolecules to traverse the epithelial barrier and initiate an appropriate immune response. Antigenic stimulation leads to a local immune response involving specific secretory IgA-producing plasma cells in the lamina propria. Dimeric IgA along with its secretory piece combines with the mucin layer to produce a mucosal immune barrier, preventing further antigenic absorption.

Mast Cells

Mast cells are present in the gastrointestinal tract and are present in increased numbers in allergic diseases (see Fig. 25.1). There are at least two populations of mast cells, designated the connective tissue mast cell (CTMC) and the mucosal mast cell (MMC).

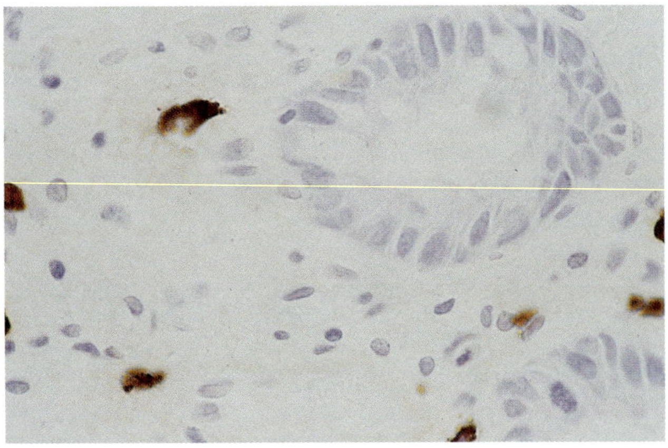

Fig. 25.1 Mast cells in normal colonic mucosa (anti-tryptase stain).

Conditions in which Circulating Non IgE Antibodies to Food are Demonstrable
infancy
immunodeficiency, e.g. IgA deficiency
ulcerative colitis
Crohn's disease
gastroenteritis (transiently)
achlorhydria/pernicious anaemia
malnutrition
food allergy

Fig. 25.2 Conditions in which circulating non-IgE antibodies to food are demonstrable. Anything which breaches the integrity of the gastrointestinal tract will lead to absorption of antigen and food antibodies. These are rarely of any pathological significance. Small amounts are detectable in normal subjects.

These can be distinguished on the basis of histamine, neutral protease, and proteoglycan content and their dependency or not on T cells (see Chapter 5).

The release of histamine and other inflammatory mediators from activated mast cells has a profound effect on gut function. There occurs an outpouring of mucus, an increase in epithelial permeability, stimulation of gastrointestinal transit and a reduction in absorptive capacity leading to diarrhoea. Mast cell activation results from cross-binding of cytophilic IgE by an allergen, but also may occur by direct stimulation by certain dietary proteins and neuropeptides.

The combination of non-immune, humoral, and cellular immune protection effectively excludes most antigens from interacting with the systemic immune system. However, absorption of antigens into the systemic circulation is so common in health that it should be regarded as a normal event. Indeed, all healthy people develop and maintain high levels of neutralizing antibodies to specific dietary antigens (Fig. 25.2). Immune complexes are formed and cleared, again without adverse effects.

If an immunizing dose of antigen reaches the small bowel and stimulates a response, this usually takes one of two non-harmful forms: a mucosal IgA response in association with systemic hyporesponsiveness (tolerance), or a mucosal IgA response accompanied by a systemic IgG or IgA antibody response. However, if the antigenic load is very large, if the local defence mechanisms are weakened, or if the immune response is inappropriate, then a damaging inflammatory reaction occurs and forms the basis of food allergic reactions. It is not clear to what extent T cells contribute to tolerance. This topic is discussed later in the chapter.

Allergy in the Gastrointestinal Tract

The great majority of antigenic determinants (epitopes) are defined by the quaternary structure of relatively small areas of the surface of the protein (see Chapter 1). With smaller polypeptides, the epitope is formed in relation to the primary amino acid sequence.

'Conformational' antigens are very readily deformed by heat or chemical degradation, and so are most unlikely to cause reactions in the gastrointestinal tract. 'Sequential' antigens, however, resist denaturation by heating, cooking, acid degradation and, to some extent, luminal digestion. Some antigenic proteins have been well characterized, for example, the immunogenic determinant in cod fish protein has a simple structure of aspartate-glutamate, one amino acid residue away from lysine. It follows that where this amino acid sequence is repeated by chance in other proteins, cross-reactivity will occur. Patients allergic to conformational antigens, e.g. occupational asthma triggered by flour in bakers, are usually able to eat their products without reacting adversely.

The hypersensitivity reactions types I to IV described by Coombs and Gell have been elucidated in the systemic immune response. However it is not clear whether both or all of these reactions are important in food allergy (Fig. 25.3).

Type I Reactions

In anaphylactic food allergy, it is proposed that the food allergen cross-links specific IgE, which triggers mast cell degranulation and causes immediate release of chemical mediators, followed by the recruitment of secondary cells of inflammation. Together, these have a profound effect in altering gut physiology. The net result is local symptoms, such as diarrhoea and abdominal pain, and increased absorption of the same or different antigens, which extends the response to systemic effects, such as mast cell activation in the bronchial tree, producing asthma, or immune complex deposition, contributing to urticaria (Fig. 25.4) and eczema.

Type II Reactions

In type II reactions - antibody-dependent cytotoxicity immunoglobulins are directed against a tissue antigen or hapten. Damage occurs if there is activation of the complement cascade to produce cell lysis, phagocytosis, or antibody-dependent cell cytotoxicity (ADCC). Food antibodies are common, both during health and in disease states. Theoretically tissue damage could occur if these were to cross-react with

Suggested Classification of Immunologically Mediated Gastrointestinal Diseases	
Disease	**Mechanism**
pernicious anaemia (autoimmune gastritis)	intrinsic factor and gastric parietal cell antibodies and cell-mediated immunity leads to atrophic gastritis
eosinophilic gastroenteritis	dense eosinophilic infiltration of stomach and small intestine
coeliac disease	? cell-mediated immunity to gluten
food allergy	type I, type III reactions?
Crohn's disease	type IV reaction
ulcerative colitis	uncertain (see text)
immune deficiency syndromes, e.g. IgA deficiency	secondary absorption of antigens
immunoproliferative syndromes, e.g. α-heavy chain disease	infiltration of gut with plasma cells producing secretory IgA or α-chains
systemic mastocytosis	mast cell proliferation – can involve liver, spleen and gastrointestinal tract

Fig. 25.3 Suggested classification of immunologically mediated gastrointestinal diseases. This classification includes gastrointestinal disease where immunological mechanisms are, or are thought to be, of primary importance.

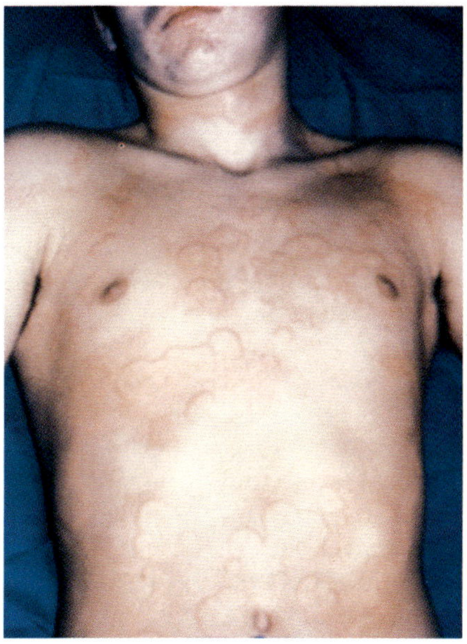

Fig. 25.4 Giant urticaria occurring immediately after exposure to certain shellfish.

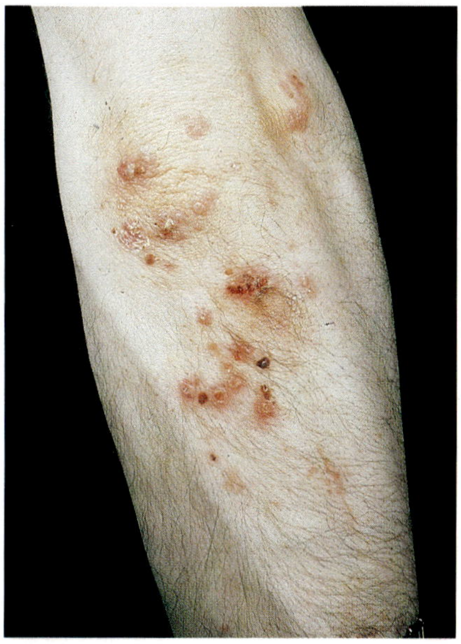

Fig. 25.5 Dermatitis herpetiformis. A blistering skin condition and a probable example of a type III reaction occurring in the skin after absorption of antigen in a patient with coeliac disease.

tissue antigens, initiating an auto-immune process, but little evidence exists to support this hypothesis. Occasional cases of thrombocytopenia in association with milk allergy may be due to type II reactions.

Type III Immune Complex-Mediated Reactions

Food antigens which are absorbed encounter specific antibodies in the circulation with the formation of immune complexes. These are normally rapidly cleared by the reticulo-endothelial system and are of no pathological significance. However, tissue damage will result if there are high concentrations of complexes, and if the antigen is present in excess (serum sickness response). In antigen excess there is usually a generalized reaction associated with large amounts of foreign proteins entering the circulation. If the complexes formed are of an appropriate size, they are deposited in vessel walls where an inflammatory reaction is provoked in the endothelium. When this occurs in the skin, kidney, and joints it leads to urticaria, albuminuria, and arthritis respectively, together with fever and lymphadenopathy.

When antibody is in excess, an Arthus-type reaction results. These are usually local reactions in the hyperimmune individual, involving deposition of antigen-antibody complexes at local sites. This type of reaction occurs in the lymphatics in response to filarial worm infestation. The skin lesions associated with dermatitis herpetiformis may be the result of a local type III reaction. Patients with dermatitis herpetiformis (Fig. 25.5) have elevated antibody levels to gluten, and both skin lesions and unaffected skin have linear deposits of IgA which bind gluten.

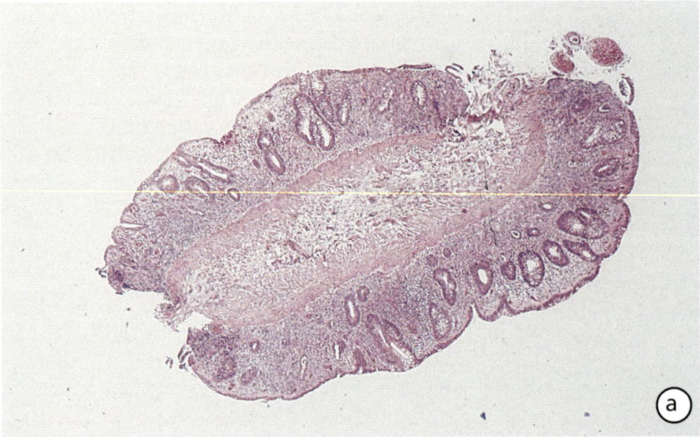

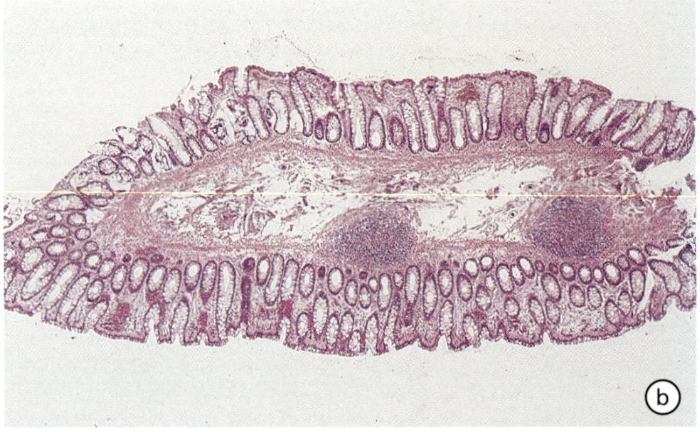

Fig. 25.6 Rectal mucosa in ulcerative colitis (a), compared with normal mucosa (b). There is an increase in acute and chronic inflammatory cells, glandular distortion and ulceration.

It seems likely that, if immune complexes are formed and cause damage after ingestion of antigen, distant organs will be affected, rather than the pathology being restricted to the gut.

Type IV Delayed Hypersensitivity (DTH)

These reactions can cause intestinal damage in animal models and there are reports of cell-mediated immune responses (DTH) to food antigens in cows' milk allergy. Type IV reactions are involved in villous atrophy which occurs in parasitic infections and graft-versus-host disease. Type IV reactions can be considered as representing cell-mediated immune damage and will be considered later in the chapter with specific regard to the diffuse lymphoid system of the human intestine.

The hypersensitivity reactions types I to IV are not intended to be mutually exclusive and, on occasions, one might expect two or more mechanisms to operate simultaneously. Other mechanisms not encompassed within this classification may occur in the gut and it is not surprising therefore that clear immunopathogenic pathways of food allergy have yet to be defined. Ulcerative colitis has elements of T cell-mediated mucosal damage, suggestive of a type IV response (Fig. 25.6).

The T-Cell Response in Normal and Pathological Intestine

The recent development of monoclonal antibodies capable of dissecting lymphocyte surface glycoprotein expression has shed light on the composition of T-cell populations in normal and inflamed human mucosa (Fig. 25.7).

The T-Cell Receptor

The majority of circulating T cells in man carry an antigen-specific receptor composed of two disulphide linked polypeptides, α and β. This receptor is responsible for specific antigen recognition, in combination with CD4 and CD8 molecules, recognizing processed antigenic peptides in association with MHC class II or MHC class I, respectively. The T-cell receptor is linked non-covalently with a series of glycoproteins collectively termed CD3. Monoclonal antibodies to the latter complex, and in particular to the CD3 ϵ-chain, provide the most reliable method for the identification of T cells in normal and pathological tissues. In conjunction with antibodies directed to various T-cell subsets, CD3 reagents provide extensive information concerning the pathological processes which occur in inflammatory bowel disease.

In addition to circulating T cells bearing the α/β heterodimer, a smaller population is known to express the γ/δ receptor. This population may be of particular significance with regard to T-cell immunity in epithelial sites. γ/δ T cells evolve by a separate route to α/β-bearing lymphocytes. Biochemically distinct forms of the γ/δ receptor exist and, at least in mice, T-cell populations bearing differently encoded γ/δ T-cell receptor forms occur at different anatomical sites.

The function of the γ/δ lymphocyte has not been determined. These cells have a limited immunological repertoire, as demonstrated by the small total number of V-region genes available for use. The proportion of these cells in the circulation and in peripheral lymphoid organs is small, but animal studies have demonstrated that γ/δ T cells may represent the major T-cell population in a range of epithelial sites, including the intestine. Cytotoxic activity has been described within the γ/δ population and one hypothesis for its presence within epithelium is that it mediates some primitive immune response. This would be compatible with the small size of the γ/δ T-cell receptor repertoire. Cells of this type could clearly be responsible for intestinal damage in coeliac disease. However, overwhelming involvement of the γ/δ T-cell population in intestinal immunity has not been successfully demonstrated in man. In the human, unlike other species, numerous α/β T-cells are present in T-lymphocyte infiltrates. These differences may reflect differences in the time course and development of lymphoid populations within the intestine in man, or differences in the form and type of antigen exposure of the intestinal T-lymphocyte population. For this reason, the precise role of γ/δ T cells in various intestinal pathologies in man has yet to be determined.

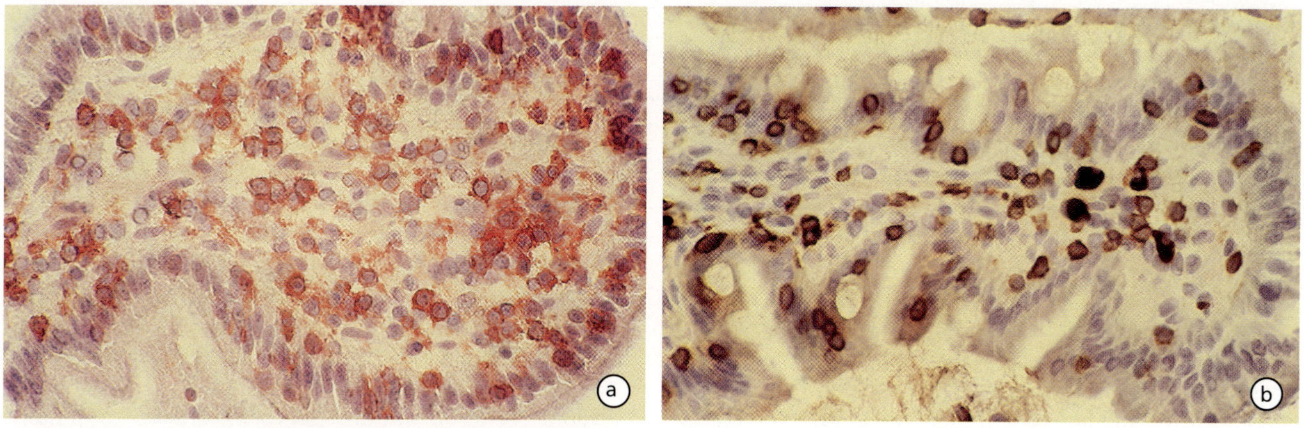

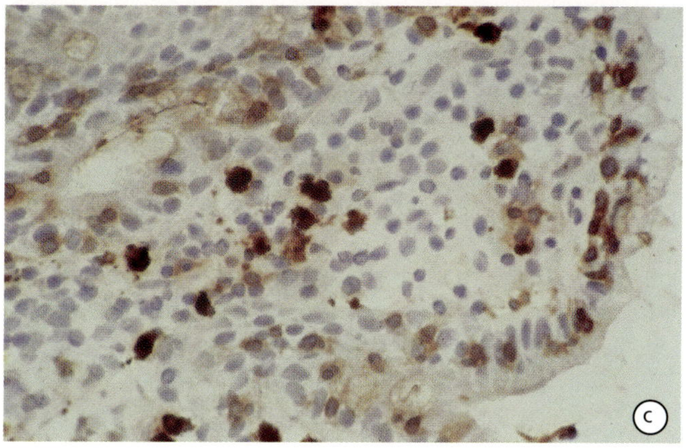

Fig. 25.7 Frozen sections of intestinal biopsies stained with monoclonal antibodies using an immunoperoxidase technique. Occasional neutrophils show dark brown staining, caused by endogenous peroxidase. (a) Staining for CD3 (red), demonstrating T cells present in both mucosa and submucosa. (b) CD45RO, demonstrating the antigen-experienced phenotype of the majority of T cells present in the intestinal mucosa. (c) Intra-epithelial lymphocytes present in the mucosa, demonstrated with the monoclonal antibody HML-1 directed against the $\alpha_4\beta_7$ integrin.

Lymphocytes Associated with Mucosal Epithelia

Lymphocytes associated with mucosal epithlia were first described morphologically and considered to have a role in the absorption of nutrients. More recent immunohistochemical studies have clearly shown that these cells are T cells. In man, mucosal T cells express CD3 and the majority are also CD8-positive (Fig. 25.7). By extrapolation from our knowledge of the peripheral immune system these cells should either represent cytotoxic or suppressor lymphocytes. With the exception of studies which have examined non-specific, or NK-like, activity, intra-epithelial T cells do not appear to be cytotoxic. Several studies have, however, claimed suppressor function for these cells. It is also clear that monoclonal antibodies which identify lymphocyte surface glycoproteins related to cytotoxic function are not found on the cell surface.

More recently, monoclonal antibodies have been produced which were initially claimed to identify specifically intra-epithelial lymphocytes, rather than cells circulating within the peripheral lymphoid compartment. Although recent work suggests that the specificity of monoclonal antibodies, such as HML-1, is not absolute with regard to T-cell populations present in epithelia, it is clear that markers such as this identify the intra-epithelial T-cell population as a specific lymphoid compartment (Fig. 25.7).

Lamina Propria T Cells

The composition of the leucocyte infiltrate present within the lamina propria is more complex than that described for the intra-epithelial lymphoid compartment. With regard to the T-cell population, the major difference is that T cells expressing the CD4-helper cell phenotype are more prominent. Approximately half of these cells carry the intra-epithelial marker, HML-1 ($\alpha_4\beta_7$), and may represent cells in transit towards intra-epithelial sites (Fig. 25.7). As with T cells in these sites, specific cytotoxic function has not been demonstrated, although various functional studies have demonstrated non-selective cytotoxicity in a range of different *in vitro* systems. A point of particular interest concerning the lamina propria T-cell population is the demonstration of selective homing receptors. It can clearly be shown with the use of monoclonal antibodies that T cells in the lamina propria express a homing receptor which is directed specifically towards mucosal high endothelial venules. This molecule (CD44) is a member of the cartilage link protein family.

Accessory Cells for T-Cell Immunity

In addition to the follicular dendritic cells associated with lymphoid follicles, it is clear that many accessory cells are present within the intestine. Two major types of antigen presenting cell are recognized within the intestinal wall.

Antigen-Presenting Cells

These large, irregular cells are specialized for the production of antigenic peptides for presentation to T cells, express abundant surface MHC Class II, but are poorly phagocytic and lack lysozomal enzymes. These cells are potent stimulators of $CD4^+$ T cells.

Histiocytes

Histiocytes or true macrophages are bone marrow-derived, have extensive phagocytic capabilities and, unlike true antigen presenting cells, are rich in lysosomal enzymes.

Both cell types are widely dispersed throughout the mucosal lymphoid tissue, intermingled with the T cells with which they are functionally associated.

Tolerance to Orally Administered Antigen

Tolerance to orally administered antigen is certainly mediated by a range of immunological effector mechanisms, It seems clear, however, that suppressor T cells can be induced in the intestine following antigenic challenge. These cells may act locally and recent evidence also suggests that the migration of suppressor populations from the intestine can reduce systemic immunity to orally administered antigen. It is certainly clear that antigen handling by accessory cells and also by epithelial cells at mucosal sites can be responsible for T-cell activation and suppression. The nature of the antigen (soluble/non-soluble or replicating/non-replicating) can determine whether local and systemic immunity or tolerance is induced. Although the experimental data is complex, it is clear that, in addition to organized elements of the intestinal immune system, T lymphocytes present in epithelia or in the lamina propria may assist in the maintenance of tolerance to orally administered antigen in the normal individual.

Heterogenous lymphocyte and accessory cell populations are present in the human intestine before birth. This observation suggests that, at least in man, colonization of the intestine with bacteria or the appearance of antigen via the oral route is not essential for specific epithelial lymphocyte homing. Therefore, the immunological apparatus necessary for antigen handling and induction of tolerance is present at birth.

Coeliac Disease

It is now well established that gliadin, a fraction of gluten which is soluble in ethanol, generates the immunopathological features seen in coeliac disease. These include lymphocyte and plasma cell infiltration, villous atrophy and crypt hyperplasia (Fig. 25.8). The administration of a gluten-free diet reverses histological changes which are present in this disease and ameliorates clinical features. Whilst the pathological events leading to the induction of coeliac disease are complicated, sufficient data exist to suggest that an immunological component plays a major part. These include the dense intra-epithelial lymphocyte and plasma cell infiltrate seen in this condition, the presence of enlarged mesenteric lymph nodes and the observation that the administration of drugs, such as steroids, cause clinical improvement.

Circulating antibodies to gliadin have been described in a significant number of patients. Autoimmune disease is claimed to be more freqrent in coeliac disease and, in a proportion of patients, T-cell lymphoma of a characteristic type appears. Theories of the pathogenesis of this lymphoma suggest evolution within chronically stimulated intestinal T lymphocytes. In addition to the well-described antibody response to gliadin, evidence for the involvement of cell-mediated immunity is also strong. Experimental induction of cell-mediated immunity in the intestine is known to cause villous atrophy and crypt hyperplasia. Further, cytokine production has been described in jejunal biopsies from coeliac patients cultured with gliadin.

More recently, gliadin has been shown to demonstrate amino acid sequence homology with an early protein of human adenovirus type 12. It is possible that an immunological cross-reaction between adenovirus and α-gliadin may initiate a cell-mediated immune response in coeliac disease. The relationship of coeliac disease to certain MHC class II loci, responsible for antigen presentation to T lymphocytes and the high frequency of previous infection with adenovirus in patients with coeliac disease, in comparison to a control group with other gastrointestinal disorders, further supports this hypothesis.

Crohn's Disease

The aetiology of Crohn's disease is obscure and whilst many studies have attempted to isolate a causative

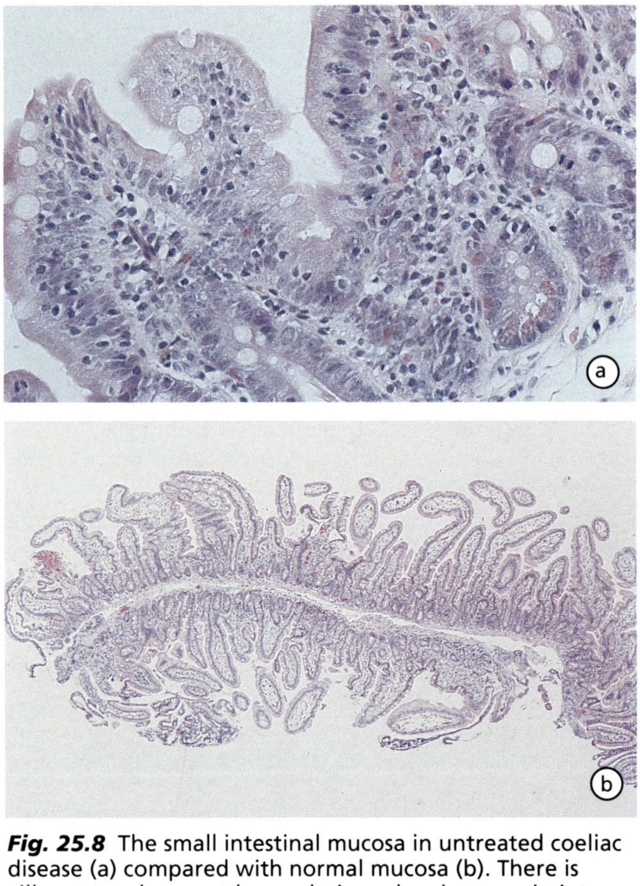

Fig. 25.8 The small intestinal mucosa in untreated coeliac disease (a) compared with normal mucosa (b). There is villous atrophy, crypt hyperplasia and an increase in intra-epithelial lymphocytes. The changes resolve on gluten withdrawal from the diet.

infectious agent, none has yet been successful. The phenotypic features of lymphoid cells and accessory cells which are found in the bowel wall in Crohn's disease have been widely studied. No consistent difference has been found between the T-cell subpopulations present in this condition and normal colon. It does appear, however, that macrophage numbers may be increased in the inflamed bowel. Whilst Crohn's disease characteristically involves the distal ileum, inflammatory changes are known to extend throughout the entire length of the bowel. The pathology of this condition classically consists of oedema, fibrosis and ulceration.

Fissures often appear, resulting in secondary infection. Of particular interest, with regard to T-cell involvement in the Crohn's disease process, is the presence of granulomatous inflammation within the intestinal wall. Imbalances in T-cell function could result in the presence of granulomas responsible for tissue damage in Crohn's disease.

Additional Lymphocyte Subset Studies in Pathological Intestine

T-cell populations infiltrating the intestine in the pathological processes described have been investigated further than simply their CD4/CD8 ratio. Exposure of T cells to antigen and the subsequent development of an 'antigen-experienced' phenotype is accompanied by a change in the molecular species of leucocyte common antigen on the surface of these cells. This switch from CD45RA to CD45R0 is accompanied by a change in the cytokine secretion profile of these cells and by the induction of various adhesion molecules on the lymphocyte surface. The demonstration that the bulk of lymphocytes infiltrating the intestine are of CD45R0 type lends further support to a role of T-cell activation in the induction of both Crohn's and coeliac disease (see Fig. 25.7).

Conclusion

The material presented clearly demonstrates the complexity of the mucosal immune system. In normal individuals this system is protective and maintains tolerance. These actions are conducted by T-cells in concert with the antibody arm of the immune response and with the organized elements of the mucosal lymphoid system. Disturbances of the delicate balances which exist between different components of this system result in the development a range of complex tissue pathologies. In coeliac disease, we know that the antigen gluten is responsible for driving the allergic response. In other cases, dietary antigens such as cows' milk can clearly be demonstrated to generate an allergic response. The evidence for the involvement of the T-cell system in Crohn's disease appears overwhelming but it is impossible to comment fully on the immunological imbalances which may initiate the process or the nature of the causative agent. Further extensive studies of mucosal immunity are required before its role in the development of disease states can be determined.

Further Reading

Brostoff, J, Challacombe SJ. *Food Allergy and Intolerance*. London: Baillière-Tindall, 1987.

Harvey J, Jones DB. Human mucosal T-lymphocyte and macrophage sub-populations in normal and inflamed intestine. *Clin Exp Allergy* 1991; **21**: 549–560.

Wright R, Hodgdson, HJF. *Gastrointestinal and Liver Immunology. Clinical Gastroenterology* (Vol. I:3). London: Ballière-Tindall, 1987.

Chapter 26

Gastrointestinal Allergic Disease – Diagnosis and Treatment

Introduction

The term 'food allergy' has often been used for a variety of adverse reactions to food, whether or not immunologically determined. However, the use of a term which implies an immunological mechanism is often inappropriate: for example, many Asian people lack aldehyde dehydrogenase and feel ill after alcohol while a large majority of African and Asian people produce very little lactase in adult life and cannot tolerate the quantities of cows' milk which are commonly consumed in North America and Europe. In such cases, a diagnostic food challenge can establish the presence of food intolerance, but an immunological approach to investigation may merely divert attention from the enzyme deficiency which is the cause of the problem.

The clinical patterns which arise are summarized in Fig. 26.1. The mouth and gastrointestinal tract are often prominently affected but dermatological, respiratory and systemic effects are not uncommon and may be the only symptoms. Highly atopic individuals sometimes report a sensitivity to two, three or more foods, with a different type of reaction to each one – for example, an asthmatic response to wine but an attack of diarrhoea followed by eczema in response to cows' milk.

Foods Involved

The foods that cause immunological reactions seem to share a number of characteristics. They usually contain heat and acid stable glycoproteins with a molecular weight in the range of 18–36 kDa. Prominent among them are cows' milk, egg, nuts, fish and shellfish, soy and wheat. Because of the different eating habits in different parts of the world, peanut hypersensitivity is relatively common in Britain and the United States but not in Sweden. Rice hypersensitivity is not uncommon in Japan but rare in Western countries. The foods which are most commonly involved have been summarized in Fig. 26.2.

When food reactions are based on an immunological mechanism, cross-reactions may occur between related food proteins. Soy bean and peanut are both legumes, and peanut-sensitive individuals may react to other legumes or to other nuts. Detailed studies have been carried out on the antigenic components of soy bean. Soy bean trypsin-inhibitor has been identified as a major antigen but there is cross-reactivity between different globulins which are present in soy bean and no single antigenic component can account for all cases. Analysis of the antigens in milk and egg has also provided evidence that several antigenic components may be present in a single food.

In contrast to the glycoproteins which cause immunological reactions, food additives are usually low molecular weight substances which act through other mechanisms – for example, through the vasodilator effects of sodium nitrite or the oesophageal irritant effects of high concentrations of monosodium glutamate.

Clinical Patterns of Food Intolerance
Food-allergic syndromes oral allergy gastric symptoms/early diarrhoea/vomiting rhinitis urticaria eczema asthma anaphylaxis late intestinal syndromes (cows' milk protein intolerance, infantile colitis, coeliac disease)
Other types of food intolerance (presenting with intestinal, cutaneous or systemic manifestations) toxic pharmacological enzyme defects

Fig. 26.1 Clinical patterns of food intolerance.

Common Foods in Allergic or Other Intolerant Reactions
milk, egg, fish and shellfish, nuts and peanuts cereal grains, flour, yeast pork, bacon, tenderized meats alcohol, chocolate, coffee, tea apple, citrus and other soft fruits celery, soya Seeds – sesame, aniseed, caraway, dill herbs and spices – cinnamon, garlic, mustard food additives – preservatives, colours

Fig. 26.2 Examples of foods that cause allergic or other intolerant reactions.

Clinical Features

When Young and colleagues carried out a postal survey which covered 30,000 people living in the High Wycombe area in the UK, 2890 (9.6 per cent) claimed that they reacted adversely to specific foods, while 1372 (4.6 per cent) thought that they were sensitive to food additives. It transpired that there was a wide discrepancy between this public perception of food-induced reactions and the medical profession's view of the problem. When a special clinic was set up to assess those individuals with a suggestive history and, in the first instance, to use challenge tests with five mixtures of food additives, only three cases of proven intolerance to food additives could be identified. While the study of foods (rather than food additives) has yet to be completed, it is clear that there is a considerable discrepancy between public perception and objective evidence of a reaction.

The wide range of symptoms which occur can make diagnosis more difficult. A relationship between food and symptoms is easily established if the lips swell, the mouth and throat tingle, and blebs of mucosal swelling develop on the inside of the cheeks in the first few minutes after eating a particular food. As Amlot has shown, this 'oral allergy syndrome' usually correlates with the presence of IgE antibodies to the food concerned, as with urticaria, asthma, anaphylaxis and (less specifically) nausea and vomiting. Many patients with immediate reactions of this kind or with perioral skin rashes (Fig. 26.3) never consult a physician because they recognize their own problem and solve it by avoiding the offending food. Late onset symptoms, however, seldom have evidence of an IgE reaction, as judged by skin prick test or radioallergosorbent test (RAST). In the case of gluten enteropathy, in which the diagnosis may be established by a jejunal biopsy, there is good evidence that other types of immunological reaction are involved, and the rather rare condition of eosinophilic gastroenteritis also involves immunological abnormalities. In most cases in which symptoms of food intolerance develop late, however, there is no clear evidence that immunological mechanisms are involved. In such cases the differential diagnosis includes the coincidental recurrence of episodes of food poisoning or an effect of toxins such as the glycoalkaloids present in some potatoes, the cyanogenic glycosides in lima beans and millet sprouts, or the toxins present in badly stored mackerel or other scombroid fish (Fig. 26.4). People who drink large quantities of coffee also suffer pharmacological effects which include irritability, tachycardia, sleep disturbance and, through its diuretic effect, a tendency towards constipation and bloating. Caffeine can also cause oesophageal reflux, nausea, vomiting and diarrhoea, possibly because of its stimulant effect on gastric secretion.

The irritable bowel syndrome has long been a rather vague diagnosis, given to patients who suffer abdominal pain, discomfort or bloating, together with a change in bowel habit, but who have no evidence of organic disease. No single explanation has been shown to account for all cases, and it is clear that these symptoms – albeit with a tendency to diarrhoea rather than constipation – can occur in patients with lactase deficiency. Levitt and colleagues have shown how the fermentation of unabsorbed food residues can lead to the formation of propionic acid in the colon which, together with the release of hydrogen and carbon dioxide, can provoke bloating, colic, nausea and intestinal hurry (Fig. 26.5). In Levitt's patient it was only by eliminating both milk and wheat products that these symptoms were controlled. It is not only unabsorbed lactose which can provoke symptoms of this kind.

Apart from those cases of the irritable bowel syndrome which are provoked by the fermentation prod-

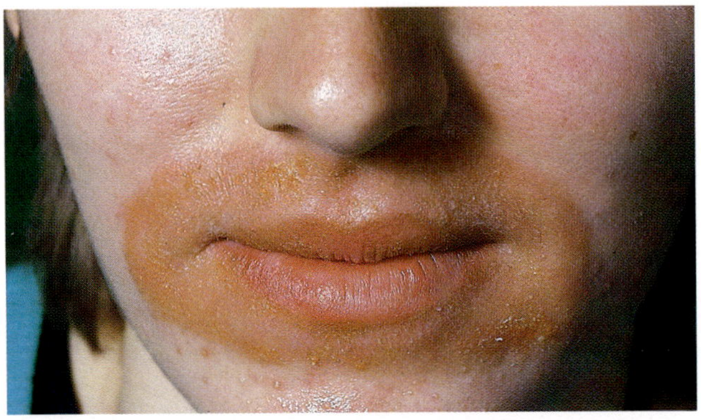

Fig. 26.3 A perioral skin rash provoked by orange juice.

Common Food Toxins

Toxin	Source
glycoalkaloids	Some varieties of potato
cyanogenic glycosides	lima beans, millet sprouts
histamine, histidine	badly stored mackerel, or other scombroid fish

Fig. 26.4 Common food toxins.

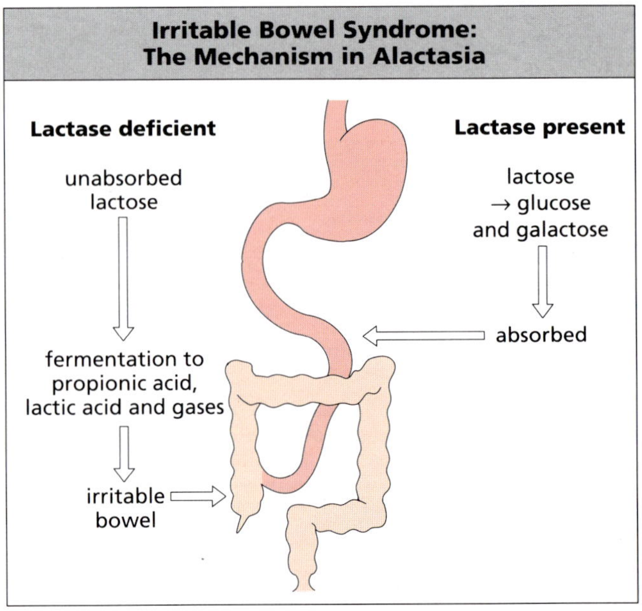

Fig. 26.5 Irritable bowel syndrome: the mechanism in alactasia.

ucts of unabsorbed food residues, transient food-intolerant symptoms are commonly reported after an attack of gastroenteritis. Among the complex factors which are involved, there is a transient loss of brush border enzymes, when the intestinal mucosa is denuded by infectious diarrhoea, giardiasis or cows' milk protein reactions. In severe cases of mucosal damage, including gluten enteropathy, it appears that lactase, sucrase and maltase may all be lost.

Coeliac Disease

Coeliac disease is the result of an intolerance to the gluten proteins in wheat, oats, rye or barley. While it is usually associated with diarrhoea, it can also cause constipation, iron deficiency anaemia, rickets and short stature. When it presents before the age of two years with abnormal stools, anorexia, vomiting and abdominal distension, or with irritability and muscle wasting, the clinical diagnosis can often be made without difficulty, but its presentation in older subjects can be much more insidious. The association with dermatitis herpetiformis may suggest the presence of this condition, but evidence of intestinal mucosal damage on biopsy is a diagnostic requirement at all ages.

The presence of circulating IgG antibodies to gliadin has been suggested as a further diagnostic test in gluten enteropathy, although this is not the only condition in which these antibodies to gliadin can be found. Furthermore, IgG antibodies are accompanied by antibodies to egg and milk proteins in coeliac patients, suggesting a reaction to a wide range of proteins which cross the damaged mucosa. Since a fall in the level of gliadin antibodies can follow gluten avoidance while antibodies to egg and milk persist, their presence may reflect exposure to food proteins rather than having any important aetiological significance.

Eosinophilic Gastroenteritis

Occasionally, patients who present with features of pyloric obstruction may be found to have an associated eosinophilia which is not due to parasites, vasculitis, neoplasm or any other recognized local cause. These patients may have diffuse eosinophilic infiltration, usually in the pyloric region, but they may also have a more generalized eosinophilic gastroenteritis (Fig. 26.6). More than half of the patients have evidence of allergic disease elsewhere in the body, ranging from allergic rhinitis to angioedema, urticaria and asthma. Jejunal mucosal biopsy can sometimes provide diagnostic evidence, but there is often minimal mucosal infiltration and predominant involvement of deeper layers of the gut wall, so that patients who fulfil the criteria may require a bowel biopsy at laparotomy before the diagnosis can be made. In some cases, subserosal changes are associated with ascites and there may be a marked eosinophilia in the ascitic fluid. Although remissions have been reported in infancy and childhood, when milk was excluded from the diet, the use of dietary restriction followed by food challenges has given disappointing results. Even when an appropriate dietary regime can be devised, corticosteroids may be needed in addition to dietary restriction before the control of symptoms can be achieved.

Other Immunological Disorders

There is still controversy over the importance of immunological reactions to food in inflammatory bowel diseases. In 1984, Jenkins and colleagues reported eight cases in which infants with continuing blood-stained diarrhoea had an associated inflammatory infiltration in the lamina propria and mild ulceration. In these babies with infantile colitis, the replacement of milk feeds with soya milk resulted in a prompt recovery. It should be noted, however, that the adverse effect of cows' milk in these infants could have had a non-immunological explanation – as in the case of infants who have an acute infective gastroenteritis and who recover more rapidly when cows' milk is withheld. The explanation is uncertain, but a transient loss of lactase and the consequent persistence and fermentation of unabsorbed lactose may contribute.

For the adult with ulcerative colitis, improvement after dietary restriction provides no evidence that foods have a causal role, and similarly, the cause of the inflammatory changes in the bowel wall remains uncertain. In Crohn's disease, too, the benefits which follow treatment with dietary restriction or corticosteroids and anti-inflammatory drugs cannot, by itself, be taken either as evidence of specific food intolerance nor of the presence of a primarily immunological disorder.

Intestinal Reactions in Subjects with Urticaria

An association between reactions in the skin and in the gastrointestinal tract has been well recognized in hereditary angioedema, in which there is a deficiency of one of the enzymes (C1 esterase inhibitor) which terminates the inflammatory cascade of the complement enzyme system. An association between urticaria and transient thickening of the wall of the

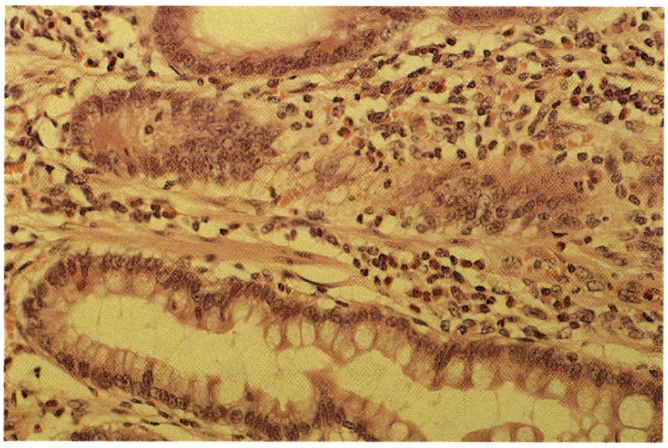

Fig. 26.6 Eosinophilic gastroenteritis.

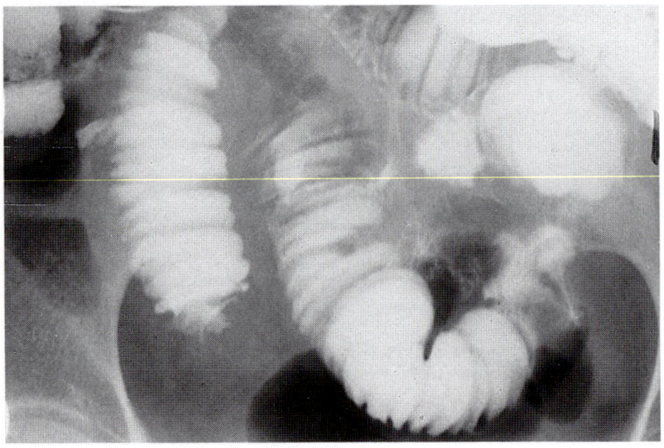

Fig. 26.7 Radiological changes in a patient with urticaria who had recurrent, transient episodes of bowel wall thickening as shown by ultrasound.

ileum has now been reported, which suggests that this might represent a food-intolerant reaction (Fig. 26.7). Current evidence suggests, however, that patients who have this association may be unable to metabolize histamine normally, either as a result of a deficiency or of the inactivation of diamine oxidase.

Remote Manifestations of Food Intolerance

The remote manifestations of food intolerance have helped to draw attention to the different mechanisms which are involved. An immediate asthmatic attack may be provoked in a fish-allergic individual by the smell of fish, and there are other examples of this kind. Nevertheless, when asthma is provoked by foods that contain sodium metabisulphite as a preservative, there is evidence that it is the irritant effect of released sulphur dioxide which causes bronchoconstriction in susceptible asthmatics rather than any immunological mechanism. Most wines contain 100–300 mg/litre of sulphur dioxide but, in 1985, when Gershwin and colleagues studied two patients with asthmatic attacks which could be provoked by 4 fl oz of white wine, one reacted to suitably flavoured alcohol solution without sulphur dioxide while the other reacted only when metabisulphite was substituted for the alcohol.

Not all cases of food-related asthma seem to be provoked by the inhalational route. Several patients with milk intolerance have been described who have asthmatic reactions one hour or more after drinking cows' milk and who have negative serum IgE tests for cows' milk allergy and low total IgE levels.

The possibility of ingested foods affecting distant organs has been reviewed elsewhere (see Further Reading). There have been well-validated reports on the effects of food on migraine, the skin and, exceptionally, on the provocation of arthralgia or of proteinuria which are beyond the scope of this chapter.

Diagnostic Procedures

Even a demonstration of IgE antibodies to a particular food cannot prove the presence of clinical sensitivity. Indeed, children who have had clinical allergic reactions to egg or milk may show a positive skin test response to these foods long after they have recovered clinically. Elimination of the suspect foods, followed by a challenge test, is therefore the main requirement for the diagnosis either of food allergy or of other food-intolerant reactions. In attempting to identify foods which are thought to be responsible for a food-intolerant reaction, it may be possible to start by excluding a single, highly suspect food together with any identifiable immunologically related substances. In the case of preservatives and colouring agents which are widely used, however, a more limited diet is needed.

Except in cases where one or more particular foods are strongly suspect, it is necessary to use exclusion diets intended to start with a regimen which is simple and well tolerated, followed by the introduction of other foods in sequential fashion. For this purpose, a number of initial diets have been recommended, the most traditional consisting of lamb, rice, pears and water. It is however essential that a regimen is recommended which can be managed by the patient without constant expert supervision. The foods which are most frequently the cause of problems include milk, egg, fish, wheat and cereal grains, spices and artificially coloured or preserved foods of various kinds. By allowing one or two fresh meats, rice, vegetables and fresh fruit (with the exception of citrus fruits and apples), dairy-free margarine, weak tea, sugar and olive oil, it is possible to begin with a diet which can be maintained for two weeks – or longer if necessary – with the understanding that a more strict diet could be imposed if there is a strong suspicion that there are harmful foods which have not yet been eliminated. An experienced dietitian's help is

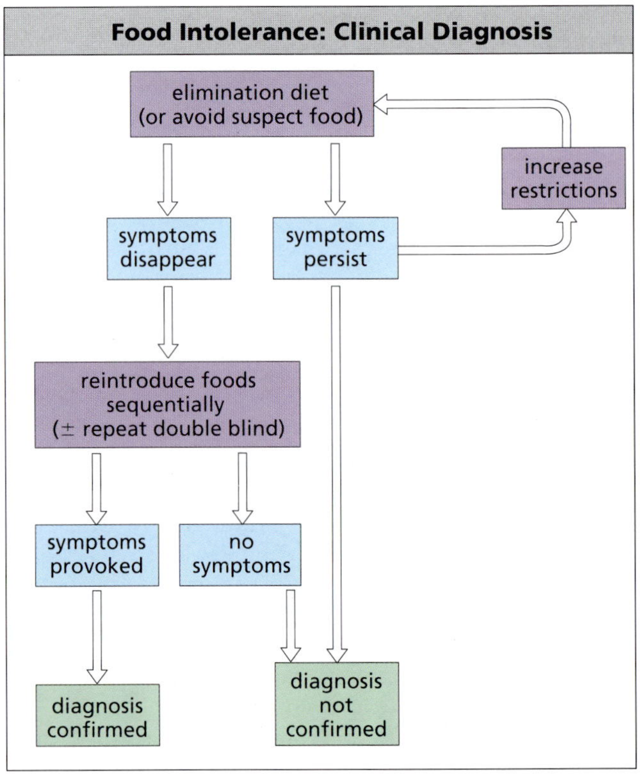

Fig. 26.8 Food intolerance: Clinical diagnosis.

strongly advisable – not only to emphasize the exclusion of common foods, such as ham, pork, bacon, sausages, wines and spirits, but also to ensure the nutritional adequacy of protein, calories, calcium and vitamins. A suggested challenge procedure is summarized in Fig. 26.8.

Open challenge procedures can only be regarded as reliable when the end-point involves one or more objective changes, such as swelling of the lip, urticaria or angioedema. Even with such changes, the potentiating role of stress cannot be ignored. A double- or single-blind placebo-controlled oral food challenge remains the only definitive procedure for an indisputable diagnosis of food intolerance. Its weakness lies in the fact that a negative response does not rule out the condition. Even in anaphylactic sensitivity associated with demonstrable IgE antibodies to a specific food, as in some well-studied cases, reactions may only occur when there are catalytic factors such as exercise (Fig. 26.9). It has also become clear that some patients who lose their symptoms on a food-restricted diet may remain symptomless until the food is given again on repeated occasions or in substantial quantities.

Food allergy is diagnosed when, in addition to evidence of food intolerance, there is evidence of an immunological response, as judged by positive skin tests or radioallergosorbent tests for IgE antibodies to the food (Fig. 26.10). Patients with the oral allergy syndrome virtually all provide such evidence. It can however be misleading to accept the clinical features of urticaria or asthma as providing confirmatory evidence of an immunological reaction. In food additive-provoked urticaria, evidence of the release of inflammatory mediators has not been shown to be associated with an immunological response and the same is true of urticaria provoked by aspirin. Since tartrazine can induce histamine release in normal subjects, it is clear that other mechanisms may be involved. Similar considerations also apply to food-provoked asthma. Nearly three-quarters of children attending a hospital asthma clinic noted that wheezing could be precipitated by at least one food, especially milk, egg, nuts and iced or aerated drinks. The potentially irritant effects of sulphites has already been noted and, in childhood asthma, food can often provoke an increase in bronchial reactivity rather than directly provoking an asthmatic episode.

Reference has been made in Fig. 26.10 to the hyperventilation syndrome as a condition which may be mistaken for food intolerance. Patients whose symptoms include giddiness, sweating, weakness, muscle stiffness, tachycardia or paraesthesia provide clinical reasons for suspecting this under-diagnosed condition. In cases of doubt, the reproduction of symptoms by one to three minutes of forced hyperventilation will establish the diagnosis beyond doubt (Fig. 26.11). In positive cases, the tests should be continued until the patient and physician recognize its validity. It should be stressed the presence of the hyperventilation syndrome does not rule out the possibility of an associated organic disease, but may be a consequence of it.

The diagnosis of coeliac disease has already been discussed. In this disorder, there have been claims that the detection of IgG antibodies to food can be of diagnostic value. Since IgG antibodies to egg and milk proteins persist in patients with coeliac disease

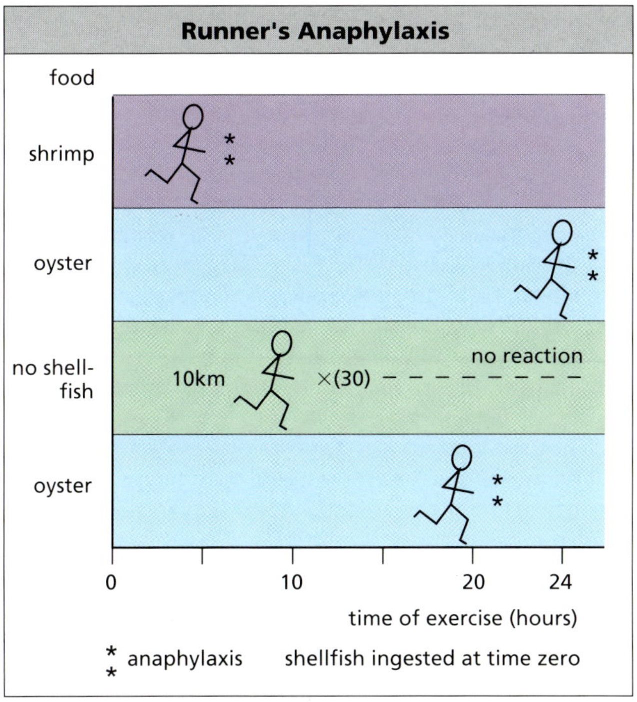

Fig. 26.9 Food-dependent exercise-induced anaphylaxis. The case of a long distance runner with IgE antibodies to shellfish, who had severe anaphylactic reactions after eating shellfish but only during exercise. (Adapted from Maulitz RM, Pratt DS, Schocket AL. *J Allergy Clin Immunol* 1979; **63**: 433–434.).

Food Intolerance Criteria for Diagnosis

	Response to challenge tests		Evidence of specific IgE antibodies
	Open	Blind	
Food allergy	+	+	+
Other forms of food intolerance	+	+	0
Food aversion or hyperventilation syndrome	+	0	0

Fig. 26.10 Food intolerance: Criteria for diagnosis.

Food Intolerance: in the Hyperventilation Syndrome

symptoms provoked by	sight, smell or ingestion of food
time course	variable
characteristic symptoms	giddiness, sweating, nausea, tachycardia, aching limbs, weakness, paraesthesia, cramps
investigation	reproduced by 1–3 minutes of forced hyperventilation

Fig. 26.11 Food tolerance in th hyperventilation syndrome.

in the absence of any clinical intolerance to these foods, such antibodies may reflect the extent to which intact food proteins have crossed the gastrointestinal mucous membrane, rather than indicate any direct association with disease pathogenesis.

The search for further diagnostic tests has yielded disappointing results, apart from some limited success in detecting the release of inflammatory mediators. It has been suggested that the basophils of children with food sensitivity release abnormal amounts of histamine spontaneously. More recently, it has been shown that peripheral blood mononuclear cells from food-allergic individuals produce a histamine-releasing factor (HRF) factor which can activate basophils from other food-allergic individuals. Nevertheless, leucocyte histamine release studies and basophil degranulation tests have not provided a useful diagnostic test. An alternative approach has been advocated using direct application of foods to the gastric mucosa of food-sensitive subjects to show that this provokes histamine release from mast cells of the gastric mucosa. Comparable results have also been obtained with tartrazine. Since the pharmacological effects of tartrazine can release histamine from white blood cells in symptomless normal subjects, it seems likely that additional factors may be involved.

Recent reports have suggested an occasional association between urticaria and a deficiency in the histamine-metabolizing enzyme diamine oxidase, and some patients with aspirin sensitivity also appear to have an enzyme deficiency, since they may have low levels of plasma cholinesterase.

Food-intolerance problems caused by enzyme deficiencies have yet to be studied in depth. Those which cause the most dramatic effects have received the most attention, including the rapidly fatal aldolase deficiency which results in infantile fructose intolerance, aminoaciduria and hepatic failure. Fructose intolerance can also be caused by diphosphatase deficiency but, since the spells of ketosis and hypoglycaemia are intermittent, this diagnosis is more easily missed. Essential fructosuria due to fructokinase deficiency is even more benign and is probably greatly underdiagnosed. Comparable diagnostic difficulties also arise in the numerous enzyme deficiencies, leading to a greater or lesser degree of protein intolerance, with aminoaciduria or hyperammonaemia. There are also cases of mental deficiency in which there is an inability to metabolize the meat-derived dipeptide, carnosine. The part played by enzyme systems therefore needs further study.

Treatment

When immediate IgE-mediated sensitivity to foods is demonstrated, the only proven method of treatment is the avoidance of the foods concerned. When anaphylactic reactions have occurred, it may also be necessary for the patient to keep a pre-loaded adrenaline syringe available in case of mishap. The main problems in this approach arise when a small child is deprived of an important food, such as cows' milk. If the child is able to tolerate protein hydrolysates or milk products from a goat or sheep, an adequate diet is easily achieved. In other cases, there is the need for a dietitian's advice so that vegetable proteins, notably soy, can be substituted, with appropriate calcium and vitamin supplementation to ensure that the diet is nutritionally adequate. It should be noted, however, that soya proteins containing sucrose and dextromaltose may themselves be prone to provoke diarrhoea. Soy-lactose formulae are much better tolerated than formulae containing sucrose or maltose.

Because of the difficulties in managing severe cows' milk protein intolerance, preventive measures have also been advocated for infants born of atopic parents. Prolonged breast feeding is usually recommended and, since sensitization cannot always be prevented by this means, it has also been suggested that the nursing mother should avoid cows' milk, and eggs, in her diet. These additional measures have had a modest success at best and, at worst, no demonstratable effect.

Food sensitivity frequently diminishes with time and some reassurance may be justified, especially in childhood. In one cohort of 67 children, one third had lost their sensitivity when challenged 1–2 years later. It was demonstrated that, after keeping to an egg-free diet for one year, 8 out of 28 children with atopic dermatitis could eat eggs freely, despite the failure of repeat skin testing to indicate any loss of specific sensitivity. A loss of clinical hypersensitivity thus occurs quite frequently with the passage of time, most often with soy and less commonly with peanut, wheat, egg and milk.

The response to dietary measures is far more difficult to establish in patients with eczema than in other conditions, possibly because of the secondary effect of scratching and the slowness with which changes occur after dietary manipulation. There are also the complicating effects of contact sensitization to other antigens. The effects of food may represent only part of a more complex clinical problem, especially in patients with eczema and asthma who are also food intolerant. Where the skin is involved, it is important to avoid non-specific irritants, including soap. It may be helpful to give non-sedating H_1-antihistamines and to use emulsifying creams to prevent dehydration or, in severe cases, to use topical corticosteroids for short periods.

Whether gastrointestinal or other symptoms are involved, dietary treatment can only begin after the identification of those foods which cause reactions or elicit a cross-reacting sensitivity. Those who are sensitive to silver birch tree pollen can have cross-reacting sensitivities to a number of soft fruits, nuts and root vegetables. Those who have ragweed allergy sometimes have an associated hypersensitivity to melon and banana. In addition, sensitivity to tenderized meat may depend not on the meat protein but on an IgE-mediated reaction to papain or other enzymes used as tenderizers. Patients who are sensitive to proteins, such as those contained in soya, may nevertheless be able to eat oils derived from the same source (for example, the commercial soya oils added to margarine). Those sensitive to nuts may tolerate nut oils: however, nut oils can be contaminated by nut proteins and have occasionally caused reactions.

Having identified those foods which can be shown to cause problems, the next objective is to broaden the diet to include as many other foods as possible. It is customary to do this in stages so that the cause of any further symptoms can be more easily identified. Patients who react to foods which are taken on two or three successive days may be able to tolerate smaller quantities at less frequent intervals. They may also be able to tolerate heat-denatured proteins – for example, cows' milk or egg incorporated in a cake – while reacting to raw or partly cooked proteins of the same origin.

Further Reading

Jenkins HR, Pincott JR, Soothill JF, Milla PJ, Harries JF. Food allergy: the major cause of infantile colitis. *Arch Dis Child* 1984; **59**: 326–329.

Lessof MH. *Food Reactions*. London: James and James, 1992.

Levitt MD, Lasser RB, Schwartz JS, Bond JH. Studies of a flatulent patient. *New Engl J Med* 1976; **295**: 260–262.

Magarian GJ. Hyperventilatory syndromes: infrequently recognised common expressions of anxiety and stress. *Medicine* 1982; **61**: 219–236.

Metcalfe DD, Sampson HA, Simon RA, eds. *Food Allergy: Adverse Reactions to Foods and Food Additives*. Boston: Blackwell Scientific Publications, 1991.

Nanda R, James R, Smith H, Dudley CRK, Jewell DP. Food intolerance and the irritable bowel syndrome. *Gut* 1989; **30**: 1099–1104.

Price JF. Paediatric allergy. In: Lessof MH, Lee TH, Kemeny DM, eds. *Allergy: An International Textbook*. Chichester: John Wiley and Sons, 1987, pp. 423–453.

Royal College of Physicians and British Nutrition Foundation Joint Report: Food intolerance and food aversion. *J R Coll Physicians Lond* 1984; **18**: 83–123.

Chapter 27

Anaphylaxis

Introduction

The clinical syndrome of systemic anaphylaxis is the most urgent and potentially serious manifestation of allergic disease. The term 'anaphylaxis' can be used to describe consequences of IgE-mediated release of potent biologically active substances upon a given target organ. Systemic anaphylaxis, in contrast to local forms of anaphylaxis (e.g. nasal, ocular, or intestinal) is a clinical entity resulting from action of such mediators upon more than one target organ and, often, upon sites distant from that of initial antigen presentation. The most dramatic and potentially lethal consequences of systemic anaphylaxis include acute upper respiratory obstruction, bronchospasm, and shock with vascular collapse; but the skin and subcutis, gastrointestinal tract, and other organs may be important sites of clinical expression. Similar clinical features may result from IgE-mediated antigen-induced release of mediators from previously sensitized mast cells and basophils, from non-IgE-mediated reactions, and from idiopathic anaphylaxis. Anaphylaxis thus denotes a clinically defined entity in which a variety of mechanisms converge in a common pathway of mast cell and/or basophil activation, mediator release, and end-organ response. The target organs may be clinically affected singly or in combination.

Successful management of systemic anaphylaxis requires prompt recognition of symptoms, aggressive therapeutic intervention, and, ultimately, efforts directed at identification of precipitating factors and prevention of future episodes.

Epidemiology

Because anaphylaxis is generally unanticipated and often overwhelming, because it requires immediate attention, and because the severity of the reaction renders intentional re-exposure to precipitating stimuli dangerous and ethically troublesome, there is little controlled clinical experience in humans. Data relating to the incidence of anaphylaxis are limited. Indeed, what limited information there is concerning the incidence of anaphylaxis relates primarily to fatalities, with less severe cases being undoubtedly under-reported. Approximately 40 deaths per year are thought to result from Hymenoptera stings in the United States. The risk of non-fatal anaphylaxis from Hymenoptera stings is estimated at just under 1 per cent of those bitten. Fatal anaphylaxis from penicillin has been estimated to have an incidence of 0.002 per cent, while the risk of non-fatal anaphylaxis has been estimated to range from 0.7–10.0 per cent. Incidence figures will be dependent not only on the rate of reporting of non-lethal episodes but also, in the case of fatalities, the recognition that sudden unexplained death was due to anaphylaxis. The true incidence of anaphylaxis will also be affected by the panoply of diagnostic and therapeutic agents used in medicine and industry. Specific sub-groups at risk within the general population have not been well identified. It remains unclear whether atopics are at greater risk of experiencing anaphylaxis, or even at risk for more severe episodes of anaphylaxis, than non-atopics. Recently, however, it has become clear that those taking β-blockers have a significantly increased risk of anaphylaxis, and that such episodes, when they do occur, tend to be more severe.

Clinical Presentation

Anaphylaxis is frequently abrupt in onset. Symptoms and signs may range from mild to severe, and involvement of various organ systems may differ from case to case. Premonitory symptoms may include cutaneous warmth or tingling and a sensation of anxiety or impending doom. Upper respiratory symptoms may include airway obstruction with manifestations of dysphonia, hoarseness, choking, or a sense of fullness in the throat. Bronchospasm may occur, with cough, dyspnoea, chest tightness, and wheezing. Rarely, respiratory arrest may ensue. Sneezing, nasal congestion, tearing, periorbital oedema, and palatal itch may form a part of the presentation. Symptoms of rhinitis and conjunctivitis are relatively common and may herald the onset of more severe manifestations. The cardiovascular findings may include presyncope or frank loss of consciousness due to hypotension, and, occasionally, overt vascular collapse with shock. Also noted may be the development of cardiac arrhythmias and, occasionally, myocardial infarction. Respiratory and vascular symptoms are usually, although not always, accompanied by the characteristic sensation of cutaneous warmth and flushing with associated pruritus. These cutaneous manifestations may progress to urticaria or angioedema, frequently with involvement of the face or pharynx. Sweating is common. Gastrointestinal manifestations include dysphagia, abdominal cramping, nausea, vomiting, and diarrhoea. Uterine cramping, urinary urgency, and urinary or faecal incontinence are sometimes associated.

The clinical findings generally follow within minutes of exposure to the precipitating agent, but they may be delayed as, for example, in the case of delayed absorption of an orally administered antigen. Mortality most often occurs early in the clinical course as a result of respiratory obstruction or vascular collapse. Respiratory events account for approximately 70 per cent of mortality from anaphylaxis, with cardiovascular manifestations accounting for most of the remaining mortality. However, significant delayed mortality and morbidity may occur due to impaired perfusion of vital organs as a result of anaphylactic shock. The occurrence of biphasic anaphylactic reactions has been reported. These may be analagous to immediate- and late-phase components of the allergic response in other forms of immediate-type hypersensitivity reactions involving skin, nose, and bronchial tree. However, information is limited, and it has not been well established that the late-phase reaction is a distinct phenomenon, as opposed to a manifestation of incomplete response to partial therapy during prolonged, severe anaphylactic episodes. Nonetheless, the possibility of a true biphasic response has implications for therapy of the acute episode and the appropriate duration of clinical observation of the patient with anaphylaxis.

Pathology

Anatomical Changes

Anatomical findings in fatal anaphylaxis in humans may include laryngeal oedema, acute pulmonary hyperinflation, pulmonary oedema, parenchymal haemorrhage, and visceral congestion. Sometimes, no significant pathological change is noted. Upper respiratory tract oedema with airways obstruction may be seen in about two-thirds of fatal cases, and acute pulmonary hyperinflation in up to half. Pathological examination of the upper airway reveals non-inflammatory oedema, while diffuse histological changes in the bronchial tree include increased secretions, submucosal oedema, and an eosinophilic infiltrate, along with vascular congestion. The lung parenchyma may reveal areas of haemorrhage, oedema, and atelectasis. Cardiovascular manifestations of anaphylaxis probably result from hypovolaemia consequent to postcapillary venule leakage with resultant shock. This may be complicated by cardiac arrhythmias. Histological evidence of myocardial necrosis is sometimes reported. Also noted in some instances is evidence of congestion of the liver, spleen, and other organs.

Laboratory Tests

There are no pathognomonic laboratory tests to establish the diagnosis of anaphylaxis. In the acute episode, haemoconcentration may result from postcapillary venule leakage. Plasma histamine

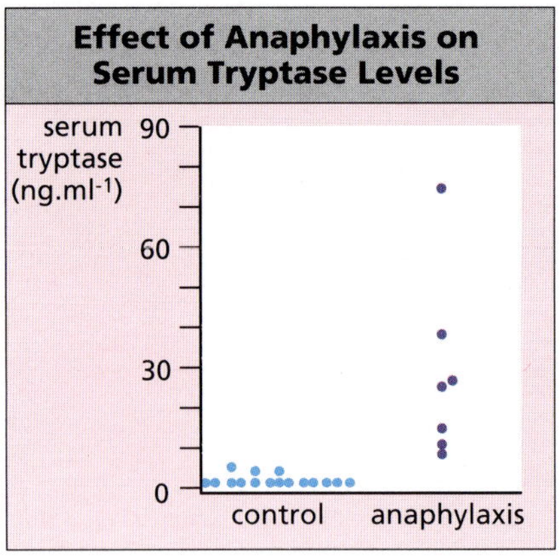

Fig. 27.1 Anaphylaxis causes an increase in serum tryptase levels. (Adapted from Schwartz LB et al. *N Engl J Med* 1987; **316**: 1622–1626.

levels may be elevated in acute attacks; and, more recently, elevation of serum tryptase levels has been described in anaphylaxis, presumably resulting from mast cell degranulation (Fig. 27.1). Occasionally, reduction of complement components or the presence of circulating immune complexes has been observed. A number of non-specific biochemical abnormalities may be seen in anaphylaxis, reflecting visceral congestion, ischaemia, or necrosis.

Pathophysiology of Anaphylaxis

Systemic anaphylaxis constitutes a clinical syndrome, and the precise pathophysiology remains incompletely understood in many instances. Much of our knowledge of the mediators involved, and their biological effects, is derived from animal studies that cannot be extrapolated with certainty to the human. Nonetheless, a pathophysiological classification of anaphylaxis has been derived which may provide a framework for our understanding of this clinical entity (Fig. 27.2).

IgE-Mediated Anaphylaxis

The most frequent mechanism in cases of anaphylaxis with a clearly defined aetiology is the IgE-dependent, immediate hypersensitivity reaction. The IgE-dependent mechanism has been implicated in anaphylaxis due to antibiotics (most frequently penicillin, in particular with antibodies to minor determinants, but numerous other antibiotic agents are well represented in the literature); other drugs or therapeutic agents (e.g. allergen extracts, vaccines, and local anaesthetics as well as ethylene oxide-altered human serum albumin in haemodialysis, and a number of hormones); foreign proteins (antisera, antitoxins, insulin and other protein hormones, enzymes including chymopapain and streptokinase, as well as Hymenoptera venoms); and some foods (especially shellfish, nuts, legumes, milk and milk by-products, egg whites, grains, and seeds) (see Fig. 27.2).

Most recently, IgE-mediated sensitivity to natural latex has become a prominent cause of anaphylaxis in medical personnel through the use of gloves, and even in patients due to intra-operative exposure to latex gloves or latex in the introduction of barium contrast material for gastrointestinal studies. All

An Operational Classification of Anaphylaxis	
Probable Mechanism	**Examples**
IgE-mediated	
Protein	
Antiserum	Tetanus and diphtheria antitoxins; antithymocyte globulin; antilymphocyte globulin
Hormones, enzymes	Insulin, adrenocorticotropic hormone; thryroid-stimulating hormone; relaxin; chymotrypsin; trypsin; penicillinase; L-asparaginase; papain
Venom	Hymenoptera
Allergen extract	Ragweed; Bermuda grass; buckwheat; egg white; cottonseed
Vaccines	Tetanus toxoid; influenza, measles, and other egg-containing vaccines
Food	Crustacea, molluscs; fresh vegetables (celery, carrots), nuts, legumes, fresh fruits
Polysaccharides	
Dextran	
Iron dextran	
Haptens	
Antibiotics	Penicillin; cephalosporins; tetracycline; demethylchlortetracycline; chlortetracycline; nitrofuantoin; streptomycin
Vitamins	Thiamine
Miscellaneous	Cisplatin; cyclophosphamide; cytosine arabinoside; ethylene oxide-altered human serum albumin
Complement-mediated	Transfusion reaction with IgA deficiency; cuprophane membrane dialysis
Arachidonate-mediated	Aspirin and other non-steroidal anti-inflammatory agents
Direct mast cell-releasing agents	Opiates; tubocurarine, polymyxin;deferoxamine; pentamidine; stilbamidine; radiocontrast media; hydralazine; doxorubicin; daunorubicin; rubidazone; teniposide
Physical	Exercise-induced anaphylaxis Cold urticaria
Idiopathic	

Fig. 27.2 An operational classification of anaphylaxis. Adapted with permission from Sheffer AL, Pennoyer DS. *J Allergy Clin Immunol* 1984; **74**: 580.

conceivable routes of administration (including oral, topical, and inhalational) have been described in association with the development of IgE-mediated anaphylaxis, but parenteral administration of antigen is the route most associated with severe anaphylaxis. Repeated exposures appear to be associated with increased frequency of the reaction.

The pathophysiology of IgE-mediated reactions has been extensively studied. Such reactions occur in those who have become allergic to the inciting antigen as a result of prior exposure. On re-exposure to the antigen, there is massive release of potent biochemical mediators from mast cells and basophils due to bridging of antigen-specific IgE molecules located on the cell surface. Similar cellular events may occur on exposure of mast cells and basophils to medium which contain anti-IgE antibodies, presumably also as a result of bridging of cell-surface IgE. Among the pre-formed and newly generated mediators released on mast cell activation are vasoactive substances, smooth muscle spasmogens, chemotactic factors, mucus glandular secretagogues, enzymes and proteoglycans. The signs and symptoms of anaphylaxis are attributable to the sum of the effects of these mediators on target organs. Reactivity of mast cells and basophils has been extensively investigated. In some atopic disorders, these cells exhibit enhanced mediator release. Histamine-releasing factors and other cytokines may induce or augment chemical mediator release. Other factors – histamine-releasing inhibitor factors – oppose cellular activation. The role of such substances in human anaphylaxis remains to be determined. Functional heterogeneity in the substances released has not been investigated, and the role of basophils in the anaphylactic event has not been identified *in vivo*. Also, the relationships between mast cell heterogeneity and anaphylactic episodes requires further study.

Nonetheless, in our understanding of the IgE-mediated mechanism of anaphylaxis, the classical model of IgE-dependent mast cell activation with subsequent release of substances (e.g. pre-formed, granule-associated substances including histamine, enzymes, proteoglycans, and chemotactic factors), and elaboration of newly-formed lipid-derived mediators (including PGD_2, LTB_4, the sulphidopeptide leukotrienes LTC_4, LTD_4 and LTE_4, and PAF) in addition to numerous cytokines remains a useful model.

In IgE-mediated hypersensitivity reactions in the skin, allergic rhinitis, and allergic asthma, the significance of the infiltration and activation of inflammatory cells in prolonging the hypersensitivity response and causing persistent symptoms is well appreciated. The influx of inflammatory cells, and the biochemical mediators and cytokines which they generate, results in persistence of clinical symptoms or their recrudescence as late-phase, IgE-mediated reactions. A general model for late-phase reactions would include initiation of the inflammatory sequence by mast cell-derived mediators with their effects on surrounding cells and on cells recruited to the area; further pro-inflammatory effects from the interactions of members of the newly developed cellular infiltrates; and, possibly, the augmentation and prolongation of the response through positive feedback of the cytokines elaborated by such newly recruited, pro-inflammatory cells on mast cells and basophils.

It remains unclear whether a late-phase reaction occurs in IgE-mediated anaphylaxis. Experimental challenge in this area has not occurred, inasmuch as it is fraught with greater hazard than experimental induction of IgE-mediated reactions in the skin test or nasal challenge models, or even in allergic asthma.

Immune Complex Complement-Mediated Anaphylaxis

Non-IgE-mediated systemic anaphylaxis is less well understood than anaphylaxis occurring as a consequence of IgE-mediated hypersensitivity, and the development of clinical manifestations is not as well correlated with mediator release in such instances. Probably the most frequent clinical scenario involving immune complex and/or complement-mediated anaphylaxis is represented by transfusion reactions, in which aggregates of immunoglobulin capable of inducing complement activation may be implicated in the development of clinical findings.

The best-studied model is that of anaphylaxis following transfusion or γ globulin administration to the IgA-deficient individual. Lacking IgA, such individuals may have pre-existing IgG–anti-IgA antibodies. On administration of IgA-containing blood products or γ globulin, complexes of IgA–IgG anti-IgA antibody form and activate the classical complement cascade. Anaphylaxis during cuprophane membrane dialysis may represent an example of alternative pathway-mediated anaphylaxis. Complement activation probably results in biologically appreciable effects through the generation of the anaphylatoxins C3a and C5a, which have direct effects upon smooth muscle tone. Thus, they influence vascular tone diffusely, vasopermeability, and bronchial constriction. They may also act as mast cell secretagogues.

Anaphylaxis due to Presumptive Abnormalities of Arachidonic Acid Metabolism

Anaphylactic reactions due to aspirin or nonsteroidal anti-inflammatory drugs (NSAIDs) may occur in up to 1 per cent of the general population. Aspirin and NSAIDs inhibit cyclooxygenase, an enzyme which occurs early in the metabolic pathway and participates in the conversion of arachidonate to prostaglandins. However, the relationship of this pharmacological effect to the clinical syndrome remains to be identified. That there is a relationship is suggested by the fact that, although idiosyncratic reactors do not manifest intolerance to agents closely related structurally to aspirin (e.g. sodium salicylate or choline salicylate), do not show negative skin test reactivity to aspirin, and do not reveal any evidence of IgE antibodies directed against aspirin and related substances, they do commonly demonstrate precipitation of symptoms with the use of structurally unrelated NSAIDs which are cyclooxygenase inhibitors. Asthmatics who are aspirin-sensitive tend to manifest their intolerance by bronchospasm, whereas nonasthmatics or patients with perennial rhinitis tend to develop urticaria or angioedema. The explanation for these varied clinical expressions of aspirin intolerance is poorly understood.

Modifying Factors in EIA

	n	Per cent of total
Warm environment	127	64
Cold environment	46	23
High humidity	63	32
Recent food ingestion	108	54
Drug ingestion (e.g. aspirin)	25	13
Menstrual cycle	25	19*
Hot shower	20	5

*Percentage of 134 women

Fig. 27.3 Modifying factors in addition to exercise in 199 patients with exercise-induced anaphylaxis. (Adapted from Wade JP, Liang MH, Sheffer AL. In. *Biochemistry of Acute Allergic Reactions*: *Fifth International Symposium*. Alan R Liss, 1989, pp. 175–182.)

Anaphylaxis Associated with Direct Mast Cell-Degranulating Agents

Numerous agents have been reported to be capable of causing direct degranulation of mast cells with histamine release. The anaphylactoid or non-immunological stimulation of primarily cutaneous mast cells is often precipitated by opiates, curariform agents, compound 48/80, dextran, pentamidine, polymyxin B and other highly charged antibiotics, and radiocontrast media. The use of such direct mast cell-degranulating agents has occasionally been reported to be associated with the development of clinical anaphylaxis. In contrast to the IgE-mediated mechanism, anaphylaxis may occur upon initial exposure to such agents. The reasons underlying the apparent sensitivity of some individuals to such substances remain unclear.

Radiocontrast medium is probably the agent in this category of greatest clinical significance, and the intravenous route of contrast medium exposure is associated with the highest risk of reactions. Anaphylaxis may occur in 1–2 per cent of unselected patients, although some signs of anaphylaxis may be appreciated in up to 10 per cent of those undergoing infusion. Patients with a history of previous anaphylaxis secondary to radiocontrast medium have a risk as high as 35 per cent of anaphylaxis upon re-exposure.

Anaphylaxis Associated with Physical Stimuli

In some instances, development of physical stimuli may be associated with development of signs and symptoms of anaphylaxis.

Cold-induced urticaria

This is generally an annoying but not a serious problem, but it may be life-threatening if there is sudden exposure to cold over a large surface area of the skin. Some cases of cold-induced urticaria appear to be IgE-mediated.

Cholinergic urticaria

Rarely, symptoms suggestive of systemic anaphylaxis may occur in cholinergic urticaria, presumably due to massive mediator release.

Exercise-induced anaphylaxis (EIA)

EIA is a form of physical allergy presenting with episodes characterized initially by pruritus, urticaria, and erythema; sometimes it progresses to upper respiratory obstruction or vascular collapse (Fig 27.3).

Episodes occur in association with physical exertion. In contrast to other forms of physical allergy, however, development of the reaction does not invariably occur following the physical stimulus, suggesting that other factors may be important (Fig. 27.4). In some patients with this disorder, exercise following ingestion of a specific food appears essential. In others, exercise occurring in association with IgE-mediated inhalant allergy may be relevant. Exercise after food appears to promote the likelihood of the reaction in many patients, and to be requisite for the development of such reactions in some. In a few patients, exercise following the administration of aspirin or NSAIDs appears essential. Elevation of plasma histamine levels and ultrastructural evidence of mast cell degranulation on skin biopsy following exercise challenge in patients with EIA have supported the hypothesis that the mast cell plays a central role in the pathophysiology of this syndrome (Fig. 27.5). However, the pathophysiology is incompletely understood.

Idiopathic Anaphylaxis

Despite intensive investigation, there remain cases of anaphylaxis for which no cause can be determined. The diagnosis of idiopathic anaphylaxis should be made only after extensive investigation. A meticulous history may reveal an unrecognized precipitating factor. Clinical evaluation and laboratory studies should exclude an underlying systemic disorder (such as hereditary angioedema, vasculitis, mastocytosis, or carcinoid syndrome). Selective use of epicutaneous skin tests or RAST may occasionally be helpful in establishing an aetiology. Surreptitious self-administration of allergenic or pharmacologically active agents may need to be considered. As understanding of the interaction of mediators, neurohumoral factors, hormonal changes, physical stimuli, and other factors participating in anaphylaxis develops, it is likely that an increasing number of cases currently labelled 'idiopathic' will be explained.

Frequency and Duration of EIA Symptoms in 199 Individuals

Symptom	n*	Per cent of total
Pruritus	183	92
Urticaria	166	83
Angioedema	157	78
Cutaneous flushing	150	75
Respiratory symptoms	117	59
Profuse sweating	86	43
Fainting (syncope)	64	32
Headache	59	30
Gastrointestinal symptoms	59	30

*Each individual presented with several symptoms.

Fig. 27.4 Frequency and duration of EIA symptoms in 199 patients. (Adapted from Wade JP, Liang MH, Sheffer AL. In: *Biochemistry of Acute Allergic Reactions: Fifth International Symposium*. Alan R Liss,1989, pp. 175–182.)

Diagnosis

The diagnosis of systemic anaphylaxis is established on clinical grounds, and is usually straightforward. A complete differential diagnosis includes virtually all causes of respiratory obstruction and vascular collapse (e.g. pulmonary embolus, arrhythmia, cardiac tamponade, myocardial infarction, sepsis, seizure disorder, insulin reaction). Most of these are easily excluded. However, several elements in the differential diagnosis may require further attention.

Vasovagal reactions may superficially resemble anaphylaxis, with the abrupt development of pallor, sweating, and presyncope or overt loss of consciousness due to hypotension. Vasovagal reactions are generally associated with bradycardia, whereas in most cases anaphylaxis is accompanied by tachycardia. Upper respiratory obstruction and bronchospasm are absent in vasovagal reactions. Nausea may be experienced during vasovagal episodes, but abdominal pain is not a feature; nor are pruritus, urticaria, or angioedema.

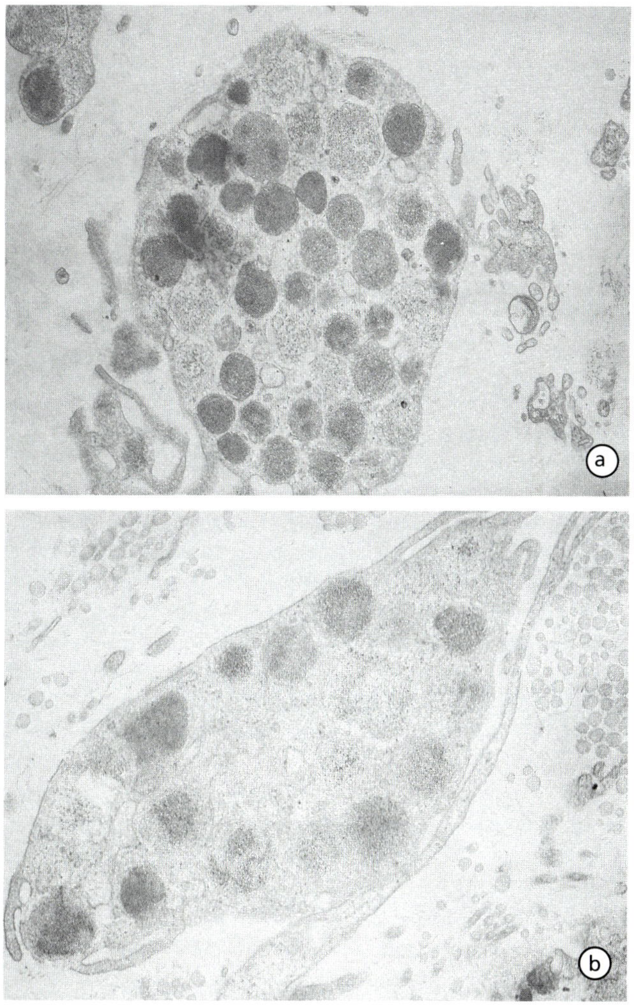

Fig. 27.5 Mast cells from patient with exercise-induced anaphylaxis. (a) Before exercise, the mast cell is indistinguishable from those of control subjects by cellular or subcellular (granules) criteria. (Original magnification × 10,000.) (b) Immediately after exercise, note loss of granule density indicative of degranulation. (Original magnification ×14,400.) (Courtesy of Professor G Murphy, additional photomicrographs from the study by Sheffer AL et al. *J Allergy Clin Immunol* 1985; **75**: 479–484.)

The diagnosis of globus hystericus must always be approached carefully, inasmuch as a patient who truly does have anaphylaxis may experience a subjective sensation of upper respiratory obstruction before the development of overt or obvious clinical findings. However, the careful evaluation of the patient with globus hystericus will reveal no anatomical evidence of upper respiratory obstruction (e.g. on X-ray or laryngoscopy), nor pruritus, urticaria or angioedema, flushing, gastrointestinal symptoms, or hypotension.

The syndromes of angioedema associated with deficiency of C1 esterase inhibitor are reminiscent of anaphylaxis, with manifestations of upper respiratory obstruction, angioedema, and colicky abdominal pain. However, pruritus, diffuse warmth, flushing, rhinitis, and vascular collapse do not form part of these syndromes. The evolution of cutaneous angioedema and of respiratory and abdominal symptoms during attacks in patients with angioedema secondary to C1 esterase inhibitor deficiency is generally slower than in patients with true anaphylaxis. Biochemically, documentation of the absence of C1 esterase inhibitor should be possible; but, as a screening test, documentation of reduction of C4 would be available more quickly. A normal C4 level essentially excludes the diagnosis of angioedema due to hereditary or acquired C1 esterase inhibitor deficiency. (By contrast, diminished C4 could be consistent with anaphylaxis on the basis of a complement-mediated process.)

Urticaria and angioedema may accompany serum sickness reactions. However, serum sickness is not associated with upper respiratory obstruction or bronchospasm, or with vascular collapse; it is by contrast associated with fever, adenopathy, arthralgias, and purpuric skin lesions.

Recurrent idiopathic anaphylaxis may need to be differentiated from mastocytosis or carcinoid syndrome. Systemic mastocytosis resembles idiopathic anaphylaxis in the occurrence of episodic attacks of flushing, urtication, rhinitis, and gastrointestinal symptoms. However, upper respiratory obstruction does not occur as part of the mastocytosis syndromes, and bronchospasm is infrequent and transient. In most patients with mastocytosis, a baseline level of symptomatology exists between acute exacerbations. The patient with mastocytosis will often have urticaria pigmentosa, and evidence of mast cell hyperplasia in skin, bone marrow, gastrointestinal tract, or other organs. It is important to remember that biochemical findings of increased plasma histamine and serum tryptase levels may be common to both conditions.

Carcinoid syndrome may be a consideration in the differential diagnosis of recurrent idiopathic anaphylaxis, given the occurrence of flushing, gastrointestinal symptoms and bronchospasm in both entities. However, urticaria or angioedema and upper respiratory obstruction do not occur as part of the carcinoid syndrome. The finding of increased plasma levels of serotonin or of increased urinary levels of 5-hydroxyindoleacetic acid (5-HIAA) will suggest the diagnosis, which can be confirmed with demonstration of the carcinoid tumour.

Scombroid poisoning results from ingestion of partially decomposed fish containing histamine that has been generated by action of histadine decarboxylase, a bacterial enzyme. Symptoms may resemble acute anaphylaxis.

Assessment of mast cell degranulation, morphologically or by assay of blood levels of released mast cell mediators, may permit the retrospective assessment of anaphylaxis. Elevated histamine levels are found in the plasma of patients with exercise-induced anaphylaxis who undergo experimental exercise challenge. Ultrastructural assessment by electron microscopy corroborates mast cell degranulation when such affected individuals undergo exercise challenge. Tryptase levels may remain elevated for up to six hours after antigen-induced anaphylaxis, with the most significant elevations occurring 1–2 hours following challenge.

Treatment

Therapy of systemic anaphylaxis may be subdivided into management of the acute episode, and subsequent evaluation and prophylaxis (Fig. 27.6).

Acute Management

Acute management of systemic anaphylaxis requires recognition of the nature of the episode. Prompt treatment is critical. Because airway obstruction and cardiovascular collapse account for most of the morbidity and mortality in anaphylaxis, initial therapy is directed at preservation of the airway, reversal of bronchospasm, and maintenance of blood pressure and tissue perfusion. Flushing, pruritus and urticaria may herald the onset of life-threatening respiratory or cardiovascular insufficiency. While mild cutaneous manifestations can usually be controlled with the use of H_1 and H_2 antihistamines, the possibility that respiratory or cardiovascular complications may develop necessitates continued observation of the patient. The use of subcutaneous adrenaline is the mainstay of treatment for more severe reactions. This agent has an inhibitory effect upon mast cell mediator release, in addition to its actions upon target organs (airway and vascular bed). Prompt administration of adrenaline (0.1%), 0.3 ml–0.5 ml (300–500 μg) adult dose, with an initial dose of 0.01 $ml.kg^{-1}$ up to 0.3 ml in children, is essential. Further antigen absorption should be reduced, if possible. For example, if antigen exposure has occurred via a sting on an extremity, a tourniquet may be applied proximal to the injection site and loosened for one minute every three minutes. Local injection of an additional dose of subcutaneous adrenaline (adult dose 0.1–0.3 ml of 0.1% dilution) to this site may also retard antigen absorption.

Readministration of subcutaneous adrenaline can be performed following the initial dose every 15–20 minutes, as clinical circumstances dictate. Intravascular volume repletion with crystalloid and, if necessary, colloid is critical in the patient with hypotension or shock. Considerable vascular pooling and third spacing may occur as a consequence of the vasopermeability and decreased vascular resistance seen in anaphylaxis. Occasionally, persistent hypotension despite administration of adrenaline and intravascular volume repletion may require the use of α-adrenergic agents. Obviously, careful monitoring of blood pressure and cardiac rhythm is critical in this setting.

Observation of the upper airway is essential in the patient with anaphylaxis. If necessary, intubation by endotracheal or nasotracheal route, or, if these are impossible, by tracheotomy, should be undertaken; and assisted mechanical ventilation may be necessary. Bronchospasm may be addressed with the use of inhalational β-agonists and intravenous aminophylline infusion. Oxygen by nasal prong or face mask is helpful.

Use of an H_1 antagonist in the clinical course is of clear benefit. Such agents may be administered intravenously, intramuscularly, or orally, depending upon circumstances and the severity of the clinical reaction. The use of H_2 antagonists is not as well documented; but on balance their administration appears warranted, particularly given that hypotension and cardiac arrhythmias appear to be secondary to effects mediated by both types of histamine receptors.

The slow onset of corticosteroids renders them of little use in the acute phase of anaphylaxis. However, the possibility of late reactions, either as a consequence of delayed antigen absorption or of the theoretically plausible late-phase reaction, probably justifies the use of corticosteroids in the treatment of anaphylaxis, although little objective evidence documents the efficacy of such drugs. Hydrocortisone is commonly administered intravenously in such situations because of the overt possibility of a biphasic or prolonged reaction, and because of its efficacy in treating idiopathic anaphylaxis.

The occurrence of bradycardia, associated with severe hypotension and a sluggish response to treatment, should alert the clinician to possible β-adrenergic blockade. Such cases may require more than the usual adrenaline therapy. However, difficulty in maintaining blood pressure and pulse may continue for several hours, and, occasionally, hypertension may complicate therapy as a result of unopposed α-adrenergic stimulation. Glucagon has not been proven consistently effective in overcoming β-adrenergic blockade in such situations.

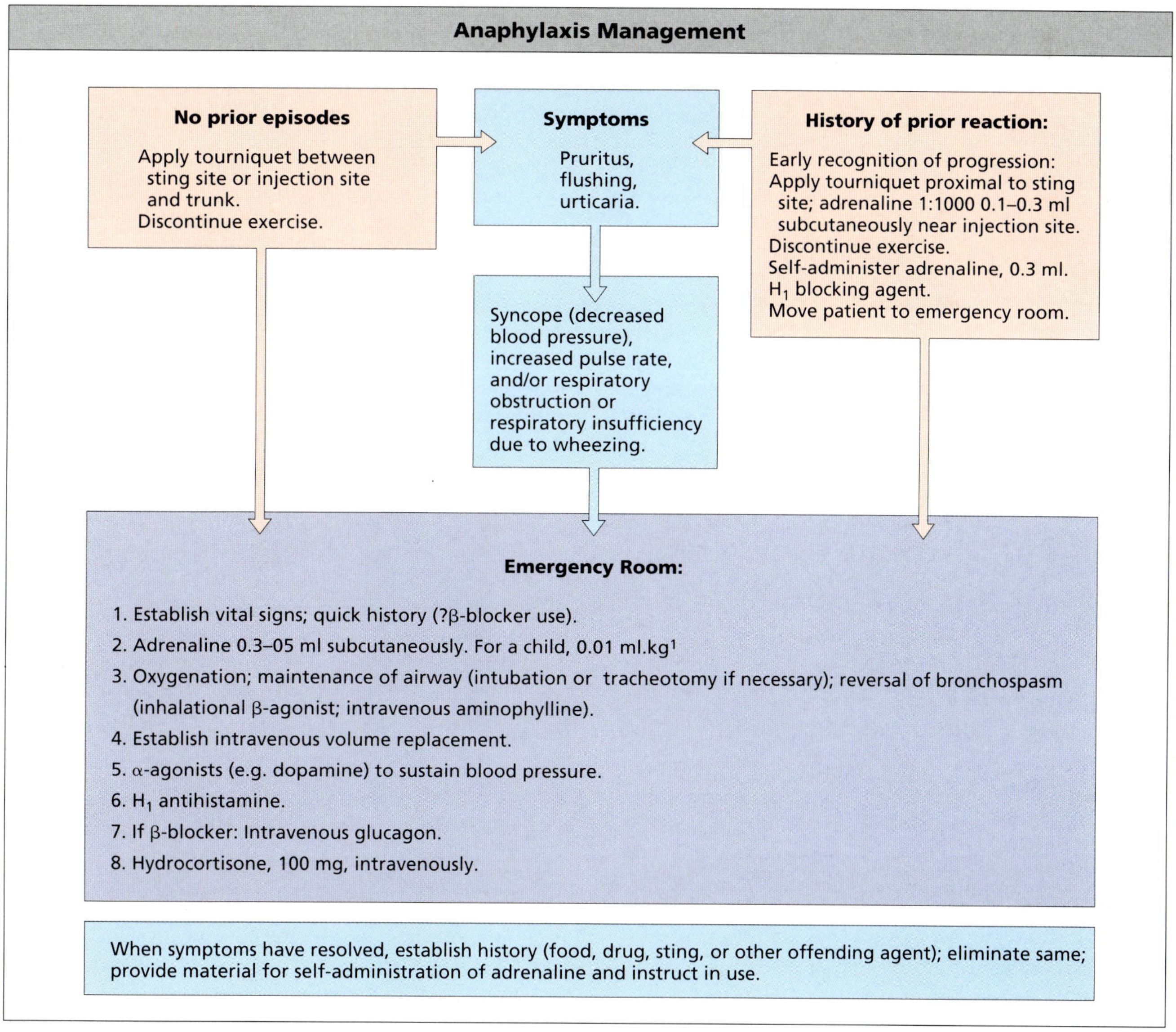
Anaphylaxis Management
No prior episodes
Apply tourniquet between sting site or injection site and trunk.
Discontinue exercise.
Symptoms
Pruritus, flushing, urticaria.
History of prior reaction:
Early recognition of progression:
Apply tourniquet proximal to sting site; adrenaline 1:1000 0.1–0.3 ml subcutaneously near injection site.
Discontinue exercise.
Self-administer adrenaline, 0.3 ml.
H_1 blocking agent.
Move patient to emergency room.
Syncope (decreased blood pressure), increased pulse rate, and/or respiratory obstruction or respiratory insufficiency due to wheezing.
Emergency Room:
1. Establish vital signs; quick history (?β-blocker use).
2. Adrenaline 0.3–05 ml subcutaneously. For a child, 0.01 ml.kg^{1}
3. Oxygenation; maintenance of airway (intubation or tracheotomy if necessary); reversal of bronchospasm (inhalational β-agonist; intravenous aminophylline).
4. Establish intravenous volume replacement.
5. α-agonists (e.g. dopamine) to sustain blood pressure.
6. H_1 antihistamine.
7. If β-blocker: Intravenous glucagon.
8. Hydrocortisone, 100 mg, intravenously.
When symptoms have resolved, establish history (food, drug, sting, or other offending agent); eliminate same; provide material for self-administration of adrenaline and instruct in use.

Fig. 27.6 A system for the management of anaphylaxis.

The possibility of prolonged, biphasic, or recrudescent anaphylaxis suggests the need for continued critical observation of the patient presenting with severe signs or symptoms. Such observation should optimally be continued for at least six to eight hours, or longer as the clinical course may require.

Prophylaxis

Prevention of anaphylaxis centres upon avoidance of known precipitating factors. Prior episodes of anaphylaxis, urticaria, angioedema, or unexplained adverse drug reactions should be carefully assessed. A thorough history, especially of recent ingestants and use of medications, including over-the-counter products, is crucial. Hypersensitivity to suspected antigens can be further evaluated by the use of selected RAST or skin tests. When extreme hypersensitivity is suspected, it may be preferable to perform RAST first; and, in performing skin testing, scratch and/or prick tests should be done in preference to intradermal tests.

Avoidance of known or suspected precipitants should be assiduously maintained. Occasionally, exposure to a known or suspected precipitant of anaphylaxis is unavoidable, while in other cases accidental exposure may occur despite rigorous efforts at avoidance. A therapeutic agent (or a closely related drug) known or strongly suspected to have been the cause of a prior episode of anaphylaxis (or of urticaria or angioedema) may be required for some compelling or even lifesaving indication. If there is no feasible alternative, evaluation of the patient's hypersensitivity by RAST or skin testing should be performed. In the case of penicillin, anaphylactic sensitivity tends to be associated with IgE antibodies directed against minor determinants.

If therapy is considered essential despite positive RAST or skin tests, the patient may undergo desensitization. The mechanism of acute desensitization is unclear, and protocols have been established for only a comparatively small number of drugs. The oral route of desensitization appears safer than parenteral routes. Patients with previous immediate-type reactions to radiocontrast media are at significant risk for anapylaxis on re-exposure. The likelihood of such a repeat reaction can be dramatically reduced by pretreatment with corticosteroids, H_1 antagonists, and ephedrine. Some therapeutic agents, e.g. heterologous serum or chymopapain are associated with a sufficiently high risk of reaction for assessment of hypersensitivity prior to their initial use to be warranted.

Latex anaphylaxis is increasingly recognized, and its incidence is particularly high in medical personnel. The process appears to represent IgE-mediated hypersensitivity to the natural latex protein (as opposed to rubber additives, e.g. mercaptobenzothiazole, thiurams, carbamates, and phenylenediamine, which appear causative in contact eczema due to rubber). Onset may be insidious, beginning with mild pruritus or urticaria on contact with latex, and progressing to full-blown anaphylaxis. Non-latex surgical and examination gloves are available and should be used by those affected. The use of latex devices in dental surgery and latex barium enema nozzles can also be associated with the development of anaphylaxis in sensitive individuals, and should be avoided.

Seminal plasma anaphylaxis is an unusual cause of anaphylaxis and is best treated by avoidance of contact with ejaculate. Spontaneous improvement begins to occur, but immunotherapy facilitates and accelerates the induction of tolerance.

Individuals with anaphylaxis due to Hymenoptera stings should be instructed to avoid settings which carry an increased chance of being stung, and they should wear dark-coloured clothes to diminish the likelihood of a sting. They should carry materials for self-administration of adrenaline on their persons, as well as a medical identification tag or bracelet. Skin testing to Hymenoptera venoms should be performed. In the sensitive patient, venom-specific immunotherapy greatly reduces the chance of a serious reaction on re-sting, and should be strongly considered in such patients.

Food-associated anaphylaxis requires identification of the specific food allergen, and then its avoidance. The history is usually revealing in such patients, and subsequent RAST or skin testing is often simply confirmatory in nature. Affected patients should scrupulously avoid the food(s) to which they are sensitive, and closely-related foods. Particular care needs to be exercised when eating away from home. It is advisable for such patients, also, to carry materials for adrenaline self-administration, and to wear a medical alert tag.

Patients with exercise-induced anaphylaxis (EIA) should be advised to discontinue exercise upon the earliest premonitory symptoms of an attack (e.g. pruritus). Although the early administration of H_1 antagonists may blunt further evolution of an incipient attack, they should not be relied upon for protection. Patients should carry materials for adrenaline self-administration in the event of more serious symptoms (upper respiratory obstruction or a feeling of faintness), and wear appropriate medical identification. If possible, they should exercise only with a companion apprised of their condition. Patients with EIA should be urged not to exercise for at least six hours following ingestion of food. Those whose attacks are dependent upon prior ingestion of a specific food should, of course, avoid that food. Rarely, exercise during the patient's inhalant allergy season may be associated with attacks, and exercise during the season should therefore be avoided or carefully limited. Exercise during periods of elevated ambient temperature is correlated with an increased likelihood of attacks, and caution should be exercised in this setting. The use of aspirin or NSAIDs should be avoided prior to exercise, and affected women should consider deferring exercise in close proximity to their menstrual period.

Patients with cold-induced urticaria should avoid situations in which sudden cold exposure of a large area of skin (such as immersion in cold water) might occur.

Patients with one or more episodes of anaphylaxis without a defined aetiology are described as having idiopathic anaphylaxis. In these cases, no clear aetiology is apparent following detailed historical review, laboratory and skin tests, ingestant diaries, and the like. The empiric avoidance of aspirin, other NSAIDs, and preservative- and dye-containing foods may be helpful in some cases. A number of patients will require maintenance therapy with H_1 and H_2 antagonists and, in some cases, daily or alternate-day corticosteroids in order to control recurrent life-threatening episodes. Such patients, as well as others at increased risk of anaphylaxis, whether from Hymenoptera stings, food allergy, exercise-induced urticaria, or patients on immunotherapy, should avoid the use of β-adrenergic blocking drugs because of the associated risk of severe or refractory anaphylaxis.

Prognosis

The prognosis after an anaphylactic attack is contingent upon early recognition and prompt institution of appropriate therapy. Often, the route of drug administration, sensitivity of the recipient, and the duration of the latent period provide some insight into the prognosis. However, patients have succumbed despite the availability of optimal therapy, and when there has been no delay in implementing maximal therapeutic manoeuvres. Cardiovascular complications often delay recovery. Once recovery has occurred, a continued asymptomatic state depends upon the patient's ability to avoid further exposure to the responsible antigen or other precipitating factor.

After the successful reversal of the symptoms of anaphylaxis, attention should be directed towards the detailed historical definition of aetiological factors provoking anaphylactic episodes. Once identified, such agents should be avoided. Finally, all individuals subject to anaphylaxis without specific contra-indication should carry adrenaline and some identification of the implicated allergen.

Further Reading

Greenberger PA, Patterson R, Radin RC. Two pretreatment regimens for high-risk patients receiving radiographic contrast media. *J Allergy Clin Immunol*, 1984; **74**: 540.

James LP, Austen KF. Fatal systemic anaphylaxis in man. *New Eng J Med*, 1964; **270**: 597.

Lang DM, Alpern MB, Visintainer PF, Smith ST. Increased risk for anaphylactoid reaction from contrast media in patients on beta-adrenergic bonders or with asthma. *Ann Intern Med*, 1991; **115**: 270.

Lieberman P. The use of antihistamines in the prevention and treatment of anaphylaxis and anaphylactoid reactions. *J Allergy Clin Immunol*, 1990; **86**; 684.

Sale SR, Greenberger PA, Patterson R. Idiopathic anaphylactic reactions. *J Am Med Assoc*, 1984; **246**: 2336.

Schwartz LB, Metcalfe DD, Miller JS, et al. Tryptase levels as an indicator of mast cell activation in systemic anaphylaxis and mastocystosis. *New Eng J Med*, 1987; **316**: 1622.

Sheffer AL, Austen KF. (1985) Exercise-induced anaphylaxis. *J Allergy Clin Immunol*, 1985; **73**: 699.

Stark BJ, Sullivan TJ. Biphasic and protracted anaphylaxis. *J Allergy Clin Immunol*, 1986; **78**: 76.

Sussman GL, Tarlow S, Dolovich J. The spectrum of IgE-mediated responses to latex. *J Am Med Assoc*, 1991; **265**,: 2844.

Szczeklik A. (1987) Adverse reactions to aspirin and nonsteroidal antiinflammatory drugs. *Ann Allergy*, 1987; **59**: 113.

Valentine MD, Lichtenstein LM. Anaphylaxis and stinging insect hypersensitivity. In: Lockey RF, Bukantz SC, eds: *Primer on Allergic and Immunologic Diseases*, *J Am Med Assoc*, 1987; **258**: 2881.

Wasserman SI, Marquardt DL. Anaphylaxis. In: Middleton E Jr, Reed CE, Ellis EF, et al. *Allergy Principles and Practice, 3rd Edition*. St. Louis: Mosby, 1988.

Wiggins CA, Dykewicz MS, Patterson R. Idiopathic anaphylaxis: Classification, evaluation, and treatment of 123 patients. *J Allergy Clin Immunol*, 1988; **82**: 849.

Wong S, Yarnold PR, Yano C, Patterson R, Harris KE. Outcome of prophylactic therapy for idiopathic anaphylaxis. *Ann Intern Med*, 1991; **114**: 133.

Chapter 28

Drug Allergy

Introduction

Adverse reactions to drugs are a significant problem in the practice of medicine. In hospitalized patients the incidence of such reactions may be as high as 30 per cent. Many of these reactions result from drug interactions or predictable side effects which are dose related. Some acute drug reactions appear to be restricted to a susceptible subset of the general population. Exaggerated side effects, often at low doses, afflict some patients because of an intolerance which may have a metabolic basis, e.g. theophylline-associated tachycardia in a patient with hyperthyroidism. In contrast, idiosyncratic reactions do not depend upon pharmacological toxicity, but rather upon drug-induced biological aberrations which may be the consequence of genetically determined metabolic disorders. The best studied example of a defined drug indiosyncracy is primaquine-sensitive haemolytic anaemia which depends upon deficiency of the enzyme G6PD. The mechanism of most idiosyncratic drug reactions remains obscure, and is the province of the new discipline of pharmacogenetics.

Immune Mechanisms of Drug Allergy

Type I Reactions

Idiosyncratic reactions to drugs are to be distinguished from allergic drug reactions. Allergic reactions to drugs depend upon a drug-specific immune reponse. The clinical manifestations can be as varied as the spectrum of immunopathology. Take penicillin allergy, for example – the most prevalent drug allergy. If penicillin administration engenders an IgE (reaginic) antibody response, primed mast cells and basophils will be triggered by subsequent treatment to degranulate, and immediate hypersensitivity reactions presenting as anaphylaxis, urticaria, or bronchoconstriction may ensue. This is the so-called Type I allergic reaction of Gell and Coombs (Fig. 28.1).

Type II Reactions

If the drug-induced antibody response is largely IgG and/or IgM, then complement-mediated cytoxicity may follow. An example is penicillin-induced Coombs positive haemolytic anaemia, in which the drug or its metabolite binds to the erythrocyte membrane, and antibody produced against the drug or the modified cell membrane binds to its target and fixes complement, resulting in cell destruction. These reactions, termed Type II hypersensitivity, may also occur via the adsorption of drug-antibody immune complexes to cell membranes, or through the induction of autoantibodies directed against blood group antigens (see Fig. 28.2).

Type III Reactions

Type III reactions are characterized by the formation of antibody/drug immune complexes. The size of the immune complex determines its site of deposition and the resultant immune injury. In the case of penicillin, drug fever is a common presentation, although serum sickness, rash, arthralgias, lymphadenopathy, palpable purpura, or urticaria also may be mediated by immune complexes.

Type IV Reactions

With improved containment of drugs during manufacture and dispersal, Type IV (cell-mediated) drug

Type I Drug Hypersensitivity

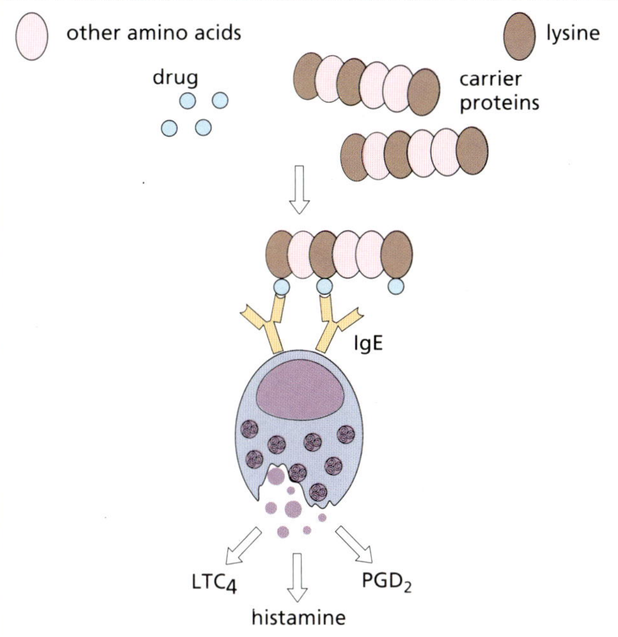

Fig. 28.1 Events of type I drug hypersensitivity. A low molecular weight drug (hapten) covalently binds to a carrier protein to form a complete antigen. This complex is able to cross-link specific IgE receptors on the mast cell or basophil membrane with subsequent degranulation and release of mediators, such as histamine.

hypersensitivity now occurs infrequently. These reactions are the result of drug interactions with T lymphocytes and they are usually associated with topically applied medications. An example is penicillin-induced dermatitis, which occurs primarily through occupational exposure in nurses, pharmacists, and those involved in antibiotic manufacture and packaging.

Risk Factors for Drug Allergy

Several risk factors for drug allergy have been identified. Host factors include age; adults have a higher incidence of allergic reactions to penicillin than do paediatric patients. Underlying genetic or metabolic factors such as the ability to mount an antibody reponse also play a role. In a study of 60 inpatients who received a high dose of penicillin, only about half of them mounted a serological IgG and/or IgE response to the major penicillin determinant. The persistence of drug-specific antibodies after their elicitation clearly increases the risk for future reactions. Among treatment-related factors the most important is the chemical propensity of a drug to serve as a hapten. Macromolecular drugs may function as complete antigens in that they are independently capable of inducing immune responses. Examples of this include horse anti-toxins, insulin, and chymopapain. Low molecular weight drugs, such as penicillin and sulphonamides, however, must first bind to a macromolecular carrier, usually a serum or cell surface protein, by forming covalent bonds. This process is known as haptenation. It is through this process that low molecular weight drugs can present multivalent signals to the immune system, an absolute requirement for immunogenicity. Drugs such as penicillin which form such multivalent complexes are relatively allergenic. Drugs which are inert in this respect are only weakly immunogenic and therefore only rarely allergenic.

Other treatment-related factors depend upon the dose and duration of treatment. Drug-induced serum sickness, interstitial nephritis and cytopenias are more frequent with high dose, long-term therapy. Longer treatment periods increase the length of exposure and therefore, the period of risk. The route of drug administration is also a risk factor. For example, a high rate of contact sensitization has been seen with topical penicillins. It has been suggested that parenteral administration of penicillin is more likely to induce adverse reactions than oral administration, but recent observations indicate that this may be more related to dose than route. Comparable doses of a parenteral and an oral penicillin produce similar rates of reaction, except for repository penicillins, such as benzathine penicillin, which elicit reactions more frequently despite being used in lower doses. The more often a drug is used, the more likely it is that an allergic reaction will be elicited, since IgE antibodies have a finite half-life in most sensitized individuals.

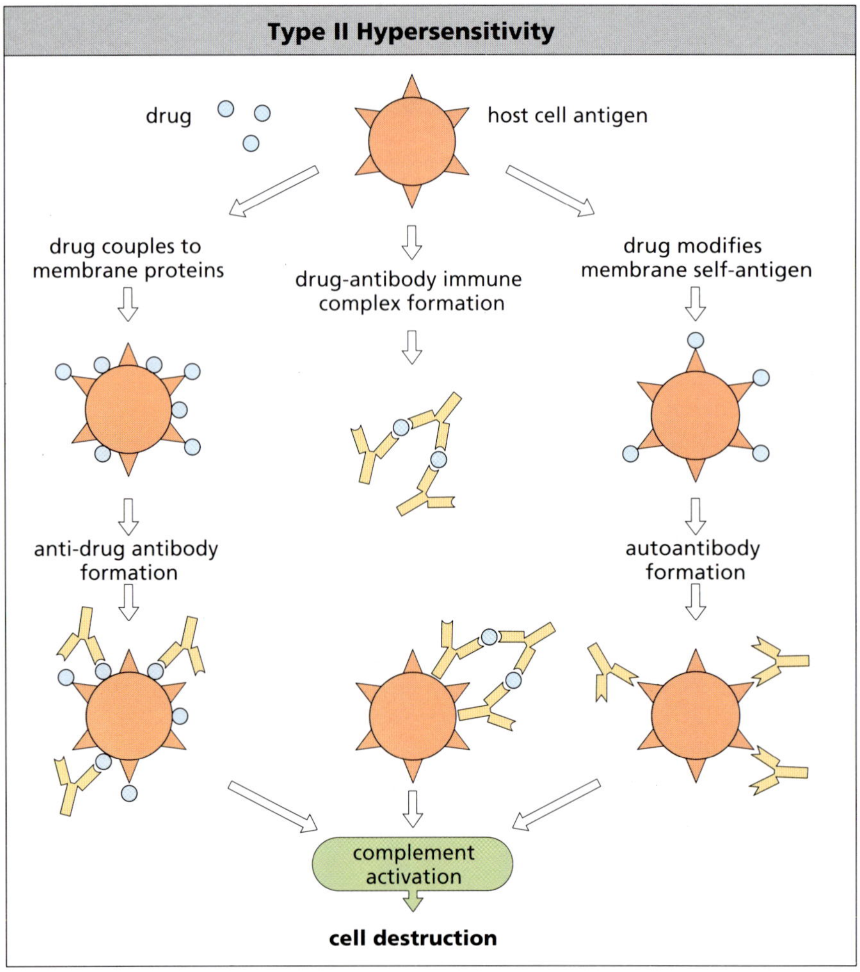

Fig. 28.2 Mechanisms of type II drug hypersensitivity. Complement-mediated cell destruction may occur via several mechanisms. [left] Drug is covalently linked to the host cell membrane. Anti-drug IgG then binds to the drug and activates complement (e.g. penicillin). [middle] Circulating drug and antibody form immune complexes which affix to cell membranes and trigger the complement cascade (e.g. cephalosporins). [right] Drug binds to the cell membrane, but the immune response is directed against the altered host cell. Auto-antibodies are produced, bind to the cell (even in the absence of drug) and activate complement (e.g. α-methyl-dopa).

Diagnosis

History and Physical Examination

A carefully elicited history is often sufficient to identify hypersensitivity reactions. All medications taken should be reviewed, whether or not they were well tolerated in the past. The routes and frequency of administration along with a history of prior exposures can be useful; for example, intermittent parental administration can predispose to allergic drug reactions. The time between the introduction of medications and the onset of symptoms is very helpful since a primary immune response often requires 10–14 days, whereas a rapid onset of symptoms may suggest an idiosyncratic reaction, especially upon first exposure. With prior sensitization, however, immune-mediated events can and often do occur promptly after the first dose. Characterization of the clinical features of the reaction, by history and physical examination if possible, is also helpful in differentiating between allergic and non-allergic drug reactions. Knowledge of the sensitizing potential of common drugs which are in common use is presented in Fig. 28.3.

Immunological Tests in the Diagnosis of Drug Allergy

Intradermal skin tests

Of the many immunological tests evaluated for drug allergy, only intradermal skin testing for IgE antibody has been shown to have strong predictive value. The role of skin testing has become most clinically relevant in the care of patients with a history of penicillin allergy. Most patients with IgE-mediated reactions demonstrate a decline in drug-specifc IgE over time, and tolerate readministration of penicillin without adverse outcome if penicillin skin test reverts to negative. Skin tests can be performed within 15 minutes and may be used to identify those patients who may safely receive penicillin when β-lactam therapy is indicated. Besides penicillin skin testing, intradermal testing has proven useful in the evaluation of allergy to other sensitizing drugs (Fig. 28.4)

Allergenic Drugs in Common Use	
Haptenic drugs	**Complete antigens**
penicillins cephalosporins sulphonamides (including antimicrobials, Sulphasalazine, oral hypoglycaemics, thiazides, and Diazoxide) muscle relaxants anti-tuberculous drugs anti-convulsants thiopental quinidine cis-platinum	insulin enzymes (chymopapain, asparaginase) foreign anti-toxins organ extracts (ACTH, hormones) vaccines

Fig. 28.3 A list of the drugs in everyday use which most commonly cause allergic reactions.

Radioallergosorbent test

Penicillin-specific IgE antibody can be measured by alternative methods which include radioallergosorbent testing (RAST) for measurement of IgE antibody in serum. The RAST detects drug-specific IgE but is less sensitive than intradermal skin tests and, therefore, less preferred. Although they are not available for routine clinical use, RAST tests have also been developed for other β-lactam antibiotics, sulphonamides, trimethoprim, isoniazid, and other drug determinants.

Leucocyte histamine release

Leucocyte histamine release can also detect specific IgE antibodies but is not diagnostically reliable for evaluation of IgE antibodies to haptenic drugs. Other cellular tests, e.g. lymphocyte proliferation and cytokine induction tests, may be useful in establishing a drug-specific immune response, but the results often correlate better with recent drug exposure than with allergic reactions.

Provocative challenge

When skin testing or RAST cannot be performed, provocative challenge may be helpful in deciding which one of concomitantly administered drugs was responsible for a reaction. This should be performed by experienced physicians under close supervision.

Patch tests

Patch testing is a skin-test modality with only occasional use in the evaluation of drug allergy; its use is confined largely to cases of reactions to topical medications and to preservatives, and for assessment of industrial contact sensitivities. Chemicals, such as neomycin sulphate or parabens, may be directly applied to the skin to induce a localized dermatitis which is interpreted 48–72 hours later. Patch testing is not recommended for the evaluation of reactions induced by orally or parentally administered drugs.

Treatment

Acute Drug Reactions

In an acute drug reaction, the offending drug should be discontinued. If the patient is on multiple medications, those drugs that are known to be most sensitizing and least necessary to the patient should be stopped empirically until the reaction abates. Symptomatic therapy may be instituted, depending upon

Drugs for which Intradermal Skin Testing may be Useful	
penicillin cephalosporins insulin chymopapain local anaesthetics muscle relaxants thiopental	foreign anti-toxins anti-tuberculous drugs anti-convulsants quinidine cis-platinum Penicillamine

Fig. 28.4 A list of the drugs for which intradermal testing has proven useful in the evaluation of allergy.

the nature of the reaction. Corticosteroids may be indicated for severe systemic reactions, including extensive exanthems accompanied by fever and/or nephritis, serum sickness, exfoliative dermatitis, or toxic epidermal necrolysis (Lyell's syndrome). Systemic anaphylaxis may require aggressive cardiovascular support with fluids and vasopressor agents.

Alternatives for Patients with Drug Allergies

Therapy with non-cross-reactive drugs

Preventive strategies for drug therapy in individuals with drug allergies are based upon the selection of appropriate substitute drugs that are not immunologically cross-reactive. If this is not possible, gradual dose escalation of potentially cross-reactive drugs may be used to minimize the risk. Acute desentitization may be performed for documented Type I allergy if medical necessity warrants it.

In the majority of clinical situations, appropriate alternative drugs exist and may be used without concern for adverse outcomes. For example, for penicillin allergic patients, one or more non-β-lactam antibiotics are usually acceptable in most infectious diseases. Drugs of similar structure may often be cross-reactive immunologically and clinically. However, such cross-reactivity is incomplete. For example, for patients allergic to insulin derived from animal sources, recombinant human insulin can usually be substituted, even though partial cross-reactivity exists. Similarly, many subjects with penicillin allergies will tolerate cephalosporins, despite the common β-lactam nuclear structure which penicillins and cephalosporins share.

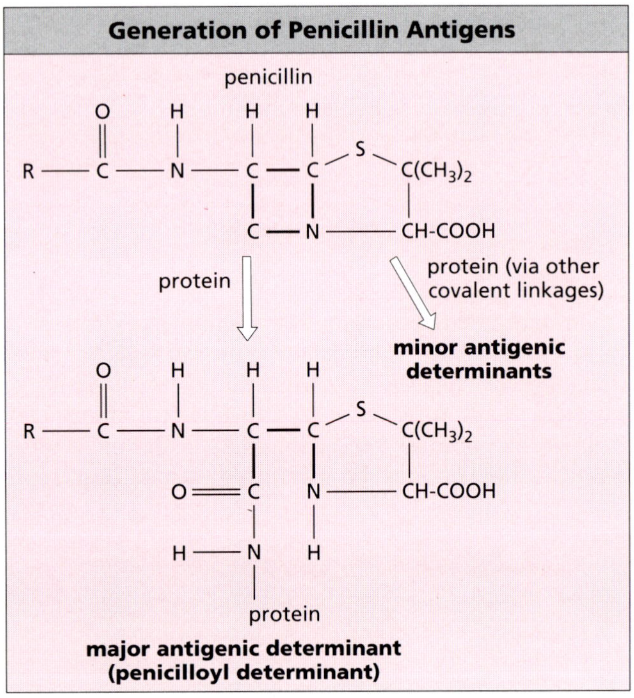

Fig. 28.5 Generation of penicillin antigens under physiological conditions *in vivo*. The β-lactam ring spontaneously opens to form a covalent bond with serum proteins. This neoantigen is known as the penicilloyl determinant. Other covalent linkages may also occur, creating minor antigenic determinants.

Drug desensitization

Infrequently, certain medical conditions cannot be successfully treated with alternative therapy. In these instances, drug desensitization is a necessary option. Standard protocols for penicillin and insulin desensitization have been developed and found to be relatively safe and effective though not without risk. They require informed consent as well as supervision by a physician, and an intensive care settng should be used whenever possible. Desensitization protocols are based upon the principal of administering gradually increasing doses of drug beginning with a very small dose and working toward a full therapeutic dose. Dose increments may be introduced as frequently as every 20–30 minutes, with full therapeutic dose tolerance achieved in 24–48 hours (see below).

The elicitation of clinical tolerance by acute drug desensitization is usually attributed to the induction by low-dose antigen of a desensitized state in IgE-primed cells, so that a higher antigen threshold is necessary for mediator release. Regardless of the mechanism, the state of tolerance is transient and must be actively maintained by continuous drug administration once achieved. If the patient has need for the sensitizing drug in the future and skin tests are still positive, desensitization must be repeated.

Special Considerations

A variety of drugs merit special mention. These are drugs in common use which have been observed to induce a variety of adverse reactions by both immune and non-immune mechanisms. Drug reactions which have clinical features of allergic reactions but have a non-immunological or idiosyncratic mechanism have been termed 'pseudoallergic' or 'anaphylactoid'.

β-lactam Antibiotics

Penicillin

Penicillins are responsible for more allergic drug reactions than any other group of drugs in common use. This high allergy profile is due both to the huge quantities of penicillins administered, and to the avid protein reactivity of this class of drugs. Under physiological conditions, the β-lactam ring in the penicillin nucleus opens to form a covalent bond with serum proteins, creating the penicilloyl determinant (Fig. 28.5). This neoantigen is termed the major determinant of penicillin allergy because more than 95 per cent of penicillin antibodies recognize this determinant. Other chemical interactions are involved in the formation of minor determinants. Most anaphylactic reactions are due to IgE antibody specific for minor determinants. Penicillin itself is an inefficient reagent for skin testing since it must conjugate with tissue proteins to form multivalent complexes to elicit IgE-dependent mast cell degranulation. To produce an active major determinant for skin tests, penicillin is coupled to polylysine to form penicilloyl-polylysine (PPL), which is commercially available. Used alone, PPL identifies between 80 and 90 per cent of patients at risk for IgE-dependent penicillin allergy. A minor determinant mixture is commercially available in Europe but currently lacks a pharmaceutical sponsor in the USA. This reagent identifies additional individuals who are at risk for acute penicillin allergy.

Methodological considerations in the application and interpretation of penicillin skin tests deserve mention. Epicutaneous (puncture testing) should precede intradermal testing, and tests should include the documentation of satisfactory positive (histamine or codeine) and negative controls. Patients who are severely ill, hypotensive, or receiving H_1 antihistamines or related drugs sometimes fail to react to the positive control and may demonstrate falsely negative Type I skin tests. Adverse reactions to properly performed skin tests are rare (less than 1 per cent), and most of these reactions are mild and resolve without treatment. Penicillin skin testing is usually indicated for those patients who are being denied penicillin because of a previous allergic reaction. Skin tests have no predictive value for non-IgE mediated reactions, including drug fever, exfoliative dermatitis, maculopapular exanthems, serum sickness, interstitial nephritis or haemolytic anaemia. Test results provide information only about the current state of Type I hypersensitivity, since drug allergy may wane with time, and repeat testing at a later date may yield a negative result.

Penicillin skin testing produces positive results in 15–65 per cent of patients with histories of penicillin allergy. This wide range for the prevalence of positive skin tests in patients with a suggestive history probably reflects differences in time elapsed since the last reaction and differing patient selection criteria. The predictive value of negative penicillin skin tests is now well established (Fig. 28.6). There are no reports of penicillin anaphylaxis in individuals with negative skin tests. Approximately 1 per cent of patients with positive histories but negative skin tests develop transient urticaria and/or pruritus. These individuals may safely receive β-lactam antibiotics again since the risk of a life-threatening IgE-mediated reaction is negligible following negative skin tests. Penicillin administration and penicillin skin testing is contraindicated in patients with a history of drug-induced exfoliative dermatitis, Stevens-Johnson syndrome, or Lyell's syndrome.

RAST is available for the measurement of anti-benzyl penicilloyl IgE antibody, but this test is less sensitive than PPL skin testing in detecting penicillin hypersensitivity and has useful predictive value only when positive. At the time of writing, RAST tests for minor determinant IgE have not been successful.

Occasionally, skin test positive individuals require penicillin therapy for the treatment of diseases such as enterococcal endocarditis and neurosyphilis. The cross-reactivity of all penicillins and most β-lactams makes the use of semi-synthetic penicillins and cephalosporins hazardous. For these situations, desensitization may be performed. Acute desensitization should by carried out with the desired penicillin using the precautions described above. The oral or parenteral route may be used following a protocol as outlined in Fig. 28.7. Once clinical tolerance to the

The Predictive Value of Penicillin Skin Tests

history of penicillin allergy	+		−	
penicillin skin test status	+	−	+	−
frequency of allergic reactions associated with penicillin administration	50–70%	1–3%	10%	0.5%

Fig. 28.6 The frequency of IgE-dependent reactions to penicillin therapy following skin testing in history-positive and history-negative subjects.

Penicillin Desensitization Protocol

Oral: Penicillin V every 15 minutes Step	Dose (units)	Parenteral: Penicillin G every 20 minutes Dose (units/ml)	Volume (ml)	Route
1	100	100	0.1	intradermal
2	200	100	0.2	subcutaneous
3	400	100	0.4	subcutaneous
4	800	100	0.8	subcutaneous
5	1 600	1 000	0.1	intradermal
6	3 200	1 000	0.3	subcutaneous
7	6 400	1 000	0.6	subcutaneous
8	12 000	10 000	0.1	intradermal
9	24 000	10 000	0.2	subcutaneous
10	48 000	10 000	0.4	subcutaneous
11	80 000	10 000	0.8	subcutaneous
12	160 000	100 000	0.1	intradermal
13	320 000	100 000	0.3	subcutaneous
14	640 000	100 000	0.6	subcutaneous
Change to intravenous Penicillin G				
15	125 000	1 000 000	0.1	intradermal
16	250 000	1 000 000	0.2	subcutaneous
17	500 000	1 000 000	0.2	intramuscular
18	1 125 000	1 000 000	0.4	intramuscular
19		1 000 000 continuous intravenous infusion		

Fig. 28.7 Recommended guidelines for penicillin desensitization in allergic subjects.

antibiotic is achieved, it may be continued with virtually no risk of anaphylaxis, although other non-life-threatening IgE-mediated reactions such as urticaria may develop intermittently during therapy.

Cephalosporins and other β-lactam antibiotics
The general structural features of β-lactam antibiotics are shown in Fig. 28.8. Cephalosporins have a similar nuclear structure to penicillin, including a common β-lactam ring. Estimates of clinical cross-reactivity vary from 10 to 50 per cent, despite clear immunologic cross-reactivity among penicillin antibodies. Skin testing is helpful when positive at concentrations which do not produce a skin response in non-allergic subjects. Because cross-reactivity cannot be definitively ruled out by skin tests, patients with positive penicillin skin tests should only receive cephalosporins with proper precautions which may include a small test dose or gradual dose escalation.

For carbapenems such as imipenem, significant skin test cross-reactivity with penicillin has been observed. Consequently, it is recommended that carbapenem therapy be withheld in penicillin allergic patients. In contrast, the monocyclic β-lactams, of which aztreonam is the prototype, may safely be given to penicillin allergic patients because aztreonam has shown negligible cross-reactivity with penicillins and cephalosporins.

Sulphonamides
One of the most commonly used sulphonamide preparations, trimethoprim-sulphamethoxazole induces a skin rash in about 3 per cent of hospitalized patients not infected with the human immunodeficiency virus (HIV). In HIV-infected individuals undergoing treatment for *Pneumocystis carinii* pneumonia, however, rash prevalence increases over tenfold. The reason for this increased morbidity is unclear, but may be related to alterations in drug metabolism, possibly leading to enhanced haptenation of proteins.

Another sulphonamide, sulphapyridine, is primarily used in the treatment of inflammatory bowel disease. Hypersensitivity reactions occur in 2 per cent of patients and consist of macular rash and/or drug fever. Clinical tolerance has been successfully induced when gradual dose escalation has been implemented by the oral route. This desensitization regimen is not useful for toxic reactions such as nausea, vomiting, and headache. Desensitization is also contraindicated in patients with a history of severe systemic reactions, including Stevens-Johnson syndrome, Lyell's syndrome, agranulocytosis, or fibrosing alveolitis.

Other chemically related sulphonamides may be cross-reactive. These include sulphon-urea oral hypoglycaemic agents, diuretics (thiazides, frusemide [furosemide], chlorthalidone, and quinethazone) and diaxozide.

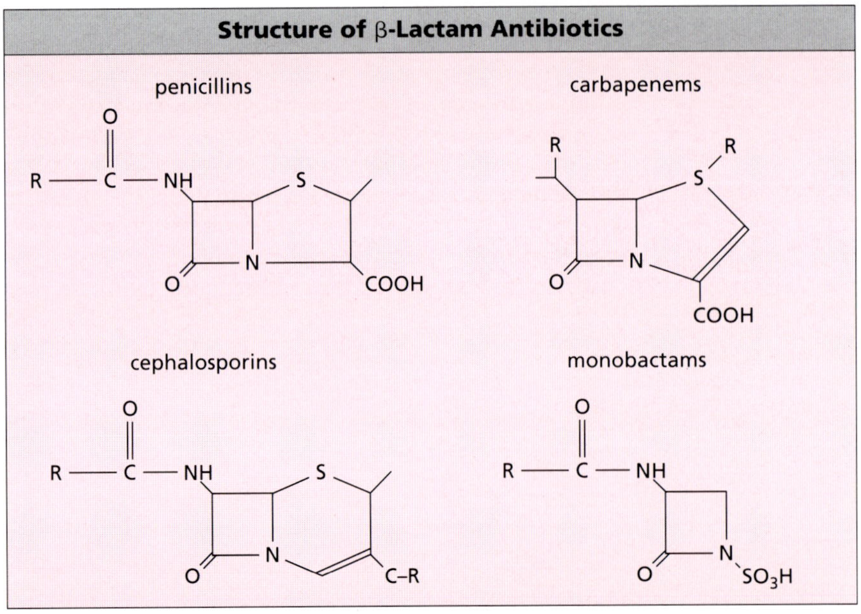

Fig. 28.8 Chemical structures of four commonly used β-lactam antibiotics.

Hypersensitivity Reactions Associated with Non-β-lactam Antibiotics

Drug	Fever	Skin rash	Eosinophilia	Other
aminoglycosides	+	+		contact dermatitis (neomycin)
Tetracycline	+	+	+	phototoxic–dermatitis
Vancomycin	+	+	+	skin rubour and flushing
Erythromycin		+		cholestatic hepatitis
Clindamycin	+	+	+	Stevens–Johnson syndrome
Chloramphenicol	+	+	+	pancytopaenia
Nitrofurantoin	+	+	+	hypersensitivity pneumonitis
anti-tuberculous drugs	+	+		lupus-like syndrome (rifampicin)

Fig. 28.9 The most common manifestations of hypersensitivity reactions to various non-β-lactam antibiotics.

Other Antimicrobials

Fig. 28.9 provides a listing of drug reactions commonly seen with the use of other antimicrobial agents.

Insulin and other Hormones

Bovine and porcine insulins differ from human insulin by three and one amino acids respectively and stimulate an IgG antibody response in most patients receiving them. Fifty per cent of them make IgE antibody early in the course of therapy. Reports of insulin allergy have decreased coincident with the introduction of recombinant human insulin. Cross-reactivity with previously induced IgE antibody as well as neoantigenic determinants such as alterations in tertiary structure may account for most residual reactions to human recombinant insulin.

Human recombinant insulin reactions occur in as many as 10 per cent of patients and consist mainly of local itching and swelling at the injection site. Such reactions occur within one to four weeks of the initiation of therapy or sooner if prior exposure has occurred. Local reactions usually resolve spontaneously in four weeks with continued insulin treatment. Treatment options are outlined in Fig. 28.10.

Systemic allergy to insulin is rare, occurring in less than 0.5 per cent of patients. The clinical history is usually notable for prior interruptions in insulin therapy, but a history of large local reactions is sometimes reported. If a mild systemic reaction occurs and continued insulin therapy is indicated, therapy should not be discontinued or interrupted. Accepted guidelines suggest that the next dose is reduced by one-third, then gradually increased by 2–5 units with each dose until therapeutic doses are tolerated. If this is not successful, insulin desensitization may be performed. Once desensitization has been completed, therapy should not be discontinued.

Other exogenous hormones of animal origin in clinical use have been associated with urticaria, angioedema and other allergic reactions. These reactions may be due to species-related structural differences or contaminants from the manufacturing process. Implicated hormones include ACTH, pituitary gland extracts, thyroxin, steroids and rarely, oestrogens and androgens.

Protamine

Derived from salmon milt, protamine is used in vascular procedures to reverse the effects of heparin and in insulin preparations to slow absorption. Adverse reactions include urticaria, bronchoconstriction, increased pulmonary artery pressure, hypotension, and death. Individuals with previous exposure during intravascular catheterization or coronary artery bypass surgery are at risk from protamine reactions, as are diabetics receiving protamine-containing insulin preparations. In insulin-treated diabetics, protamine-specific IgE and IgG antibody in serum have been shown to be significant risk factors for severe systemic reactions. We have found that protamine skin tests and basophil histamine release may not be reliable tests for protamine IgE antibody. Acute treatment of protamine reactions should follow guidelines for treatment of anaphylaxis. Prevention depends upon obtaining a thorough history with respect to any previous adverse reactions or exposure, and implementing appropriate precautions.

Management of Insulin Allergy

Local reaction:
1. Administer antihistamines 30 minutes before insulin
2. Substitute recombinant human insulin
3. Split dose into multiple sites

Systemic reactions:
1. Treat acute reaction appropriately
2. Do not stop insulin therapy. Reduce subsequent dose by one-third, then increase by 2–5 units per dose until therapeutic dose is achieved
3. Desensitization may be performed as follows:

Day	Time	Insulin (units)	Type	Route
1	morning	0.00001	reg	intradermal
	noon	0.0001	reg	intradermal
	evening	0.001	reg	intradermal
2	morning	0.01	reg	intradermal
	noon	0.1	reg	intradermal
	evening	1.0	reg	intradermal
3	morning	2	reg	subcutaneous
	noon	4	reg	subcutaneous
	evening	8	reg	subcutaneous
4	morning	12	reg	subcutaneous
	noon	16	reg	subcutaneous
5	morning	20	NPH	subcutaneous
6	morning	25	NPH	subcutaneous

Proceed by increasing by 5 units per day until therapeutic level is reached.
Lente may be used in place of NPH.

Fig. 28.10 A plan for the management of insulin allergy.

Other heparin antagonists are not generally available for clinical use but may be obtained in special circumstances.

Chymopapain

A proteolytic enzyme derived from the papaya tree, chymopapain has been used for chemonucleosis in the treatment of disc herniation. It is also a constituent of commonly used products such as contact lens solutions, toothpaste, meat tenderizer, and as a clarifying agent in beer. Anaphylaxis has been observed in 1 per cent of patients. Generally, allergic reactions occur upon first injection, suggesting that prior sensitization has occurred. Prior to the planned procedure, patients at risk should be identified through skin testing; if skin tests cannot be done, chymopapain-specific IgE antibody may be measured *in vitro* but this test may be insufficiently sensitive to detect all high-risk patients. It is also recommended that chemonucleosis procedures be performed under local rather than general anaesthesia so that early signs of anaphylaxis may be recognized.

Local Anaesthetics

A variety of reactions have been associated with local anaesthetics. The majority are toxic or vasovagal in nature with cardiovascular and psychomotor effects. Less than 1 per cent of reactions are immunologically mediated; most of these are contact dermatitis, but pruritus, urticaria, angioedema, and anaphylaxis have been reported.

In patients with hypersensitivity to local anaesthetics, a detailed history is helpful in distinguishing toxic and vasovagal reactions from possible allergic reactions. The drug formulation used for skin testing should be free of adrenalin, which will block a positive reaction. Lignocaine is usually used since it is rarely associated with allergic reactions. True positive skin tests are very rare, though occasional skin test reactions have been well documented in the literature and confirmed by passive-transfer testing. A successful RAST has not been developed. Skin tests should be followed by subcutaneous incremental challenge culminating in a full strength (1–2 per cent) challenge. If this is uneventful, the patient may receive local anaesthetics without risk of an IgE-mediated reaction.

Muscle Relaxants and other Drugs used in General Anaesthesia

Succinylcholine and most other muscle relaxants used in general anaesthesia have bifunctional quaternary ammonium determinants which render them complete allergens. Skin testing is valid at appropriate concentrations which do not elicit a response in non-allergic subjects (Fig. 28 .11).

Guidelines for General Anaesthetic Skin Testing

Drug	Maximal concentration for intradermal testing
d-Tubocuranine	300μg/ml
Pancuronium	200μg/ml
Suxamethonium (succinylcholine)	200μg/ml
thiopental sodium	2.5mg/ml

Fig. 28.11 Guidelines for skin testing of drugs used in general anaesthesia.

Immunizing Agents

Vaccines for active immunization have multiple potential antigenic determinants, including the infectious agent itself, additives including antibiotics and preservatives used in the manufacturing process, and materials derived from the culture media (e.g. egg protein).

Tetanus toxoid and diphtheria vaccine may cause fever or local reactions within 12 to 24 hours, but serum sickness, severe local reactions, and anaphylaxis are rare. If the need for a booster arises in a patient with a prior reaction, the antibody titre should be measured to verify need. A level greater than 0.01 IU/ml is protective. If a booster dose is needed, graded incremental dosing may be performed. Skin testing may be misleading as there are numerous false positive results.

Bacterial vaccines, such as pertussis (in DPT) and pneumococcus typically induce mild, local reactions but systemic reactions including anaphylaxis, serum sickness, encephalopathy and death have been reported following vaccination.

Because agents for viral immunization are often grown in tissue culture or eggs, certain atopic individuals have a higher incidence of allergic reactions, including anaphylaxis. Grown in embryonated chicken eggs, influenza and yellow fever vaccines may cause reactions in individuals allergic to eggs. Rubeola and mumps vaccine are grown in chick embryo tissue culture and contain little host protein so that patients who can eat eggs without any problems may receive these vaccines normally. Other immunological reactions seldom occur, but include thrombocytopenia (rubella and rubeola vaccines), erythaema multiforme, Stevens–Johnson syndrome, Lyell's syndrome and encephalomyelitis (rubeola, polio, rabies, and vaccinia vaccines).

Pre-treatment Guidelines for the Prevention of Anaphylactoid Radiocontrast Media (RCM) Reactions

Drug (dose)	Route	Instructions
Prednisone (50mg)	oral or intramuscular	Administer 13, 7, and 1 hour before RCM procedure
Diphenhydramine (50mg)	oral or intramuscular	Administer 1 hour before RCM procedure
Ephedrine sulphate (25mg)*	oral	Administer 1 hour before RCM procedure
* withold if history of coronary artery disease or arrhythmia		

Fig. 28.12 Guidelines for pre-treatment to prevent anaphylactoid reactions to radiocontrast media.

Passive immunotherapy can also be associated with allergic reactions. Heterologous immune serum is primarily associated with two types of immune reactions: anaphylaxis, which is frequently seen in patients allergic to that particular animal dander, and serum sickness, which appears to be dose related. Foreign antisera are still used in the treatment of snake bite, rabies, botulism, organ transplantation, and autoimmune disease. Prior to use, patients should be skin tested following the guidelines in the package insert. Skin testing is predictive for anaphylaxis but not for serum sickness. For those skin test positive individuals in whom treatment is necessary, desensitization may be performed.

Human immune serum globulin is prepared from a large donor pool. Antibody formation or anaphylaxis may ensue, especially if globulin is administered intravenously or for a prolonged period of time.

Anaphylactoid Reactions to Radiocontrast Media

Often clinically indistinguishable from true anaphylaxis, radiocontrast media reactions are called anaphylactoid or pseudoallergic, since there is no evidence of a specific immune reaction against these materials. Conventional radiocontrast agents are hypertonic, water soluble, iodinated aromatic compounds that are usually administered in large volumes as a salt preparation. Metrizamide is non-ionic and thereby isotonic, but its high cost has prevented widespread use, despite clear evidence of fewer reactions.

Most anaphylactoid reactions to radiocontrast media are mild and consist of pruritus, focal urticaria, rhinitis, conjunctivitis, or bronchoconstriction. These are usually self-limited and easily treated with anti-histamines. Approximately 0.1 per cent of radiocontrast procedures result in serious reactions, characterized by generalized urticaria, angioedema, bronchoconstriction, or hypotension. These are potentially fatal and should be treated promptly with fluids and adrenalin as for anaphylaxis.

Prevention is the cornerstone of long-term management. Anaphylactoid reactions occur most often following intravenous administration; alternative routes are much safer. Skin testing is not useful since the reactions are not IgE dependent. A history of atopic disease, such as rhinitis or asthma, increases the risk of reaction between three and four times, probably because of increased releasability of the atopic effector cells. Iodine sensitivity is irrelevant since the iodine in radiocontrast media is tightly organically bound. Consequently, a history of shellfish allergy is not predictive for radiocontrast media reactions.

Those patients who have had an anaphylactoid reaction are at increased risk for future reactions and must be medicated for subsequent radiocontrast studies. Premedication with H_1 antihistamines and corticosteroids has been shown to reduce not only the severity of anaphylactoid reactions but also their incidence. A recommended approach is shown in Fig. 28.12. Addition of 25mg ephedrine by mouth at the time of diphenhydramine administration has been found to further reduce the risk in a single non-concurrently controlled study, so its use cannot be generally recommended especially for elderly patients or those with cardiovascular disease.

Aspirin Sensitivity

Pseudoallergic reactions to aspirin are usually manifest as urticaria or asthma. Based upon positive oral aspirin challenge, the prevalence of asthmatic reactions may be as high as 30 per cent of asthmatic children or steroid-dependent adult asthmatics. The mechanism has not been elucidated but clearly does not involve an immunological mechanism, since identical reactions are triggered by first exposure to structurally unrelated analgesics as seen in Fig. 28.13. Since all reactive drugs are cyclooxygenase inhibitors, a possible explanation is the shunting of arachidonic acid metabolites from the cyclooxygenase pathway to the lipoxygenase pathway such that leukotriene production is increased. Recent reports of increased urinary LTE_4 levels following oral challenge of aspirin-induced asthmatic subjects supports this hypothesis. The typical clinical presentation of aspirin-induced asthma occurs in middle-aged adults

Anti-inflammatory Drugs

Cross-reactive with aspirin	Generally not cross-reactive with aspirin
amidopyrine	paracetamol (acetaminophen)
antipyrine	choline magnesium trisalicylate
diflunisal	choline salicylate
ditazole	chloroquine
fenoprofen	corticosteroids
flufenamic acid	propoxyphene
ibuprofen	salicylamide
indomethacin	salsalate
ketoprofen	sodium salicylate
meclofenamate	
mefenamic acid	
naproxen	
noramidopyrine	
oxyphenbutazone	
phenylbutazone (variable)	
piroxicam	
sulindac	
tolmetin	
zomepirac	

Fig. 28.13 Anti-inflammatory drugs, divided according to their cross-reactivity with aspirin.

with a history of non-allergic rhinosinusitis, nasal polyposis and asthma (usually of intrinsic variety and steroid-dependent). The elicitation of rhinitis, cough, chest tightness, or wheezing generally occurs within two hours of ingestion. Urticarial reactions to aspirin also occur, but rarely in those who experience asthma. Aspirin may aggravate chronic urticaria and occasionally causes hives or angioedema in patients without underlying skin disorders.

Avoidance of aspirin-containing products as well as most non-steroidal anti-inflammatory agents constitutes the general recommendation for such patients. Paracetamol (acetaminophen), sodium salicylate, and choline magnesium trisalicylate are acceptable and safe alternatives. Occasionally, coexisting medical conditions require the regular use of aspirin or non-steroidal anti-inflammatory agents in patients with a history of aspirin sensitivity. There is no role for skin testing since an IgE-dependent mechanism has not been established. The first step is to confirm aspirin intolerance by provocative challenge, preferably double-blinded and placebo controlled and undertaken by experienced personnel. Clinical tolerance may be induced in most challenge-positive patients by a desensitization regimen requiring between two and three days. Thereafter, a chronic state of desensitization may be maintained indefinitely with regular daily aspirin administration.

Summary

The general approach to management of drug allergy is based upon several principles. When possible, the offending agent and potentially cross-reactive drugs should be avoided. If the need for the drug becomes clinically important, allergy testing using skin tests, RAST or provocative challenge may be performed. If the patient is indeed sensitized, a non-cross-reactive alternative agent should be administered. In those cases in which a suitable alternative is not available, desensitization may be performed to induce clinical tolerance. Thus, drug allergy should be viewed as a manageable problem for most patients. The variety of diagnostic and preventive strategies available allows the vast majority of drug allergic patients to receive the appropriate medicines which they require.

Further Reading

Adkinson NF. Risk factors for drug allergy. *J Allergy Clin Immun* 1984; **74**:567–572.

DeSwarte RD. Drug Allergy. In: *Allergic Diseases: Diagnosis and Management* ed: Patterson R. Philadelphia: JB Lippincott, 1989:505–661.

Sullivan TJ. Drug Allergy. In: *Allergy: Principles and Practice* ed: Middleton E, et al. St Louis: CV Mosby, 1988:1523–1536.

Weiss ME, Adkinson NF. Immediate hypersensitivity reactions to penicillin and related antibiotics. *Clin Allergy* 1988; **18**:515–540.

Glossary

Acute phase proteins: Serum proteins whose levels increase during infection or inflammatory reactions.

Adhesion: The 'sticking' of migratory leukocytes to endothelial or structural cells by the interaction of complementary adhesion proteins.

Adhesion proteins: Complementary cell surface molecules expressed on leukocytes, endothelial and structural cells which allow leukocyte adherence.

Adjuvant: A substance that non-specifically enhances the immune response to an antigen.

Agretope: The portion of an antigen or antigen fragment which interacts with an MHC molecule.

A-kinase (cAMP dPK): Cyclic AMP dependent protein kinase; a family of enzymes activated by cyclic AMP which catalyse intracellular phosphorylation reactions.

Allergen: A foreign protein or hapten which induces the formation of anaphylactic antibodies and which may precipitate an allergic response.

Allergenic: Behaving like an allergen.

Allergy: Initially embraced immunology, but now focussed on the host tissue-damaging or irritation effects of immunological responses.

Anaphylactoid reaction: An allergic-like reaction but produced by non-immunological mechanisms.

Anaphylatoxins: Complement peptides C3a and C5a which cause smooth muscle contraction, increased microvascular permeability, leukocyte migration and activation, and degranulation of some types of mast cell.

Anaphylaxis: The consequences of an allergic reaction in an isolated organ or systemically.

Antibody: A molecule produced by the immune system in response to antigen which has the property of combining specifically with the antigen which induced its formation.

Antidromic reflex: *See* axon reflex.

Antigen: A molecule which induces the formation of antibody.

Antigen presentation: The process by which certain cells in the body (antigen-presenting cells) express antigen on their cell surface in a form recognizable by lymphocytes.

Antigen processing: The conversion of an antigen into a form in which it can be recognized by lymphocytes.

Antiserum: Serum containing antibodies to a specific antigen.

APCs (antigen-presenting cells): A variety of mobile or tissue-fixed cells, usually of the monocyte-macrophage family, which present antigen to lymphocytes through MHC class II molecules.

Apoptosis: Programmed cell death in which one cell engulfs another, usually senescent, cell in order to prevent liberation of its potentially toxic constituents.

Arachidonic acid: A 20-carbon fatty acid liberated from membrane phospholipid which may be converted into prostaglandins of the 2 series and leukotrienes of the 4 series.

Atopy: The ability to produce IgE antibodies to common allergens; demonstrable by RAST or skin prick tests.

Axon reflex: Local propagation of a nerve reflex by retrograde or antidromic stimulation of nerve axons resulting in the release of neuropeptides.

Bradykinin: A vasoactive nonapeptide which is probably the most important mediator generated by the kinin system.

C1-C9: The components of the complement classical and lytic pathways which are responsible for mediating inflammatory reactions, opsonization of particles and lysis of cell membranes.

C domains: The constant domains of antibodies and T cell receptors. These domains do not contribute to the antigen-binding site and show relatively little variability between receptor molecules.

CD markers: Surface molecules of cells, usually leukocytes and platelets, that are identified with monoclonal antibodies and may be used to distinguish cell populations.

CD3+ cells: Lymphocytes with pan-T cell marker CD3 on their surface.

CD4+ cells: T-lymphocytes with CD4 surface marker, usually equatable with helper T-cells.

CD8+ cells: T-lymphocytes with CD8 surface marker, usually equatable with suppressor T cells.

CD23: A cell membrane molecule associated with the low affinity receptor for IgE ($Fc_\epsilon R2$).

Cell line: A collection of cells which divide continuously in culture. May be either monoclonal or polyclonal and may have been transformed naturally or be an artificial hybridization.

Challenge: Administration of an implicated allergen to an allergic subject, in order to provoke an allergic response.

Charcot-Leyden crystal: Lysolecithin crystals found in sputum of asthmatic subjects.

Chemokinesis: Increased random migratory activity of cells in response to a chemical stimulus.

Chemotaxis: Increased directional migration of cells particularly in response to concentration gradients of certain chemotactic factors (chemotaxins).

Chymase: A neutral protease of the mast cell granule found in only the MC_{TC} sub-population of human mast cells.

Class I/II/III MHC molecules: Three major classes of molecule within the MHC. Class 1 molecules have one MHC encoded peptide associated with β2-microglobulin. Class II molecules have two MHC encoded peptides which are non-covalently associated, and Class III molecules are other molecules including complement components.

Class switching: The process by which an individual B cell can link new immunoglobulin heavy chain C genes to its recombined V gene to produce a different class of antibody with the same specificity. This process is also reflected in the overall class switch seen during the maturation of an immune response.

Clone: A family of cells or organisms having a genetically identical consititution.

CMI (cell-mediated immunity): A term used to refer to immune reactions that are mediated by cells, usually lymphocytes, rather than by antibody or other humoral factors.

Complement: A group of serum proteins involved in the control of inflammation, the activation of phagocytes and the lytic attack on cell membranes. The system can be activated by interaction with the immune system.

Conjugate: A reagent which is formed by covalently coupling two molecules together such as fluorescein coupled to an immunoglobulin molecule.

Constant regions: The relatively invariant parts of immunoglobulin heavy and light chains, and α, β, γ and δ chains of the T cell receptor.

CR1, CR2, CR3: Receptors for activated C3 fragments.

CSFs (colony stimulating factors): A group of cytokines which control the differentiation of haemopoietic stem cells.

Cyclosporin: An immunosuppressive drug with an action primarily on CD4+ lymphocytes.

Cytokines: A generic term for soluble molecules which mediate interactions between cells.

Cytophilic: Having a propensity to bind to cells.

Cytostatic: Having the ability to stop cell growth.

Cytotoxic: Having the ability to kill cells.

DAG (diacylglycerol): A potent protein kinase C activator usually generated from the action of phospholipases on membrane phospholipids.

Degranulation: Exocytosis of granular products from inflammatory cells, usually mast cells, basophils, eosinophils and neutrophils.

Dendritic cells: A set of antigen-presenting cells present in epithelial structures and in lymph nodes, spleen and at low levels in blood, which are particularly active in presenting antigen and stimulating T cells.

Desensitization: A protocol of repeated injections of allergen or modified allergen with the aim of reducing a patient's allergic responsiveness to that allergen.

Desetope: The part of an MHC molecule which links to antigen or processed antigen.

Diapedesis: The movement of a blood leukocyte through a blood vessel wall into the extravascular compartment.

Domain: A region of a peptide having a coherent tertiary structure. Both immunoglobulins and MHC Class I and Class II molecules have domains.

DTH (delayed type hypersensitivity): This term includes the delayed skin reactions associated with Type IV hypersensitivity.

ECP: Eosinophil chemotactic protein released following eosinophil degranulation.

EDN: Eosinophil-derived neurotoxin released following eosinophil degranulation.

Eicosanoids: Group name of products derived from 20-carbon fatty acids which includes prostaglandins, leukotrienes, thromboxanes and lipoxins.

ELAM-1: Endothelial leukocyte adhesion molecule-1, expressed on vascular endothelial cells, and involved in neutrophil recruitment.

ELISA (enzyme-linked immunosorbent assay): Technique used to quantitate small amounts of material by use of specific monoclonal antibodies.

Endothelium: Cells lining the blood vessels which contract to allow extravasation of plasma proteins and which express endothelial adhesion proteins.

Epitope: A single antigenic determinant. Functionally it is the portion of an antigen which combines with the antibody paratope.

EPO: Eosinophil peroxidase released following eosinophil degranulation.

Fab: The part of antibody molecule which contains the antigen combining site, consisting of a light chain and part of the heavy chain.

Fc: The portion of antibody that is responsible for binding to antibody receptors on cells and the C1q component of complement.

Flare: The red area of neurogenic origin, surrounding a skin weal response to allergen, histamine or like substance.

G-CSF (granulocyte-colony stimulating factor): A cytokine involved in the proliferation and maturation of granulocytes.

Genetic association: A term used to describe the condition where particular gene associations are found with particular diseases.

Genome: The total genetic material contained within the cell.

Genotype: The genetic material inherited from parents; not all of it is necessarily expressed in the individual.

Giant cells: Large multinucleated cells sometimes seen in granulomatous reactions and thought to result from the fusion of macrophages.

GM-CSF (granulocyte-macrophage-colony stimulating factor): A cytokine involved in the proliferation and maturation of granulocytes and macrophages.

G-protein: A guanosine triphosphate-dependent membrane protein complex which transduces many receptor-dependent events.

Granulocytopoiesis: Production of granulocytes in the bone marrow.

H_1, H_2 and H_3 receptors: Subtypes of the histamine receptor family which transduce the action of histamine.

Haplotype: A set of genetic determinants located on a single chromosome.

Hapten: A small molecule which is incapable of inducing an antibody response by itself but can, when bound to a protein carrier, act as an epitope, e.g. penicilloic acid.

Heavy chain: Larger molecules of the bi-heterodimer which comprises an immunoglobulin. Heavy chains are characteristic for each antibody class. Each heavy chain is composed of constant domains at the C-terminal (Fc end) and variable domains at the N-terminal (Fab end). *See also* light chain.

HETE: Hydroxyeicosatetraenoic acids, lipoxygenase products of arachidonic acid. Often preceded by a number, e.g. 5- or 15-, which identifies individual chemical structures.

Histamine: A major vasocative amine released from mast cell and basophil granules.

Histocompatibility: The ability to accept grafts between individuals.

HLA: The human major histocompatibility complex.

Humoral: Pertaining to the extracellular fluids, including the serum and lymph.

Hybridoma: Cell line created *in vitro* by fusing two different cell types of which one is a tumour cell. Lymphocyte hybridomas are usually used for making monoclonal antibodies.

5-Hydroxytryptamine (5-HT, serotonin): A vasoactive amine present in platelets and some rodent, but not human, mast cells.

Hyperreactivity: A state of increased reactivity to a provoking stimulus, e.g. bronchial hyperreactivity in asthma. Specifically, a greater magnitude of response to a given concentration of stimulus.

Hyperresponsiveness: A state of increased responsiveness to a provoking stimulus, e.g. bronchial hyperresponsiveness in asthma. Specifically, the ability to respond, either in magnitude or in sensitivity, to a lower concentration of stimulus.

Hypersensitivity: Synonymous with allergy (by usage).

ICAM-1: Intercellular adhesion molecule-1 expressed on endothelial and other cells which interacts with LFA-1 (CD11b/CD18) expressed on leukocytes.

Idiotype: A single antigenic determinant on an antibody V region.

IFNs (interferons): Members of the cytokine family originally associated with resistance to viral infections. IFN-γ is now recognized as a pluripotent cytokine, particularly associated with cell-mediated immunity.

ILs (interleukins): Members of the cytokine family which were originally conceived as intercellular messengers between leukocytes but are now perceived as having wider immunological and inflammatory effects.

Immune complex: An aggregate of antibody and antigen which may induce a hypersensitivity response, often by stimulating the complement cascade.

Immunoblotting: A technique of contact transference of proteins from SDS polyacrylamide gel to nitrocellulose so that they may be identified by monoclonal antibodies.

Immunocytochemistry: A technique used to identify cellular constituents by use of specific monoclonal antibodies.

Immunofluorescence: A technique used to identify particular antigens microscopically in tissues or on cells by the binding of a fluorescent antibody conjugate.

Integrin: A family of cell-adhesion molecules most frequently found on leukocytes, consisting of a common β-chain, but different α-chains, and involved in leukocyte recruitment.

IPs (inositol phosphates): Intracellular messengers (e.g. inositol 1, 4, 5-trisphosphate) involved in elevation of intracellular calcium from intracellular or extracellular stores.

Isoelectric focusing: Separation of molecules on the basis of charge. Each molecule will migrate to the point in a pH gradient at which it has no net charge.

J chain: A monomorphic polypeptide present in, and required for the polymerization of polymeric IgA and IgM.

Kinins: A group of vasoactive peptides comprising bradykinin, kallidin (lysyl-bradykinin) and des-arg-bradykinin.

Langerhans' cells: Antigen-presenting cells of the skin which emigrate to local lymph nodes to become dendritic cells; they are very active in presenting antigen to T cells.

LFAs (leukocyte function antigens): A group of leukocyte adhesion proteins composed of CD11/CD18 heterodimers.

Ligand: A linking or binding molecule, usually used to define a specific antigenic determinant to which an antibody binds.

Light chains: Smaller molecules of the bi-heterodimer which comprises an immunoglobulin. They may be of κ or λ subtypes, regardless of immunoglobulin class. Present only in the Fab end of the immunoglobulin and composed of both variable and constant domains. *See also* heavy chain.

LPS (lipopolysaccharide): A product of some gram-negative bacterial cell walls which can act as a B cell mitogen.

LTs (leukotrienes): Members of the eicosanoid family, lipoxygenase products, usually of arachidonic acid, with potent myogenic, cardiovascular and inflammatory effects.

Lymphokines: A generic term for molecules other than antibodies which are involved in signalling between cells of the immune system and are produced by lymphocytes (cf. interleukins).

MALT (mucosa-associated lymphoid tissue): Generic term for lymphoid tissue associated with the gastrointestinal tract, bronchial tree and other mucosae.

MBP (major basic protein): A basic arginine-rich protein making up the electron-dense core of the eosinophil granule and which may be released during eosinophil degranulation.

M-CSF (macrophage-colony stimulating factor): A member of the cytokine family, involved in the proliferation and maturation of macrophages.

MC_T and MC_{TC}: Mast cell subtypes defined by their granular content of tryptase (MC_T) and tryptase and chymase (MC_{TC}).

Mediator: A chemical substance released by one cell which stimulates another, e.g. mast cell mediators.

MHC (major histocompatibility complex): A genetic region found in all mammals where products are primarily responsible for the rapid rejection of grafts between individuals, and function in signalling between lymphocytes and cells expressing antigen.

MHC class II: The histocompatibility antigens expressed on cells of the monocyte/macrophage family which present antigen to the T-cell receptor on T-lymphocytes.

MIF (migration inhibition factor): A group of peptides produced by lymphocytes which are capable of inhibiting macrophage migration.

Mitogen: A substance which causes cells, particularly lymphocytes, to undergo cell division.

Monoclonal: Derived from a single clone, for example, monoclonal antibodies, which are produced by a single clone and are homogenous.

Myeloma: A lymphoma produced from cells of the B cell lineage.

Neuropeptide: Peptides released from nerves following stimulation. The many neuropeptides now recognized include substance P, vasoactive intestinal polypeptide (VIP), neurotensin and bombesin.

NK (natural killer) cells: A group of lymphocytes which have the intrinsic ability to recognize and destroy some virally infected cells and some tumour cells.

Nude mouse: A genetically athymic mouse which also carries a closely linked gene producing a defect in hair production.

Oedema: Tissue swelling due to extravasation of plasma proteins.

Opsonization: A process by which phagocytosis is facilitated by the deposition of opsonins (e.g. antibody and C3b) on the antigen.

PAF (platelet activating factor): A lipid-derived product generated by many inflammatory cells which activates platelets and induces bronchial hyperresponsiveness.

Paratope: The part of an antibody molecule which makes contact with the antigenic determinant (epitope).

Pathogen: An organism which causes disease.

PCA (passive cutaneous anaphylaxis): The technique used to detect antigen-specific IgE, in which the test animal is injected intravenously with the antigen and dye, the skin having previously been sensitized with antibody.

PGs (prostaglandins): members of the eicosanoid family, cyclooxygenase products usually of arachidonic acid, including PGA_2, PGD_2, PGE_2, $PGF_2\alpha$.

Phagocytosis: The process by which cells engulf material and enclose it within a vacuole (phagosome) in the cytoplasm.

Phagolysosome: A phagosome containing proteolytic enzymes capable of degrading the ingested particles.

Phagosome: An intracellular vacuole containing material ingested by phagocytosis.

Phenotype: The morphological characteristics of a cell or animal resulting from genetic expression.

Pinocytosis: The process by which liquids or very small particles are taken into the cell.

PK reaction (Prausnitz-Küstner reaction): The passive transfer of allergic responsiveness to an unresponsive recipient by intradermal injection of serum from an allergic donor.

Plasma cell: An antibody-producing B cell which has reached the end of its differentiation pathway.

Polyclonal: A term which describes the products of a number of different cell types (cf. monoclonal).

Primary lymphoid tissues: Lymphoid organs in which lymphocytes complete their initial maturation steps; they include the foetal liver, adult bone marrow and thymus, and the bursa fabricius in birds.

Primary response: The immune response (cellular or humoral) following an initial encounter with a particular antigen. Synonymous with sensitization.

Promyelocyte: A precursor cell of the myleocyte family.

RAST (radioallergosorbent test): A laboratory technique for the detection of circulating IgE with specific allergen determinants.

Receptor: A specific protein or group proteins, usually on the cell surface, capable of recognizing and binding a specific ligand.

Respiratory burst: Increase in oxidative metabolism following stimulation granulocytes, usually by phagocytosis.

RIA (radioimmunoassay): A technique for the laboratory assay of small amounts of materials by competition for antibody binding with known amounts of radioactive substance.

RMCP I and II (rat mast cell proteases I and II): Chymotryptic proteases of rat mast cell granules. Used in the immunocytochemical differentiation of mucosal- and connective-derived mast cells.

Rosetting: A technique for identifying or isolating cells by mixing them with particles or cells to which they bind (e.g. sheep erythrocytes to human T cells). The rosettes consist of a central cell surrounded by bound cells.

SCF (stem cell factor): A cytokine released by stromal cells which interacts with the c-kit receptor on mast cells to stimulate cell maturation and activation.

SDS-PAGE (sodium dodecyl sulphate polyacrylamide gel electrophoresis): A method of separating proteins by gel electrophoresis.

Secondary response: The immune response which follows a second or subsequent encounter with a particular antigen.

Sensitization: The stimulation of allergic antibody production usually by an initial encounter to a specific allergenic substance. Synonymous with primary response.

Serotonin: *See* 5-hydroxytryptamine.

Skin prick test: The detection of allergen to specific allergens through the production of a weal-and-flare response by pricking the skin through droplets of allergen or injecting them intradermally.

SLE (systemic lupus erythematosus): An autoimmune disease of humans usually involving anti-nuclear antibodies.

Substance P: A common neuropeptide which is likely to be involved in the neurogenic spread of the skin flare response.

TCR (T cell receptor): The T cell antigen receptor consisting of either an α/β dimer (TCR2) or a γ/δ dimer (TCR1) associated with the CD3 molecular complex.

T-dependent/T-independent antigens: T-dependent antigens require immune recognition by both T and B cells to produce an immune response. T-independent antigens can directly stimulate B cells to produce specific antibody.

TGF-β (transforming growth factor β): A cytokine involved in the stimulation of fibroblasts for collagen synthesis.

T_H cell (helper T cells): A functional subclass of T cells which can help to generate cytotoxic T cells or cooperate with B cells in production of antibody response. Helper cells recognize antigen in association with class II MHC molecules.

T_{H1}-cells: A subdivision of TH-cells involved in cell-mediated immunity and characterized by their production of IFN-γ, TNF-β and IL-2.

T_{H2}-cells: A subdivision of TH-cells involved in allergy by their influence on B-cells to produce IgE and pro-inflammatory effects. Characterized by their production of IL-3, IL-4 and IL-5.

TNF (tumour necrosis factor): A multifunctional cytokine initially identified for its effects on tumour cells.

Tolerance: A state of specific immunological unresponsiveness.

Tryptase: The major neutral protease of the mast cell granule found in all human mast cells.

TxA_2 (thromboxane A_2): A member of the cyclooxygenase product family of eicosanoids from arachidonic acid. Synthesized by platelets and other cells, its many actions include platelet aggregation, bronchonstriction.

VCAM-1 (vascular cell adhesion molecule): An adhesion molecule expressed on vascular endothelial cells.

V domains: The variable N-terminal (Fab) domains of antibody heavy and light chains and the α, β, γ and δ regions of the T-cell receptor which are responsible for antigen recognition.

VLA (very late antigen): A series of integrins expressed on the surface of leukoctyes involved in cell recruitment, especially T-cells and eosinophils.

Weal: An area of oedema produced at the site of intradermal introduction of allergen, histamine or similar provocant. Stimulation of axon reflexes in the weal area gives rise to the larger flare response.

Amino Acid Abbreviations

Alanine	Ala	A
Arginine	Arg	R
Asparagine	Asn	N
Aspartic acid	Asp	D
	Asn and/or Asp	B
Cysteine	Cys	C
Glutamine	Gln	Q
Glutamic Acid	Glu	E
	Gln and/or Glu	Z
Glycine	Gly	G
Histidine	His	H
Isoleucine	Ile	I
Leucine	Leu	L
Lysine	Lys	K
Methionine	Met	M
Phenylalanine	Phe	F
Proline	Pro	P
Serine	Ser	S
Threonine	Thr	T
Tryptophan	Trp	W
Tyrosine	Tyr	Y
Valine	Val	V

Index

B

I

J

K

L